Contributors

Carol Chapman, CDA, RDH, MS
Clinical Coordinator
Department of Dental Hygiene
Florida SouthWestern State College
Fort Myers, Florida

Mary Govoni, CDA, RDA, RDH, MBA
Speaker, Author, Consultant
Mary Govoni & Associates
Okemos, Michigan

Rebecca A. Nagy, BA
Rebecca Editing and Creative Services
Perry, Michigan

Pamela Zarkowski, JD, MPH, BSDH
Provost and Vice President for Academic Affairs
University of Detroit Mercy
McNichols Campus
Detroit, Michigan

Kathy J. Zwieg, CDA, LDA
Editor-In-Chief
Inside Dental Assisting
Aegis Communications
New Town, Pennsylvania;
Principal
KZ Consultants
Lino Lakes, Minnesota

Reviewers

Cynthia Baker, DDS, MA
Department Head
Dental Assistant Program
Greenville Technical College
Barton Campus
Greenville, South Carolina

Cindy Bradley, BA, CDA, CDPMA, CPFDA, EFDA
Instructor
Dental Assisting Program
Orlando Tech
Orlando, Florida

Jennifer Kelly, BA, MA
Instructor
Dental Assisting Program
Heald College
Honolulu, Hawaii

Loretta Mason, BASc
Practice Manager
Redwood Dental Group;
Practice Manager
American Dental Partners
Pinckney, Michigan

Leeann Simmons, BS, MS
Instructor
Allied Health/Science Department
Dental Hygiene
Delaware Technical Community College
Wilmington, Delaware

Kathy Zwieg, CDA, LDA
Editor-in-Chief
Inside Dental Assisting
Aegis Communications
New Town, Pennsylvania;
Principal
KZ Consultants
Lino Lakes, Minnesota

To

Phyllis Bonk Grzegorcyzk, RN, PhD

Phyllis has been a professional colleague, mentor, former Dean, Health and Public Service Division, and Interim Vice President for Instruction at Washtenaw Community College. As a colleague, she has always been available to us to influence our teaching and, as a personal friend, to face life's many challenges.

And to

Linda Collins, RDH

A friend and caring dental hygienist.

Preface

Dentistry is a dynamic profession, and this edition of the textbook continues to display how the profession functions as a healthcare system while being a business for profit. The business office in today's dental practice functions as a vibrant technological facility and, with the use of skilled personnel, can increase service to the patient while being a highly productive component of the dental practice.

BACKGROUND

This textbook evolved from a course team taught by the authors of the first edition, Jerry Crowe Patt and Betty Ladley Finkbeiner. When Jerry retired, Charles Allan Finkbeiner, Betty's spouse, assumed the second author's role, as they team-taught a practice management course at Washtenaw Community College in Ann Arbor, Michigan. The resultant benefits of two faculty members with working experience in both dentistry and business continue to be evident in this eighth edition.

AUDIENCE

This textbook is intended to be used by dentists, dental students, dental assistants, dental hygienists, and dental therapists as a primer and reference guide for the new employee in the dental business office. For the newly practicing dentist, this textbook is an excellent resource on how to set up the business office and select staff, equipment, and supplies to maintain this vital part of the practice. For the inexperienced person, this book provides a broad overview of the dental business operation, as well as technical information about patient charts, tooth nomenclature, insurance billing information, ethics, and infection control as it relates to the business office. For the more experienced employee, this book becomes an adjunct reference for those times when one may be needed.

IMPORTANCE TO THE PROFESSION

This is a time of exploding technology, both in the business office and in clinical treatment areas within the dental practice. Dentistry as a business must face the same issues as other healthcare and business systems and realize that the world is changing. There is diversity in race, ethnicity, gender, and age, and today's dental professional must be able to address these issues.

The authors believe that the business office needs to take its rightful place in the dental practice; that is, it should not be just the "front office" or a pass-through but rather a place where communication, organization, and skillful management concepts can enhance the success of the practice. This textbook provides suggested answers and comments for new employees to use in patient communication when they otherwise might appear not to know how to respond to a patient. It also provides working solutions to many of the common day-to-day tasks in the business office.

ORGANIZATION

The book introduces the reader first to the concepts of the business of dentistry as a service profession, dental team and patient management, legal and ethical issues, technology in the office, and design and equipment placement in the office. Chapters within the second portion of the book discuss communication, the key to patient success. This section includes document management and storage, as well as written and electronic communication, telecommunications, and social media. The third section of the book introduces business office systems that include appointment management, recall, inventory, dental insurance, accounts receivable, and accounts payable. The final section of the book places emphasis on the dental professional in the workplace and aids in the planning and management of a career path for all members of the dental team. The back pages of the book provide the reader easy access to grammar, numbers, prefixes and suffixes, common abbreviations, and dental terminology—common points of reference.

Throughout the book emphasis is placed on technology, using computer technology as the primary mode for records management. The reader has access to common practices using the computer to maintain maximum productivity and efficiency.

KEY FEATURES

- *Comprehensive Coverage:* This textbook covers all aspects of the business of managing a dental practice, information that is vital to its success. Although the emphasis is often on the administrative dental assistant, all members of the dental team are highlighted in specific areas. Also included is a look at the emerging dental workforce models. In addition,

special attention is given to the impact of infection control in not only the clinical area of the dental office but also the business office.
- *Practice Management Software:* Screen shots throughout the book supplement text discussions and paperwork examples to illustrate how processes and procedures can be properly and efficiently performed through the use of practice management software. Examples are provided from EagleSoft, one of the most widely used programs in dental offices.
- *Expert Authorship:* Betty Ladley Finkbeiner is a leading authority in dental assisting education, with many years of experience and many publications to her credit. She has been writing this text for more than 35 years. Charles Finkbeiner is an experienced instructor in the areas of business and computer information systems. Their combined experience and teamwork provide students with the tools they need to become successful members of the dental office team.
- *Need-to-Know Content:* Some highlights include the following:
  - Foundational chapters present truly practical discussions of ethics and legal issues.
  - Information on management companies in dental practice is provided.
  - Patient and staff communication resolutions are highlighted throughout.
  - Chapters incorporate information on a wide spectrum of practices involving documentation and technology to suit the needs of a variety of office settings.
- *Art Program:* Chapters incorporate plenty of illustrations to supplement text descriptions with examples of paperwork, office software, technology, and processes.
- *Key Terminology:* Key terms are bolded throughout the text, with definitions provided in a listing at the end of each chapter to help familiarize readers with unfamiliar new vocabulary.
- *Learning Activities:* End-of-chapter exercises involve a mixture of review questions that encourage readers to assimilate chapter information and learn to think critically about day-to-day office situations.
- *Summary Tables and Boxes:* Concepts are summarized throughout chapters in boxes and tables, calling readers' attention to important nuggets of information and providing easy-to-read recaps of text discussions that serve as useful review and study tools.
- *Chapter Outlines and Objectives:* Each chapter begins with an outline of content to be presented and a listing of learning outcomes, setting the stage for chapter coverage and serving as checkpoints readers can use for reference or study.
- *Spiral Binding:* The spiral makes for easy lay-flat reading and improves the usability of the book as an office reference.

NEW TO THIS EDITION

- *Focus on the Paperless Dental Office:* Emphasis throughout is placed on the use of the computer technology as a replacement for paper records; examples of computer-generated documents highlight each chapter, with suggestions on how manual documents reflect similar content.
- *Emphasis on Technology:* Chapters incorporate information on the latest technology used in dentistry so that readers remain current with the increasingly important role of electronics.
- *Updated Art Program:* Many new illustrations help readers visualize current paperwork and new technologies. Plenty of examples demonstrate the efficiencies that can be realized through the use of practice management software.
- *New Content:* Additions include the following:
  - Updated management styles
  - New management concepts in organizational culture
  - New concepts in cultural competency
  - Factors that motivate employees
  - Use of social media in patient marketing
  - Additional information on understanding patient needs
  - The use of a management company
  - Electronic banking and payroll
  - Tax forms
  - Updated infection control concepts
  - Updated insurance management techniques
  - Career planning for all members of the dental health team

ANCILLARIES

Student Workbook

An accompanying workbook provides practical exercises, as well as those that promote critical thinking. A CD-ROM of the latest version EagleSoft practice management software is provided in the back of the workbook, and original exercises are included throughout.

Evolve Website

A companion Evolve website has been created specifically for this book and can be accessed directly at http://evolve.elsevier.com/Finkbeiner/practice. Resources are available for free to all students and for instructors who have adopted the book.

Instructor Resources

- TEACH Instructor's Resource Manual
  - Lesson Plans: Detailed 50-minute plans with in-class and take-home assignments, activities, and discussion points, all mapped to chapter objectives and content
  - Lecture Outlines: PowerPoint presentations with talking points and discussion questions
  - Answer Keys: Answers and rationales for textbook Learning Activities and workbook exercises
- *Test Bank:* Approximately 500 objective-style questions—multiple-choice, true/false, and matching—with accompanying rationales for correct answers and page-number references for remediation
- *Image Collection:* All the book's images available for download into PowerPoint or other presentation formats

- *Critical Thinking Exercises:* Mini-case scenarios followed by thought questions that deal with typical office situations and dilemmas

Student Resources

- *Exclusive EagleSoft Screen Shot Exercises:* Scenarios that incorporate actual screen shots from the EagleSoft program and are followed by questions and instant feedback for student practice.
- *Practice Quizzes:* Approximately 290 self-assessment questions for student practice, separated by chapter. Each question includes rationales for correct and incorrect answers, as well as page number references for remediation.
- *Glossary Exercises:* Flashcards are created from chapter key terms and from dental vocabulary.

Betty Ladley Finkbeiner
Charles Allan Finkbeiner

Acknowledgments

This eighth edition has continued to expand the evolving communication technology in dentistry today. As we prepared the manuscript, we recognized the need to incorporate some very bright minds who are currently involved in dental education, and thus we have garnered input from a variety of contributors for this edition, including Carol Chapman, Mary Govoni, Loretta Mason, Rebecca A. Nagy, Pamela Zarkowski, and Kathy J. Zwieg. In addition, the use of the Internet and technology made the task much easier.

John Donne's quote, "No man is an island" from *Devotions,* could be transposed into a statement that "No book is written by the authors alone." This book has culminated into its published state with the tremendous support of the staff behind the scenes at Elsevier, including Kristin Wilhelm, Content Strategist, and Joslyn Dumas, Content Development Specialist; support was provided by Project Manager, Lisa A. P. Bushey.

The authors have been supported by many professionals who have lent their expertise to this edition. For support during this time, we thank our friends who were always listening to our latest challenges and to our professional colleagues who provided us with materials to enhance the textbook and ancillary materials. We thank the following for their expertise in many areas: Carol Chapman of Florida SouthWestern State College for providing her educational expertise; Dr. Sarah Shoffstall-Conel and Dr. Mary Williard for their updates on the Alaska Native Tribal Health Consortium; Kevin Henry, Group Editorial Director, Advanstar Dental Media, for his help with professional contacts and dental materials; Theodore Schumann, a noted CPA, for his input on scheduling productivity; Deborah Anderson for her production of QuickBooks materials; and Cindy Durley, Executive Director, DANB and the DALE Foundation, for her continued personal support on professional updates.

In addition, one must always thank those who daily helped the authors maintain their equipoise and remain calm through many storms. They are the ones who provided the coffee hours, meals, or entertainment when we needed a break. These are just a few to whom we owe our gratitude: Marianne Kollasch, Pat and Jack Keavney, Carol Gross, Barbara Coady, Ron Leonard, Lois and Ron Toth, Joyce Divirgilius, Suzan Harden, Mark Ladley, Pat Neil, Mary Mills, and Vonnie Winklepleck.

Finally, we owe a debt of gratitude to the staff at EagleSoft, a Patterson Company, for making it possible to include the interactive CD-ROM that accompanies every copy of the workbook. There is simply no way to give the thanks necessary to Jana Berghoff, Technology Marketing Manager, for all of the input she provided the authors. Her consistent interest in the project and her willingness to provide us advice, guidance, and the needed materials was overwhelming. In addition, we are indebted to Jenny Allen, Level III Technology Advisor, for the time and work she spent on developing the needed illustrations in the records chapters.

Betty Ladley Finkbeiner
Charles Allan Finkbeiner

Contents

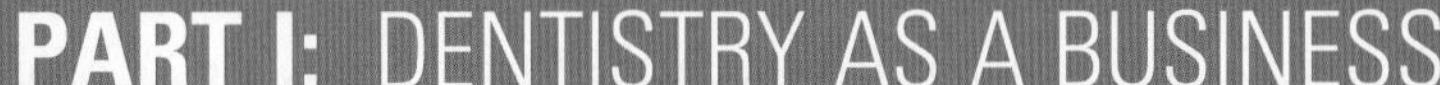

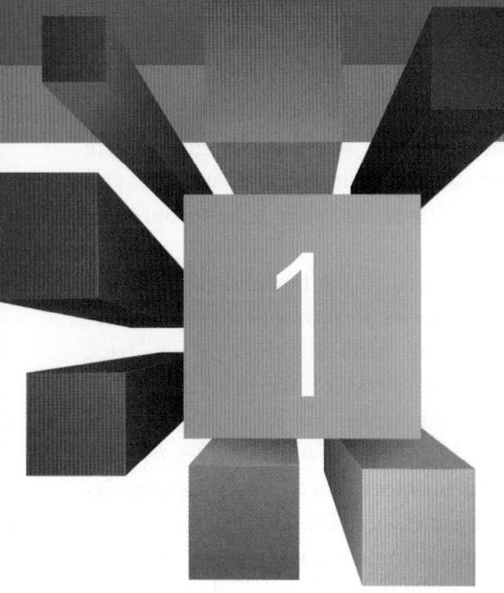

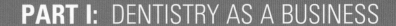

1 The Business of Dentistry

 http://evolve.elsevier.com/Finkbeiner/practice

LEARNING OUTCOMES

1. Define the key terms in this chapter.
2. Explain the dual role of dentistry as a business and a healthcare provider.
3. Describe the importance of identifying dentistry as a service profession, including:
   - Describe the importance of communication in patient service.
   - Explain cultural competency.
   - Describe the application of the Lewis Model of reactions to dentistry.
4. Discuss organizational culture and describe common organizational cultures that could be applied to a dental practice.
5. Define various types of dental practices.
6. Explain how a dental management company can benefit a dental practice.
7. Differentiate between leadership and management and discuss the importance of both in the twenty-first century.
8. Discuss characteristics of an effective leader.

KEY TERMS

Business An enterprise in which one is engaged to achieve a livelihood.

Communication The process of transmitting information from one person to another.

Competence The ability of an individual to do a job properly. Competence is a combination of practical and theoretical skills, cognitive skills, behaviors, and values that are used to improve performance.

Culture Culture is a shared, learned, symbolic system of values, beliefs, and attitudes that shapes and influences perceptions and behaviors.

Cultural competency In dentistry, cultural competency refers to the ability of the system to provide care to patients with diverse values, beliefs, and behaviors, including adapting treatment delivery to meet the patients' social, cultural, and linguistic needs.

DDS Doctor of Dental Surgery; a degree granted to a dentist upon graduation from a university dental school. A DDS is essentially the same degree as a DMD.

Dental management company An outside agency designed to affiliate itself with a group of professionals to manage the business component of a dental practice.

Dentistry A healthcare profession concerned with the care of the teeth and surrounding tissues, including prevention and elimination of decay, replacement of missing teeth and structures, aesthetics, and correction of malocclusion.

DMD Doctor of Dental Medicine; a degree granted to a dentist upon graduation from a university dental school. A DMD is essentially the same degree as a DDS.

Intelligence sourcing (I-sourcing) Transferring jobs from people to virtual programmers.

Leadership A method of influencing others for good, rousing others to action, and inspiring others to become the best they can be as a group works together toward a common goal.

Management The act or art of leading a team to accomplish goals and objectives while using skill, care, and tactful behavior.

Organizational culture The sum of the attitudes, experiences, beliefs, and values of an organization. It is the specific collection of values and norms that are shared by people and groups in an organization and that control the way they interact with each other as well as with those outside of the organization or dental practice.

Service In dentistry, service is the process of providing quality care for patients while following standards of care established by governmental agencies and by the profession itself.

Dentistry is a dynamic profession. In the United States, the dental profession is changing as it is faced with an aging and diverse population. This textbook focuses on the roles of the members of the dental staff as they relate to the dental business office. It is important to remember that, although one person may be assigned as the overall manager of the business office, every person who is an employee of the practice must devote some portion of his or her day-to-day activities to business-related duties.

Dentistry is a healthcare profession that has a twofold role: (1) to provide healthcare service and (2) to make a profit as a small business. As a healthcare service, dentistry provides quality care for the patient by following the standards of care established by governmental agencies and by the profession itself. As a healthcare profession, dentistry embraces the following objectives:

- Promote optimal oral health in a culturally sensitive manner.
- Provide oral health education.
- Promote prevention.
- Emulate the highest standards of patient-centered care.
- Acquire the most advanced knowledge and skills to meet the changing needs of a diverse patient population.
- Exhibit a willingness to share knowledge.
- Participate in professional activities.

As a business—an enterprise in which one is engaged to achieve a livelihood—the dental practice must meet the following criteria:

- Practice ethically.
- Operate efficiently.
- Operate safely.
- Be productive.
- Use technology.
- Make a profit.

Personnel titles in the dental practice may vary from office to office. Within the business office, there may be multiple staff assigned to a variety of tasks, including an administrative assistant, an office manager, a treatment coordinator, an insurance coordinator, an appointment coordinator, receptionists, and clerks. For the purpose of simplicity, in this textbook, the person who is primarily assigned to the management of the dental business office will be referred to as the *administrative assistant* or the *business manager.*

The administrative professional's role in the dental office of the twenty-first century is one that will be continually changing and challenging. Although projections by futurists tell us that nearly all purchases will be made virtually and that numerous jobs will be transferred from people to virtual programmers—a phenomenon known as *intelligence sourcing* or *I sourcing*—the dental practice will remain a people-oriented health profession. The person assigned to the administrative role in the dental office must have the ability to achieve the mission of the practice, increase productivity, demonstrate skills in computer technology, and effectively use the most important asset of the practice: its human resources. Indeed, this is a time of rapid technological change, both in the business office and in the clinical treatment areas within the practice. Dentistry as a business must face the same issues as other healthcare and business systems and realize that the world is changing. There is diversity in the areas of race, ethnicity, gender, and age, and today's dental professionals must be able to appropriately address any issues that arise.

For years dentists have referred to the business office as the *front office.* This terminology serves to promote division rather than to create a cohesive team. After all, there is no "back office." Dentists refer to other areas of the dental practice according to the work that takes place in them. The clinical areas of the office are referred to as *treatment, laboratory, hygiene,* or *radiographic rooms.* The business office should assume its rightful name, because all business activities of the practice take place there, including financial transactions, patient and staff communication, appointment management, recall, inventory, insurance management, and records maintenance.

The traditional education of the dentist has placed great emphasis on developing a highly competent diagnostician and clinician, but it has often left a noticeable void in the area of practice management. Dentistry in the twenty-first century faces an ever-changing population, a culturally diverse workforce and patient clientele, heightened consumer rights, a changing economy, increased state and federal regulations, an aging population, managed care, satellite offices, expanding group practices, the redefinition of dental assistant and dental hygienist use and credentialing, and even an expansion of personnel (e.g., the dental therapist). Futuristic-thinking dental practitioners will embrace change as a lifelong, ongoing process for both the individual and the practice. The successful dental practice will be led by individuals who look at all situations as opportunities to create excitement and enthusiasm when meeting new challenges. These individuals will realize that technology alone cannot drive the practice and that employees are major assets. Therefore, a greater emphasis must be placed on practice leadership and management. The administrative assistant or business manager becomes a vital professional by maintaining records, implementing business systems, managing business operations, and maintaining communication—transmitting information from one person to another—with the dentist, the staff, the patients, and the community.

As modern dentists accept the roles of dentist and entrepreneur, they also accept the responsibility of delegating expanded intraoral duties to the appropriate clinical assistants, dental hygienists, and dental therapists; certain extraoral duties to the laboratory technician; and additional responsibilities to the administrative assistant, the business manager, or an external management group.

DENTISTRY AS A SERVICE PROFESSION

Today it is evident that the industrial age that dominated the society of our parents and grandparents has given way to a service-oriented age, and dentistry is a major healthcare service. Dental treatment may be the objective for the patient; however, the dental staff must be constantly aware that, when patients

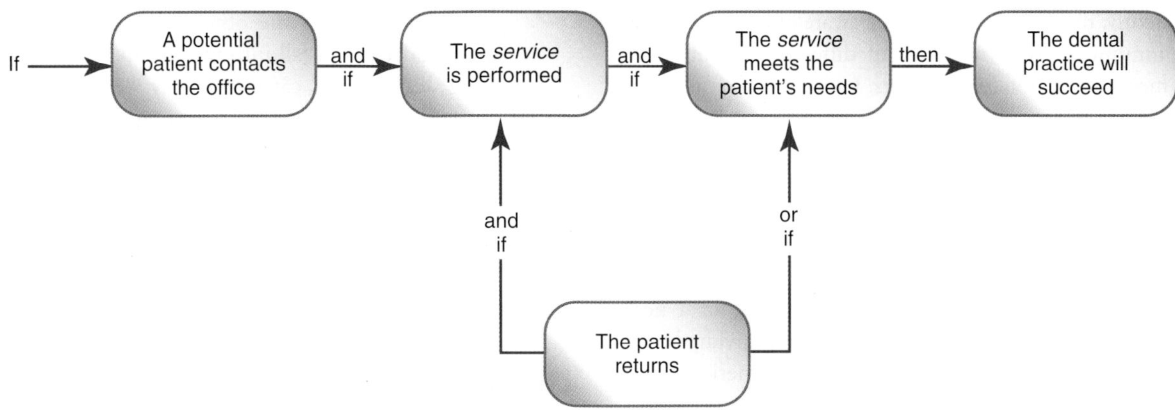

FIGURE 1-1 The service concept.

come to the office to seek treatment or perhaps a restoration (a tangible product), they are also seeking the most important product: service, an intangible product in the form of care. Service is a system of accommodating or providing assistance to another person.

Patients remain with a dental practice only if they are satisfied with the services rendered. Figure 1-1 illustrates the many "ifs" that the dental staff will encounter during the process of retaining a patient in a practice. It is important to remember that patients have choices. If patients choose to come to the office as a result of either a recommendation or random selection and if they are satisfied with their treatment and care, they may return. If patients are still satisfied at the return visit, they may continue to return. However, if there is dissatisfaction at any stage of their service, patients may opt not to return to the office.

The basis for patient retention is communication that involves the ability to understand and be understood. A patient seldom leaves a dental practice because of dissatisfaction with the margins of his or her composite restoration. However, the patient may leave because a staff member made it difficult to obtain a completed insurance claim form, was too busy to listen to a concern, made frequent errors on financial statements, or did not communicate the treatment plan in advance.

PRACTICE NOTE

The basis of patient retention is communication.

Service is not a result of clinical and cognitive skills but rather of attitudinal skills that evolve into a commitment to the welfare of others. Box 1-1 lists a variety of activities that indicate a service-oriented office.

BOX 1-1

Activities That Promote Service

- Maintaining regularly scheduled office hours
- Providing emergency care during the dentist's absence
- Maintaining the appointment schedule without delays
- Maintaining professional ethics
- Practicing quality care
- Recognizing the patient's needs
- Taking time to listen to the patient's concerns
- Respecting the patient's right to choice
- Informing patients of alternative treatment plans
- Allaying fears
- Hiring qualified employees
- Assigning only legally delegable duties to qualified staff
- Seeking staff input during decision making
- Encouraging an environment of caring
- Updating procedural techniques, equipment, and office decor regularly
- Maintaining office equipment
- Maintaining professional skills routinely
- Operating safely
- Maintaining quality assurance
- Attending risk-management seminars
- Participating in community services
- Being genuine and honest

Cultural Competency

The word culture comes from the Latin root *colere,* which means "to inhabit, to cultivate, or to honor." In general, it refers to human activity. Culture is a shared, learned, symbolic system of values, beliefs, and attitudes that shapes and influences perception and behavior as an abstract "mental blueprint." Cultural competency in dentistry refers to the ability of the system to provide care to patients with diverse values, beliefs, and behaviors, and it includes adapting treatment delivery to meet the patients' social, cultural, and linguistic needs.

The dental professional's work in the dental office is affected by culture when working with both patients and staff. People who grew up as part of a certain generation experience different situations during their formative years than do people who grew up in a different generation. Likewise, individuals who grew up in different cultures and with different languages often attach meaning to verbal communication in vastly different ways.

Consequently, the dental staff must be aware of how to successfully communicate with members of different generations as well as members of different cultures. Culture makes a significant difference in communication. We learn to speak and give nonverbal cues on the basis of our culture. There are several issues that affect communication in the dental office.

First is the use of nonequivalent words. It is difficult to find a word in one language that is exactly equivalent to a word in an unrelated language. The use of technical dental terms makes this activity even more difficult. A good example of a nonequivalent word is demonstrated by an Eskimo individual, who has several names for snow, whereas a North American individual has only one: *snow.*

Another factor that affects communication within various cultures is silence. The United States is referred to as a *talk* or *verbal society.* For a North American, silence is often uncomfortable, and it is usually not considered appropriate in the American workplace. For example, if an American is criticized in the workplace, the person is allowed to respond verbally to show that the criticism has been understood and to explain how he or she will avoid making the mistake again. In the Philippines, however, the worker more likely would apologize with an action such as extending a favor to the one who has been offended but saying nothing.

Mexico is geographically close to the United States, but culturally it is much different from its northern neighbors. Mexico has a separate history and thus a different culture and different ways of doing and looking at things. The beliefs, expectations, ethics, etiquette, and social conduct of Mexicans are so different from those of Americans that Mexicans may almost seem to be from a different world. Thus, when treating Mexican patients or communicating with a Mexican staff member, one must be aware of the cultural differences and seek to understand how to most appropriately explain the method of practice in the dental office.

Many references are available for translating information into the languages of patients or staff members within the office. For instance, if the office has a significant number of Spanish-speaking patients, all efforts must be made to provide literature, health forms, questionnaires, and other communication in both English and Spanish. *Spanish Terminology for the Dental Team* is a small book published by Elsevier to help in this scenario. It is worth the effort, too, for the staff to enroll in a short course in the language that the patients or staff may speak.

British linguist Richard Lewis plots the culture of different countries as it applies to the following three categories:

Linear-actives: Those who plan, schedule, organize, and pursue action chains, and do one thing at a time. Germany and Switzerland are in this group.

Multi-actives: Those lively, loquacious peoples who do many things at once and who plan their priorities not according to a time schedule but according to the relative thrill or importance that each appointment brings with it. Italians, Latin Americans, and Arabs are members of this group.

Reactives: Those cultures that prioritize courtesy and respect, listening quietly and calmly to their interlocutors, and reacting carefully to the other side's proposals. China, Japan, and Finland fall into this group.

Thinking about these categories may be helpful for the dental professional who is presenting proposed treatment to a patient or discussing job tasks with a staff member; it will help him or her to better understand the potential reaction of the person to whom he or she is speaking. Figure 1-2 demonstrates how you may be able to examine the reactions of persons of various ethnic backgrounds using the Lewis model of linear-active, multi-active, and reactive variations (Box 1-2).

ORGANIZATIONAL CULTURE

The term organizational culture has become well known in business. Many authors have defined organizational culture, but, perhaps for the purpose of dental management, it can best be defined as something that an organization or dental practice "is" rather than what it "has." Organizational culture comprises the attitudes, experiences, beliefs, and values of an organization. It has been defined as the "specific collection of values and norms that are shared by people and groups in an organization

BOX 1-2

Suggestions for Communicating With a Diverse Population

- Be nonjudgmental. Do not judge an individual's values, culture, appearance, intelligence, attitudes, or other characteristics.
- Respect the other person's time by being prompt. Hard as it may be, demonstrate patience with patients who do not understand the American value of time. In some countries, the concept of "time is money" is not common. After you become familiar with a patient, try to make adjustments in the schedule so that you can be productive if you have to wait for this patient. You may even list an earlier time on their appointment card than you do on your own schedule to ensure that they will arrive to the office on time.
- Speak standard English. Avoid using slang terms.
- If the office is located in a multicultural area, consider having bilingual signs and business cards. This idea can extend to health questionnaires or other educational materials to be given to patients.
- A smile is a generally acceptable gesture in most cultures.
- Several cultures are offended by people standing with their hands in their pockets.
- Be aware of your gestures. Cultures vary with regard to the interpretation of many gestures, including the following:
    - In China and Japan, hugging and kissing when greeting are uncommon.
    - Persons from both China and Japan avoid prolonged direct eye contact.
    - In the Philippines, shaking hands is a common custom for both men and women.
    - Filipino and Taiwanese individuals consider speaking in a loud voice to be rude and ill mannered.
    - The Taiwanese society is not touch oriented, and public displays of affection are rare.
    - In Taiwan, the open hand is used to point.

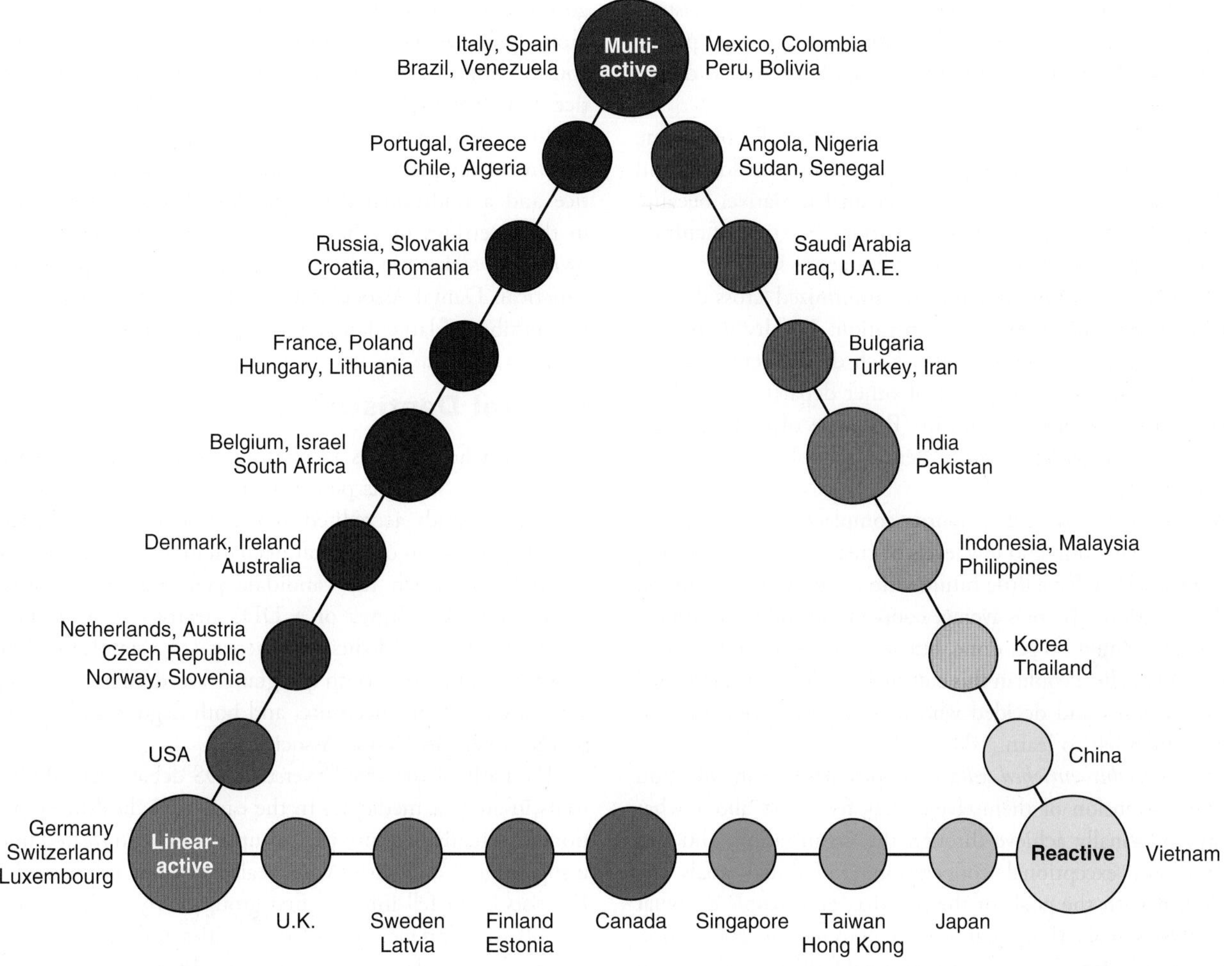

FIGURE 1-2 Lewis model of cultural types. (Copyright © 2014 Richard Lewis Communications.)

and that control the way they interact with each other and with others outside the organization or dental practice." Some authors even add to this definition the physical location of the organization, its dress codes, and the office arrangement and design.

Organizational culture can become very complex. However, the following list describes common organizational cultures that can be applied to a dental practice:

- A *power culture* concentrates the power among a few. Control radiates from the center like a web. Power cultures have few rules and little bureaucracy, but swift decisions can ensue. This could be compared with an authoritarian leadership style. In this culture, one person—the dentist or the practice owner—makes the decisions and seeks little or no input from the staff.
- In the *role culture,* people have clearly delegated authority within a highly defined structure. Typically these organizations form hierarchical bureaucracies. Power is derived from the individual's position, and little scope exists for expert power. This term could be applied to a large organization or a clinic in which there are several different specialty clinics, each of which has a specific person in charge.
- In the *task culture,* teams are formed to solve particular problems. Power comes from expertise as long as the team requires expertise. These cultures often feature multiple reporting lines and a matrix structure.
- A *person culture* exists when all individuals believe themselves to be superior to the organization. Survival can become difficult for such organizations, because the concept of an organization suggests that a group of like-minded individuals are pursuing the organization's goals. Some professional partnerships, such as dentistry, can operate as person cultures, because each partner brings a particular expertise and clientele to the office.
- The *work-hard/play-hard culture* is characterized by few risks being taken, all of which involves rapid feedback. This is typical in large organizations, which strive for high-quality customer service. These organizations are often characterized by team meetings, jargon, and buzzwords.
- The *process culture* occurs in organizations in which there is little or no feedback. People become more concerned with how things are done rather than with what is being achieved; this feeling is often associated with bureaucracies. Although it is easy to criticize these cultures for being overly cautious

or bogged down in red tape, they do produce consistent results, which is ideal in certain circumstances (e.g., public services). This type of culture may apply to public dental clinics.

- The *blame culture* cultivates distrust and fear. People blame each other to avoid being reprimanded or put down, and this results in no new ideas or personal initiative, because people do not want to risk being wrong. This type of culture can be very detrimental to a dental practice staff.
- *Multidirectional culture* cultivates minimized cross-department communication and cooperation. Loyalty is only to specific groups or departments. Each department becomes a clique that is often critical of other departments, which in turn creates a lot of gossip. This type of culture could exist in a large clinic or a dental school with multiple departments.
- A *live-and-let-live culture* spurns complacency. It manifests mental stagnation and low levels of creativity. Staff members in this culture have little future vision and have given up on their passions. There is average cooperation and communication and things do get done, but staff members do not grow professionally. People in this culture have developed personal relationships and decided who to stay away from; there is not much left to learn.
- In a *leadership-enriched culture*, people view the organization as an extension of themselves. They feel good about what they personally achieve through the organization, and this promotes exceptional cooperation. Individual goals are aligned with the goals of the practice, and people do what it takes to make things happen. As a group, the organization is more like family; it provides personal fulfillment that often transcends ego so that people are consistently bringing out the best in each other. In this culture, every individual in the organization wants to do a good job. This is an ideal culture to promote in a dental practice. In dentistry, it is likely that a multifaceted culture could develop (e.g., leadership-enriched culture combined with task culture).

What does organizational culture mean for a new employee or an interviewee looking at a prospective job? It is not easy to identify the type of culture during an hour-long interview, but, if a working interview is possible, the type of culture may soon be identified. This allows prospective employees to see whether the "hum" is there and whether the ethos of the practice fits with his or her individual values, beliefs, attitudes, and emotions.

TYPES OF DENTAL PRACTICES

In a *solo practice*, a dentist practices by himself or herself and is responsible for both the business and clinical components of the practice.

Alternatively, a *group practice* may be formed by more than one dentist either via a legal agreement with each other and managed by themselves, or it may be formed with a dental management company that manages the business aspect of the practice. In this case, the clinical portion of the group is governed by the dentists themselves. It is also possible for a group practice to be managed by an outside company that controls both the business and clinical components of the practice. However, each state does have responsibility for specifying the limitations of practice under that state's dental practice act.

One of the primary differences between a large group practice and a traditional dental practice is ownership. Dentists in these settings may have an ownership stake or part of an ownership stake, but many are employees of the practice. The American Dental Association noted that, from 2010 to 2011, the number of large dental group practices had risen 25%.

General Dentistry

A dentist who practices all phases of dentistry is referred to as a *general dentist*. This person will have completed a specified program of study accredited by the American Dental Association's Commission on Dental Accreditation. Depending on the school from which the candidate graduates, he or she will receive a DMD degree or a DDS degree. *DMD* stands for "Doctor of Dental Medicine," whereas *DDS* stands for "Doctor of Dental Surgery." Both programs are designed to prepare general dentists for licensure, and both degrees are recognized by the American Dental Association.

The basis of the DMD versus DDS debate actually has its roots in ancient medicine. In the early days, healthcare practitioners were divided into two groups: those who treated injuries using surgery and those who healed diseases using medicine. Dentists often fell into the first group. Early American dental schools were independent of universities and functioned more like trade schools, granting their graduates DDS degrees to perform clinical procedures. Dentistry has certainly changed since then, and today's dentists are respected members of the medical community who assume responsibility for the diagnosis and treatment of diseases, perform surgical procedures, and educate the public about dental health.

Upon completion of a program of study, the graduate is eligible to take the state board dental examination to obtain licensure in a specific state and then practice as a general dentist. The dentist is responsible for maintaining this licensure in accordance with the rules of his or her state board of dentistry and for completing the specified continuing education requirements.

Specialties of Dentistry

With additional education as specified by the individual states through each state's board of dentistry, a dentist may obtain additional education and pass a specialty board examination that qualifies the person to become a dental specialist. The American Dental Association recognizes nine specialties. The suffix *-ics* identifies the name of the specialty (e.g., *orthodontics*), and the suffix *-ist* identifies the name of the specialist (e.g., *orthodontist*).

The specialties recognized by the American Dental Association are as follows:

1. *Dental Public Health:* Dental public health is the science and art of preventing and controlling dental diseases and promoting dental health through organized community efforts. It is the form of dental practice that considers the community—rather than the individual—as its patient. This specialty is concerned with public education, applied dental research, the administration of group dental care programs, and the prevention and control of dental diseases within communities. A specialist in this field is referred to as a *public health dentist.*
2. *Endodontics:* Endodontics is the specialty concerned with the morphology, physiology, and pathology of the dental pulp and its associated tissues. This specialty is concerned with the biology of the normal pulp; common diseases of the pulp and their causative factors; the diagnosis, prevention, and treatment of these diseases; and common injuries of the pulp and its associated tissues. A specialist in this field is referred to as an *endodontist.*
3. *Oral and Maxillofacial Pathology:* Oral pathology is the specialty of dentistry that deals with the nature, identification, and management of diseases that affect the oral cavity and its adjacent structures. It is a science that investigates the causes, processes, and effects of these diseases. This specialty will include the research and diagnosis of diseases using clinical, radiographic, microscopic, biochemical, and other examinations. A specialist in this field is referred to as an *oral and maxillofacial pathologist.*
4. *Oral and Maxillofacial Radiology:* Oral and maxillofacial radiology is the specialty concerned with the production and interpretation of images and data produced by all forms of radiant energy used for the diagnosis and management of diseases, disorders, and conditions of the oral cavity and the maxillofacial region. A specialist in this field is referred to as an *oral and maxillofacial radiologist.*
5. *Oral and Maxillofacial Surgery:* Oral and maxillofacial surgery is the specialty of dentistry responsible for the diagnosis and surgical treatment of diseases, injuries, and defects of the oral and maxillofacial region that involve function and aesthetics. A specialist in this field is referred to as an *oral and maxillofacial surgeon.*
6. *Orthodontics and Dentofacial Orthopedics:* Orthodontics and dentofacial orthopedics is the dental specialty that includes the diagnosis, prevention, interception, and correction of all forms of malocclusion and of neuromuscular and skeletal abnormalities of the developing or mature orofacial structures. This specialty includes the design, application, and control of functional and corrective appliances and the movement of the dentition and its supporting structures to achieve an optimal occlusal relationship that provides improved function and aesthetics. A specialist in this field is referred to as an *orthodontist.*
7. *Pediatric Dentistry:* Pediatric dentistry is an age-defined specialty that provides both primary and comprehensive preventive and therapeutic oral healthcare for children from infancy through adolescence; it also includes the care of patients with special healthcare needs beyond the age of adolescence. A specialist in this field is referred to as a *pediatric dentist.*
8. *Periodontics:* Periodontics is the specialty of dentistry that encompasses the prevention, diagnosis, and treatment of diseases of the supporting and surrounding tissues of the teeth or their replacements and the maintenance of the health, function, and aesthetics of these structures and tissues. Dentists in this specialty work closely with their patients' general dentists to ensure the success of restorative dentistry, which is dependent on good periodontal health. A specialist in this field is referred to as a *periodontist.*
9. *Prosthodontics:* Prosthodontics is the dental specialty that involves the diagnosis, treatment planning, rehabilitation, and maintenance of the oral function, comfort, appearance, and health of patients with conditions associated with missing or deficient teeth or other oral and maxillofacial tissues. Replacements that include artificial devices are referred to as *dental prostheses.* A specialist in this field is called a *prosthodontist.*

DENTAL MANAGEMENT COMPANIES

As stated previously, dentistry is not only a healthcare profession; it is also a business. With today's changing population and economy there is an emergence of dental management companies. The management company is typically designed to affiliate itself with professional corporations. These are doctors who already have incorporated and display their names as "Joseph W. Lake, DDS, PC." The management company does just what its name implies: it manages the business component of the practice, whereas the clinical portion of the practice remains solely with the dentist owners.

A typical management company owns the assets of the office, including the building and the equipment. The doctors determine their mission as it relates to patient care, office hours, staffing, philosophy, and mode of delivery of services. A contract is made with the dentist and the staff for salary, hours, uniforms, and benefits. Malpractice insurance is made available to the staff for purchase through the management company, but they may opt to choose other insurance.

There are several advantages to using a management company. These include but are not limited to the following:

- The clinician can focus totally on clinical treatment and not worry about business forms, statements, and so on.
- The business company is skilled in running a business and is aware of all business regulations, tax laws, and so on.
- The company can provide benefit programs that may be more beneficial than what could be offered in a solo practice.
- The company can provide opportunities for the growth of the staff, including advancement into a greater number of positions in management.
- The company can provide educational programs that a small solo practice may not be able to afford for its staff.

As with any change in the dental practice, when choosing a management company, the dentists' group should research the company thoroughly to ensure that its mission, ethics, and procedures adhere closely to their own mission and practice philosophy. Emphasis should be placed on choosing a company that maintains its role in the business aspect of the company and that does not interfere with the clinical domain of the practice.

LEADERSHIP AND MANAGEMENT IN THE TWENTY-FIRST CENTURY

Traditionally, a dentist may have managed the office using an authoritative, free-reign, or participatory leadership style. Today, the effective leader or manager must have skills that include change mastery, technology, and virtual office systems that extend beyond the local domain.

Leadership and **management** are related but different in concept and definition. The leader in a dental practice is commonly the dentist. The manager is often the administrative assistant. To be a good leader, one must possess the characteristics of a manager or administrative assistant, and the administrative assistant may find a situation in which he or she must assume a leadership role.

To be an effective leader, a person must possess a certain set of personal traits. These are described in the following sections.

Live by a Set of Values

In the modern dental practice, ethical behavior is the accepted and expected. The difficult task is ensuring that this ethical behavior is present in the entire practice. The leader of the dental practice—the dentist employer—must work within the office to identify and define those principles of ethics and acceptable behavior and ensure that these are carried out during routine daily practice. Effective leaders must often make difficult decisions to stand on their values and understand that the set of values they identify for the practice must begin at the top and permeate throughout all levels of the practice.

Build a Shared Vision

The ethical dental office has a visionary leader, and it may even have more than one. This persons—the dentist—must be able to build on the shared vision and involve employees at all levels. It is wise for the dentist to determine a practice mission statement that speaks to the way the practice is to be managed and the role of the staff and the patients. Chapter 3 provides a sample of an office policy that can be distributed to patients in which this mission statement defines the practice.

To successfully build an organizational vision, employees at all levels must be involved. An effective leader works with the staff to determine how the practice's vision and individual goals and objectives meet the vision of the practice. As this vision takes shape, the leader and the employees need to determine the following:

- What are the dental practice's values? What values should it have? Does some modification need to be made?
- What contributions should the dental practice make to the community? Which staff members should be involved?
- Who are the patients? What are the demographics and needs of these individuals?
- What is the dental practice's reputation? What reputation should it have? Are changes needed in this reputation?
- How do people work together within the practice?

Maintain a Commitment to Service

A dentist has made a commitment to service when choosing dentistry as a career. However, sometimes this commitment can be overshadowed by the need to make a profit and build a career. There can be a successful balance if the dentist, as a leader, understands how a successful business can be achieved and at the same time makes a commitment to helping people grow in the workplace. Thus, the commitment to service is not only to the patients but also to the staff.

Empower Others

Power is the capacity to influence others. Power can flow in any direction within the dental practice, and it can apply to an individual or a group. Empowerment can be defined as "putting power where it is needed." An effective leader can empower the staff by taking actions such as the following:

- Providing employees with access to information that will help them increase their productivity and effectiveness
- Allowing staff members to take on more responsibility, including assigning them all legal tasks delegated to them in a given state
- Giving staff members a voice in decision making

Empowered employees feel a sense of ownership in the practice and become confident in their jobs. They are enthusiastic, and they take responsibility for getting their jobs done efficiently. Usually empowered employees are happier individuals; they feel they are part of the practice, and they enjoy the job's rewards.

The empowered leader has a basic trust in people and believes that the members of the staff are good, honest, and trustworthy. This leader believes that the staff will accomplish more if given the right resources as well as the responsibility for accomplishing the assigned tasks.

Reward Risk Taking

Leaders of successful dental practices are willing to seek new answers to problems, to try new approaches, to use technology, and to be flexible. Successful dentists know that not all risk taking is successful, but they are willing to take calculated risks, knowing that the status quo can also result in failure. This type of leader encourages the staff to take some risks as well. For instance, one of the staff may be considering taking an online educational program to become a registered dental assistant. The dentist encourages the assistant to do this, but the employee is fearful of failure. The assistant indicates that she has children at home, that she has never taken such a course online, and that she is unsure whether she will succeed. She must take a risk. The dentist employer needs to reward this risk taking. Encouragement from the dentist to take such a course followed by the dentist rewarding this risk-taking employee with increased responsibility and compensation can ensure a confident employee. Keys to successful risk taking include the following:

- Trusting in one's own abilities
- Being open-minded
- Overcoming the fear of mistakes
- Developing a support system

Manage Chaos

Crises occur during the daily routine of the dental office. The effective leader can practice the art of meeting individuals where they are in a conflict situation and then move them forward to bring about desired outcomes.

Know How to Follow

A good leader is also a good follower. The effective leader knows the importance of stepping back and being a follower when a situation demands it. A good leader also has trust in others and knows that others can also be leaders if they are given the proper opportunities and training.

Today's Leader

The leader in the modern dental office must embrace trust, a willingness to understand change, humility, commitment, focus, compassion, integrity, peacemaking, and endurance (Box 1-3).

As a business, the dentist/leader of the twenty-first century strives to achieve practice goals by doing the following:

- Considering long-term results over short-term results
- Stressing effectiveness over efficiency alone
- Thinking strategically rather than operationally
- Being proactive rather than reactive to situations
- Being driven by plans rather than problems

Members of an effective dental office may think and act independently but must always keep the dental practice as the main priority. Marketing the services of a dental practice involves the consideration of human, financial, and technical resources in a worldwide market. Patients seen in the dental office come from diverse backgrounds and present with complex and diverse conditions. Likewise, the dental materials and technologies used in all areas of the office come from the worldwide market. The dental office of today must also be a virtual office that serves the local community and that recognizes its role in the global community.

BOX 1-3

Elements That Build Effective Leadership

- *Trust* promotes good relationships and confidence with the staff as expanded duties are delegated to clinical staff and advanced management techniques are assigned to business staff.
- *A willingness to understand change* and to recognize that disruptions are inevitable is part of effective leadership; the willingness to shift gears paves the way for change.
- *Humility* involves a focus on being open, teachable, and flexible.
- *Commitment* seeks to develop vision and values in a leader and moves leaders to stand for something greater.
- *Focus* gives leaders the ability to achieve and direct their time and energy toward important goals and objectives.
- *Compassion* is the desire to understand and care for others, such as staff members, family members, patients, or the community as a whole.
- *Integrity* demands that leaders be responsible for quality assurance in their service of patients as well as in all of their relationships.
- *Peacemaking* leaders bring calmness to the office by listening, learning from others, and seeking good solutions rather than making quick decisions.
- *Endurance* refers to courage, perseverance, and strength when situations, people, or the environment become chaotic or difficult.

PERSONAL CHARACTERISTICS OF AN EFFECTIVE LEADER

Generally the first contact that a patient has with the dental office is with a staff person in the business office, the administrative assistant, the office manager, or the receptionist. It is difficult to identify a job today that does not include interaction with people. Whether you have a job in education, custodial services, law, science, religion, office technology, or architecture, you will find that productivity is greatly enhanced by an ability to communicate. In fact, it is difficult to find any job today in which communication is not important. It has been found that 80% of the people who fail at their jobs do so not because of a lack of technical skills but because they do not relate well to people.

The staff member's attitude either gives the patient a positive impression or convinces the patient to seek dental care elsewhere. Whether communicating with patients, staff, or friends, basic "people skills" must be developed for successful communication. In addition to the elements found in a leader that were discussed earlier in this chapter, the administrative assistant must have skills that include self-confidence, competence, genuineness, enthusiasm, assertiveness, honesty, acceptance of others, the ability to be a good listener, and a willingness to be a team player.

Self-Confidence

Self-confidence is an individual's belief that he or she can do a job well. To have self-confidence, a person must accept herself or himself. This requires a healthy mental personal picture and the accentuation of positive attributes. Having self-confidence means identifying strengths and building on them as well as accepting weaknesses and not dwelling on them.

An administrative assistant with self-confidence assumes responsibility, adapts to change, accepts challenges, and provides input during decision making. For instance, administrative assistants who are self-confident initiate marketing needs, make suggestions for changes, and implement new procedures without hesitation because they are confident that they know what is going on. They are willing to take risks and able to recommend changes in a routine or procedure with the confidence that their ideas are worthwhile and merit consideration.

Competence

Competence differs from confidence. Competence refers to the ability of an individual to do a job properly. Competence is a combination of practical and theoretical skills, cognitive skills, behaviors, and values that are used to improve performance. Competence is what a person needs to be successful on the job. A person may be competent but lack the self-confidence needed to take on the responsibilities and challenges of the job.

Genuineness

Being genuine means being oneself. A person who is genuine is sincere and straightforward. This is important when dealing with people in a healthcare profession. A genuine caring person is not afraid to reach out and touch someone. Placing a hand on the shoulder of a frightened patient or holding a frightened child's hand (Figure 1-3) shows caring and displays a genuine concern for another person's feelings. It requires putting yourself in the patient's place and showing the kind of concern you would like to receive if the roles were reversed.

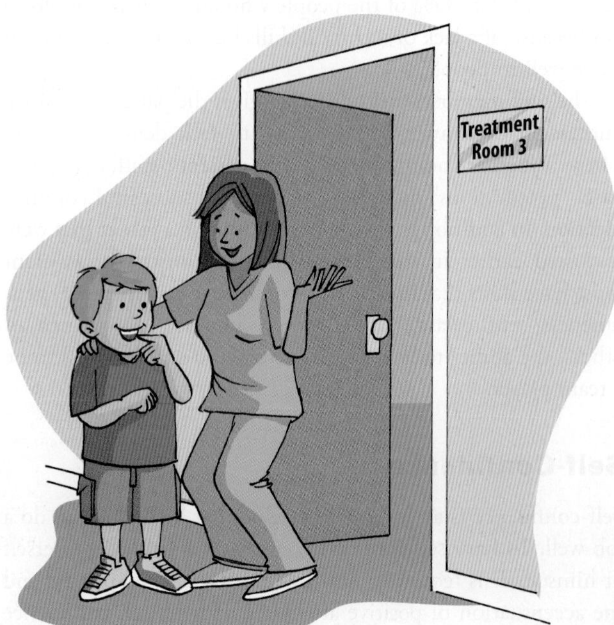

FIGURE 1-3 An arm resting on a child's shoulder displays caring.

Patients feel comfortable with a genuinely caring administrative assistant, and they are also more likely to open up and share their innermost feelings with this type of person. When patients express fear or frustration, an assistant with genuine concern says, "I'm sorry to hear you feel this way. Is there anything I can do to help you?" Patients may simply need a person to listen, a friendly smile, or a comforting pat on the shoulder. Care should be taken to avoid such gestures if the patient indicates that they do not want you to enter their personal space.

Acceptance of a Culturally Diverse Population

As discussed previously, today's administrative assistant must communicate with people who speak English as a second language. It may be necessary to use another dictionary or reference (e.g., *Spanish Terminology for the Dental Team*) if an interpreter is not available. Such references help one to communicate with patients to obtain basic information for clinical and financial records as well as answers to clinical questions.

Each person's values are established as a result of his or her background and previous experience. To accept others, one must be willing to accept them as worthy human beings without a desire to change them to fit into a preconceived value system. Accept them for who they are; do not try to make them be what a certain value system states that they ought to be. Communication is often difficult when a person acts or appears different from what is perceived as the norm. For instance, when a patient with a prosthesis replacing his or her right arm visits the office, the prosthesis may attract attention, and a staff member may even stare at the device. The focus is on the disability rather than the patient. In the healthcare profession, it is important to concentrate on seeing the patient and not just his or her disability.

Enthusiasm

Being enthusiastic means being interested in work, being expressive, and leaving personal problems at home. Being enthusiastic does not mean being phony or a constant chatterbox; it means having a sincere interest in work and the greater world. A dental assistant who is enthusiastic about work is likely to read professional journals, to seek knowledge about new technology or specific areas of interest, to participate in community activities or professional organizations, and to become an involved professional. To be enthusiastic, one must act enthusiastically.

PRACTICE NOTE

To be enthusiastic, you must act enthusiastically.

An enthusiastic dental assistant takes time to learn about patients and their interests. When patients ask questions, the dental assistant seeks the answers. An enthusiastic dental assistant is happy to get to work, enjoys sharing others' experiences, appreciates good humor, and finds job satisfaction at the end of the day. Enthusiastic people have a positive outlook on life.

Assertiveness

Being assertive does not mean the same thing as being aggressive. An assertive person is bold and enterprising in a nonhostile manner. An administrative assistant is often called on to assume new responsibilities, and he or she must take the initiative to get the job done. Consider the following situation: Staff members in the office where the administrative assistant has been employed for 3 years have been complaining about salaries, often among themselves at lunchtime. Everyone feels awkward about discussing it with the dentist, because they are not sure what to say. An assertive person will take the initiative to research salaries in areas that represent comparable responsibilities, determine the production and value of each staff member, and present the data to the dentist in a nonthreatening manner. To be assertive often requires tact, initiative, and willingness to take a risk.

Effective Listening

Listening is more than hearing. A good listener hears not only the facts but also the feeling behind the facts. Good listening is a combination of hearing what a person says and becoming involved with the person who is talking. Sometimes a hearing loss or preoccupation with one's own problems, goals, or feelings can make it difficult to hear what is really being communicated. In a busy dental office, what the patient is really saying may be ignored because a staff member is too preoccupied with work, deadlines, or future activities to listen effectively to the patient's needs. Often only what one wants to hear or has time to hear is actually heard.

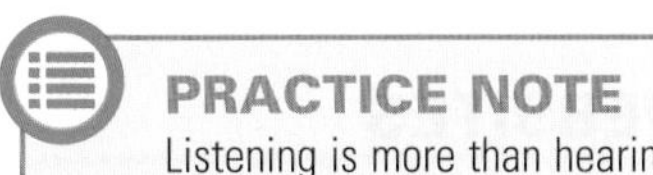

PRACTICE NOTE
Listening is more than hearing.

Sometimes a listener forgets to listen with the eyes. To see what a person is saying, it is necessary to look at the speaker when he or she is talking (Figure 1-4). When observing a person's body language, it is important to observe his or her facial expressions, gestures, and posture, which all give clues about that person's feelings. Consequently, it is possible to better hear what people are saying by observing the emotions that they display.

During reflective listening, the listener absorbs what has been said, reflects on it, and restates or paraphrases the feeling or content of the message in a way that demonstrates understanding and acceptance. This type of listening is beneficial to a healthcare professional; the dentist and the patient interact to create a better understanding of the situation. A scenario in a dental office might go something like the following:

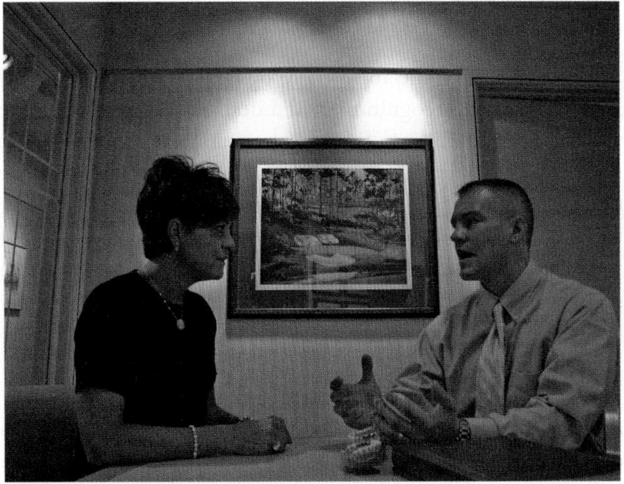

FIGURE 1-4 A dentist listens with her eyes during a consultation with a patient. (Courtesy Shane McDowell, DMD [Snyder McDowell LLC] and Staci DiRoma, Fort Myers, FL.)

Patient: "I just don't know whether to have a porcelain crown on this front tooth or not. My family has always accepted me like this, but every time I have my picture taken I always worry that this gray tooth will show, so I keep my mouth closed."

Assistant: "So you have considered having the crown done, but sometimes you feel you shouldn't do it? Is that how you feel?"

Patient: "Uh huh."

The assistant has restated the basic statement of the patient. The message was given in the assistant's own words, and it was not judgmental. When they have been correctly paraphrased, patients generally respond in the affirmative. If not, the paraphrasing needs to be repeated until the message is clear to both parties.

Another example of this listening style and paraphrasing is given here:

Dentist employer: "I don't understand why we haven't received the new impression material that we ordered."

Assistant: "You seem concerned about the order. Let me check on the order I placed and see if it has been shipped."

Dentist employer: "Okay, thanks. I was just wondering if maybe the supply house isn't stocking that material anymore."

This conversation could have ended with the dentist's original statement, which would have left the assistant becoming upset and thinking that the dentist's words had a hidden meaning. Instead, the assistant queried the dentist to determine the true meaning of the statement.

At first using these techniques may seem cumbersome or artificial. Practice them, and soon the benefits of reflective listening will become clear. Good listening skills require that the listener truly understand the speaker before formulating a response. Such action results in improved relationships with patients and staff and often in fewer conflicts.

Recognition of Others' Needs

All people need some form of recognition. Office colleagues need friendship, recognition, and a desire to feel that they are valued for their contributions to the team's success. However, this does not mean that office colleagues have to socialize outside of the office. It simply means that they should be willing to work cooperatively together to accomplish the objectives of the practice. Ignoring another person's needs does not facilitate good interpersonal relations.

Sense of Humor

A dental office can be a stressful setting for staff members who clamor to meet the demands of the daily schedule and of the patient who is filled with fear about potential treatment. How one interprets a crisis situation, however, is more important. Look at the situation with a sense of humor, and lighten up. However, always be careful to laugh at the situation and not at the person. Patients and colleagues should not be made the brunt of jokes.

Consider adding humor to the office with cartoons on the bulletin board. Remember that humor lessens conflict and eases tension. It is perhaps the best medicine prescribed in any dental office.

Willingness to Be a Team Player

Dentistry is a team-oriented business. Building a team is a simple concept when it is realized that teams are made up of individuals with diverse skills and talents. Each team member must have clearly defined skills that need to be identified and measured against the skills of other team members. After a person realizes his or her role on the team and how best to accomplish specific tasks, achieving team goals can be accomplished and eagerly anticipated. Offices that are committed to building a team can achieve results more effectively than offices in which each individual works independently.

These characteristics should be present when working with staff members as well as with patients. In other words, coworkers should be afforded all of the same collaboration and courtesies that are shown to patients.

LEARNING ACTIVITIES

1. Define cultural competence.
2. Explain how organizational culture applies to the function of a dental practice.
3. Choose a culture from a country such as Asia, India, or Somalia and research the cultural characteristics that may become issues in a dental practice.
4. Research the different treatments that could be completed by members of each of the nine dental specialties.
5. Explain the role of a leader and a manager in a dental practice.
6. Describe common organizational cultures that could exist in a dental practice.
7. Describe situations in a dental office that are more effective when they are performed as a team.
8. Describe the role of a dental management company within the dental practice.

Please refer to the student workbook for additional learning activities.

BIBLIOGRAPHY

Alvesson M, Sveningsson S: *Changing organizational culture: cultural change work in progress*, New York, 2008, Routledge.

Bruch H, Wass DL, Covey DR, et al: *Habits of highly effective managers*, ed 2, New York, 2009, Simon & Schuster.

Drucker PF: *On leadership*, Boston, 2011, Harvard Business School Publishing.

Fulton-Calkins PJ, Rankin DS, Shumack KA: *The administrative professional*, ed 14, Mason, OH, 2011, South-Western Cengage Learning.

Green KA, Lopez M, Wysocki A, et al: *Diversity in the workplace: benefits, challenges, and the required managerial tools*, Gainesville, FL, 2012, University of Florida.

Hesselgrave D: "Verbal and nonverbal communication," http://home.snu.edu/~hculbert/verbal.htm.

Mosby: *Spanish terminology for the dental team*, ed 2, St Louis, 2011, Mosby.

Rath T, Conchie B: *Strengths based leadership*, New York, 2008, Gallup Press.

RECOMMENDED WEBSITES

www.masterycompany.com
www.amdpi.com
www.edis.ifas.ufl.edu

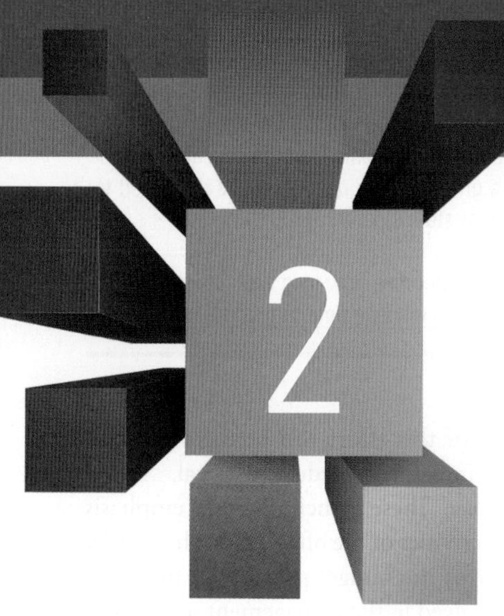

2 Dental Team Management

http://evolve.elsevier.com/Finkbeiner/practice

LEARNING OUTCOMES

1. Define the key terms in this chapter.
2. Discuss the importance of establishing goals and objectives for a dental practice.
3. Discuss factors that motivate employees and the importance of business office etiquette.
4. Identify members of a dental practice and discuss the emerging dental workforce model.
5. Discuss the shifting role of the administrative assistant in a dental practice and list the various duties involved with the position.
6. Discuss the importance of staff management, including:
   - Identify the five *Rs* of good management.
   - Identify the functions of an administrative assistant.
   - Identify characteristics of an effective administrative assistant.
   - Discuss the attributes of an ethical administrative assistant.
7. Discuss the importance of staff communication, including:
   - Describe the channels of communication
   - Explain employee empowerment.
   - Discuss the procedures for conducting a staff meeting.
   - Discuss the management of staff conflict and barriers to staff communication.
8. Explain the importance of hiring a skilled administrative assistant.
9. Describe how to manage time efficiently.
10. Explain the purpose and components of an office procedural manual including the contents of a personnel policy.
11. Describe recruitment and hiring practices, including:
    - Explain the use of pre-employment testing.
    - Discuss the interview process.
    - Describe new employee orientation.

KEY TERMS

Administrative assistant A person whose role is often defined as secretary, receptionist, business assistant, or "front-desk person" and whose responsibilities include the day-to-day management of the dental practice.

ADT Advanced Dental Therapist; a dental professional who can formulate an individualized treatment plan authorized by the collaborating dentist and who can perform nonsurgical extractions of permanent teeth. This person is identified in dental laws in limited areas of the country.

Certified Dental Assistant A credential granted by the Dental Assistant National Board and received after successful completion of the Certified Dental Assistant examination.

CDHC Community Dental Health Coordinator; an individual trained to provide basic preventive care and patient education and to help those patients with unmet dental care needs to access dental services. These specialists only practice in certain areas of the United States.

Communication The ability to understand and be understood. It is the act or process of using words, sounds, signs, or behaviors to express your ideas, thoughts, feelings, etc., to someone else.

DDS Doctor of Dental Surgery; a degree granted upon graduation from a university dental school. The graduate is eligible to take a state Board of Dentistry licensure examination as specified by the given state. A DDS is essentially the same degree as a DMD.

Dental Therapist A mid-level dental provider who can perform limited restorative and therapeutic services and who works under a collaborative management agreement with a dentist in accordance with the rules of the Board of Dentistry in certain states.

DMD Doctor of Dental Medicine; a degree granted to a dentist upon graduation from a university dental school. A DMD is essentially the same degree as a DDS.

DT Dental Therapist; a mid-level dental provider who can perform limited restorative and therapeutic services and who works under a collaborative management agreement with a dentist. This person is identified in dental laws in limited areas of the country.

EFDA Expanded Functions Dental Assistant; a person with an advanced level of education in dental auxiliary treatments who can, under the specified level of supervision, perform the placement and finishing of restorations after the dentist has prepared the tooth and perform other advanced intraoral functions.

Licensed Dental Assistant A credential granted to a dental assistant by a specific state after the successful completion of the educational requirements needed to perform additional clinical duties in a dental office.

Manager A term that is often used to refer to an administrative assistant.

Registered Dental Assistant A credential granted to a dental assistant by a specific state after the successful completion of the educational requirements needed to perform additional clinical duties in a dental office.

Registered Dental Hygienist
A licensed dental staff member who has completed the educational and testing requirements of a given state to perform duties delegated to the dental hygienist per that state's dental laws.

Time management
The ability to prioritize tasks, to determine how long each project will take, and to work effectively to manage time to production.

ESTABLISHING PRACTICE GOALS AND OBJECTIVES

Before opening a dental practice, the dentist should define a practice philosophy, establish specific objectives, and create a mission statement for the practice. A lack of goals and objectives results in a lack of direction for the dentist and staff, which may result in poor relationships with patients. As the practice grows, these goals and objectives will need to be revised and the mission statement updated. It is vital that the dentist in a healthcare practice seek input from the staff when establishing these objectives. If a dental management company is used in the practice, it is essential that the role of this company be included in the objectives and that the relationship between the various staff members be well defined.

A common sequence for establishing objectives includes the following steps:

- *Develop a practice philosophy.* In a broad statement, the dentist identifies the practice's basic feelings toward patient care, business management, auxiliary use, health and safety, and continuing education.
- *Develop practice objectives.* During this stage, each broad goal is broken into a series of specific objectives for the practice. These objectives should be specific positive action statements that indicate the expected results. As the dentist and staff work through the development of objectives for the practice, these objectives become rules by which the office is managed. As the practice expands and new technology is developed, it will be necessary to review and revise these goals and objectives. Most important to participatory management is the involvement of the entire dental team in the development of these objectives.
- *Determine a mission statement.* This is a statement that speaks to the way the practice is to be managed and the roles of the staff and the patients. It is provided to the staff and the patients so that they may have a better understanding of the mission of the practice.
- *Develop practice policies.* These are statements of basic policy that will affect both staff members and patients. These statements may be covered by broad headings that are followed by specific policies. It is wise to share these with both the patients (as shown in the office policy in Chapter 3) and the staff (as shown in the procedural manual later in this chapter).
- *Develop procedural policies.* Each broad statement can be broken down again into specific objectives and further defined as specific tasks for all of the common office procedures. The results of this effort will be most valuable when they are inserted into the procedural manual.
- *Develop business principles.* These principles place emphasis on the actual business activities of the office. Here the dentist outlines in numeric terms the budget process for the practices and procedures involved in the management of business activities.
- *Develop practice standards.* It is necessary for the dentist to identify a quality standard that defines his or her own self-performance level as well as the performance level expected of the staff. The dentist should provide the staff with an explanation of how these standards will be maintained. Plans should be made regarding how to periodically validate that the practice standards are being met.
- *Develop a staff recognition program.* As previously stated, the staff is the greatest asset that a dentist can have in his or her office. Specific guidelines should be established for hiring a qualified staff, selecting a wide range of creative benefits, and establishing a competitive salary scale that reflects productivity and cost-of-living increases.

FACTORS THAT MOTIVATE EMPLOYEES

Most employees work hard if they are compensated well and recognized for their efforts. However, a common complaint of dental staff members is a lack of recognition. An employee must be given challenging responsibilities, and salaries must be commensurate with the accomplishment of these responsibilities. Frequently saying "thank you" helps to improve rapport, but profit sharing, gift certificates, and travel must not be overlooked as real incentives for a recognition program. Box 2-1 contains a list of suggestions that may help to motivate employees.

BUSINESS OFFICE ETIQUETTE

The term *office etiquette* refers to business manners. Rules that applied to social graces 25 years ago or even 10 years ago may no longer work in our society. Many former rules of etiquette were formal and rigid and often do not apply to the more casual lifestyles of today's society. However, in a professional business office, the fact still remains that one's actions and behaviors are observed by clients, patients, visitors, and those who have the potential to promote.

For a dentist employer, the potential for practice growth and patient acceptance depends on the etiquette of the staff. Good

BOX 2-1

Suggestions for Motivating Employees

- Keep work assignments interesting and challenging.
- Provide recognition when a job is well done.
- Be open, friendly, and professional with staff.
- Respect the employee for their skills and work.
- Encourage communication and involvement in setting goals.
- Provide job security.
- Listen when an employee has an idea about how to do things better.
- Allow employees to think for themselves.
- Provide employees with a chance to develop skills.
- Assign a job that is not too easy.
- Provide good pay.
- Provide good benefits.

manners can lead to promotions over equally qualified persons with less poise; they create a self-confident, successful, and professional person. They also help professionals to handle their superiors, and they lessen awkwardness among people. These behaviors are essential to the building of good relationships. Specific applications of etiquette are applied to different phases of business activities in many of the chapters in this book.

Etiquette or the application of good manners can be applied to daily interactions with each member of the staff as well as with all of the patients. Good etiquette must be practiced on a daily basis, and it cannot simply be turned on and off when patients are around. The statement "Good manners begin at home" can be adapted to the dental office by remembering that good manners begin with the dentist and staff. The failure to promote good manners with each other can be detrimental. Employers subconsciously take the pulse of relationships among their employees and staff. If such readings reveal poor relationships among the staff or with patients, action needs to be taken to modify behavior to ensure the success of the practice. Furthermore, as discussed later in this chapter, poor relationships relate directly to productivity. Box 2-2 lists several suggestions for implementing good professional business etiquette.

BOX 2-2

Tips for Professional Etiquette in the Dental Office

- Determine the office code of behavior.
- Extend a friendly greeting to coworkers each day.
- Make introductions when individuals are not acquainted.
- Extend friendly greetings to people who enter the office; stand when you greet the person.
- Introduce yourself.
- Extend a cordial "thank you" or "goodbye" when someone leaves the office for the day.
- Maintain good relations with your peers.
- Learn how to handle your rivals with tact.
- Be a team player.
- Avoid becoming a do-gooder who seeks constant recognition.
- When conflict exists, learn to mend fences.
- Dress and act professionally when representing the office at conferences or seminars.
- Use correct grammar, pronounce words correctly, and expand your vocabulary.
- Explain technical terms in understandable language without being demeaning.
- Make patients feel important; discuss issues that are of interest to them.
- Introduce yourself to a new patient; shake hands heartily to extend a warm welcome.
- If a person is engaged in a conversation with another person, avoid standing within hearing range. If you wish to talk to one of them, leave the area and return later.
- Do not eat or drink in front of patients.
- Say "thank you" when a patient or staff member is helpful, has cooperated during treatment, or has complimented you.
- Send thank-you notes for referrals or other thoughtful acts.
- Respect the privacy of both patients and colleagues.
- If the telephone rings while you are talking to a patient, excuse yourself to answer it. If a lengthy conversation is expected, ask the caller if you can return the call, and then complete the business with the patient.

THE MEMBERS OF THE DENTAL TEAM

The traditional dental team includes one or more of the dental professionals listed below. Although each in-office clinical staff person has specific clinical duties, it should be noted that all staff must assume certain business-related responsibilities.

Dentist

The dentist, a DDS or a DMD, has primary responsibility for the clinical treatment of the patients in the dental office. He or she is the person responsible for the diagnosis and treatment of the patient. The dentist must maintain a close relationship with the business office or the management company to ensure that all the business activities are closely monitored. The professional organization for the dentist is the American Dental Association (ADA; www.ada.org). A dentist is licensed to practice in every state.

Dental Hygienist

The dental hygienist is responsible for the preventive care of patients in the dental practice. The dental hygienist is also responsible for recall and must work with the business staff to ensure that this practice is carried out. In some offices, recall is maintained by the business staff; see Chapter 12 for a discussion of the benefits of the hygienist assuming this responsibility. In addition, the hygienist must communicate inventory needs to the business staff so that supplies can be ordered regularly. The dental hygienist may also be an independent contractor and work for himself or herself. At this time, only a few states allow unsupervised practice in all settings for a licensed dental hygienist. The professional organization for the registered dental hygienist is the American Dental Hygienists' Association (ADHA; www.adha.org). A dental hygienist is licensed to practice in every state.

Dental Assistant

The dental assistant may be a clinical assistant or a business assistant. A clinical assistant performs chairside duties, whereas the business assistant performs business duties at a variety of levels. The professional association for dental assistants is the American Dental Assistants' Association (ADAA; www.dentalassistant.org).

A dental assistant may take one or more of the certification examinations offered by the Dental Assistant National Board (DANB): Certified Dental Assistant (CDA), Certified Orthodontic Assistant (COA), Certified Preventive Functions Dental Assistant (CPFDA), and Certified Restorative Functions Dental Assistant (CRFDA). The national certifications each consist of two or more component exams. In some states, these certifications or their individual component exams meet state requirements for dental assistants to qualify to perform specified functions. Information about these examinations can be found at www.danb.org.

State laws vary widely with regard to the duties that a dentist may delegate to dental assistants and are related to registration, licensure, or other types of dental assistant credentialing. In some states, a clinical assistant may become licensed or registered and may use the title Registered Dental Assistant (RDA), Licensed Dental Assistant (LDA), or another similar title as prescribed by that state's dental practice act. In other states, dental assistants are not registered or licensed, but they may earn certificates or permits to perform specific functions such as radiography, coronal polishing, placing sealants, or monitoring patients who are receiving nitrous oxide analgesia. In many states, there is an "unlicensed" level of dental assistant, who may be trained on the job to perform basic supportive procedures, as well as a higher credentialed level of dental assistant, who must meet specific education and exam requirements as defined by state regulations and who is authorized to perform specified intraoral duties under a dentist's supervision. One resource for more detailed information about dental assisting duties and requirements for each state is the "Meet State Requirements" area of the DANB website (www.danb.org). For authoritative information about dental assisting regulations for a specific state, contact the board of dentistry for that specific state.

Within the business office, the dental assistant may become an administrative assistant, office manager, insurance coordinator, or a treatment coordinator, or he or she may perform a variety of other specific business activities. Often a dentist or management company will hire a person with an extensive business background for one of these positions and then provide them additional education in dentistry. The American Association of Dental Office Managers (AADOM; www.dentalmanagers.com) is a supportive organization for this staff person.

Dental Laboratory Technician

A laboratory technician works in a commercial laboratory or in a private dental practice. This person may take a national certification examination to become a Certified Dental Technician (CDT). The dental laboratory technician does not perform any intraoral duties. For more information about dental laboratory technicians, visit the website of the National Board for Certification in Dental Laboratory Technology at www.nbccert.org.

Emerging Dental Workforce Models

In recent years, various groups within the dental community have looked for ways to increase access to dental care for underserved populations, and some have proposed the addition of new types of dental healthcare providers and auxiliaries to the dental workforce. Some states have established an advanced level of dental auxiliary, often called an Expanded Functions Dental Auxiliary (EFDA), who can, under the specified level of supervision, perform the placement and finishing of restorations after the dentist has prepared the tooth and carried out other advanced intraoral functions. Using EFDAs for the performance of advanced functions may help a dental office to reduce costs and treat more patients.

The ADA has piloted a program in which Community Dental Health Coordinators (CDHCs) are trained to provide basic preventive care and patient education and to assist those with unmet dental care needs to access dental services. CDHCs are recruited from the communities that they will serve; this helps to eliminate obstacles such as language or cultural barriers that interfere with access to care. New Mexico is the first state to establish a state certification for CDHCs, and pilot project participants have provided services in communities in six other states.

A number of states have been considering the addition of mid-level dental providers who can perform limited restorative and therapeutic services and who work under a collaborative management agreement with a dentist. Minnesota became the first state to authorize a mid-level provider when it established licensure for Dental Therapists (DTs) and Advanced Dental Therapists (ADTs). The scope of practice for the Minnesota DT is broad and includes cavity preparation, the restoration of primary and permanent teeth, and the extraction of primary teeth; Minnesota ADTs can also formulate individualized treatment plans that are authorized by the collaborating dentist, and they can perform the nonsurgical extraction of permanent teeth. In Minnesota, DTs and ADTs must work in practice settings that serve low-income, uninsured, and underserved patients.

In 1999, an oral health survey of American Indian and Alaska Native (AI/AN) dental patients found that 79% of the 2- to 5-year-old members of this population had a history of tooth decay. The Alaska Native Tribal Health Consortium (ANTHC), in collaboration with Alaska's Tribal Health Organizations (THOs), developed a new and diverse dental workforce model to address AI/AN oral health disparities.

The ANTHC began working on bringing Dental Health Aide Therapists (DHATs) to Alaska during the early 2000s. The first DHAT began practicing there in 2004. The first DTs working in the United States were the Alaskan DHATs. DHATs are different from the Minnesota DTs and ADTs in that DHATs are federally authorized and regulated. The Dental Health Aide (DHA) program includes four types of dental care providers. The Primary Dental Health Aide (PDHA) concentrates on delivering preventive services at the village level. The Expanded Function Dental Health Aide (EFDHA) has an elevated skill set that enables him or her to function under the direct or indirect supervision of a dentist and to perform simple to complex tooth restorations and supragingival dental cleanings. The Dental Health Aide Hygienist (DHAH) is able to administer local anesthetic. The highest level of provider is the DHAT; the DHAT is a dental provider who is similar to a Physician Assistant in the field of medicine. Although the DHAT is a new type of provider in the United States, DHAT-like providers work in more than 50 countries worldwide, including Canada and New Zealand. These new Alaskan dental team members work with the THO dentists and hygienists to provide preventive, basic restorative, and urgent care services. The DHAT completes a 2-year course of study followed by a 3-month or 400-hour preceptorship under the supervising dentist. After completion of the preceptorship, a DHAT can apply for certification through a federal board. After becoming certified, the DHAT can practice under general supervision remotely from his or her supervisor. The DHAT scope of practice is very similar to that of the ADT. These individuals are providing care in AI/AN communities in which access to dental care has historically been very difficult.

The scopes of practice of the four different DHA providers vary widely, and so do their training and education requirements in Alaska. DHAs are certified but not licensed providers. Recertification occurs every 2 years and requires the completion of 24 hours of continuing education and continual competency evaluation.

As other states consider the addition of advanced dental auxiliaries or mid-level dental providers to the dental workforce, it is likely that these models will continue to evolve. For information about scope of practice or qualifications for advanced auxiliaries or mid-level providers in a particular state, contact that state's board of dentistry.

THE SHIFTING ROLE OF THE ADMINISTRATIVE ASSISTANT

For many years, the administrative assistant's role has been defined by various terms, including *secretary, receptionist, business assistant*, and even *front-desk person*. Many of these titles are still used today, but the changing role of this important staff person has resulted in the more appropriate title of *administrative assistant*. The duties of the administrative assistant are varied and may be assigned at different levels. As the dental team expands, the dentist is likely to delegate more management duties to the administrative assistant. In a large dental practice, a dentist may employ several staff members in the business office, each with separate responsibilities. However, in a smaller practice, these duties may be delegated to one person. The **administrative assistant** title in this text refers to the person whose primary responsibility involves the business activities of the dental office. If a management company is used, many of the business office tasks will be assigned to that company's staff. In general, the duties of an administrative assistant include many of the tasks identified in Box 2-3.

STAFF MANAGEMENT

The term *management* was defined in Chapter 1. However, as this chapter looks more specifically at the business office, it is important to realize that management in the dental office may be defined as the process of getting things accomplished with and through people by guiding and motivating their efforts toward common objectives.

Some people say that "managers are born, not made." However, **managers** can develop their natural skills into sound management skills through experience, effort, and learning. As a person advances into an administrative position, he or she will make mistakes, but remember that learning comes from mistakes as well as successes.

The "Five Rs" of Management

Successful management can be attributed to five basic "Rs": responsibility, respect, rapport, recognition, and remuneration.

PRACTICE NOTE

Individuals can develop their natural skills into sound management skills through experience, effort, and learning.

An employee should be delegated all tasks that are legally delegable to his or her role and for which he or she is properly qualified. Employees cannot work to achieve their maximum productivity if they feel that they are not given responsibility for which they are answerable.

Responsibility denotes duty or obligation. It also denotes follow-through and the completion of a project. An employee who is to become a valuable member of the dental health team must be delegated responsibility. If responsibility is withheld, then it is assumed that the administrative assistant or employer does not feel that the employee is capable of the task; the retention of this employee should be carefully considered.

Respect is consideration or esteem given to another person. Each member of the dental health team must respect the others' education, skills, and values. To not have respect indicates a lack of confidence and again reflects a poor attitude toward another person's capabilities. Each member has a major role on the team and should possess expert skills and credentials that warrant respect.

Rapport is a mutually trusting or emotional relationship that exists among the office staff members. Each dentist sets the tone

BOX 2-3

Basic Job Responsibilities of the Administrative Assistant

Maintain Patient and Staff Relations

- Schedule appointments.
- Set up meetings and conferences.
- Obtain information for and maintain all patient clinical and financial records.
- Prepare consultation materials.
- Communicate both verbally and in writing with patients and staff both within and outside of the office.
- Administer computer networks.
- Set up and administer financial arrangements with patients and other parties.
- Maintain recall and inventory systems.
- Implement marketing strategies.
- Design office manuals and pamphlets.
- Arrange for and conduct staff meetings and other conferences.
- Solve day-to-day problems within the role of the administrative professional.
- Provide support for patients and professional staff.
- Make travel arrangements.
- Implement state and federal regulations.
- Initiate job advertisements, conduct interviews, and make recommendations regarding the employment of office personnel.
- Set up training and evaluation processes for employees.
- Organize, assign, and evaluate workloads.
- Arrange for risk management and Occupational Safety and Health Administration (OSHA) seminars.
- Supervise appropriate office support staff.

Operate Electronic Office Equipment

- Use telecommunication technology (e.g., telephone, voicemail, e-mail, fax machine).
- Manage the practice's websites.
- Help to upgrade and recommend office software.
- Provide computer and software training.

Manage Records

- Manage patient records, including clinical charts, insurance forms, laboratory requisitions, Health Insurance Portability and Accountability Act of 1996 (HIPAA) forms, and other financial and clinical data.
- Maintain employee records.
- Maintain OSHA records.
- Maintain Safety Data Sheets.
- Prepare state and federal forms.
- Maintain an accounts payable system.
- Use a credit bureau and a collection agency as appropriate.
- Order and receive supplies and verify invoices.

Manage Communication

- Manage incoming and outgoing mail.
- Maintain an e-mail system.
- Maintain United States Postal Service mail.
- Assist in maintaining current website.

for the rapport in the office. A good rapport in the office is effused into the patients who recognize how well the team members work together during tense times and how they enjoy each other's professional friendship.

Recognition is a type of achievement. A person can be recognized for a task well done or for special achievements. Recognition can come in the form of verbal praise, a sign placed in the office that recognizes an individual's employment and credentials, a monetary gift, or a gift certificate.

Remuneration is a monetary recognition of achievement. Most employees say that they are willing to work hard if they are compensated for their efforts. Remuneration should be based on education, merit performance, longevity, and cost of living. Dentist employers who affirm that their employees have worked with them for many years with repeated job satisfaction reviews are those who delegate responsibility; who create good rapport in the office; who respect, trust, and recognize their employees; and who provide compensation commensurate to other small business and allied health employers.

Functions of an Administrative Assistant

Because this textbook deals primarily with practice management, the role of the administrative assistant will be discussed in detail.

The basic functions of an administrative assistant in a dental office are shown in the schematic drawing in Figure 2-1. Some assistants may interpret this diagram to mean that their job is "a vicious circle." In actuality, many of these functions overlap, and the basis for each depends on planning. Sound planning before beginning an activity may eliminate the need for crisis management or handling one crisis after another.

Planning involves identifying what is to be done in the future. The goals and objectives discussed earlier are vital to planning. The administrative assistant will be involved in long-range planning as well as daily planning.

Organizing involves determining how the work will be divided and accomplished by members of the dental team. After procedures have been identified and tasks enumerated for each procedure, the administrative assistant is required to assign the duties to specific staff members. It is essential that the dentist give this authority to the administrative assistant. Without this authority, the administrative assistant cannot manage effectively.

Staffing includes the recruiting, selecting, orienting, promoting, paying, and rewarding of employees. Cooperation among staff members will be necessary as new employees are integrated into each technical area of the office. Staffing also involves instructing, evaluating, and educating employees as well as providing opportunities for their future development. In addition,

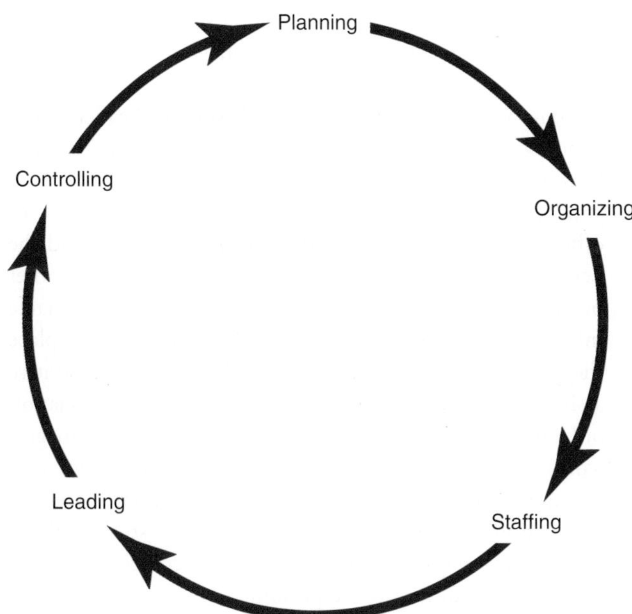

FIGURE 2-1 Functions of an administrative assistant.

the administrative assistant is responsible for recommending an appropriate system of pay and a benefit package.

Leading involves directing, guiding, and supervising the staff during the performance of their duties and responsibilities. It consists of exercising leadership; communicating ideas, orders, and instructions; and motivating employees to perform their work effectively and efficiently. This is really the "people" function of management.

Controlling is the function of management that deals with determining whether or not plans are being completed and, when necessary, making decisions to modify plans to achieve specific objectives.

Basic Skills of an Administrative Assistant

At this point, one may wonder what basic skills are required to function as an administrative assistant and to perform the administrative role effectively. Although many skills are needed, a few of the most important ones are the following:

- Conceptual skills
- Human relations skills
- Administrative skills
- Technical skills

The relative importance of these skills varies according to the type of office; the type of practice (i.e., general or specialty); the job being performed; the staff being managed; and the involvement of a practice management company if one is used.

Conceptual skills involve the ability to acquire, analyze, and interpret information in a logical manner. These skills help one to put an idea or concept into perspective and to perceive how this idea would affect the whole practice.

Human relations skills help with the understanding of people and with effectively interacting with them. These skills are vital in a health profession and include communication, motivation, and an ability to lead.

Administrative skills are those that help you to use all of the other skills effectively when performing administrative functions. These include the ability to establish and follow policies and procedures, to process paperwork in an organized manner, and to coordinate activities in the dental office.

PRACTICE NOTE

Human relations skills help you to understand people and allow you to interact with them.

Technical skills include understanding and being able to effectively supervise the specific processes, practices, and techniques required of specific jobs in the business office. This is the use of all of the knowledge of dentistry and business, so that the day-to-day operations of the office may flow smoothly.

The Ethical Administrative Assistant

In Chapter 1, several characteristics of an effective leader were listed. In addition to these characteristics and the basic skills that the administrative assistant should possess, the professional attitude and ethics of this person have a significant influence on the staff. The following suggestions may identify some attributes of an ethical and caring administrative assistant:

- *Respect the dentist and the practice concepts.* Being respectful of a dentist employer means not circumventing him or her with issues or concerns. If an administrative assistant has an idea to improve the practice, discuss it with the employer. If there are problems with a task or a staff member, share these concerns. Believe in the dentist and the practice, and support the objectives that have been defined. If a person stays in a practice in which unethical conduct occurs, he or she is essentially supporting this type of practice; thus, one's personal ethics become questionable.
- *Maintain frequent communication.* For people to follow someone, they must know who that person is, what he or she represents and can do, and what his or her vision is. To do this, the administrative assistant must tell and show the other members of the staff what he or she is about. In other words, the administrative assistant should disseminate ideas in meetings and during day-to-day interactions with the staff and cultivate relationships outside of the office to have a network of contacts from whom to draw information when a task needs to be performed. Written and verbal communication must be continuous and supportive. These individuals must take time to communicate positive responses to the staff. The attitude presented to others affects their performance both positively and negatively. The staff must know that the administrative assistant possesses the skills and knowledge necessary to lead them in their daily workload and that the administrative assistant is also capable of performing the assigned tasks. Frequent communication does not relate to staff interaction only; it must also be practiced

with patients. Patients need to understand relevant issues that relate to their dental care, and they must receive frequent communication from and about the office.

- *Utilize feedback.* Administrative assistants must be able to recognize nonverbal cues, use feedback as a positive source of communication, and transmit feedback between management and staff.
- *Make ethical decisions.* To do this, one must gather facts and analyze problems, develop alternatives, determine the ethical issues involved, brainstorm with staff members, determine what actions should be taken and whether they are practical, and evaluate the results of the decision that was made.
- *Avoid unnecessary delays in decision making.* Sound decisions should be made as soon as possible; if conflicts go unresolved, greater problems may be created.
- *Delegate authority.* The administrative assistant can demonstrate his or her confidence in the staff members by allowing them to assume responsibility and provide freedom for them to work.
- *Identify constraints within which work must be done.* Time limits on production needs must be established, and staff members must be allowed to develop their own approaches within the defined framework.
- *Exercise self-control.* Emotional outbursts do not lead to constructive management. The administrative assistant should never "talk down" to staff members.
- *Make time available to staff.* The administrative assistant should not be too busy to listen to a staff person. This does not mean dropping everything to listen, but time should be made available for staff input.
- *Build and develop strong followers.* One of the hallmarks of a successful administrative assistant is that he or she surrounds himself or herself with action-oriented, dedicated followers. By showing confidence in the followers' abilities, providing challenging assignments, and being genuinely concerned, the administrative assistant garners respect, loyalty, and commitment while inspiring high-quality performance. In essence, the administrative assistant makes it easier to delegate and free himself or herself to devote more energy to issues that require his or her time. The key to this characteristic is for the administrative assistant to be genuine and honest in his or her delegation rather than only delegating duties that involve no challenge or that are not recognized.
- *Be visible.* An administrative assistant cannot hide behind a desk and be a leader. There is nothing arrogant or inappropriate about letting others know what the administrative assistant and other members of the staff have accomplished. The administrative assistant should share a complimentary memo with the staff or patients when significant achievements have been made. He or she should participate and encourage staff members to participate in activities that place the people and the office in the spotlight. He or she should be cautious to not take on too much, and he or she should complete what is taken on with quality and panache.
- *Learn from mistakes.* Everyone makes mistakes, so they should not be agonized over. However, it is important to find ways to avoid making the same mistake again or assigning the blame to others. Some individuals consistently blame others for their mistakes. This characteristic will not be present in a good administrative assistant. Leadership is about accepting the mistake, moving forward, and not wallowing in the past.
- *Expand the leadership role.* An administrative assistant or office manager must extend the leadership role beyond the dental office. Make an effort to become involved in other professional or business groups that will provide valuable information for the office and offer the opportunity to place the office in the spotlight. Specifically, the administrative assistant will want to participate in the American Association of Dental Office Managers, AADOM (www.dentalmanagers.com). This organization provides an opportunity for networking and support with educational webinars, access to foundations of dental practice management, study clubs, a newsletter, a magazine, and an annual conference specifically designed for business office personnel.

STAFF COMMUNICATION

Communication is an essential element of management, and it becomes a vital link for establishing meaningful relationships among the administrative assistant, the dentist, other members of the staff, and the patients. The basic definition of **communication** is understanding and being understood by another person. As Bob Adams states in his book, *Streetwise Managing People: Lead Your Staff to Peak Performance,* "Quality Communication = Positive Interaction." When an office staff employs positive, constructive communication, it is sending a consistent message. The relative success of a dental practice is measured by the ability of the staff members to communicate with each other and with their patients.

Communicating with staff members is in many ways like communicating with patients. Information is being transmitted between people and therefore understanding should occur. However, when communicating with staff members, the status of the individuals involved have changed, and thus the channels of communication may be more complex. To achieve quality communication, consider following the simple steps suggested in Box 2-4.

Channels of Communication

As a dental practice increases in size, the channels of communication become more complicated. Both formal and informal communication exist. A formal communication channel is dictated by the type of management that exists in the practice. Formal communication may be downward, upward, or horizontal.

Downward communication is exemplified when a dentist issues an order or mandate that is disseminated to the staff member at the next level. Downward communication includes instructions, explanations, and communications that help the employee to perform his or her work. These instructions may be given to the business or clinical staff. If a management

BOX 2-4

Suggestions for Creating Positive Staff Interactions

- Help others to be right rather than wrong.
- Whenever possible, have fun.
- Be enthusiastic.
- Seek ways for new ideas to work rather than reasons why they will not.
- Be bold and courageous; take chances.
- Help others to achieve success.
- Maintain a positive mental attitude.
- Maintain confidentiality.
- Verify information given to you before you repeat what you hear; avoid gossip.
- Speak positively about others whenever the opportunity arises.
- Say "thank you" for kind gestures or a job well done.
- Express a happy attitude in your nonverbal communication.
- If you do not have anything positive to say, then do not say anything.

company exists, there may be two-way downward communication from the dentist to the management company and from the management company to the dentist. In this case, too, the management company may give instructions to the business staff within the office.

Upward channels of communication are vital in a formal setting. Employees should be free to express their attitudes and feelings. This type of communication reverses the flow of information and is generally of a reporting nature. It may include suggestions, complaints, or grievances. A lack of upward communication may result in dissatisfied employees.

Horizontal communication is essential for a larger organization. This type of communication involves the transmittal of information from one department to another. This type of communication exists within large offices, clinics, hospitals, and dental schools. Likewise, it could occur in a dental office between the management company and the dentist.

Informal channels of communication can also be referred to as the "grapevine." This form of communication is often feared by administrative assistants; however, if it is handled effectively, it can provide the assistant with insight into staff emotions. Frequently the grapevine carries rumors, personal interpretations, or distorted information. Fear often causes an active grapevine. It becomes the responsibility of the administrative assistant to listen to the grapevine and to eliminate rumors by explaining the actual facts. Thus, the administrative assistant develops skill in the handling of tension created by the grapevine.

Empowering Employees

In Chapter 1, *empowerment* was defined as "putting power where it is needed." Just as the dentist leader has empowered the administrative assistant or office manager, this person should also provide the staff working in the business office with the power and authority to accomplish office objectives.

The dentist who gives employees the power, ability, and permission to accomplish office objectives and to perform legal tasks independently will have the edge over the competition. To be successful, the dentist must be able and willing to recognize the value that each employee brings to the office. In Bob Adams' book, *Streetwise Managing People: Lead Your Staff to Peak Performance*, the author declares that "empowered employees attempt to work above and beyond their anticipated capabilities." To empower employees, he recommends the creation of an environment in which staff members do the following:

- Behave as owners of the job and the company
- Behave in a responsible manner
- See the consequences of the work they do
- Know how they are doing and how they are valued in the practice
- Are included in determining solutions to problems
- Have direct input into the way in which the work they do is done
- Spend a good deal of time smiling
- Ask others if they need help

PRACTICE NOTE

To be successful, the dentist must be able and willing to recognize the value that each employee brings to the office.

Many concepts that Adams introduces seem to show common sense. When applied to a dental practice, these concepts seem to fit like a glove. Box 2-5 lists concepts that can be adapted easily to any dental practice to empower each member of the staff to become a meaningful member of the dental team.

Conducting a Staff Meeting

Two types of staff meetings commonly occur in the dental office: (1) morning "huddle" meetings and (2) routine team or staff meetings, which occur at least monthly.

The "huddle" meeting occurs once a day, most often in the morning, before the day begins. It lasts about 10 to 15 minutes and serves as a time to review all of the patients for the day and to discuss preventive and restorative work that needs to be done, emergency times, patient concerns, and any radiographs to be taken. During this time, patient management problems can be addressed, staff assignments can be made for assorted expanded duties, and business activities can be reviewed. Some offices have such a meeting twice a day and review the morning patients before beginning the afternoon assignments. Such meetings provide the opportunity to adequately prepare for patient treatment and to ensure that the entire team is tuned in to rendering patient care.

Regularly scheduled staff or team meetings should become a routine part of the dental practice, and they should occur at least once a month. These meetings are an effective means of

BOX 2-5

Concepts to Empower Employees

- Create a communication process that is complete, consistent, and clearly understood by all members of the staff.
- Ensure that all employees understand what is expected of them in their respective job positions.
- Provide each employee with the appropriate training, information, and materials to successfully accomplish their job duties.
- Clearly define and establish evaluation instruments for the responsibilities for each job.
- Create controls that are guidelines that allow flexibility.
- Encourage and practice behaviors that promote encouragement, support, and clear feedback to employees.
- Encourage and promote a sense of responsibility in each employee.
- Encourage and promote continuing education and credentialing.
- Create opportunities for staff members to work together in teams.
- Make it easy for people to praise each other. Make the office one that recognizes and acknowledges praiseworthy actions.
- Listen to employees at all times. Make the office systems listen to the employees.
- Trust the employees.

keeping communication channels open. The staff meeting provides an opportunity to define and review the goals of the practice and to help motivate the staff. Although criticism may be part of a staff meeting, such a meeting should not be designed as a gripe session. The time and length of the staff meeting will vary according to the needs of the staff. Some offices schedule an hour per week or month, others close the office for a half or a full day for a retreat session, and still others find breakfast or lunch meetings to be effective. It may be worthwhile to consider having a different staff member head the meeting so that all persons may take responsibility for planning and executing the meetings.

PRACTICE NOTE

The staff meeting provides an opportunity to define and review the goals of the practice.

An agenda may be used when planning a staff meeting. The agenda, in combination with the list of rules presented in Box 2-6, expedites the business objectives of the staff meeting.

Managing Conflict

Some administrative assistants become defensive and irritated when confronted with a complaint. These individuals may feel that a complaint reflects on them personally. Conflicts are normal between an administrative assistant and an employee or between a patient and a member of the staff; however, concern should be raised if numerous complaints arise, because this may indicate a serious problem.

BOX 2-6

Guidelines for Holding Effective Team Meetings

- Notify each staff member of the time and place of the staff meeting. The use of e-mail will ensure that all parties are sent the information.
- Request a return reply for attendance.
- Determine the priority of agenda items.
- Obtain suggestions for these items from staff members.
- Provide a copy of the agenda to each staff member, and adhere to the agenda items.
- Review accomplishments.
- Determine goals and things that need to be changed.
- Establish a method for accomplishing these goals.
- Review outcomes of the meeting.
- Provide keyboarded minutes to the staff.
- Maintain a strict meeting schedule.
- Do not allow one person to monopolize the meeting.
- Do not turn the meeting into a gripe session.

Regardless of the nature of the complaint, the administrative assistant should review the details of the complaint and seek to resolve the problem quickly. Steps taken to resolve the problem may include the following:

- *Make time available* as soon as possible to discuss the problem. A delay may result in additional conflict, or it may be interpreted to mean that the administrative assistant is not interested in listening to the problem.
- *Listen patiently* to all of the issues, and keep an open mind. The administrative assistant can gain the staff member's confidence by encouraging the staff member to talk and by indicating that there is an intention to provide fair treatment.
- *Determine the real issue.* Frequently a complaint is made about a problem when in reality a deeper concern is the real issue. For example, a person may be complaining about unfair work assignments when actually the source of the problem is a personality clash between two staff members.
- *Exercise self-control.* Avoid arguments or expressions of personality conflicts between the complaining parties. Emotional outbursts generally do not lead to a constructive resolution of the problem. Should such an outburst result, it is wise to terminate the meeting until a future meeting can be scheduled so that the problem can be discussed in a calm manner.
- *Avoid a delay in decision making.* A dental office is a relatively small business organization, and allowing a conflict to go unresolved can cause undue stress on the entire staff. If it is necessary to delay a decision, let the persons involved know the status of the problem.
- *Maintain a record.* Documentation of meetings or discussions is helpful should future conflicts arise over the same problem. It is impossible to recall all of the issues about an

incident; therefore, information should be retained in an employee file or another appropriate area for future reference. This memorandum should be presented to the employee, and the employee will then sign it to ensure credibility.

It is not easy to resolve conflict, and most of us wish to avoid it. However, conflict will arise whenever two or more people are working together. The administrative assistant must try to be fair and objective. If these suggestions are followed, at least an attempt to resolve the complaint in a professional manner will have been made; this may avoid minor conflicts that can escalate into major crises.

Barriers to Staff Communication

Barriers that exist in patient communication are prejudice, poor listening, preoccupation, impatience, diversity, and even impaired hearing. These barriers all exist within the staff. Additional barriers, such as status or position, resistance to change and new ideas, and attitudes about work compound communication difficulties with coworkers. Because these barriers exist, administrative assistants should never assume that the message being sent will be received as it was intended. They should be aware of potential misinterpretations and work to overcome such barriers to improve channels of communication with the staff.

Periodically, the staff should evaluate its exchange of information and determine whether all channels of communication are open to everyone. During a staff meeting, an agenda item to consider may be the completion of a questionnaire that would indicate each staff member's feelings about office communication.

ADVANTAGES OF HIRING A SKILLED ADMINISTRATIVE ASSISTANT

A dentist today cannot afford the risk of hiring inexperienced personnel to manage the business office. In addition to having a broad knowledge of dentistry, the administrative assistant should be curious, highly organized, and able to accept responsibility and make decisions; he or she should have an understanding of computers and other automated business equipment, possess skills in management, and communicate well with people.

Few statistics are available, but it seems that, in the past, dentists have hired persons with little knowledge of dentistry and minimal experience, or they have promoted chairside or clinical assistants to roles as administrative assistants. Because administrative assistants need a broad background in dentistry, it appears that the last arrangement mentioned would have a distinct advantage if the assistant were willing to accept the transition. Many dentists today are hiring administrative assistants with strong backgrounds in business and then providing a rigorous training program in dental terminology and concepts. If a clinical assistant is transitioned to an administrative role, this will require the clinical assistant to become more involved in the financial systems of the office and to become familiar with common business concepts. The administrative assistant of today is responsible for many dental, financial, and governmental forms. Therefore, a strong business background is highly desirable. Regardless of the door through which the administrative assistant arrives to this position, it is desirable to hire a person with education in both business and dental assisting. The advantages of hiring an educated administrative assistant are listed in Box 2-7.

In addition to hiring an educated administrative assistant, it behooves the dentist or management company to retain an effective office manager in place for the long term, because this provides the stability that many patients are looking for in a dental practice. When an administrative assistant has worked with the dentist for a long time, he or she becomes familiar with the dentist's practice philosophy and is able to provide a solution to minor problems without involving the doctor.

BOX 2-7

Advantages of Hiring an Educated Administrative Assistant

An educated administrative assistant has the following attributes:

- Understands basic dental terminology
- Understands interpersonal communication
- Understands clinical data
- Is able to turn clinical data into financial data
- Is able to explain treatment procedures to a patient
- Can promote or sell dental care
- Understands the consequences of dental neglect
- Practices infection-control procedures
- Implements Occupational Safety and Health Administration regulations
- Understands appointment sequencing for various dental procedures
- Is able to manage emergency procedures
- Is less likely to make common errors

TIME MANAGEMENT

Learning to Use Time Efficiently

A vital aspect of the administrative assistant's job is time management. There is more to working efficiently than just knowing how to perform a specific task. Administrative assistants also need to know when to perform each task, how to choose which job to do first, and how long each project will take. Understanding the relationship of time to production is also important. All of these together make up time management.

Much research has been done over the years on time and motion studies in the dental treatment room. These studies have resulted in the dental profession implementing the concepts of four-handed dentistry and the use of a chairside or clinical assistant to increase productivity and reduce stress. Less emphasis has been placed on production in the dental business office. However, much can be learned from the research that general business has done on time management. Remember, although dentistry is a healthcare system, it is still a small business, and it still has profit as an objective. Thus, time management is a vital component in the dental practice.

Time management in the dental business office involves planning, scheduling work, and avoiding wasted time. The behaviors that waste time in the business office are failing to plan and budget time, giving in to interruptions, failing to follow through and complete a task, slowness with regard to reading and making decisions, performing unnecessary work, and failing to delegate. Other time wasters include a lack of privacy and desk clutter. Solutions to many common time wasters are suggested in Box 2-8.

To determine the effectiveness of time management, the way that work is currently being performed must be assessed. Ways to use time more effectively can be determined, or it may be confirmed that time is already being used efficiently. Evaluation of time management is an ongoing process and can be done routinely by recording the way time is being spent; analyzing how it is spent; determining what activities can be adjusted to make a worker more effective; scheduling activities on a daily, weekly, monthly, and long-range basis; and adhering to the schedule. Efficient time management requires organizing individual tasks, maintaining daily schedules, analyzing daily tasks, scheduling major projects, establishing deadlines, and organizing workflow.

BOX 2-8

Solutions to Eliminate Time Wasters

Time Wasters

- Lack of goals
- Telephone interruptions
- Procrastination
- Feeling tired, stressed, or irritable
- Lack of future plans
- Disorganized work area
- Accepting too many jobs
- Waiting for information or return calls
- Incomplete work
- Socializing with coworkers
- Unnecessary work

Solution

- Prepare a to-do list and use it.
- Use an answering machine or voicemail during specified work times.
- Do it first!
- Schedule a thorough physical examination, develop a wellness plan, and enroll in a stress-management course.
- Develop short- and long-range goals.
- Purchase organizers, put away work when it is finished, and do not begin a new project until the one currently being worked on is complete.
- Learn to say "no."
- Plan time to finish projects with no interruptions.
- Avoid certain situations, and restrict others from too much socializing.
- Analyze the task, and eliminate it if it is not necessary.

Maintaining Daily Schedules

To efficiently maintain a daily schedule, it is necessary to use a calendar of activities and tasks and a "to-do" list that helps to determine priorities, incorporate flexibility, and make use of free time. The proposed schedule can then be reviewed with the dentist.

The use of a calendar and a personal appointment book as well as an office appointment book is necessary for the maintenance of a daily schedule. A desk or electronic calendar provides a method for keeping track of the daily schedule, and it can be used for both short- and long-range scheduling. Handwritten entries should be neat and consistent; confidential entries should not be made in an electronic calendar that is accessible to others.

A to-do list should provide a summary of all pending tasks and not just those to be performed on a specific day. This list need not include routine daily tasks, such as opening and closing the office or opening mail. However, times of the day should be considered for each task. For instance, the bank deposit should not be made until after the mail has arrived, because checks may be received in the mail that could be included in the deposit. Delete each task after it is completed, and transfer tasks that were not completed to a list for the following day.

Determine priorities by ranking each task on the list by its level of urgency and importance. Items on the list can be ranked as follows: (1) tasks that must be completed immediately, (2) tasks that must be completed that day, and (3) tasks that must be done whenever there is time.

Be flexible when making plans for the day, because emergencies arise, and new priority tasks will be identified. For instance, the dentist may need the administrative assistant to immediately produce an important document. At this point, it may be necessary to seek help from other staff members to complete other pressing tasks. With total team effort, a reprioritizing of previously identified tasks can be accomplished quickly when unplanned needs must be met.

In addition to the routine to-do list, another list could be kept to detail various tasks that should be completed when time permits. Such a list provides tasks that can be done when there is a slow time or when there are no patients scheduled.

DESIGNING A PROCEDURAL MANUAL

The procedural manual is a valuable instrument for maintaining maximum efficiency in the dental office while providing a means of communication. It includes the dentist's philosophy for the practice, and it defines the job responsibilities of each team member. The manual also states in specific detail the techniques to be implemented for each procedure in both the business and clinical areas of the office. Although the manual should be written under the direction of the dentist, each member of the team should contribute equally to the development of the manual to provide a total team effort. This manual should be made available to each staff member; it may be posted for the staff on a computer in a public in-house location.

The following list of guidelines provides subjects to be included in an office procedural manual. A basic office manual format can be purchased and inserts added to address the dentist's philosophy and specific duties related to the practice. Templates are also available for manuals in Microsoft Office Templates online. Individual tabs can be made as needed.

Guidelines for a Procedural Manual

I. Statement of purpose or objective of the manual
II. Statement of philosophy of the practice
III. Table of contents
IV. Office communications
  A. Vocabulary
  B. Telecommunications
  C. Reception techniques
  D. Written communication
  E. Patient education
  F. Confidentiality
V. Staff policies
  A. Conduct
  B. Grooming and appearance
  C. Dress codes: clinical and business office attire
  D. Staff meetings
    1. Daily
    2. Regular
  E. Use of office phones for personal needs
  F. Personal cell phone usage
VI. Employment policies
  A. Probationary period
  B. Promotion
  C. Hours of work
  D. Overtime
  E. Holidays
  F. Vacations
  G. Absences and leaves
  H. Salaries
  I. Insurance
  J. Additional benefits
  K. Use of telephones
  L. Use of social media
  M. Termination of employment
VII. Office records
  A. Infection control
    1. Clinical
    2. Records handling
  B. Patient records
  C. Occupational Safety and Health Administration (OSHA) records
  D. Safety Data Sheets (SDSs)
  E. Employee records
  F. Transfer of records
  G. Accounts receivable
  H. Accounts payable
  I. Use of electronic records
VIII. Infection-control policy
  A. OSHA guidelines
    a. Infection control policy
      1. Steps to take after exposure to bloodborne pathogens
  B. Health risk categories
  C. Nomenclature
  D. Disinfection and sterilization guidelines
  E. Waste management
  F. Medical history procedures
  G. Standard precautions
  H. Preventive vaccinations
IX. Clinical procedures
  A. Assignments
  B. Emergencies
  C. Tray setups
  D. Sterilization
  E. Prescriptions
  F. Inventory system
X. Continuing education
XI. Professional organizations

Writing a Personnel Policy

As part of the office procedural manual, a well-defined personnel policy must be established. A fair and equitable personnel policy may help to eliminate conflicts that could arise among team members. The material in Box 2-9 illustrates a suggested personnel policy. This policy may be altered to satisfy the needs of an individual office.

HIRING PRACTICES

Writing a Job Description

A current and accurate job description should exist for each position in the dental office. These job descriptions help employees who are telling prospective employees what will be expected of them on the job, and they also assist with the training of new staff members.

Before an accurate job description can be written, a job analysis must be performed. A job analysis involves observing the employee and gathering information about the job. List the tasks that make up the job, and then determine the skills, personality characteristics, and educational background needed for the employee to perform this job satisfactorily. The staff then reviews the job description. It is revised as necessary and then placed in the procedural manual. An outline for a job description is shown in Figure 2-2.

BOX 2-9

Personnel Policies for the Office of Joseph W. Lake, DDS, and Ashley M. Lake, DDS

Probationary Period

Your first 3 months will be considered a probationary period, during which Drs. Joseph and Ashley Lake will see how you progress with the new work. During this period, your employment may be terminated without notice. The dentist will create a Merit Rating Report at the termination of the probationary period and quarterly thereafter. This report will be used as the basis for salary increases and promotions.

Promotion

Your demonstrated ability to perform your job well, your attendance and punctuality record, and your relationships with employees will all have a bearing on your opportunities for promotion and advancement in salary. Any outside courses of study that result in skills in addition to those noted on your application will be added to your record to ensure complete information when reviewing your record for advancement. All employees will be reviewed every 6 months.

Hours of Work

The office is open from 8:00 AM to 5:00 PM Monday and Wednesday and from 8:00 AM to 9:00 PM on Tuesday and Thursday. On Fridays, the office is closed. Lunch hour is from 12:00 PM to 1:00 PM. The basic week totals 35 working hours that will be assigned by each dentist.

Overtime

Overtime salary is paid in half-hour units. Fractions of less than a half hour of overtime are not reported. If your salary is less than $3520 per month, compensation for work authorized by the dentist is paid at the rate of time and one half beyond 35 hours during any week or for work performed on Saturdays and holidays.

Staff meetings are held daily before patients are seen. You are expected to attend each of these meetings to plan for the day's activities. Each month, at an announced time, a staff meeting is held for a minimum of 1 hour to plan for practice development. All staff must be in attendance unless otherwise excused.

Holidays

You will have the following legal holidays off with pay: New Year's Day, Memorial Day, Independence Day, Labor Day, Thanksgiving Day, and Christmas Day. When the office is closed for a religious holiday or other holiday, an announcement will be made in advance.

Vacations

Requests for vacation time in excess of 1 day must be made 30 days in advance. You will be entitled to 2 weeks of vacation after completing 12 months of continuous employment and to 4 weeks of vacation after 10 years of employment. A legal holiday that falls within the vacation period adds 1 day to your vacation. When a staff member's vacation falls within a vacation period, salary will be paid in advance to the latest regular salary payment date falling within the vacation period.

Absences and Leaves

Regular attendance and punctuality are necessary for smooth functioning of the dental office, and your record in this respect will be considered when determining your advancement and salary adjustment. However, there are certain absences that are unavoidable and for which provision will be made. In each case, the dentists should be notified in advance, when possible, or before 7:30 AM on the day of your absence. If you fail to make proper notification, the unadvised absence will be counted as absence without salary.

Sick Leave for Your Own Confining Illness

When an absence is for your own illness, salary is paid for up to 1 day for each month of employment, cumulative to 30 days. If you need sick leave in addition to the above, such a request should be made to Dr. Lake for additional time without pay.

Court Duty

If you are required to serve as a juror or witness, your absence is considered as a leave with salary.

Death in the Immediate Family

If there is a death in your immediate family, up to 3 days of leave may be granted with salary.

Leave of Absence for Other Reasons

If you request a leave of absence for other reasons or for a longer period than is provided with salary, various factors will be taken into consideration, including your previous work and attendance records, the length of leave you are requesting, the work needs of the office, and any other pertinent factors.

Salaries

Payment of your salary is by check on a weekly basis, covering salary through Wednesday of the current week. Salary checks are distributed each Friday. Salary increases are considered every 6 months. The quality of your work, the amount of responsibility you assume, your attendance and punctuality records, your attitude toward the staff and patients, and your length of service are factors that enter into the consideration. Deductions from salary regularly include withholding tax and Social Security. Deductions for group insurance, hospital care, and other benefits are made only on written request.

Insurance

To help provide security in times of sickness and hospitalization, health insurance is available as follows: membership in a group health insurance plan is available to all those employed more than 1 year on a payroll deduction basis.

Staff members may select this insurance at their own expense for the first 12 months of employment. Deductions for hospital care are made the first payday of each month. At the end of 12 months, Dr. Lake will pay this coverage upon a successful merit rating evaluation. Coverage of your spouse and dependent children under 19 years of age may be included in your hospital care contract.

Social Security is provided through payments by you and Dr. Lake to the US government. Your share of the cost is deducted from each salary payment.

Additional Benefits

In addition to regular salary increases, the members of the staff are eligible for several additional benefits.

BOX 2-9—cont'd

Personnel Policies for the Office of Joseph W. Lake, DDS, and Ashley M. Lake, DDS

Uniform Stipend

Dr. Lake will provide a uniform stipend as follows:

- Chairside or clinical assistants and hygienists will wear surgical scrubs with outer laboratory coats provided by the office and for which all laundry will be provided. At the end of 6 months of successful employment, Dr. Lake will issue an additional $100 a month for shoes.
- Administrative assistants will receive a dress stipend not to exceed $1200 at the end of 6 months. At the end of 12 months, an additional dress or uniform stipend will be issued not to exceed $2000. Thereafter, a stipend will be issued annually not to exceed $2750.

Professional Organizations

At the end of 12 months of successful employment, the dues of your professional organization will be paid by Dr. Lake. The statement and proof of membership must be submitted to Dr. Lake for payment.

Education and Travel

You are encouraged to increase your skills at all times. To ensure your exposure to current changes in dentistry, Dr. Lake will provide the following benefits: after 6 months of employment, payment not in excess of $450 for any educational seminar; after 12 months of employment, 3 days absence with pay and $1200 applicable to coursework or educational travel; after 5 years of employment, 5 days absence with pay and $2500 applicable to coursework or educational travel.

Profit Sharing

After the completion of 2 full years of successful employment, Dr. Lake will provide the following profit-sharing bonus to each staff member: 2% of total business in excess of $350,000 plus 2% of total receipts in excess of $350,000.

Infection-Control Policy

An effective infection-control program has been implemented in the office for the protection of staff members, patients, and family members. It is recommended that you adhere to the *Infection Control Policy Handbook* and that you are aware of all updates of this manual as they occur. The cost of hepatitis B vaccination and tuberculosis vaccination will be covered by the office.

It is highly recommended that you receive other protective vaccines for childhood diseases not previously contracted. You will be compensated for such immunization. Each employee is expected to follow the basic guidelines of the Occupational Safety and Health Administration's Bloodborne Pathogens Standard as follows:

- A written exposure control plan must be updated annually.
- Standard precautions must be used.
- Consideration, implementation, and the use of safer needles and sharps must occur.
- Use engineering and work practice controls, including appropriate personal protective equipment (e.g., gloves, face and eye protection, gowns).
- Use labels and color-coding for sharps disposal boxes as well as proper containers for regulated waste, contaminated laundry, and other specimens.
- Employee training will be provided.
- Decontamination of surfaces must occur.
- Recommended decontamination and processing of all dental instruments and equipment must be performed.

Exposure Incident Protocol

In the case of an exposure incident, immediate action must take place in accordance with the protocol posted in all clinical areas and provided in the *Infection Control Policy Handbook,* which includes the following:

- Provide immediate care to the exposure site.
- Determine the risk associated with exposure by the type of fluid and the type of exposure.
- Evaluate the exposure source.
- The exposed employee is referred as soon as possible to a healthcare provider who will follow the current recommendations of the US Public Health Service Centers for Disease Control and Prevention for testing, medical examination, prophylaxis, and counseling procedures.

The employer must send all of the following with the exposed employee to the care provider:

- A copy of the bloodborne pathogen standard
- A description of the exposed employee's duties as they relate to the exposure incident
- Documentation of the routes of exposure and the circumstances under which the exposure occurred

The healthcare provider will then do the following:

- Evaluate the exposure incident.
- Arrange for the testing of the employee and the source individual (if his or her status is not already known).
- Notify the employee of the results of all tests.
- Provide counseling and postexposure prophylaxis.
- Evaluate reported illnesses.
- Send a written opinion to the employer limited to documentation that the employee was informed of his or her evaluation results, whether the hepatitis B vaccine was indicated, and whether it was received.

Termination of Employment

Resignation

You are asked to give 2 weeks written notice of resignation. If you have been employed for 6 months or more and you resign during the vacation period having given 2 weeks notice, you will be compensated for your vacation according to the vacation schedule.

Release

If you are released from your position for reasons other than misconduct, in which case no notice is given, you will have notice or salary in lieu of notice as follows: if you have been employed for at least 6 but less than 12 months, 1 week; if you have been employed for 13 months or more, 2 weeks.

Use of Telephones and other Social Media

Telephone traffic is heavy at this dental practice. Personal telephone calls affect the workload in two ways: (1) they prohibit incoming calls from patients, and (2) they take time away from your job. Limit your number of personal calls, and receive incoming calls only in an emergency. The use of all social media must be turned off or set on "silent" mode during office hours.

Continued

BOX 2-9—cont'd

Personnel Policies for the Office of Joseph W. Lake, DDS, and Ashley M. Lake, DDS

Definition of Social Media

For the purposes of this policy, social media should be understood to include any website or forum that allows for open communication on the Internet, including but not limited to the following:

- Social networking sites (e.g., LinkedIn, Facebook);
- Microblogging sites (e.g., Twitter);
- Blogs (including company and personal blogs);
- Online encyclopedias (e.g., Wikipedia); and
- Video- and photo-sharing websites (e.g., YouTube, Flickr).

Think Before Posting

In general, each member of the staff should think carefully before posting anything online, because most online social platforms are open for all to see. Despite this policy, employees cannot always be sure who will view, share, or archive the information that is posted. Before posting anything, employees should remember that they are responsible for what is posted online. Employees should carefully consider the risks and rewards with respect to each posting. Employees should remember that any conduct—online or otherwise—that negatively or adversely impacts the employee's job performance or conduct or the job performance or conduct of coworkers or that adversely affects the employers' clients, customers, colleagues, associates, or legitimate business interests may result in disciplinary action up to and including termination. If employees have any doubt about what to post online, it is probably better not to post; after something has been placed in cyberspace, it is often very difficult to retract that information. Employees should use their professional judgment and exercise personal responsibility when posting to any social media websites.

Staff members should attempt to limit their use of social media during working hours or on equipment provided by the dental practice unless such use is related to work or authorized by a supervisor. Likewise, staff members should avoid using their office-provided e-mail addresses to register on social networks, blogs, or other websites for personal use.

Employees should note that this provision is not meant to prohibit them from engaging in the use of social media; rather, it is intended to maintain the professional image of the office.

Job Title __________________
You will report to ______________

GENERAL OBJECTIVES:

The administrative assistant will manage the day-to-day activities of the business office.This person will be responsible for maintaining office documents, patient, employee, and governmental records; scheduling patients; interviewing and managing staff; managing accounts receivable and payable; managing inventory; managing recall and assist hygienist as needed in managing the recall systems; operating electronic office equipment; and maintaining various types of telecommunications systems.

SPECIFIC OBJECTIVES:

Maintain office documents
- Select and complete patient clinical records
- Manage insurance claim forms
- Assist in maintaining recall system
- Maintain employee records
- Complete and maintain governmental forms

Maintain an accounts receivable system
- Maintain accounts receivable activity
- Prepare bank deposits
- Prepare statements
- Follow up delinquent accounts

Perform accounts payable activities
- Verify invoices with monthly statements
- Write checks
- Reconcile the bank statement
- Prepare materials for the accountant

Supervise staff personnel
- Prepare job descriptions
- Interview and screen potential employees
- Determine staff needs and schedules
- Orient new staff
- Evaluate staff

Perform support duties
- Establish equipment maintenance program
- Plan for update and risk management seminars
- Implement state and federal regulations
- Help support staff as needed

JOB CRITERIA:

Education
- Certified/Registered Dental Assistant, Certified Dental Office Manager, or a minimum of 5 years experience in business management
- Knowledge of electronic office automation
- Formal business courses
- Knowledge or experience in management

Personal requirements
- Must be able to work with any employee and be able to resolve conflicts between employees
- Must be able to discuss all dental/financial needs with patients and be objective and pleasant to them
- Must be able to cooperate with other dental office staff personnel
- Must be able to work with the doctor and convey needs to the staff in a participatory manner

SALARY:

$52,000 - $89,500 plus benefits
Salary based on the salary chart in the office procedure manual

Date prepared:01/25/--

FIGURE 2-2 A sample job description.

Dental Administrative Assistant
No experience necessary. Will train on the job. Must possess good people skills and some knowledge of basic bookkeeping. Send a resume to: Box 5679, Grand Rapids Press, Grand Rapids, MI 49502

A

FIGURE 2-3A A sample newspaper advertisement for a Dental Administrative Assistant.

Registered Dental Assistant who is ambitious and skilled in ergonomic four-handed dentistry. Duties require clinical, laboratory, and business office management skills in a general practice. Must have expanded functions credential. Attractive salary and benefits. Write to: Joseph W. Lake, D.D.S., 611 Main St. S.E., Grand Rapids, MI 49502

B

FIGURE 2-3B A sample newspaper advertisement for a Clinical Assistant.

Writing a Job Advertisement

The content of an advertisement for a new staff member should be the result of a well-thought-out job description. List the skills that the person is expected to have, ask for a résumé, and identify attractive features of the job (e.g., benefits, salary, working conditions). To attract highly qualified candidates, the advertisement cannot be a mundane, brief statement about seeking inexperienced people. Periodically look at the classified ads in the local paper for ideas from other allied health professions. Compare the three advertisements in Figure 2-3A-C. Which advertisements present a greater challenge for a prospective employee? The ad in Figure 2-3A seeking an inexperienced person will probably get more responses, but that is not the purpose of placing a job advertisement. Figures 2-3 B and C set specific parameters for potential candidates. For jobs discussed in the advertisements, the dentist is looking for candidates who display the criteria requested for an administrative assistant, clinical assistant, and dental hygienist. The procedure of advertising should seek to screen potential candidates. A request for an educated person cuts down on potential training costs for the dentist and can ensure a minimal level of education.

Interviewing Prospective Employees

Part of the management role of the administrative assistant may be interviewing applicants for a position on the staff. This is an important responsibility, and it requires a great deal of skill. The suggestions in Box 2-10 may be helpful when an interview is being conducted.

Legal Considerations in Hiring

There are several legal factors to be considered when hiring an employee. These include application forms, citizenship status, and testing.

An employer must ensure that application forms avoid any questions about race or ethnic background. Furthermore, each applicant who completes an application form must be provided with the same type of form. Be certain that the application form used in the office does not violate any state requirements. For example, a state may deem it unlawful to use a lie-detector test. Thus, a question on an application asking the applicant to take a lie-detector test could be in violation of state law.

Our established dental office staff is looking for an experienced Dental Hygienist. Must be a motivated self-starter! Applicants must be friendly, possess excellent communication skills and have the ability to deliver exceptional patient service. Bi-Lingual a plus. Dentrix knowledge helpful. Compensation: based on experience. Write to Box 1334 Grand Rapids Press, 228 Fulton St., E., Grand Rapids, MI 49502

C

FIGURE 2-3C Job advertisement for an experienced Dental Hygienist.

BOX 2-10

Suggestions for Job Interview Preparation

- Perform a task analysis of the proposed job.
- Determine the competencies needed to fulfill the job requirements.
- Prepare a well-defined job description.
- Have the applicant complete a job application.
- Determine how to measure an applicant's abilities. Tests may be used to measure certain abilities, such as keyboarding speed and accuracy.
- Explain the requirements of the job completely.
- Determine key questions to ask during the interview.
- Review your reactions to the applicant. Were you comfortable? Was the applicant an active participant in the conversation? Was the individual shy or domineering?
- Make accurate observations about the applicant's answers, grammar, and nonverbal cues during the interview. Use a checklist to ensure that each candidate is evaluated on the same basis.
- Record evaluations as soon as the interview is completed to ensure that you do not forget the responses.
- Investigate any references that the applicant has provided. This confirms the accuracy of the applicant's statements.

It is illegal to discriminate against any individual (other than an alien who is not authorized to work in the United States) when hiring, discharging, recruiting, or referring for a fee because of that individual's national origin or citizenship status. It is illegal to discriminate against work-eligible individuals. It is in violation of federal law to hire an unauthorized (illegal) alien. An employer must require proof of an applicant's legal status, and the Immigration and Naturalization Service (INS)

Form I-9 (Employment Eligibility Verification form) must be filled out before employment. Documents accepted for verification can be found in the Lists of Acceptable Documents available on the Form I-9 website (www.formi9.com). See Figure 2-4 for a sample of Form I-9 and the Lists of Acceptable Documents needed to establish employment eligibility.

Pre-employment Testing

A variety of employment testing may include standardized tests, polygraph tests, and drug and alcohol tests. Although a small dental office seldom uses all these tests, it is possible that an institution or a larger corporation with dental facilities may take advantage of them all.

Businesses such as dental practices may legally use professionally developed standardized tests to verify knowledge, aptitude, and skills during a selection process. Tests used to screen applicants can become discriminatory when they serve to disqualify members of a minority culture who are unfamiliar with the language or concepts but who are fully qualified for the job. Dentistry can avail itself of standardized tests developed by the DANB and various state regulatory agencies. To create a new test when many such tests already exist can place a practitioner at potential legal risk.

Many private-sector employers are considering drug and alcohol testing as a pre-employment requirement. The main type of test is a urinalysis, which is likely to be part of a pre-employment physical examination.

Employment Eligibility Verification

Department of Homeland Security
U.S. Citizenship and Immigration Services

USCIS
Form I-9
OMB No. 1615-0047
Expires 03/31/2016

►START HERE. Read instructions carefully before completing this form. The instructions must be available during completion of this form.

ANTI-DISCRIMINATION NOTICE: It is illegal to discriminate against work-authorized individuals. Employers **CANNOT** specify which document(s) they will accept from an employee. The refusal to hire an individual because the documentation presented has a future expiration date may also constitute illegal discrimination.

Section 1. Employee Information and Attestation *(Employees must complete and sign Section 1 of Form I-9 no later than the **first day of employment**, but not before accepting a job offer.)*

Last Name *(Family Name)*	First Name *(Given Name)*	Middle Initial	Other Names Used *(if any)*

Address *(Street Number and Name)*	Apt. Number	City or Town	State	Zip Code

Date of Birth *(mm/dd/yyyy)*	U.S. Social Security Number	E-mail Address	Telephone Number

I am aware that federal law provides for imprisonment and/or fines for false statements or use of false documents in connection with the completion of this form.

I attest, under penalty of perjury, that I am (check one of the following):

☐ A citizen of the United States

☐ A noncitizen national of the United States *(See instructions)*

☐ A lawful permanent resident (Alien Registration Number/USCIS Number): ____________

☐ An alien authorized to work until (expiration date, if applicable, mm/dd/yyyy) ____________. Some aliens may write "N/A" in this field. *(See instructions)*

*For aliens authorized to work, provide your Alien Registration Number/USCIS Number **OR** Form I-94 Admission Number:*

1. Alien Registration Number/USCIS Number: ____________

OR

2. Form I-94 Admission Number: ____________

If you obtained your admission number from CBP in connection with your arrival in the United States, include the following:

Foreign Passport Number: ____________

Country of Issuance: ____________

Some aliens may write "N/A" on the Foreign Passport Number and Country of Issuance fields. *(See instructions)*

3-D Barcode
Do Not Write in This Space

Signature of Employee:	Date *(mm/dd/yyyy)*:

Preparer and/or Translator Certification *(To be completed and signed if Section 1 is prepared by a person other than the employee.)*

I attest, under penalty of perjury, that I have assisted in the completion of this form and that to the best of my knowledge the information is true and correct.

Signature of Preparer or Translator:	Date *(mm/dd/yyyy)*:

Last Name *(Family Name)*	First Name *(Given Name)*

Address *(Street Number and Name)*	City or Town	State	Zip Code

STOP ***Employer Completes Next Page*** STOP

Form I-9 03/08/13 N

Page 7 of 9

FIGURE 2-4 Federal Employment Eligibility Verification form (Form I-9). (From the US Citizen and Immigration Services, Department of Homeland Security, Washington, DC.)

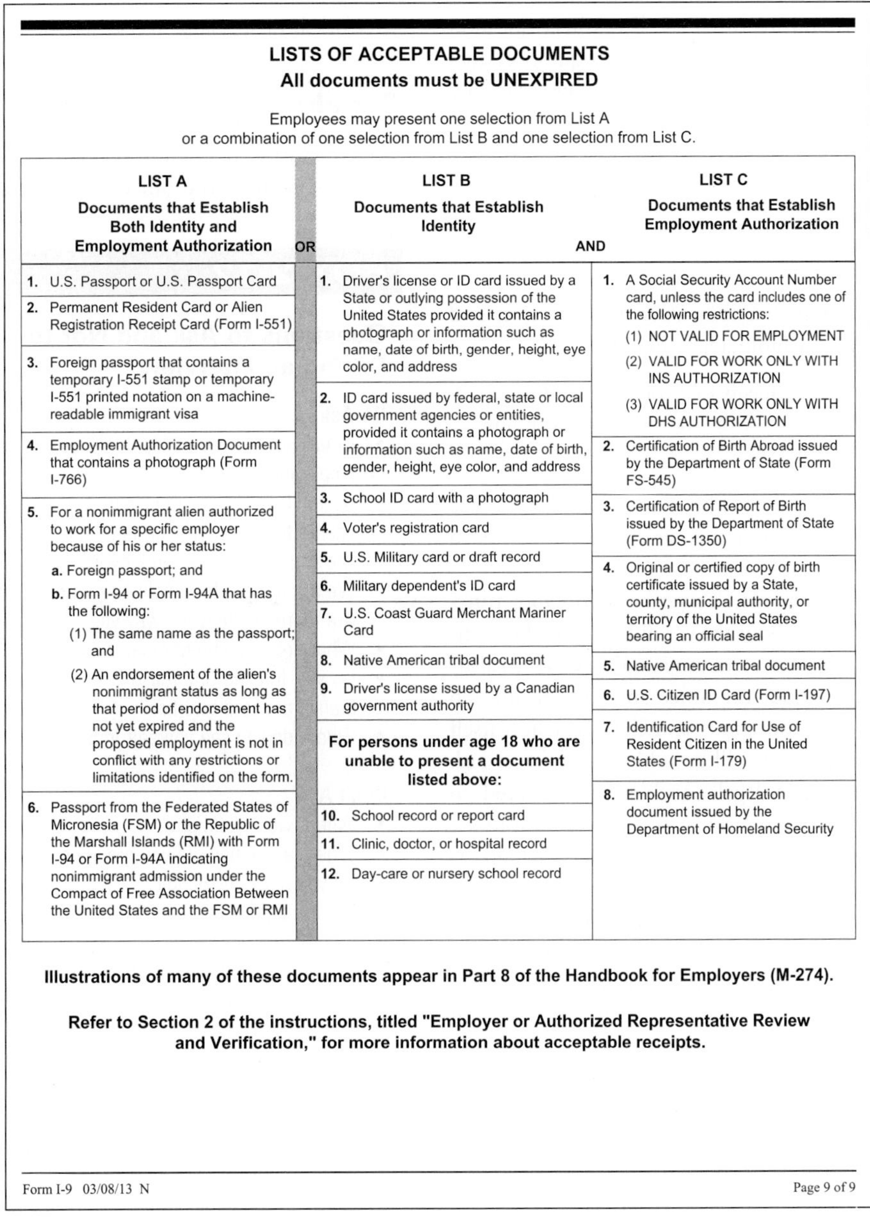

LISTS OF ACCEPTABLE DOCUMENTS
All documents must be UNEXPIRED

Employees may present one selection from List A
or a combination of one selection from List B and one selection from List C.

LIST A **Documents that Establish Both Identity and Employment Authorization**	OR	LIST B **Documents that Establish Identity**	AND	LIST C **Documents that Establish Employment Authorization**
1. U.S. Passport or U.S. Passport Card		1. Driver's license or ID card issued by a State or outlying possession of the United States provided it contains a photograph or information such as name, date of birth, gender, height, eye color, and address		1. A Social Security Account Number card, unless the card includes one of the following restrictions: (1) NOT VALID FOR EMPLOYMENT (2) VALID FOR WORK ONLY WITH INS AUTHORIZATION (3) VALID FOR WORK ONLY WITH DHS AUTHORIZATION
2. Permanent Resident Card or Alien Registration Receipt Card (Form I-551)		2. ID card issued by federal, state or local government agencies or entities, provided it contains a photograph or information such as name, date of birth, gender, height, eye color, and address		2. Certification of Birth Abroad issued by the Department of State (Form FS-545)
3. Foreign passport that contains a temporary I-551 stamp or temporary I-551 printed notation on a machine-readable immigrant visa		3. School ID card with a photograph		3. Certification of Report of Birth issued by the Department of State (Form DS-1350)
4. Employment Authorization Document that contains a photograph (Form I-766)		4. Voter's registration card		4. Original or certified copy of birth certificate issued by a State, county, municipal authority, or territory of the United States bearing an official seal
5. For a nonimmigrant alien authorized to work for a specific employer because of his or her status: a. Foreign passport; and b. Form I-94 or Form I-94A that has the following: (1) The same name as the passport; and (2) An endorsement of the alien's nonimmigrant status as long as that period of endorsement has not yet expired and the proposed employment is not in conflict with any restrictions or limitations identified on the form.		5. U.S. Military card or draft record		5. Native American tribal document
6. Passport from the Federated States of Micronesia (FSM) or the Republic of the Marshall Islands (RMI) with Form I-94 or Form I-94A indicating nonimmigrant admission under the Compact of Free Association Between the United States and the FSM or RMI		6. Military dependent's ID card		6. U.S. Citizen ID Card (Form I-197)
		7. U.S. Coast Guard Merchant Mariner Card		7. Identification Card for Use of Resident Citizen in the United States (Form I-179)
		8. Native American tribal document		8. Employment authorization document issued by the Department of Homeland Security
		9. Driver's license issued by a Canadian government authority		
		For persons under age 18 who are unable to present a document listed above:		
		10. School record or report card		
		11. Clinic, doctor, or hospital record		
		12. Day-care or nursery school record		

Illustrations of many of these documents appear in Part 8 of the Handbook for Employers (M-274).

Refer to Section 2 of the instructions, titled "Employer or Authorized Representative Review and Verification," for more information about acceptable receipts.

Form I-9 03/08/13 N — Page 9 of 9

FIGURE 2-4, cont'd

An employer who refuses to hire someone with AIDS violates federal and state disability discrimination laws. Protection under Title VII of the 1964 Civil Rights Act has been extended to disabled persons, including those infected with the AIDS virus or who have tested positive for the HIV virus. An employer probably would not be justified in refusing to hire an individual with AIDS unless the employer could establish that the prospective employee would endanger the health and safety of others. This issue is controversial for the dental care profession; it must be met with a thorough understanding of both the legal and ethical ramifications.

Conducting an Interview

Before conducting an interview, gather all of the information about each candidate, develop an outline of questions, and determine the physical setting for the interview. Often a neutral location such as a lounge or a conference room will make the candidate feel more at ease.

As the interview begins, establish rapport with the candidate with a personal introduction, and create a sense of pleasantness with the candidate. Explain the purpose of the interview, and generate a relaxed atmosphere. During the interview, motivate the candidate to participate.

The main part of the interview consists of asking questions, listening to responses, answering questions, and providing a transition from one discussion topic to another. Gain confidence in questioning the applicant to reflect each facet of the individual's background. Ask questions such as, "Tell me about your previous job experiences," "What is your attitude toward your previous working experience?," and "What do you feel your strengths and weaknesses are for the position available in this office?"

Common types of questions asked during an interview include direct, indirect, and hypothetical. The direct question generally elicits an expected response. An indirect question does not imply a "yes" or "no" response. The following examples illustrate the differences in these types of questions.

Direct: "Would you be opposed to traveling to a satellite office?"

Indirect: "How would you feel about traveling to a satellite office?"

A hypothetical question describes an actual situation and elicits a response from the candidate, as follows:

Hypothetical: "If one of our patients told you he refused to pay his account because he didn't like the way he was treated, how would you respond?"

This type of question is valuable because it is as close as the interviewer will get to observing the candidate's behavior in such a situation.

During the discussion, the interviewer has two major functions: to gather information about the candidate's qualifications for the job in a nondiscriminatory manner and to convey information to the candidate about the office and the specific job responsibilities. By keeping questions and the discussion itself relevant to the job, the first task will be achieved. The first task requires awareness of certain legal considerations related to interviewing. Rules of thumb for asking interview questions are shown in Box 2-11. Guidelines provided by the US Department of Labor and the US Equal Employment Opportunity Commission (EEOC) prohibit discriminatory hiring on the basis of race, creed, color, gender, national origin, handicap, or age. Questions related to any of these as well as to marital status, children, ownership of a house or car, credit rating, or type of military discharge can also be considered discriminatory. Questions that should and should not be asked during an interview include many of those shown in Box 2-12, and topics that should be avoided are listed in Box 2-13.

The second task of the interview can be met if all of the following areas are included in the discussion:

- Specific job responsibilities
- Orientation procedures
- Opportunities for advancement
- Management procedures
- Professional responsibilities
- Work hours, salary, and fringe benefits

BOX 2-11

Three Rules of Thumb for Interviewing

When asking interview questions, consider the following rules of thumb:

1. Ask only for information that you intend to use to make hiring decisions.
2. Know how you will use the information to make the decision.
3. Recognize that it is difficult to defend the practice of seeking information that you do not use.

Concluding an Interview

The conclusion of the interview is a good opportunity for the applicant to tour the office. This is also a good time, if it is

BOX 2-12

Questions to Ask and Not to Ask During an Interview

Do Ask

- What was your absentee record at your prior place of employment?
- Do you know of any reason (e.g., transportation) why you would be unable to get to work on time and on a regular basis?
- Are you available to work overtime?
- We are looking for employees with a commitment to this position. Are there any reasons why you might not stay with us?
- What are your career objectives?
- Do you foresee any reasons why you could not be assigned to a branch or satellite office?
- Where do you see yourself in 5 years?

Don't Ask

- Where were you born?
- Where and when did you graduate from high school?
- Do you have any handicaps?
- What religious holidays do you practice?
- Are you married?
- Do you plan to have children? How many?
- Do you own a home?
- Do you own a car?
- Do you have any debts?
- Can you provide three credit references?
- Is your spouse likely to be transferred?
- Is your spouse from this area?
- How old are you?
- How do you feel about working with members of a different race?
- What languages do your parents speak?

BOX 2-13

Topics to Avoid During the Interview Process

- Arrest records
- Marital status
- Maiden name
- Spouse's name
- Spouse's education
- Spouse's income
- Form of birth control
- Childcare arrangements
- Lawsuits or legal complaints
- Ownership of car or residence
- Loans
- Insurance claims
- National origin
- Mother's maiden name
- Place of birth
- Disabilities
- Weight
- Age
- Date of high school graduation
- Religion
- Social organizations

BOX 2-14

Factors to Avoid When Making Staff Selections

When making a selection or recommendation for hiring a staff person, avoid making assumptions such as the following:

- The dentist or staff members might prefer employees of certain ethnic or racial origins.
- Those who come in contact with your employees might not want to deal with women or minorities.
- Coworkers might object.to some personal characteristic; school attended, dress, area where they live.
- The job might involve unusual working conditions that would disqualify the applicant.

convenient, for the rest of the staff to meet the candidate. Inform the applicant about the plans for arriving at a decision and a date by which the decision will be made. Factors to avoid when making a decision are listed in Box 2-14.

After all of the candidates have been interviewed and a decision made about each, the person to be hired should be promptly contacted. A letter of confirmation should be sent to the new employee stating the conditions of employment: wages, hours, promotions, beginning date, and other conditions agreed on during previous discussions. The letter should identify the probationary period, which allows either party to terminate employment within an established period of time without fear of penalty. It is wise to have the employee sign and return a copy of the letter. A copy is then retained by the employee, and the signed copy is placed in the employee's file. A letter should also be sent to candidates who are not being hired, and their applications may remain on file if desired.

New Employee Training

A well-organized dental team provides a smooth transition for the new employee into the practice. The time frame for the new employee to become well established in the office will vary according to the individual office. The many activities involved in new employee training include the following:

- Describe how the practice is run and what standards are required of the staff.
- Explain the organizational chart and job descriptions.
- Complete employee documents, including federal and state tax forms.
- Review procedural techniques.
- Allow time for observation, but let the skills and responsibilities of the new employee be used as soon as possible.
- Identify areas of strength and weakness. Positive reinforcement is necessary to create confidence. However, poor performance should be altered to avoid the reinforcement of less-than-quality work. It is easier to correct poor performance early during training rather than later, when it seriously affects office production.
- Provide additional training beyond the educational experiences already achieved. This may be accomplished within the office, or it may require a more formal setting in a nearby school.
- Evaluate the performance of the new employee regularly. This allows changes in performance to be made, and it provides the staff person with knowledge of his or her status.
- Review progress with adequate promotion via benefits or a pay increase.
- Terminate an employee if substandard performance continues. If all efforts to improve the employee's performance have failed, it is wise to terminate the employee promptly rather than to continue with substandard performance.

LEARNING ACTIVITIES

1. Write job descriptions for a chairside or clinical assistant, an administrative assistant, and a dental hygienist. What tasks should be identified for each of these jobs in a job analysis? Review the classified advertisements in a local paper for ideas.
2. Compare the content of ads for various health occupations. What characteristics appeal to you in these ads? Why?
3. Create an interview outline that lists the sequence of events of an interview.
4. Develop a series of questions that will determine whether a candidate has the appropriate skills for a job.
5. After creating a list of questions that could be asked during a job interview, form a small group to practice interview skills. Identify an administrative assistant, a dentist, and a candidate to perform this task.

Please refer to the student workbook for additional learning activities.

BIBLIOGRAPHY

Adams B: *Streetwise managing people: lead your staff to peak performance*, Holbrook, MA, 1998, Adams Media Corporation.

Drucker PF: *On leadership*, Boston, 2011, Harvard Business School Publishing Corporation.

Fulton-Calkins PJ, Rankin DS, Shumack KA: *The administrative professional*, ed 14, Mason, OH, 2011, Thomson South-Western.

Ishimoto C: Unlocking teamwork potential, Dental Economics 99(September):1, 2007.

Keyton J: *Communication and organizational culture*, Thousand Oaks, CA, 2005, Sage Publications.

Miles L: *Dynamic dentistry: practice management tools and strategy for breakthrough success*, Virginia Beach, VA, 2003, Link Publishing.

Perkins PS: *The art and science of communication: tools for effective communication in the workplace*, New York, 2008, John Wiley & Sons.

Potter BA: *Medical office administration*, St Louis, 2014, Elsevier.

Radz G: The biggest benefits of having a long-term dental office manager, Dentistry IQ 2013.

Shoffstall-Cone S, Williard M: Alaska Dental Health Aide Program, Int J Circumpolar Health 2013.

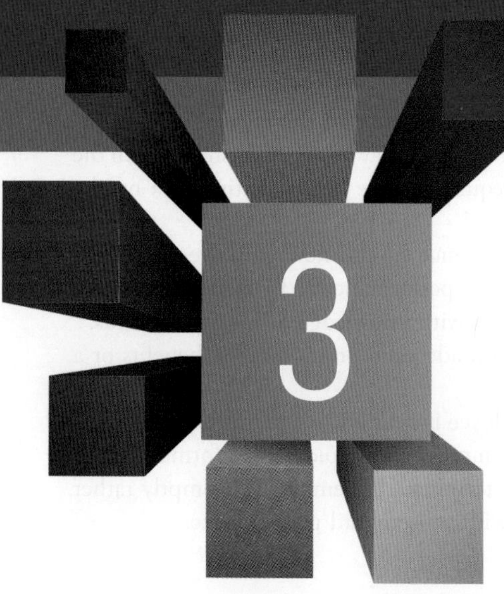

3 Practice Management

 http://evolve.elsevier.com/Finkbeiner/practice

LEARNING OUTCOMES

1. Define the key terms in this chapter.
2. Discuss the importance of understanding patient needs.
3. Identify barriers to patient communication and the importance of recognizing nonverbal cues.
4. Explain how improving verbal images in the patients mind can allay fears and identify phrases that promote successful patient management.
5. Discuss the special needs of patients and their inherent rights, as well as ways to recognize abuse.
6. Describe reception room techniques, the role of the receptionist, and the importance of an appealing reception area.
7. Discuss the contents of an office policy and design an office policy statement.
8. Explain marketing techniques in dentistry, including:
    - Describe use of social media in patient marketing.
    - Describe internal and external marketing.

KEY TERMS

Client-centered therapy A form of therapy that, when applied to dentistry, encourages listening to patients to learn about their feelings, desires, and priorities.

Hierarchy of needs Five basic levels of needs described by Abraham Maslow that are used to aid in the understanding of how a person's needs motivate behavior. They are as follows: physiologic or biologic, safety or security, social or love, esteem, and self-actualization.

Locus of control A theory that refers to an individual's perception of the underlying main causes of events in his or her life.

Marketing A form of advertising. In dentistry, it is what one does within the office to retain patients.

Nonverbal cues Gestures and body movements that a person makes in a given situation to denote a feeling.

Office policy A form of written communication that identifies the dentist's philosophy and policies and that defines the responsibilities of the patient and the dental staff.

Patients' rights The inherent rights of a patient to be informed about services being performed, their costs, and the consequences of such treatment.

Website A location on the World Wide Web that provides information about an office and its staff and services.

The most important person in the dental practice is the patient. Recall that each patient has a different background and different needs. The dentist and the staff must be able to project a helpful attitude. While communicating with patients, it is important to recognize each person as an individual with specific needs and to determine how to be sensitive to those needs. Every effort must be made to alleviate patients' discomfort, and patients must be taught to help themselves.

UNDERSTANDING PATIENT NEEDS

Each staff member who comes in contact with patients should have an understanding of the basic drives involved in motivating patients. Unless the dentist and staff have a basic understanding of these drives, they will become discouraged after numerous attempts fail to motivate patients to appreciate good dental health and quality dentistry.

As a result of the concern for humanism inherent in this healthcare profession, it is appropriate to be aware of the contributions of two humanistic psychologists: Abraham Maslow and Carl Rogers.

PRACTICE NOTE
The most important person in the dental practice is the patient.

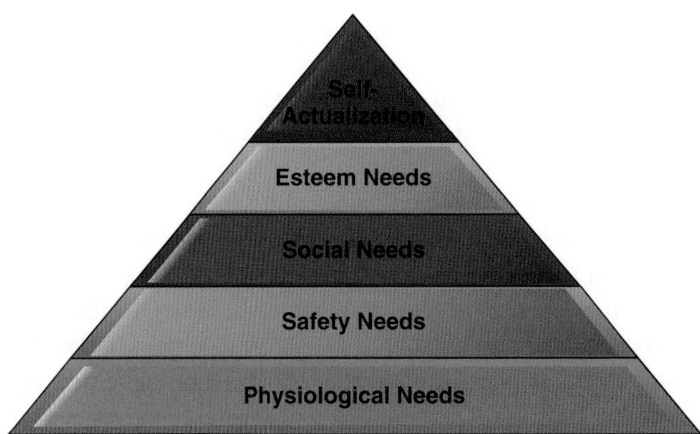

FIGURE 3-1 Maslow's hierarchy of needs. (From Black BP: *Professional nursing*, ed 7, St Louis, 2014, Saunders.)

Maslow's Hierarchy of Needs

Dr. Abraham Maslow has described a hierarchy of needs (Figure 3-1) that aids in the understanding of how a person's needs motivate his or her behavior. Maslow identified the following five basic levels of needs, which range from basic biologic needs to complex social or psychologic drives:

1. *Physiologic or biologic needs:* These are bodily needs, and they are the first to be satisfied. You must satisfy these physical needs, or you will not live long enough to satisfy any social or psychologic needs. If you are healthy, eat regularly, and housed adequately, you can advance to the next level of the hierarchy with a sense of well-being.
2. *Safety or security needs:* When the basic biological needs are met, you are ready for the second level of the hierarchy. This level allows you to explore your environment. Just as small children begin to explore their environment after their food and comfort needs have been met, you as an adult begin to explore. This is the level at which you feel safe and free from danger, threats, or other deprivation. If you have a job that is nonthreatening and live in a safe environment, you will feel secure and will be able to advance to the next level.
3. *Social or love needs:* If you are secure in your environment, you can advance to the level of social interaction. The poet John Donne wrote, "No man is an island, complete to itself." Donne realized that to be human means to interact with others. At this level of the hierarchy, Maslow realized the need to interact with others with whom you share similar beliefs and who provide you with reinforcement to continue your social relationships. This love or social interaction gives you confidence to advance to the next level on the hierarchy.
4. *Esteem needs:* From interaction with others at the previous level, you will generate goals for yourself. Your peers often consider these needs as ego needs that relate to your self-esteem, reputation, and recognition. Here, you look forward to achieving your goals; from accomplishment, you will receive self-esteem. Typically the self-satisfaction that you receive from accomplishing these goals provides an impetus to establish new goals and begin the cycle again.
5. *Self-actualization:* Self-actualized people are motivated by the need to grow. To achieve this need, you must have achieved self-esteem and have confidence in yourself. Later in life, Maslow expanded his thoughts about the self-actualized person and explained that, to achieve this level, people must be relatively free of illness, sufficiently satisfied in their basic needs, positively using their capacities, and motivated by some existing or sought-after personal values. A person at this level often wants to help others achieve their goals by teaching them lessons that he or she learned during the earlier stages. Some people never reach this level because they have not aspired to its recognition.

Relating this hierarchy to dentistry means getting to know the patients and the individuals with whom one is associated. Before a dentist can motivate a patient to accept a certain type of dental treatment, it must be understood where the patient is on the hierarchy of needs.

To help realize the application of these needs to dentistry, consider the following situation. One of the practice's patients is a bank president who is respected for his civic activities and who has a warm, loving family and a fine home. The patient develops severe pain in the maxillary anterior area that is sudden, sharp, and excruciating. It is difficult for him to eat, and there is a great deal of swelling in his upper lip. This person has dropped from the esteem level to the physiologic or biologic level, and the dentist must satisfy the pressing physiologic need immediately before attempting to suggest any further treatment.

Setting up a payment plan for a patient often exposes a conflict of needs. A patient must ensure that his or her basic needs of food, housing, and clothing are met, yet there may be a desire to meet social needs by improving his or her appearance with some form of dental treatment. A conflict arises during the decision-making process when the patient is confronted with a conflict involving how to satisfy all of these needs with a specified income. The dentist and staff must make an effort to determine the patient's needs, to realize the patient's potential conflict, and to consider presenting an alternative treatment plan so that the patient has some options.

This theory need not only apply to relationships with patients; it can also be applied to interactions among staff members. The dentist, the assistant, and the hygienist all have the same needs, and each is concerned—like the patient—about his or her security today and in the future. Often conflict arises when a person becomes fixed at one level. There may appear to be no change in motivation, and the person remains unchanged in his or her perspective. This is often evidenced when a person has an interest in making money or increasing his or her social status without regard for other people's levels of motivation.

Perhaps one of the best lessons to be learned from Maslow's theory is that an individual has a choice in determining his or her behavior. Although basic physiologic and environmental needs have strong influences, an individual makes his or her choices voluntarily.

Rogers' Client-Centered Therapy

Dr. Carl Rogers, another humanistic psychologist, believed that "it is the client who knows what hurts, what directions to go, what problems are crucial, what experiences have been deeply buried." Rogers also suggests accepting the patient or the other person as a genuine person with his or her own set of values and goals and states that these people must be treated with "unconditional positive regard." Client-centered therapy assumes that patients know how they feel, what they want, and their priorities. When applied to dentistry, this philosophy encourages the dentist and staff to listen to the patient. In addition, this concept suggests respecting patients as human beings and not just as numbers, case studies, or research projects. Patients have needs, and their desires should not be repressed. The combined concepts of Maslow and Rogers provide the groundwork for a humanistic, caring attitude that should be a requisite for all healthcare providers.

Locus of Control

A person's locus of control is the degree to which that person feels that he or she has control over the events that occur in his or her life. At one end of the spectrum are individuals who believe that life events "just happen" or are determined by destiny, fate, or chance (external locus of control). At the other end of the spectrum are people who believe that life events are determined by their own actions (internal locus of control).

The locus of control theory was developed in 1954 by psychologist Julian Rotter. He suggested that our behavior is controlled by rewards and punishments, and it is the consequences of our actions that determine our beliefs. Rotter published a scale designed to measure and assess a person's external and internal loci of control.

A health-specific version of Rotter's scale, The Health Locus of Control, was developed in 1976 by Wallston and colleagues. It examines the degree to which individuals believe that their health is controlled by internal and external factors. Individuals who have had successful attempts at health control are more likely to have internal loci of control than individuals who have been unsuccessful in their attempts.

A person with an external locus of control is more likely to believe that the dentist has control over his or her oral health or that his or her oral health has been predetermined by fate. This type of patient may state, "I'm sure I will need dentures, because my mother and father both had dentures."

The patient who is proactive in the care of his or her mouth is more likely to have an internal locus of control. An example of this would be the patient who follows directions and applies new techniques to improve his or her oral health. This type of patient may say, "I'll try that electric toothbrush and see if I have less plaque at my next visit," or "I want to get that implant placed before I lose any more bone."

Specific questions that can be asked at chairside can help to determine a patient's personality orientation toward an external or internal locus of control:

- "Do you believe brushing twice a day keeps your mouth healthy?"
- "Do you believe you can prevent cavities?"
- "Do you believe that no matter what you do you will lose your teeth?"

Box 3-1 lists the range of personality characteristics demonstrated by individuals on the spectrum from an external locus of control to an internal locus of control.

For the dental professional, this study becomes helpful when motivating staff and patients to perform various tasks. For instance, if a patient insists that he or she is not able to brush his or her teeth more than once a day, then alternatives need to be presented to encourage that patient to use techniques that will help him or her to remove plaque and maintain a healthier mouth. If a staff member insists that he or she is not capable of placing an intraoral sensor in a patient's mouth, then some practice could be provided on a typodont or manikin to help him or her improve this skill.

An internal locus of control is often associated with the concepts of self-determination and personal agency. Research has suggested that males tend to be more internally focused than females. As people age, they tend to become more internal, and people with higher organizational structures also tend to be more internal.

However, it is also important to remember that internal does not always imply "good" and external does not always equate to "bad." In some situations, an external locus of control can actually be a good thing, particularly if a person's level of competence in a particular area is not very strong. There are cautions that need to be considered when using this model, and, within the limited space of this text, it is not possible to discuss all of

BOX 3-1

Locus of Control

External Locus of Control

- Believe that outcomes are outside of their control
- Often credit luck or chance for any successes
- Doubt that they can change their situation through their own efforts
- Frequently feel discouraged or powerless in the face of difficult situations
- Often are more prone to experiencing learned helplessness

Internal Locus of Control

- Believe that outcomes are within their own control
- Feel that success is determined by hard work, attributes, and decisions
- Likely to take responsibility for their actions
- Tend to be less influenced by others' opinions
- Often do better at tasks when they are allowed to work at their own pace
- Usually have a strong sense of self-confidence
- Tend to be physically healthy
- Often display a happier attitude and are more independent
- Often achieve greater success in the workplace

Adapted from http://wilderdom.com/psycology/loc/LocusofcotnrolWhatIs.html.

the factors involved in considering the internal and external loci of control without being overly simplistic. For more information about this concept, it would be wise for the reader to consult some of Rotter's research.

BARRIERS TO PATIENT COMMUNICATION

Common Obstacles

Often practitioners are unable to communicate with patients because barriers have been established. One of the first barriers that may be created is prejudging a patient. A dentist may hesitate to present an extensive treatment to a patient because of the way the patient dresses or the type of car he or she drives. As a result, the patient is never told about alternative forms of treatment, because his or her economic status has been prejudged. Often a person with a disability is prejudged. When a patient who has an artificial limb, who is in a wheelchair, or who has a visible birthmark on his or her face enters the dental office, frequently the first noticeable feature is the disability. If this patient is with a spouse or another person, the patient may go unnoticed while questions are directed to the accompanying person. As a dental healthcare worker, it is important to treat people with disabilities as you do any other patients and to direct all communication to the patient himself or herself.

Another barrier occurs when one *hears* but does not *listen*. A dental professional should never be too busy to listen with understanding to a patient. It is important to do more than just listen to the words; one must listen to the *meaning* of the words and the feeling behind the meaning. Before presenting a personal point of view, you must be able to restate what the patient has said to the patient's satisfaction. This may sound easy, but often it is not. People are frequently too eager to present their own point of view, and they fail to understand the real meaning of what the other person is attempting to say. What is the patient really saying when he or she says, "I think I'll wait to have that treatment done"? If the dental professional responds, "Oh, that's okay, Mrs. Gates, I understand," then he or she will not know what the patient is really saying and may cut off communication. The patient may really be saying, "I'm scared," "I can't afford it," or "I don't like the way you treat me." The best way to arrive at the real meaning is to continue the dialogue until the patient's true feelings are discerned. The following example demonstrates this idea:

> *Assistant:* "Mrs. Romano, do you feel that you want to wait to have the treatment?"
>
> *Patient:* "Yes."
>
> *Assistant:* "Do you want to wait because you are too busy now?" *(The patient may say yes and terminate the conversation at this point, or the conversation may continue.)*

If the patient says "Yes," the assistant may reply as follows:

> *Assistant:* "Mrs. Romano, we understand busy schedules, and we do value your time. We can custom design your appointments just as we design a personalized treatment plan. Why don't we take a look at your schedule and see if we can work together to find time for your treatment?"

Alternatively, there may be a financial reason behind the patient's decision:

> *Patient:* "No, it's just that I don't know if I should spend that much money, because I have so many other expenses right now."
>
> *Assistant:* "Mrs. Romano, we know how budgets can be stretched today, and we can work with you to help you afford this investment, which is going to pay dividends over the next 10 to 20 years."

At this point, the assistant could explain the financial arrangements that can be made in the office.

Notice in this dialogue that the assistant offered a solution to the problem so that it could be discussed further.

However, the dialogue may have continued along different lines, as shown in the following example:

> *Patient:* "Well, it's not that I can't afford it. I guess what it boils down to is that I've never had that type of treatment, and I'm not sure what it's going to involve."
>
> *Assistant:* "In other words, you don't understand the procedure?"
>
> *Patient:* "Yes, I guess that's it. I'm really a bit skeptical about what's going to happen." *(At this point, the hidden meaning becomes evident.)*

In this case, the assistant rephrased what the patient said to arrive at the real meaning.

A third barrier is preoccupation. During daily routines, many demands are placed on one's time, and it is easy to begin to suddenly think about other activities while trying to communicate with a patient. Everyone has been in that position at one time or another. A patient is trying to explain why an appointment time is not convenient, and suddenly the dental professional realizes that she or he has not heard a word that was said because of his or her concentration on another problem. This often happens in an office that is understaffed. Each staff member has so much work to accomplish that listening to a patient sometimes just becomes an additional burden. Unfortunately, patients are quick to recognize such preoccupation, and they may suddenly stop talking, or eventually they may even stop coming into the dental office. This type of situation reemphasizes the service model illustrated in Chapter 1. As mentioned previously, the patient is the most important person in the dental office and should be given complete attention.

Unawareness of importance, impatience, and even hearing loss are barriers to communication. How important the problem is to the patient may not be realized, and the patient's concern may simply be ignored as a whim. Likewise, one may inadvertently become impatient with a chatty young child or an older person who is slow. It is also possible that a dental staff member may not hear everything a patient says because of an unrealized hearing loss.

It is not beneficial just to know about these barriers: the dental professional must be willing to evaluate his or her own behavior as it relates to them. Before each contact with a patient, the staff member must decide to ignore extraneous activities and be willing to listen to and understand the patient's problem before offering a solution.

Recognizing Nonverbal Cues

In recent years, many books have been written to define and guide the reader toward recognizing nonverbal communication cues. Nonverbal cues refer to the gestures and body movements that a person makes in a given situation.

Every member of the dental staff should have some awareness of this area. Just as "a picture is worth a thousand words" so may a gesture give meaning to a person's inner feelings. Nonverbal communication provides feedback regarding the patient's true reactions.

The alert assistant is able to pick up these cues and interpret them while communicating with the patient. Care should be taken to not be misled by one gesture. A series of gestures generally gives a more realistic indication of a person's attitude. A dental office presents many opportunities for the use and receiving of nonverbal cues.

Nervousness

A patient who enters the reception room and sits down, locks his or her ankles together, and clenches his or her hands may be expressing fear by holding back emotions (Figure 3-2). This may occur in the dental chair, when a person clenches the armrests and locks the ankles together (Figure 3-3). When the patient relaxes, he or she will automatically unlock the ankles.

Defensiveness

A patient or staff member may use a gesture of crossed arms and clenched fists as signals to indicate disagreement or defensiveness. This gesture may even indicate that the person has withdrawn from the conversation (Figure 3-4). This may occur when a patient is being ignored by the dentist and the assistant as they communicate with each other (Figure 3-5).

Touching

An assistant has many opportunities to use this gesture, which indicates caring or interest in a patient (Figure 3-6). A hand on a small child's shoulder may show concern, or an arm around the shoulder of a senior citizen may provide reassurance (Figure 3-7). Care should be taken not to invade the patient's personal space, however.

Openness

During a consultation with a patient, the dentist should express openness rather than assume an authoritative posture behind a desk. Having the patient seated beside the desk removes this barrier and allows the dentist an opportunity for more open gestures, as shown in Figure 3-8.

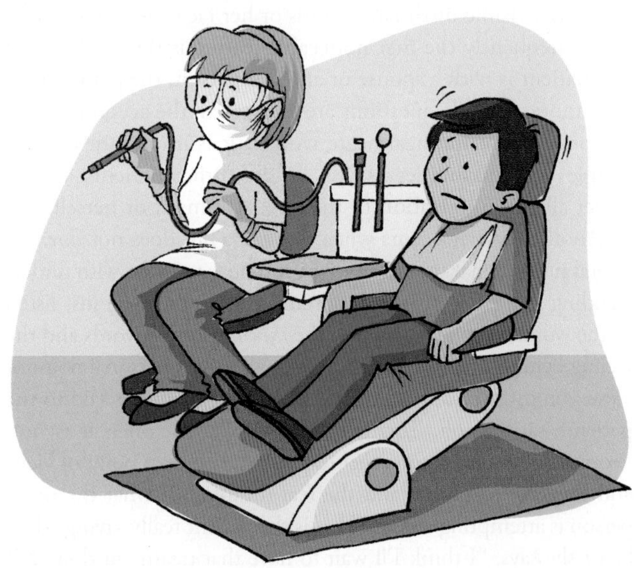

FIGURE 3-3 A patient displaying nervousness in the dental chair.

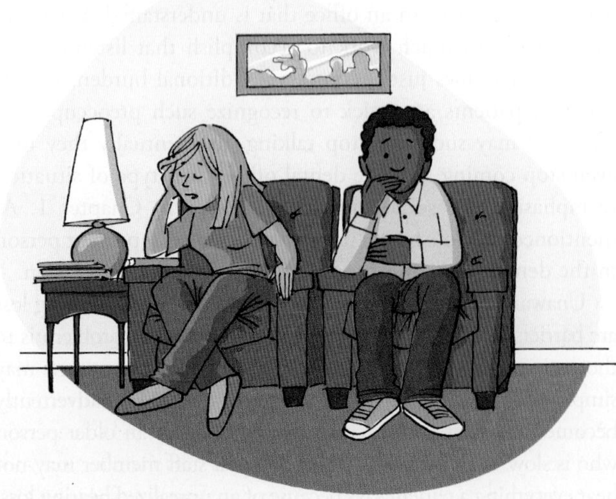

FIGURE 3-2 The difference between a bored patient and a "scared-to-death" patient.

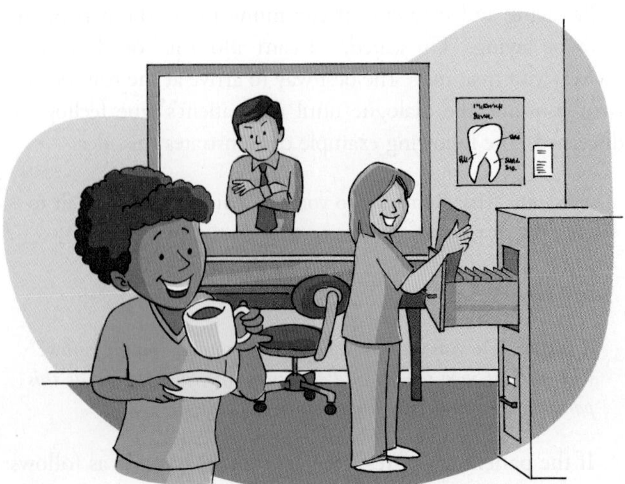

FIGURE 3-4 A patient who is being ignored crossing his arms defensively.

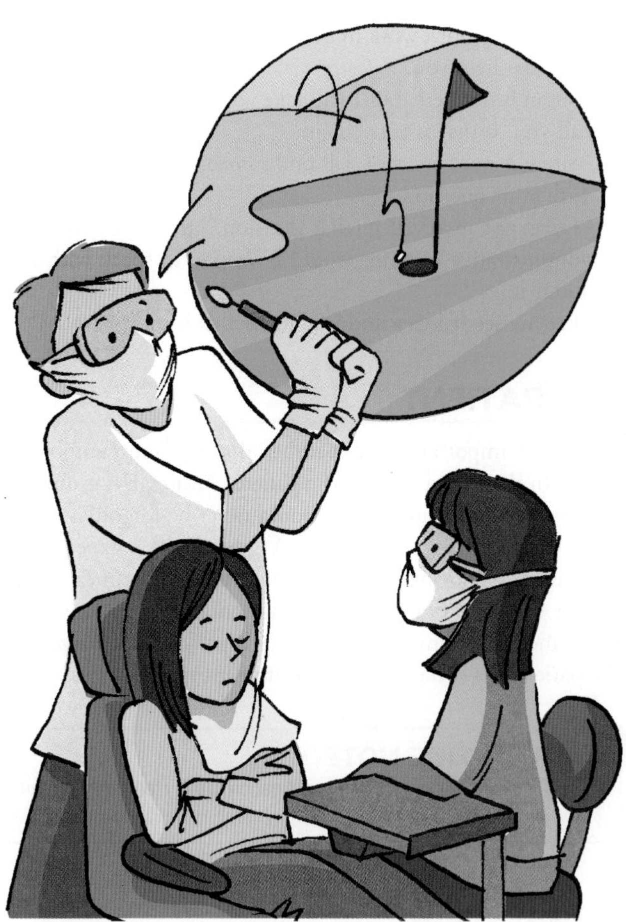

FIGURE 3-5 A dentist and an assistant ignoring a patient.

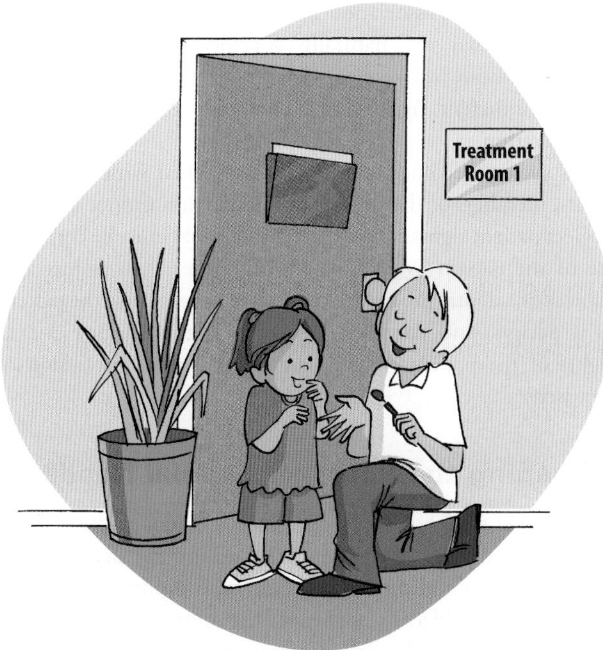

FIGURE 3-6 An assistant displaying caring by showing interest in a child.

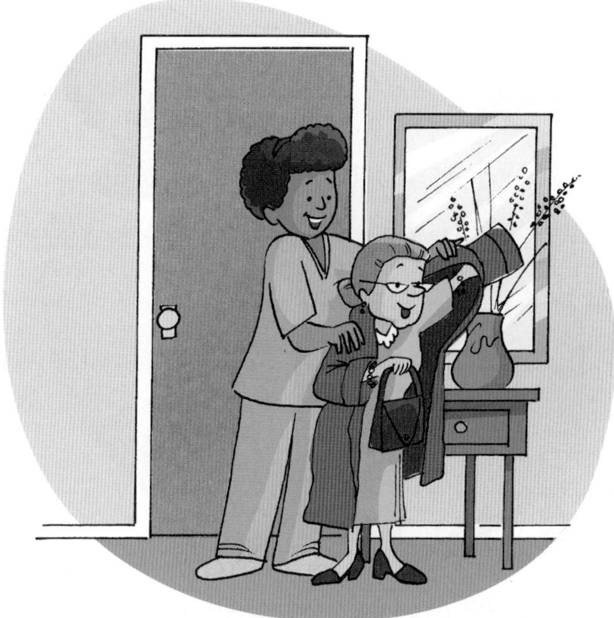

FIGURE 3-7 Assisting an older adult patient with her coat indicates caring.

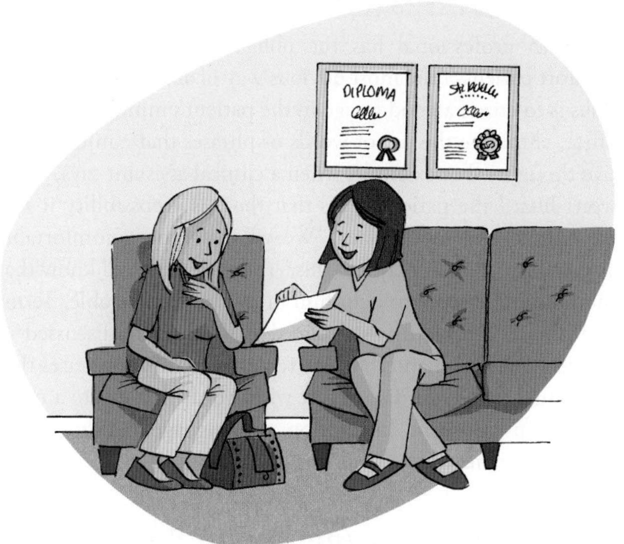

FIGURE 3-8 A dentist in consultation with a patient.

Embarrassment

A patient's hand covering his or her mouth may indicate that he or she wishes to avoid the embarrassment of exposing an unsightly oral condition. A similar signal may be the tightening of the upper lip to conceal the teeth (Figure 3-9).

Many more nonverbal cues exist. It is vital to become aware of the meaning of these valuable tools for communication. No one tool or technique will ensure successful communication. Rather, communication is based on a leader who has well-defined goals and a staff working as a team. These efforts, in combination with a sincere interest in satisfying a patient's needs, provide a successful communication system in the dental office.

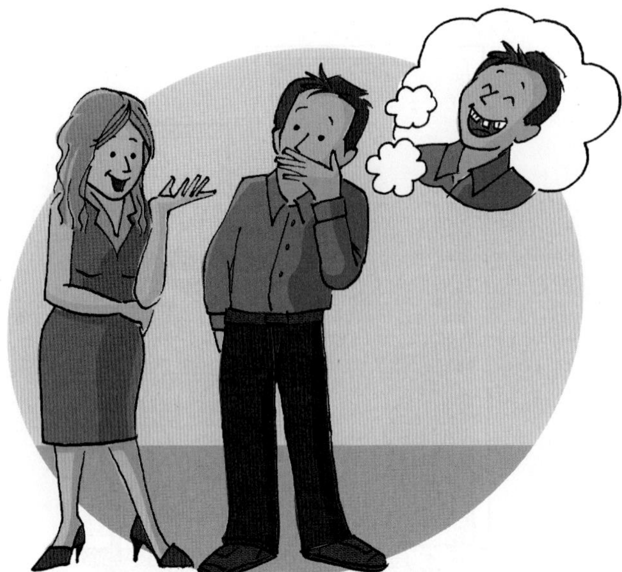

FIGURE 3-9 A patient covering his mouth to indicate embarrassment.

IMPROVING VERBAL IMAGES

A health professional has the obligation to allay fears and comfort patients. The most obvious way of accomplishing these tasks is to create a good image in the patient's mind. In a dental office, eliminate the use of words or phrases that conjure negative thoughts. For example, when a clinical assistant says, "This won't hurt," the patient hears that there is a possibility it *will* hurt. If the assistant had said, "We will make you as comfortable as possible" or "You may feel this," the patient would know that the assistant is there to help him or her be comfortable. Terms and phrases frequently used in a dental office are discussed in greater detail in Chapter 10. Try replacing terms or phrases that may cause images of discomfort with words that create a more positive environment. In addition, use language that the patient will understand when discussing treatment.

Be Positive in Responses to Patients

Another factor to consider when creating a good verbal image is to be positive in your responses. When a patient or another person asks about an issue, avoid phrases such as the following:

- "I don't know about that."
- "I don't deal with that type of record."
- "That is not my job."
- "Susan takes care of that, and she is not here."
- "It's not my fault."
- "I didn't do it."

These phrases indicate to a patient you do not and that you are not willing to help.

Try saying something like this instead:

- "Let me find out about that issue."
- "I will find someone who can help you with that record, if you will wait for just a few minutes."
- "I generally don't work in that area, but let me find someone who can help you."
- "Susan is not here, but I will take your inquiry and have her call you, if that is convenient."
- "Susan is not here, so I will find someone who can help you with your question."
- "I was not involved in that decision, but I know that the administrative assistant would be happy to speak with you about it."
- "Let me see if I can find out about this issue."

THE PATIENT

It remains important to remember that the most important person in the dental office is the patient. Although it is obvious that dentistry is a business, it should never be forgotten that it is first a healthcare profession. A great deal is expected of the patient: following directions, keeping appointments, and paying the fee promptly. In return, dental professionals must take time to recognize the patient as a person and realize that the patient has special needs and inherent rights.

PRACTICE NOTE

A health professional has an obligation to allay fears and comfort patients.

Patient Rights

The phrase *patient rights* is much used today. The result has been action on the part of most healthcare professions to design a patients' bill of rights. It is unfortunate that, in some healthcare agencies, the care has become so impersonal that it is necessary for a professional association or agency to formally document the things that are naturally considered patients' rights. Some healthcare workers see this action as confirmation of a patient's inherent rights rather than the result of a lack of consideration.

As society becomes increasingly concerned with individual rights, members of the dental healthcare team cannot afford to neglect patient rights. The dental professional must be considerate of the patient as a human being rather than as just as a subject of a dental procedure. Take time to recognize the patient as a person, and consider the list of rights in Box 3-2 as rights of the patient rather than threats to the profession of dentistry.

Managing the Patient's Special Needs

Many patients with special needs enter a dental practice. Some of these needs were reviewed earlier during the discussion of barriers to communication. A patient who is physically or psychologically disabled or challenged, an older adult, a child, a single parent, or a homeless person may visit the office for various types of treatment. The terms *physically challenged* and *disabled* are both acceptable today. Although *physically*

BOX 3-2

Patient Rights

Patients in a dental practice are entitled to the following:

- Being treated with adequate, appropriate, and compassionate care at all times and under all circumstances
- Being treated without discrimination on the basis of race, religion, color, national origin, gender, age, handicap, marital status, sexual preference, or source of payment
- Being informed about all aspects of treatment
- Being informed of appointment and fee schedules
- Being able to review their financial and clinical records
- Obtaining a thorough evaluation of their needs
- Being treated as a partner in care and decision making related to treatment planning
- Receiving current information about treatment and being assured of quality treatment
- Being able to refuse treatment to the extent provided by law and being informed of the medical and dental consequences of that refusal
- Expecting that all records pertinent to their dental care will be kept confidential
- Being informed if the dentist participates in different third-party payment plans
- Requesting and expecting appropriate referrals for consultation
- Being taught how to maintain good oral health for a lifetime
- Receiving treatment that will prevent future dental or oral disease
- Expecting continuity of treatment
- Being charged a fair and equitable fee
- Having appointment schedules and times maintained
- Being treated by a staff of professionals who maintain their own good health and hygiene
- Being respected for requesting a second opinion
- Being respected as a human being who has feelings and needs

challenged is used less, it should be realized that not all persons may be disabled.

The Americans with Disabilities Act of 1990 (ADA) sets specific guidelines for businesses. Several issues involving the structural design of a building are discussed in Chapter 6. Other factors that this law addresses require the dentist to not discriminate against a person who needs dental care. For most disabled persons, if they can get into a treatment room, they can receive treatment. Perhaps the biggest problem a dentist faces when treating a challenged patient is when the patient cannot mentally or physically cooperate. For example, a dentist faces several compromises when a patient has cerebral palsy and the mouth is moving uncontrollably or when the patient is a quadriplegic whose high neck injuries make moving from a wheelchair to a dental chair dangerous. Although there are some dental treatments that can be done with the patient in a wheelchair, the law allows a dentist to make referrals for the patient's safety.

It may be necessary to make a special effort to communicate with some patients. For instance, if the disabilities include vision or hearing impairments or if the patient uses a wheelchair or a walker, it may be necessary to take special care when communicating. When speaking, the dental professional may need to stand in front of patients who have hearing difficulties to ensure that these patients are able to read the speaker's lips. For patients with poor vision, the dental professional may need to read questions or have a guardian review materials that require a response, such as a health questionnaire. For people using wheelchairs, walkers, or crutches, it may be necessary to take extra time when asking them to move about, or it may even be necessary to go to them directly with forms that need to be signed.

Recognizing Abuse

Abuse is evident in many forms in today's society, and the most common forms are child abuse and adult abuse. Each year, more than 3 million children are abused or neglected by caregivers, relatives, or strangers. More than 11200 children die annually as a result of this abuse. Child abuse may be classified as physical, sexual, emotional, or overall neglect. Adults, elderly individuals who are dependent on others for care, and people in volatile relationships may also be victims of abuse.

Dentists are faced with abuse in two ways. The forensic dentist may be presented with a postmortem case of a victim who has bite marks or tooth marks present on his or her body. In addition, a dentist may treat victims of abuse in the office.

Abused children or adults may show overall signs of neglect, abnormal fears or neuroses, or evidence of extraoral or intraoral anomalies, such as bite marks, scars, lacerations, fractured teeth, burns, and bruises of varying colors on exposed areas of the body.

The dentist has an obligation to examine the patient thoroughly, ask reasonable questions about existing conditions, and document the injuries on the dental record. Reports of suspected abuse should be made to the state or county social services office. In most states, failure to report suspected abuse is a misdemeanor.

RECEPTION ROOM TECHNIQUES

Because the duties of the administrative assistant include many facets of communication, continual awareness of communication barriers is necessary.

The impression that the administrative assistant makes on patients is usually lasting, and, of course, it should be favorable. Remember to represent the dentist and the practice; a patient who feels comfortable with the administrative assistant will probably feel comfortable with the dentist.

The Role of the Receptionist

The receptionist will be the first person to greet patients as they enter the office. The receptionist should appear neat and professional. In many business offices today, the administrative assistant wears professional businesslike clothing rather than a uniform. The receptionist should be certain that his or her clothing or uniform is clean, that shoes are well polished, and that hair is neatly styled. The positive image created by the receptionist indicates a clean and well-organized office. The image portrayed in this role must remain with the patient, so this is no place to try out new clothing styles, to experiment with garish jewelry, to show visible tattoos, or to wear facial and oral piercings.

As the patient enters the office, the receptionist should be seated, acknowledge the patient immediately with a pleasant smile and cheerful "Hello," and call him or her by name. Everyone likes the feeling of being known and recognized. Although the receptionist may be busy with a telephone call, he or she should at least look up and smile. This will inform the patient that the receptionist is aware of his or her presence.

Reception Room Appeal

A bright, cheerful, and pleasantly decorated office usually makes a favorable impression on the patient. If the room appears to have a warm and friendly atmosphere, the patient will relax. (The design of the reception room for the patient's comfort is discussed in Chapter 6.) Offering a cup of coffee, tea, or another beverage may also help to put the patient at ease.

Reading material in the reception room should be current and geared toward a wide variety of interests. A good selection may include gourmet cooking, sports, travel, community and world news, and health magazines. Recipe cards can be placed in an attractive holder (Figure 3-10) to help patients copy information from magazines and assorted health-related cookbooks (Figure 3-11). This will prevent them from tearing pages out of books and magazines. Avoid dirty carpet, frayed furniture, and unsightly plants. In addition, children's books as well as quiet games and toys should be available. An area designated as a children's play area is helpful. If background music is played in the office, be sure to select music that has a soothing effect rather than loud rock or heavy concert music.

Waiting Patients

One of the responsibilities of the receptionist is to keep patients informed of delays and to indicate the waiting time. Unexpected delays or emergencies should be explained honestly. Be careful not to make excuses or say that the dentist is running late (Figure 3-12). Be honest about the length of time that the patient will have to wait to be seen.

The answer to...

What's for dinner?

COMPLIMENTS OF

JOSEPH W. LAKE, D.D.S
616-101-9575

RECIPE		SERVES

FIGURE 3-10 A recipe card for copying information from magazines.

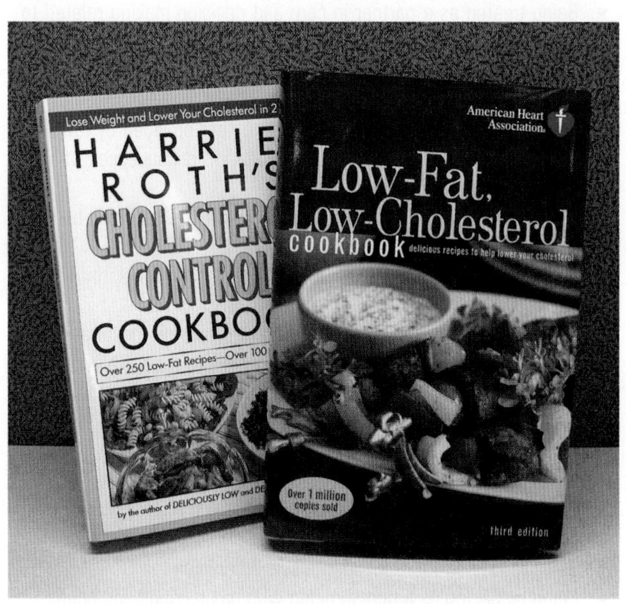

FIGURE 3-11 Cookbooks related to health.

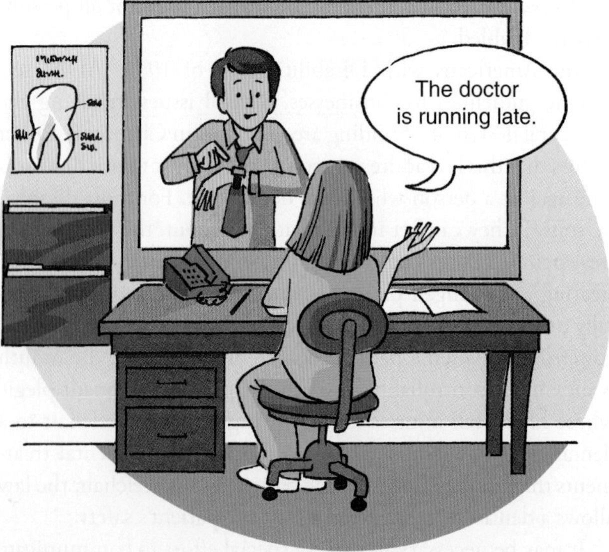

FIGURE 3-12 Team members should avoid telling patients that the dentist is running late. Instead, they should be honest about the expected wait time.

OFFICE POLICY

The office policy brochure is the key to establishing communication and understanding between the patient and the office staff. The office policy should be a written statement of the dentist's philosophy, mission statement, and policies that defines the responsibilities of both the patient and the dental office staff. It is given to a new patient at the first visit, and it serves not only as an informational device but also as a good public relations tool. Some of the policies in this brochure may be included on the office website, if one is available.

Often a new practitioner neglects to establish an office policy only to be confronted with misunderstandings with patients at a later date. The office policy should be implemented when the office is first opened and revised as the practice grows and changes. However, such a policy can be integrated into an established practice with minimal effort.

Contents of an Office Policy

Each practice has its own specific needs, but every policy should include the following elements:

- *Philosophy:* This is a statement of the dentist's attitude toward the practice of dentistry and, more specifically, his or her moral and ethical obligation to the patient. It is in this section that the dentist can make a statement about how the practice is unique and what gives it something special that will attract and retain patients.
- *Office hours:* Although these may occasionally vary, specific hours should be listed for the patient's benefit. It is advisable to inform patients of times available for emergency appointments. This will avoid a congested schedule and unnecessary calls at inconvenient times.
- *Appointment control:* A statement should be included to designate the person who controls appointment making. It should also be noted that patients are seen by appointment only to discourage "drop-ins." A broken appointment policy should be included in the office policy and adhered to consistently.
- *Payment policy:* The dentist should outline specific acceptable payment plans. These plans should be described in detail, and the person responsible for implementing them should be identified. In addition, a statement should be made regarding parental responsibility for the treatment of minors.
- *Hygiene:* The value of hygiene, self-care, and preventive dentistry through the periodic recall system should be emphasized. The system used in the office should be explained thoroughly to each patient.
- *Attitude toward children:* The roles of the dentist, staff members, and parents in the treatment of children must be explained. The preparation of a child before treatment and the management of the parent and child during treatment should be well defined to avoid future conflicts.
- *Auxiliary use:* The dentist has the responsibility to define the relationship of each staff member to patients, thereby explaining the value of team dentistry for quality care and maximum efficiency. The dentist should identify the credentials and responsibilities of each staff member.
- *Infection-control policies:* Such policies can be explained to assure patients that the latest barrier techniques and the most current preventive concepts are being used for their protection.
- *Quality assurance:* This is an explanation of efforts taken to ensure that procedures and techniques used in the office are routinely evaluated to maintain good quality.
- *Staff continuing education:* This explains the efforts that the dentist makes to continuously update himself or herself and the staff in the areas of life support, infection control, and other technological advances.
- *Office data:* The dentist's name, address, phone number, fax number, and e-mail address should appear on the cover or be easy to find within the policy for the patient's convenience.

Designing an Office Policy Statement

The administrative assistant can be invaluable to the dentist for designing the office policy statement. After the basic policy has been established, the assistant makes the final draft and then helps by designing several styles from which the dentist can make a final selection. The final style is the dentist's choice, but it should be attractive, well organized, brief, and sized to be easily handled by patients. Many offices prefer to use a professional printer to achieve a professional-looking pamphlet. In Figure 3-13, the policy has been designed to be printed on both sides of heavy 8½ × 11-inch bond paper and then folded in half. A simpler and less expensive statement printed on office letterhead is shown in Figure 3-14. Remember that the office policy has two primary purposes: it is a practice builder, and it informs the patient about office procedures and the dentist's philosophy. When it achieves both of these purposes, the office policy becomes a valuable public relations device.

MARKETING

When advertising a dental practice was first legalized in 1977 via the action of the Supreme Court, many dentists perceived this action to be demeaning to the profession. Today, dentists across the country have come to realize that, in a competitive and consumer-oriented society, they must become involved in marketing to increase their practice loads.

The use of a website can be very helpful for the marketing of a dental practice. A website can contain vital information about the dentist and the staff, including their names, titles, degrees, and functions. The site can also explain the types of services that the dentists in the practice offer, and it may also contain educational materials. It can include games, crafts, health tips, and other interesting information that a user may enjoy just for fun. It is wise to include an e-mail address so that the user can interact with the office. In addition, provisions can be made for the creation of a page through which patients can make appointments.

Creating a Website

One of the most popular and successful marketing tools has become the professional website (see Figure 3-16). It is possible to design this type of site within the office if a staff member or someone on the management staff has the appropriate skills. If not, businesses are available that offer reasonable fees for the creation of a website on the Internet. Before creating a website, the dental staff should consider the following:

- Identify objectives for the use of the website.
- Create a logo or trademark.
- Design the pages.
- Identify a web server to which the pages can be uploaded.
- Upload the pages to the server.
- Determine when and by whom the website will be updated.
- Update the website regularly to maintain its currency.

Identifying Objectives

When defining the objectives of the practice, reference should be made to the original objectives as discussed in Chapter 1. This would also be a good place to include the mission of the practice.

The objectives can be stated on the website, and any content related to these objectives can be explained.

The objectives should be written in a patient-oriented style. For example, a dentist may sum up the office's identity by using words such as *thorough*, *caring*, or *leading edge*. The word *thorough* denotes that each patient will be given quality time. *Caring* suggests old-fashioned commitment to the patient, regardless of business pressure. The phrase *leading edge* indicates that the dentist and staff are progressive and keep abreast of new materials and techniques. These messages must be driven home at every opportunity. For instance, when a patient contacts the

Welcome to our office…

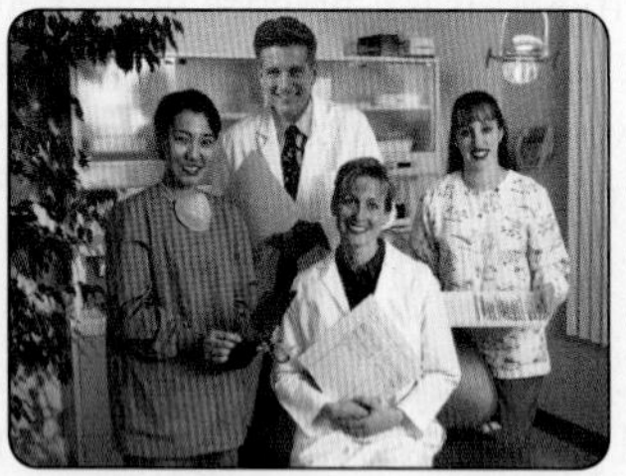

Joseph W. Lake, DDS
Ashley M. Lake, DDS

611 Main Street, SE
Grand Rapids, MI 49502
Phone: 616-101-9575
Fax: 616-101-9999
e-mail: office@dapc.com

INITIAL EXAMINATION…

Each patient that we have the privilege to serve is entitled to and will receive a thorough examination. This examination includes necessary x-rays, diagnostic models, and an oral examination as required to make an accurate analysis of your mouth. An estimate of the fee involved will be given.

OFFICE HOURS…

Office hours are from 8 to 12 and 1 to 5 on Monday and Wednesday and 9 to 12 and 1 to 7 on Tuesday and Thursday. There are no office hours on Friday or Saturday, though on those days a recorder will answer your call, take messages, and refer you to an on-call doctor.

APPOINTMENTS…

The administrative assistant has complete charge of appointments in the office. We will reserve a time that is convenient for you. We will make every effort to keep our schedule on time.

When a change of appointment is necessary, 24 hours advance notice is required.

EMERGENCY TIME…

Time is specifically reserved for emergency care at 10:15 A.M. and 3:45 P.M. We will treat your immediate problem and re-schedule you for further necessary treatment.

MINORS…

Parental approval of the dental treatment is necessary. For a child 15 years old or younger, the dentist or hygienist will notify the parent, guardian, or caretaker that they have a right to have an adult chaperone present when it is necessary to close the door while treating the child.

Small children are more receptive to dental care in the morning. We will request cooperation in having them excused from school.

FIGURE 3-13 An example of an office policy intended to be printed on heavy letter-sized paper and folded in half.

PAYMENT POLICIES...

When extensive treatment is necessary, an estimate of the fee will be presented before services are rendered. The administrative assistant will explain our payment policies and make financial arrangements that are mutually satisfactory.

The fee for treatment requiring a single office visit is payable at the conclusion of the appointment. Other treatment is billed monthly and payable upon receipt of the statement.

Please feel free to make inquiries about our fees, or your dental treatment. You will find the staff most capable, sympathetic, and courteous in providing this information.

Our fees are related directly to the cost of office operation and to strict attention to office efficiency.

INFECTION CONTROL POLICY...

In this office we use a variety of barrier techniques for your individual protection. These techniques include gloves, masks, protective eye shields and coverings, protective clothing, and when necessary specialized intraoral devices. Our staff regularly attends meetings on safety standards and we implement all of the latest OSHA standards and recommendations of the American Dental Association.

DENTAL STAFF...

The administrative and clinical assistants in this office are Certified or Registered Dental Assistants and they are highly skilled in the areas of office management and clinical assisting. The administrative assistant is in charge of all payment arrangements, insurance forms, billing, and appointment scheduling. The clinical assistants are the doctor's operative assistants and with the utilization of these skilled assistants is able to increase efficiency in treatment, thus enabling you to receive complete and thorough dentistry.

While all assistants may assume responsibility for patient education, the Registered Dental Hygienist is in charge of dietary analysis and the oral prophylaxis. After the defective areas are charted, the doctor will do a complete oral examination. The extensive education and experience of our hygienist establishes this professional as an authority in the field of oral hygiene.

PERIODIC EXAMINATION...

We share the desire of all of our patients to minimize the need for extensive dental treatment. This can only be done by regular examinations which detect dental disease before it becomes extensive.

At the conclusion of your treatment, you will be placed on our Preventive Recall Program, which requests you to return at a specified time for a re-examination. Your current dental treatment will be inspected, your home care program reviewed, and your teeth cleaned and polished.

The goal of this program is to:
- Maintain your attractive appearance
- Provide good dental comfort and health
- Prevent unnecessary loss of teeth

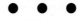

To keep abreast of new techniques, our staff enrolls in four to eight days of continuing education each year. During the time that the doctor and the staff attend meetings, a recorder will direct you to a colleague who will take emergency calls for this office.

Our office is always receptive to suggestions that might be useful to improve our services to you.

FIGURE 3-13, cont'd

office for the first appointment, the administrative assistant can take the opportunity to promote the thoroughness of the practice. Instead of first asking what time of day is most convenient, he or she can start the conversation with the following statement: "Mrs. Timmon, let me be the first to welcome you to Dr. Lake's practice. She is a very caring and thorough dentist who takes time to be current with all of the leading technology and materials. I promise you that all members of our team will go out of our way to provide you with dental care and to make your visits pleasant."

The website should be made "you" oriented rather than "I" oriented. In other words, the statements on the site should let the patient know how important they are to the dentist and how the treatment plan is designed to promote quality care for the patient. The dentist should avoid the use of "I can," "I will," "I am certain," or "I guarantee." It is important to place the patient first and to direct the message toward the patient's needs and satisfaction.

Creating an Office Trademark or Logo

The dentist needs to create an identity. Large corporations such as 3M, Sony, Starbucks, Microsoft, and Amazon all have an identity. The dentist can carry the logo throughout the practice. It should be placed on stationery, appointment cards, or any other written materials. It is an identity that the patients will recognize.

Designing the Pages. The pages of the website must be eye appealing to the reader. Care should be taken to choose colors that are easy to view, especially to prospective patients who may be visually challenged. For instance, the use of light yellow or light teal on white may be difficult to read. Animation and font style and size can enhance a page and make an impression on the reader.

Text materials should be succinct and clear, and they should include the use of headings and titles to define different sections of the narrative. Care should be taken to be certain that the basic rules of grammar are followed and that there is no repetition in the messages.

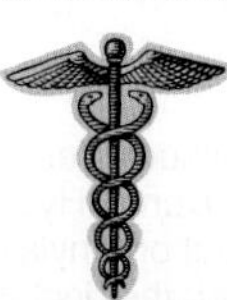

Dental Associates, PC

Joseph W. Lake, DDS - Ashley M. Lake, DDS

Dear Patient:

On behalf of the staff and myself, I welcome you to our office. You are important to us. We pride ourselves in making dentistry a pleasant experience for our patients. You can always expect to be treated as a guest when visiting us.

It is our desire to provide the most thorough and efficient treatment possible. Complete oral health care comprises not only the elimination of existing dental disease but also the prevention of future disease. Except in emergency cases, new adult patients receive a thorough dental examination consisting of the following:

1. Record of medical/dental history
2. Visual mouth examination
3. Complete x-ray examination
4. Prophylaxis (preventive cleaning)
5. Any other diagnostic aids necessary to render a thorough diagnosis
6. Oral hygiene instructions

The requirements for children vary according to age and dental needs.

After the examination is completed, an appointment will be made to discuss the conditions present and the most thorough treatment plans for you. Also at this visit, appointments will be scheduled, estimated fees given, payment plans presented, and all financial arrangements completed. The practice depends upon reimbursement from patients for the costs incurred in their care and financial responsibility on the part of the patient must be determined before treatment. If you require a consultant at this time, we require that he or she accompany you for this important appointment. The responsible adult must be present at a consultation involving children.

We sincerely believe that one of the most important services that we have to offer is a plan for preventive dentistry. All patients are notified at periodic intervals for preventive examinations and the oral prophylaxis.

Except for emergency cases, you may expect us to be on time. Likewise, we will expect the same courtesy. Should it be necessary for you to reschedule an appointment, we require 24 hours notice, except in case of an emergency. This allows us to use your reserved time for another patient.

It is our hope that your dental visits will be prompt and pleasant so that in the future you will want to help increase our fine family of patients through your recommendations.

To continue improving our service, we invite your comments and suggestions at all times.

Sincerely,

Joseph W. Lake, DDS

611 Main Street, SE – Grand Rapids, MI 49502 Phone: 616.101.9575 Fax: 616.101.9999
E-mail: office@dapc.com or Visit us at: www.Lakedental.com

FIGURE 3-14 An example of an office policy statement printed on letterhead.

Graphics, photographs, music, and videos can be added to the website to make it more interesting. Care should be taken not to overload the site with too much activity but rather to keep it simple and thorough. Remember, persons of all ages will be reading this website, so it needs to have universal appeal. Web development software is available for purchase and will help with the creation of the website. Menus should be designed so that the viewer may navigate easily through the site.

The use of hyperlinks, which are words or graphics on a web page that take a user to another page or another website, may be used. These will enable the viewer to go to another destination that has been identified to seek further information.

Identifying a Web Server. After the pages have been designed, the files are stored on a computer hard drive. It is then time to upload or publish the pages to the Internet. The Internet service provider (ISP) that the office uses for e-mail and online services may offer free web space to the doctor. If not, a number of companies provide web space at no charge, but they may require some form of advertising of the ISP to which the pages have been uploaded. If the doctor does not want to have banner ads on the website, then a paid provider may be used.

Uploading the Pages to the Server. When using a free web server, the instructions and passwords are sent to the user with directions for how to upload files to the server. Password protection is important, because it ensures that no one else can alter the website. Copying the files from the office hard drive to the web server is relatively simple.

After the files have all been uploaded, run a test of the website to ensure that it functions well, that all of the files have been uploaded, and that they are in the appropriate order for presentation.

Determine When and By Whom the Website Will Be Updated. At this point, it should be determined who will assume responsibility for updating the website, and a schedule should be established to determine when this will be done. At the original time that the website is created, the staff may feel it necessary to do an update soon rather than waiting for several weeks. This can provide an opportunity to make any necessary corrections as soon as possible.

Update the Website Regularly. To maintain its currency, the website should be updated regularly. There is nothing worse than a patient finding stale news or inaccurate information. Set a schedule and adhere to it to ensure an accurate website that will encourage patients and staff to view it frequently.

Enthusiastic Attitude

The single most important characteristic of a staff member is an enthusiastic attitude. The employee with an enthusiastic attitude shows up for work every day on time; he or she is willing to help others, maintains a cheery disposition all day, and ensures that patients come first. This enthusiastic attitude means that the "no whining" rule is always in place, because whining is contagious. The enthusiastic attitude means that the patient's problems come first and that personal problems are kept to oneself or shared only with friends in private.

PRACTICE NOTE

The single most important characteristic of a staff member is an enthusiastic attitude.

Seizing Opportunities

There are many ways to get the word out about a practice. For instance, when a new patient makes an appointment, say, "Mrs. Timmons, we are looking forward to seeing you at 3 PM on Wednesday. By the way, would you like to make an appointment for any other members of your family at this time?" This is also a good opportunity to refer them to the office website, to give them instructions for how to reach the website, and to suggest that they look at it thoroughly because it contains information about the staff and the educational goals of the office as well as directions to the office.

Practice Ambassadors

Each member of the staff is expected to be an ambassador for the practice. He or she should be provided with his or her own business cards, and he or she should promote the practice to family and friends. It may even be possible to suggest that the office be used after hours for community group meetings if office space is adequate. When a new staff member joins a practice, the dentist should prepare an announcement that can be sent to the new team member's family, friends, or other professional associates.

Internal Marketing

Marketing can be divided into two types: internal and external. Internal marketing is what one does within the office to retain patients and includes the crucial first impression. It involves how patient perceptions regarding the dental staff's level of caring and enjoyment of their work; it is the patient's feeling that the dentist is willing to learn more about his or her individual dental problem. Internal marketing influences how patients are retained after they have been attracted to the practice.

As mentioned in Chapter 2, one of the most important assets that a dentist has in his or her office is the dental staff. When staff members are committed to the practice, highly motivated, and enthusiastic, they become the impetus for a successful internal marketing program. Look at Figure 3-15, and note that most of the ideas for internal marketing for patient retention are staff oriented. Staff members should be given specialized duties that they perform as part of an internal marketing program. For instance, a staff person who writes well could manage written communication, whereas another who has a good understanding of insurance could explain insurance benefits to patients.

Patients who know that the dentist and staff care about them and do not consider them merely case numbers or blank checks will return to the practice and, more important, will refer friends and colleagues.

External Marketing

Some dentists view external marketing with skepticism, but, if it is used, it must be presented in an ethical form. The key to successful external marketing is to determine prospective patients and the best method of attracting them. The dentist must identify his or her objectives, define the strengths of the practice, determine the budget, and review all of the sources for external advertising. Some forms of such marketing can be as simple as offering lectures to local organizations or as complex as media advertising. A review of Figure 3-16 illustrates other potential sources of external marketing. When using any source of advertising, the dentist must realize that the results will not be immediate and that a consistent and repetitive message must be directed to prospective patients to obtain results.

The most important factor to remember in any form of marketing is to produce what you claim. No matter where or how much the dentist advertises, if quality dental care is not delivered in a caring and sensitive manner, the patient will not return. A good motto for a dentist to remember is, "You may attract them, but you won't keep them."

Newsletters as Marketing Devices

As dentistry seeks to address the consumer market, newsletters have become a major asset for the dental practice. Newsletters may be considered for the internal market by sending them to current patients, or they may be used for the external market by sending them out to the nearby community addressed to the resident of a given address. The use of e-mail allows for the sending of newsletters to patients with no mailing costs. If done ethically and with concern for the values of the community and the education of the public, this form of marketing can be a

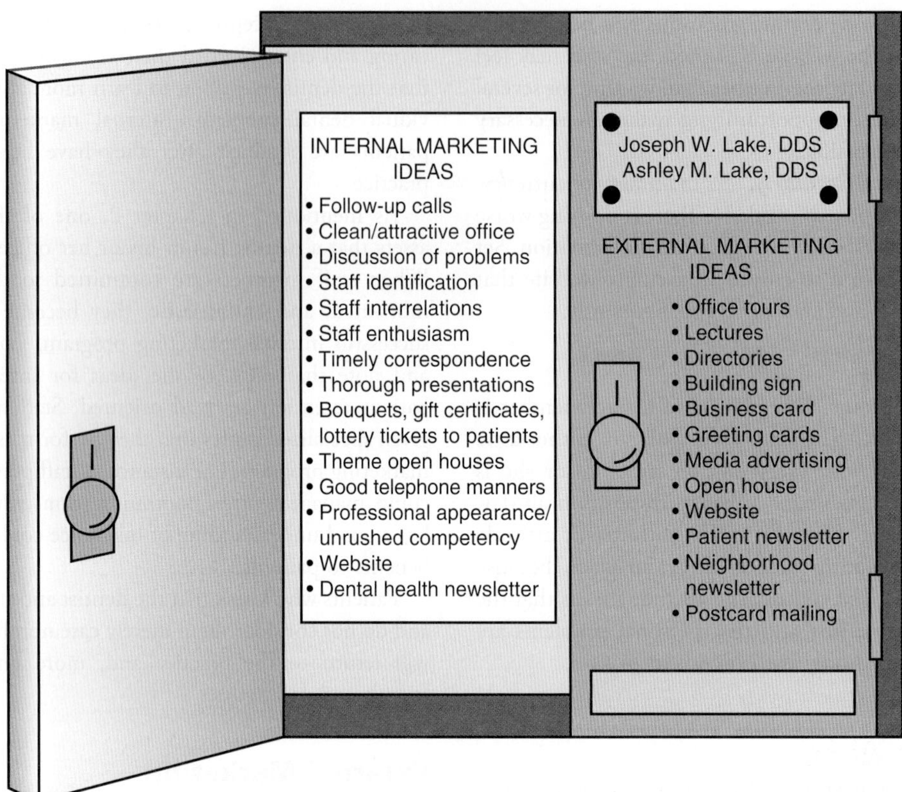

FIGURE 3-15 Internal and external marketing ideas.

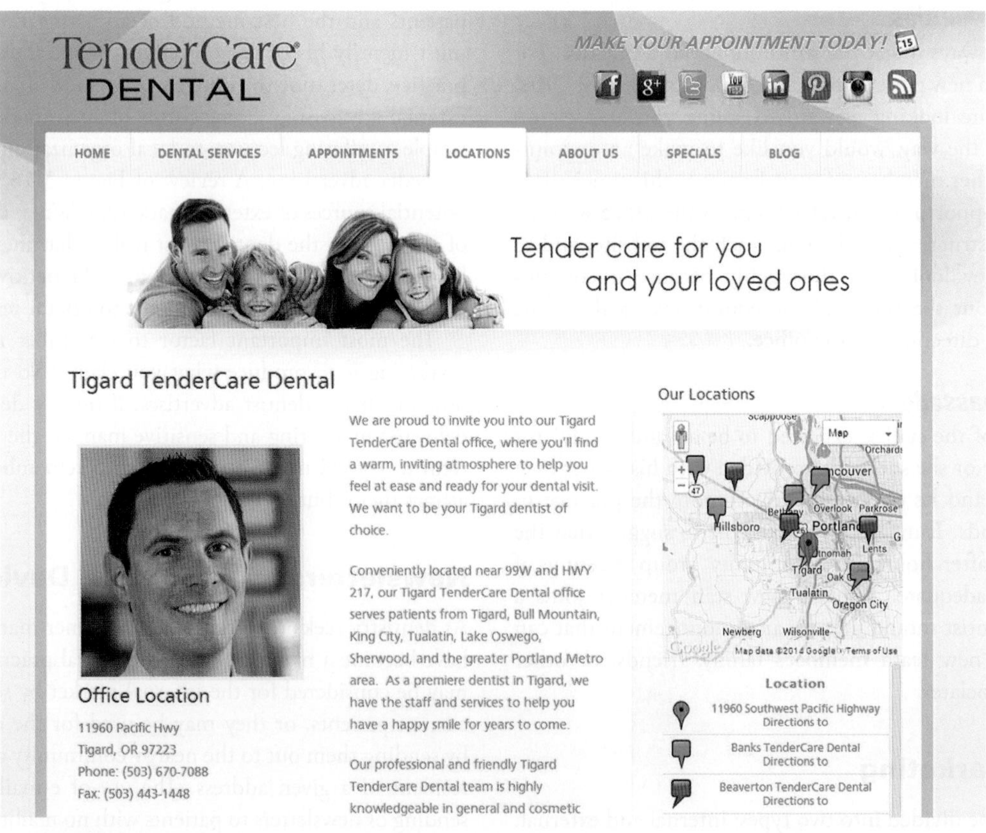

FIGURE 3-16 An example of a website to be used for both internal and external marketing. (Courtesy of Catlin Dental, Fort Myers, FL.)

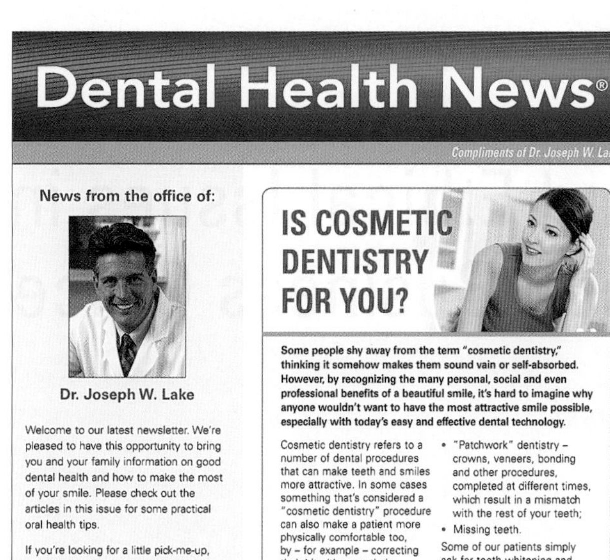

Dental Health News®

Compliments of Dr. Joseph W. Lake

News from the office of:

Dr. Joseph W. Lake

Welcome to our latest newsletter. We're pleased to have this opportunity to bring you and your family information on good dental health and how to make the most of your smile. Please check out the articles in this issue for some practical oral health tips.

If you're looking for a little pick-me-up, consider the benefits of teeth whitening. Quick, easy, safe and effective, teeth whitening can result in a brighter smile and a younger, more vibrant appearance.

Enjoy this newsletter, and please feel free to pass it on to a friend or family member who may be interested in reading up on the latest dental health news.

Thank you for your continued patronage. We look forward to seeing you again soon!

All the best,

Joseph Lake

Dr. Joseph W. Lake and Team

IS COSMETIC DENTISTRY FOR YOU?

Some people shy away from the term "cosmetic dentistry," thinking it somehow makes them sound vain or self-absorbed. However, by recognizing the many personal, social and even professional benefits of a beautiful smile, it's hard to imagine why anyone wouldn't want to have the most attractive smile possible, especially with today's easy and effective dental technology.

Cosmetic dentistry refers to a number of dental procedures that can make teeth and smiles more attractive. In some cases something that's considered a "cosmetic dentistry" procedure can also make a patient more physically comfortable too, by – for example – correcting their bite (the way their teeth come together).

Ask us about solutions to these common tooth imperfections:

- Gaps or spaces between teeth;
- Yellow or discolored teeth;
- Uneven, chipped or broken teeth;
- Small or short teeth, or teeth that are too long;
- Crooked, crowded or rotated teeth;
- Too much, or not enough gum tissue (making teeth seem too short or too long);
- An abundance of unsightly metal fillings;
- "Patchwork" dentistry – crowns, veneers, bonding and other procedures, completed at different times, which result in a mismatch with the rest of your teeth;
- Missing teeth.

Some of our patients simply ask for teeth whitening and perhaps some minor tooth-shaping or gum contouring, while others require a full smile makeover. You may have seen from "Extreme Makeover" or similar shows what a difference a smile makeover can make in a person's overall appearance and wondered if some of those procedures might correct your own dental imperfections. Why not pick up the phone and make an appointment for a no-obligation discussion on all your options now?

We look forward to creating your perfect smile!

COS

VOLUME 12, ISSUE 1

FIGURE 3-17 An example of a dental practice newsletter, which can be used as a marketing tool to help promote the business. (Courtesy Market Connections, Inc., www.dentalhealthnews.org, Toronto, Ontario, Canada.)

valuable tool. Of course, the newsletter can also be posted on the website.

There are several companies that create newsletters for dental practices, as shown in Figure 3-17. Such services can provide customized educational articles and photographs that can be personalized for the individual office. These newsletters can promote the practice in addition to establishing rapport with existing patients and the community. Most companies provide mailing services for the office for patients who do not have e-mail. The newsletter can also be sent to a new patient with a "get acquainted" packet of information before the patient's first appointment. It is possible for a newsletter to be created in the office using one of a variety of software packages available for the creation of such forms of written communication.

LEARNING ACTIVITIES

1. Identify and give examples of barriers in communication.
2. Describe the duties of a receptionist for communicating with patients and putting them at ease.
3. Explain how Maslow's hierarchy of needs, Carl Rogers' client-centered therapy, and locus of control theory can be applied to dentistry.
4. What is marketing?
5. With a colleague, create an outline for a website that could be used as a marketing device.
6. List five rights of the patient that should be considered during a treatment procedure.
7. With a colleague, make up a conversation that may occur in a dental office, and indicate how you can use positive phrases instead of negative ones to interact with the patient.

Please refer to the student workbook for additional learning activities.

BIBLIOGRAPHY

Adam AP: *Kinn's the administrative medical assistant*, ed 8, St Louis, 2014, Elsevier.

Frazier GL: *Connecting with customers*, ed 2, Upper Saddle River, NJ, 2004, Prentice Hall.

Fulton-Calkins PJ, Rankin DS, Shumack KA: *The administrative professional*, ed 14, Mason, OH, 2011, Thomson South-Western.

Griffin J: *How to say it at work: power words, phrases, and communication secrets for getting ahead*, ed 2, Upper Saddle River, NJ, 2008, Prentice Hall.

Locker KO, Kaczmarek S: *Business communication: building critical skills*, ed 6, New York, 2013, Irwin/McGraw-Hill.

Miles L: *Dynamic dentistry: practice management tools and strategy for breakthrough success*, Virginia Beach, VA, 2003, Link Publishing.

Perkins PS: *The art and science of communication: tools for effective communication in the workplace*, New York, 2008, John Wiley & Sons.

Rotter J: Generalized expectancies for internal versus external control of reinforcement, Psychol Monogr, 80, Whole No. 609, 1966.

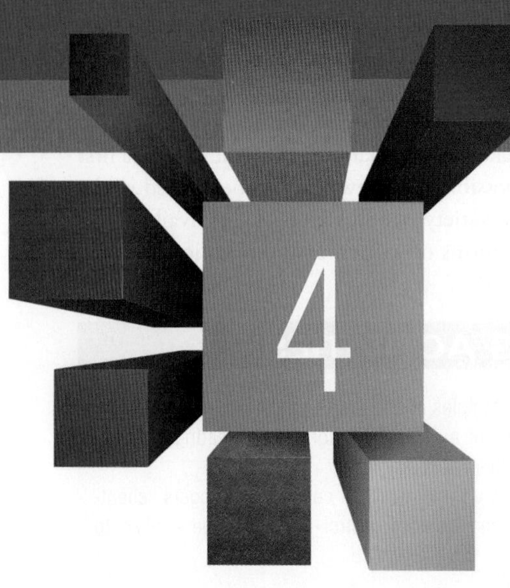

Legal and Ethical Issues in the Dental Business Office

Pamela Zarkowski

 http://evolve.elsevier.com/Finkbeiner/practice

LEARNING OUTCOMES

1. Define the key terms in this chapter.
2. Understand the definition and classifications of law in relation to dentistry and the important terms involved with litigation.
3. Discuss crimes and torts with regard to the standard of care in a dental office.
4. Understand the dental practice act.
5. Discuss professional standards that dental assisting uses including accreditation, certification and licensure.
6. Describe the code of ethics of professional dental organizations.
7. Discuss the ethical and legal considerations for the administrative assistant.
8. Explain various types of consent.
9. Understand managed care and risk management programs as they relate to dentistry.
10. Understand the legal responsibilities of a dental practice and list business office activities that could lead to potential litigation, including abandonment, fraud, records management, defamation of character, negligence, invasion of privacy, Good Samaritan Law, American with Disabilities Act and computer security.
11. Identify 12 steps in making ethical decisions.

KEY TERMS

Abandonment The severance of a professional relationship with a patient who is still in need of dental care and attention without giving adequate notice to the patient.

Americans with Disabilities Act (AwDA) A federal law that affects the dental office by prohibiting employee discrimination and by requiring facilities to be accessible to physically and mentally compromised patients.

Assignment A term that refers to the dentist assigning to a dental assistant or dental hygienist a specific procedure that is to be performed on a designated patient of record.

Beneficence The principle of ethics that refers to "doing good." The dental professional has a duty to promote the patient's welfare.

Civil law A law that relates to duties between persons or between citizens and their government.

Common law A law that relates to judicial decisions.

Computer security Protection of computer systems and information from harm, theft, unauthorized use, manipulation or piracy.

Consent The voluntary acceptance or agreement to what is planned or done by another person.

Crime A wrongdoing against the public or an unlawful act that is prosecuted by a public official.

Criminal law A law that refers to wrongs committed against the public as a whole.

Defamation of character The communication of false information to a third party about a person that results in injury to that person's reputation.

Defendant The person or party that is being sued in a lawsuit.

Dental practice act The law in each state that defines the scope of dental practice and the requirements necessary to practice as a dental professional.

Ethics The branch of philosophy that identifies a systematic and intellectual approach to the standards of behavior.

Expert witness A witness who is called to testify, to explain what happened based on the patient's record, and to offer an opinion as to whether the dental care as administered met acceptable standards.

Fact witness A witness who describes what he or she saw or did during a specific act.

Felony A serious crime that is punishable by imprisonment, generally for more than 1 year.

Fraud A deliberately practiced deception that is committed to secure unfair or unlawful gain.

Informed consent Consent for treatment that is given by a patient of sound mind after being informed in understandable language about such treatment by the healthcare provider.

Invasion of privacy Publishing, making known, or using information related to the private life or affairs of a person without that person's approval or permission.

Justice The concept of fairness and integrity.

Lawsuit A legal action in court.

Litigation The judicial process used in a lawsuit.

Malpractice Intentional or unintentional professional misconduct, evil practice, or illegal or immoral conduct.

Managed care A cost-containment system that directs the use of health benefits by restricting the type, level, and frequency of treatment; limiting access to care; and controlling the level of reimbursement for services.

Misdemeanor A crime of a less serious nature than a felony.

National Practitioner Data Bank (NPDB) An agency that was implemented as a central repository for information about paid malpractice claims and adverse reports of healthcare licensees.

Nonmaleficence A term that refers to the "do no harm" clause in the principle of ethics. The dental provider has a duty to refrain from harming the patient.

Negligence An act of omission (neglecting to do something that a reasonably prudent person would do) or commission (doing something that a reasonably prudent person would not do).

Patient of record A patient who has been examined and diagnosed by a licensed dentist and whose treatment has been planned by that dentist.

Plaintiff The person or party that institutes a lawsuit.

Standard of care Treatment that a reasonably prudent professional would perform in similar circumstances.

Supervision A term that refers to the conditions under which a patient of record may be treated by an assistant or hygienist and the protocol to be followed after the treatment is rendered.

Tort A civil wrongdoing that is a breach of legal duty owed to the plaintiff by the defendant and that must be the primary cause of harm to the plaintiff.

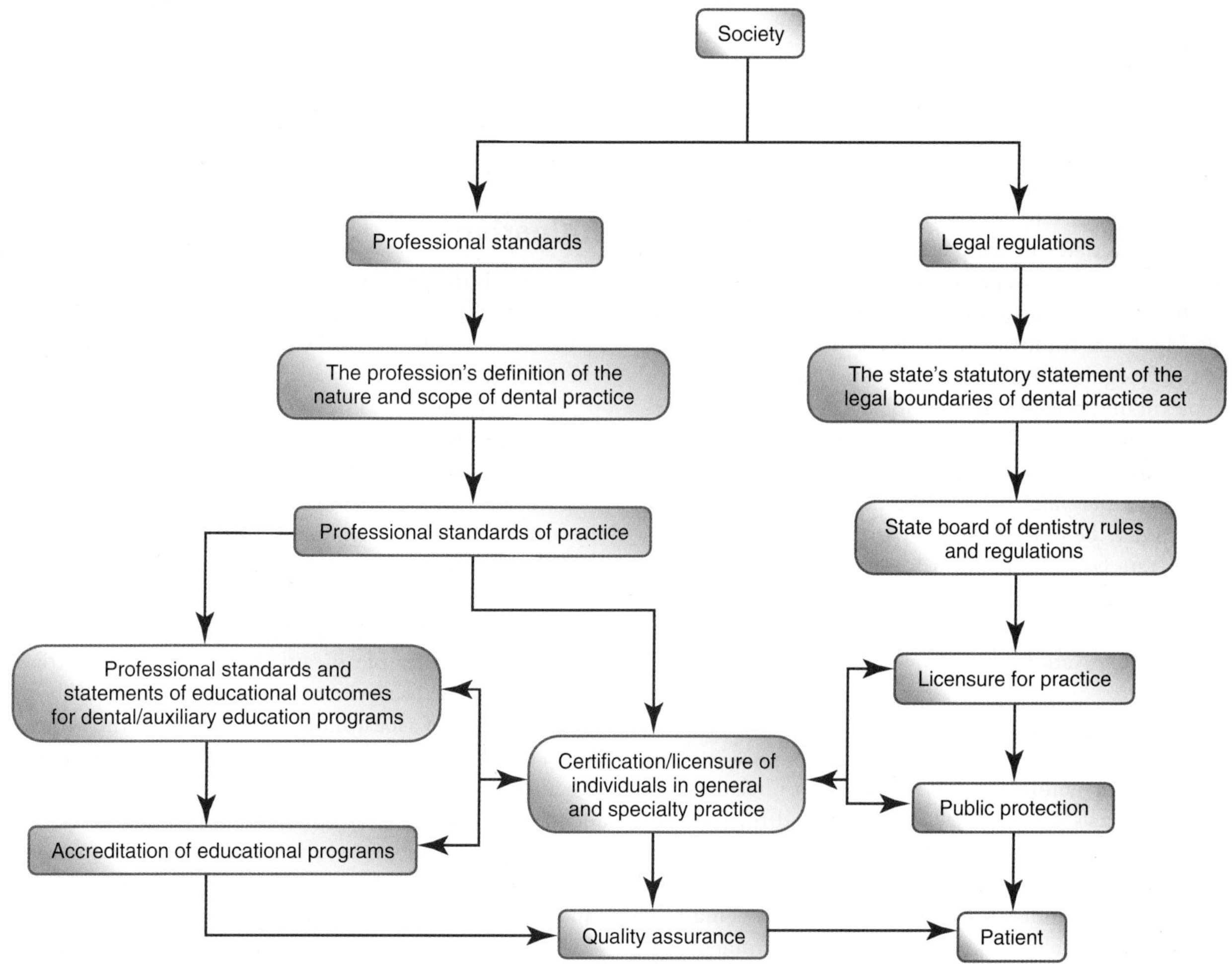

FIGURE 4-1 Diagram of the professional and legal regulations of dentistry.

Each day, dental professionals are faced with issues involving the legal requirements and standards of care—both voluntary and involuntary—related to the delivery of dental treatment. The dental practice act of each state defines the requirements necessary to practice dentistry and the scope of dental practice for each member of the dental team for that particular state. Standards for dental care may arise from both common law (judicial decisions) and statutory law (enacted by a legislative body), such as the state dental practice act. The dental professional is also governed by voluntary standards, such as the principles of ethics, developed and implemented by the dental profession itself. Both legal and voluntary requirements and standards are implemented for the protection of society and, ultimately, the patient. This process of regulation is illustrated in Figure 4-1.

An administrative assistant practicing in a dental office today needs to have an understanding of the effect of law on the dental practice and an awareness of its importance on his or her performance of daily duties. Each member of an office or dental business entity should be familiar with the code of ethics for its professional group and its colleagues.

Membership in a professional organization is voluntary, and thus the principles and guidelines of these organizations are also considered voluntary. However, these standards may be used as guidelines for peer review or other quality assurance activities. Professional organizations continually assess their standards and the qualifications of their members. The standards of professional health entities are a reflection of a combination of factors, including current oral healthcare needs and the public's expectations for dentists and the dental team to appropriately meet those needs. Examples of voluntary standards are illustrated in the profession's code of ethics, professional standards for the accreditation of educational programs, standards for credentialing, and standards of various service organizations. Legal standards for dental care are determined through common law and result in standards such as the Informed Consent Doctrine, which is discussed later in this chapter. In addition, federal and state legislation may create other legal obligations, such as the confidentiality of patient information. Legislative action, which is reflected in a state's dental practice act, establishes the legal requirements and the scope of practice for dental providers within the state. This action establishes education, credentialing, and licensure requirements for the dentist and any dental auxiliaries recognized in the state dental practice act.

Copies of the principles of ethics for any of the dental professional organizations may be obtained from their national offices or their official websites. Copies of dental practice acts may be available from the state's board of dentistry or online. In addition, there may be other resources pertinent to dental professionals that are available online, such as guidelines for requesting medical or dental records and public health codes or obligations. A *State Fact Booklet* may also be purchased from the Dental Assisting National Board website at www.danb.org.

DEFINITION OF LAW

Law consists of enforceable rules that govern relationships among individuals and between individuals and their society. A broad definition of the law implies that there must be established rules, such as a state constitution, statutes, administrative agency rules, and judicial decisions. Rules of law must be enforceable and establish limits of conduct for governments and individuals in society.

Law Relative to Dentistry

In many states, the board of dentistry is an administrative agency at the state level. The executive officers of an administrative agency perform specific functions, including enforcing laws within their agency. The state boards have the power to make rules and regulations that conform to enacted laws, such as the dental practice act. Rules and regulations adopted by the board are components of the body of law referred to as *administrative laws.* State statutes must conform to the state's constitution and the federal constitution. The dental practice act is an example of state statutory law.

Classifications of Law

Law can be divided into two classifications: civil and criminal. Civil law relates to duties between persons or between citizens and their government. Criminal law deals with wrongs committed against the public as a whole.

In a civil case, one party (the plaintiff) tries to correct an interference with his or her interest—such as the protection of his or her person (bodily harm), privacy, or property—by another party (the defendant). The defendant may have failed to comply with a duty or otherwise breached an acceptable standard of conduct. The defendant may be required to pay for the damages caused by the failure to comply with that duty. In criminal law, the interests of society are at stake; the government may seek to impose a penalty, such as a fine or imprisonment, on the guilty person.

Litigation

Litigation is the process of a lawsuit. A lawsuit is a legal action in a court. The person or party that institutes the suit in court is the plaintiff. The person being accused of the wrongdoing is the defendant.

During malpractice litigation, the patient may be the plaintiff. The dentist or the person who is being sued is the defendant. It is likely that other individuals in the dental office (e.g., dentist associate, dental assistant, dental hygienist) may be named as defendants or as fact witnesses in the legal proceedings. A fact witness, when placed under oath, must provide only firsthand knowledge and not hearsay. Fact witness testimony consists of the recitation of facts or events. This is different from the role of an expert witness in a trial. For example, if the fact witness is being questioned about the administration of a local anesthetic to a patient, the witness may be asked if he or she was told what type of anesthetic to prepare, whether he or she prepared the anesthetic and passed it to the dentist, how much anesthetic was administered to the patient, and what the patient's reaction was after the anesthetic was administered. If the fact witness only received the directions and prepared the anesthetic for the setup but did not participate in its administration, only the initial questions can be answered. To describe any further action not observed would be inappropriate and may be considered speculation or hearsay.

An expert witness is called to testify and explain to the judge and jury what happened based on the patient's record and to offer an opinion as to whether or not the dental care as administered met acceptable standards. Such standards may vary by state. Often a dentist may be called as an expert witness to testify in malpractice litigation because of his or her educational background and clinical expertise. A strong knowledge of the laws and rules that guide dental care and dental standards as well as an understanding of malpractice liability is beneficial in such cases.

CRIMES AND TORTS

Overview and Definitions

A crime is a wrongdoing against the public at large, and it is prosecuted by a public official. In most cases in which a crime is committed, there is intent to do wrong. However, a person or entity that violates certain laws may be guilty of a crime whether there was intent or not. Criminal liability typically involves both the performance of a prohibited act and a specified state of mind or intent on the part of the actor. In some cases, the omission of an act can be a crime if the person or entity has a legal duty to perform the act; an example of this would be the failure to file a federal income tax return.

A crime can be classified as a misdemeanor or a felony. A misdemeanor is less serious than a felony, and it is punishable by a fine or imprisonment of up to 1 year. A felony is a more serious crime, and generally it is punishable by imprisonment for a longer period of time.

A tort is a civil wrongdoing. It is an interference with a recognized interest or a breach of a legal duty owed by a defendant to a plaintiff. The plaintiff in most instances must show that the defendant's action or omission was a cause of loss or harm to the plaintiff. A tort is generally resolved through a civil trial and results in a monetary settlement for damages. There are two types of torts: intentional and unintentional.

If the wrongdoing is classified as an intentional tort, this indicates that the person committing the tort intended to commit the wrongful act. Intentional torts for which a dental assistant could be held liable include assault and battery, defamation of character, invasion of privacy, misrepresentation, inflection of mental distress, and false imprisonment. An unintentional tort includes negligence, which is sometimes referred to as *malpractice.*

Unintentional torts do not require a particular mental state. Failure to exercise a standard of care, such as performing a treatment that a reasonably prudent professional would perform in similar circumstances, is an example of an unintentional tort. Thus, even if a dental professional neither wishes to bring about the consequences of the act nor believes that they will occur, negligence may be alleged: someone suffered injury because another person failed to live up to a particular standard of care. Questions related to the failure to exercise a standard of care must be answered. If an individual is accused of a negligent act, the plaintiff's attorney must prove that the defendant failed to satisfy the following four elements:

1. There is a duty to follow a standard of care.
2. The duty was breached.
3. As a result of the breach of duty, the plaintiff suffered an injury.
4. The injury was a direct result of the breach of duty.

Strict liability is an unintentional tort. It relates to a person having the legal responsibility for damages or injury, even if the person found strictly liable was not at fault or negligent, regardless of the care exercised. Negligence is the performance of an act that a reasonably careful person under similar circumstances would not do or the failure to perform an act that a reasonably careful person would do under similar circumstances. Professionals usually consider malpractice a form of negligence, but it can mean, in a broader sense, any wrongdoing by a professional. Malpractice can refer to any professional misconduct, evil practice, or illegal or immoral conduct, not just negligence. Malpractice can be either unintentional or intentional. Box 4-1 contains a list of negligent acts that might occur in a dental office.

PRACTICE NOTE

Failure to exercise a standard of care can occur during patient assessment, treatment planning, treatment, and patient referral. The standard of care may be influenced by the dental practice act, which defines the scope of practice for dental professionals. In addition, the standard is influenced by individuals who have the same training and experience.

BOX 4-1

Negligent Acts That Could Occur in a Dental Office

- Abandonment
- Physical injury
- Mistaken identity
- Foreign objects left in a patient after a surgical procedure
- Use of defective equipment
- Failure to observe patient reactions and take appropriate action
- Medication errors
- Drug administration errors
- Failure to take an adequate health or dental history
- Failure to exercise good judgment
- Failure to communicate
- Loss of or damage to patient's personal property
- Failure to obtain informed consent
- Failure to obtain informed refusal
- Failure to refer a patient to a physician or another dental provider
- Disease transmission

PRACTICE NOTE

Professionals usually consider malpractice to be a form of negligence, but it can mean, in a broader sense, any wrongdoing by a professional.

DENTAL PRACTICE ACT

The legal requirements necessary to practice dentistry as well as the scope of what can be practiced are developed through legislative action within the state and identified in the state dental practice act. This act defines the minimum educational standards; the requirements for credentialing; and the criteria for license revocation or suspension for a dentist, a dental hygienist, and, in several states, a dental assistant. The act may describe supervision requirements, required content of a dental record, and specific guidelines concerning the continuing education required to maintain a license. Other legal requirements are enacted by the government in the form of rules and regulations; like the dental practice act, these also regulate the practice of dentistry. An example of a government agency that creates requirements that affect the practice of dentistry is the state Department of Labor.

A state's dental practice act is periodically reviewed and updated. However, as changes take place in technology and as standards of dental care are modified, dental practice acts may be modified to reflect those changes. An administrative assistant should regularly obtain a copy of the state's dental practice act to determine if there are modifications to the rules and regulations that guide oral health providers and that govern the scope of dental practice. For example, a dental practice act may be modified when the scope of practice for a dental assistant is expanded. Dental practice acts are available online for easy access and review.

Many state dental practice acts define conditions under which a dental assistant or dental hygienist may perform specific duties. Each state provides a list of definitions within the law, and the descriptive language may vary significantly from state to state. Examples of such terminology include *patient of record, assignment,* and *supervision. Patient of record* refers to a patient who has been examined and diagnosed by a licensed dentist and whose treatment has been planned by that dentist. *Assignment* commonly refers to the dentist assigning a specific procedure to a dental assistant or dental hygienist that is to be performed on a designated patient of record. In some jurisdictions, for certain procedures, the dentist does not need to be physically present in the office or in the treatment room at the time that the procedure is being performed. *Supervision* refers to the conditions under which a patient of record may be treated by an assistant or hygienist and the protocol to be followed after the treatment is rendered. One type of supervision is referred to as *direct supervision;* this generally means that the dentist has designated a patient of record on whom services are to be performed and has described the procedure to be performed. The dentist examines the patient before prescribing the procedures to be performed and again after the completion of the procedure. According to the definition of direct supervision, the dentist generally must be physically present in the office at the time that the procedures are being performed.

It is important to remember that the legal standards within dental law are for the protection of the public, and requirements for the protection of the public may differ in each state. Terminology and the interpretation of a term used in a dental practice act may vary from state to state. The term *assignment* may be used in one dental practice act; however, in another state, the term *general supervision* may have a description that is similar or identical to that of *assignment.* It is important to carefully read all definitions and descriptions found in a dental practice act to completely understand the dental professional's scope of practice and supervisory requirements.

PROFESSIONAL STANDARDS

Over the last half century, the dental assisting profession has taken several steps to ensure the competence of its practitioners through such means as the credentialing process. *Credentialing* is a generic term that refers to the ways in which professionals can measure and maintain their competence.

The processes used in credentialing include accreditation, certification, and licensure. Accreditation generally is the process by which an entity or educational program is evaluated and recognized by an outside agency for having attained a predetermined set of standards. These standards are identified by professional and educational organizations as well as by peer groups. In dentistry, the Commission on Dental Accreditation of the American Dental Association (ADA) is responsible for accrediting educational programs in dentistry, dental assisting, dental hygiene, and dental laboratory technology. When a program is accredited by the ADA's Commission on Dental Accreditation (CODA), the program makes public its accreditation status. Such accreditation validates that a specific educational program has met a set of standards to address the needs of the profession and the public. Information about accreditation standards for educational programs can be found at www.ada.org/117.aspx. In many instances, a criterion for obtaining a credential such as certification or licensure is contingent on the individual seeking the certification to provide evidence that the person successfully completed an ADA-accredited educational program.

National certification in dental assisting is a voluntary procedure, and it may be achieved through the Dental Assisting National Board. This organization provides credentialing for the clinical dental assistant, the orthodontic assistant, and the administrative assistant as described in Chapter 2. The process of credentialing requires satisfying prerequisites that include educational and clinical experiences, and it measures whether the person has met certain criteria established by the nongovernmental organization for the dental assisting profession.

Licensure is the credential granted to a candidate by the state after the individual provides appropriate documentation to prove he or she has met the state's designated requirements to practice in the profession. Generally this license is granted after the person has satisfied specific educational requirements and successfully completed some form of designated state testing, such as a clinical or written examination.

CODE OF ETHICS

Ethics is the branch of philosophy that involves a systematic and intellectual approach to the standards of behavior. The purpose of a professional code of ethics is to help members of the profession achieve high levels of behavior through moral consciousness, decision making, and practice by members of the profession. Ethics in daily professional practice challenges a practitioner to differentiate between right and wrong. Morals are considered voluntary personal commitments to a set of values. Values are the standards used for decision making that endure over a significant period of time. The expected behaviors of the dental professional are based on a set of standards derived from aspired to acceptable behaviors. Every health professional must realize that there are both right and wrong actions that can be taken and that there is no right way to do a wrong thing.

American Dental Association Principles of Ethics and Code of Professional Conduct

Each organized group within the profession of dentistry, including the ADA, the American Dental Assistants Association (ADAA), and the American Dental Hygienists' Association (ADHA), has developed a code of ethics for its members. These codes are based on ethical principles that reflect a concern for the patient's protection during all aspects of care. The codes may also address professional practice, record keeping, service to the community, research, and other practice-related topics.

PRACTICE NOTE
There is no right way to do a wrong thing.

Dentistry as a profession enjoys a certain level of independence with regard to decision making and self-governance as a result of the training and education of its members. However, this right carries with it an obligation to maintain quality standards and to be responsible to one's patients and peers. This right does not allow a member of the profession to disregard professional standards or the laws that govern the practice of dentistry. The profession's primary goal is to provide quality care to patients in a competent and timely manner. To maintain high standards of care, the dental professional can continue to improve the quality of care through education, training, research, and adherence to a stringent code of ethics and professional conduct. The *ADA Principles of Ethics and Code of Professional Conduct* can be found on the ADA website at www.ada.org/sections/about/pdfs/code_of_ethics_2012.pdf

This document identifies five basic categories of ethics and professional conduct for a dentist. An overview of these principles is included in Box 4-2.

American Dental Assistants Association Principles of Ethics

Like the American Dental Association, the ADAA has addressed the issue of ethics by preparing the following statement regarding the principles of ethics for its members:

BOX 4-2

Overview of the American Dental Association Principles of Ethics and Code of Professional Conduct

SECTION 1 — Principle: Patient Autonomy ("Self-governance")
The dentist has a duty to respect the patient's rights to self-determination and confidentiality.

This principle expresses the concept that professionals have a duty to treat the patient according to the patient's desires, within the bounds of accepted treatment, and to protect the patient's confidentiality. In accordance with this principle, the dentist's primary obligations include involving patients in treatment decisions in a meaningful way, with due consideration being given to the patient's needs, desires, and abilities, and safeguarding the patient's privacy.

SECTION 2 — Principle: Nonmaleficence ("Do no harm")
The dentist has a duty to refrain from harming the patient.

This principle expresses the concept that professionals have a duty to protect the patient from harm. Under this principle, the dentist's primary obligations include keeping knowledge and skills current, knowing one's own limitations and when to refer to a specialist or other professional, and knowing when and under what circumstances the delegation of patient care to auxiliaries is appropriate.

SECTION 3 — Principle: Beneficence ("Do good")
The dentist has a duty to promote the patient's welfare.

This principle expresses the concept that professionals have a duty to act for the benefit of others. Under this principle, the dentist's primary obligation is service to the patient and the public at large. The most important aspect of this obligation is the competent and timely delivery of dental care within the bounds of clinical circumstances presented by the patient, with due consideration being given to the needs, desires, and values of the patient. The same ethical considerations apply whether the dentist engages in fee-for-service, managed care, or another practice arrangement. Dentists may choose to enter into contracts governing the provision of care to a group of patients; however, contractual obligations do not excuse dentists from their ethical duty to put the patient's welfare first.

SECTION 4 — Principle: Justice ("Fairness")
The dentist has a duty to treat people fairly.

This principle expresses the concept that professionals have a duty to be fair in their dealings with patients, colleagues, and society. Under this principle, the dentist's primary obligations include dealing with people justly and delivering dental care without prejudice. In its broadest sense, this principle expresses the concept that the dental professional should actively seek allies throughout society for specific activities that will help improve access to care for all.

SECTION 5 — Principle: Veracity ("Truthfulness")
The dentist has a duty to communicate truthfully.

This principle expresses the concept that professionals have a duty to be honest and trustworthy in their dealings with people. Under this principle, the dentist's primary obligations include respecting the position of trust inherent in the dentist/patient relationship, communicating truthfully and without deception, and maintaining intellectual integrity.

Codes of professional conduct can be found for each section in the *ADA Principles of Ethics and Code of Professional Conduct* (an ADA publication) or on the ADA website at www.ada.org/sections/about/pdfs/code_of_ethics_2012.pdf.

Each individual involved in the practice of dentistry assumes the obligation of maintaining and enriching the profession. Each member may choose to meet this obligation according to the dictates of personal conscience based on the needs of the human beings the profession of dentistry is committed to serve. The spirit of the Golden Rule is the basic guiding principle of this concept. The member must strive at all times to maintain confidentiality and exhibit respect for the dentist/employer. The member shall refrain from performing any professional service that is prohibited by state law and has the obligation to prove competence prior to providing services to any patient. The member shall constantly strive to upgrade and expand technical skills for the benefit of the employer and the consumer public. The member should additionally seek to sustain and improve the local organization, state association, and the ADAA by active participation and personal commitment.

This statement as well as a code of professional conduct for assistants can be found at www.dentalassistant.org/Content/Details/ADAA_Code_of_Professional_Conduct.pdf

American Dental Hygienists' Association Code of Ethics

The purpose of the American Dental Hygienists' Association's (ADHA) code of ethics was created to provide guidance for the achievement of high levels of ethical consciousness, decision making, and practice by the members of the profession. Sections found within the code include key concepts, basic beliefs, core values, and standards of professional responsibility. The ADHA code can be found at www.adha.org/bylaws-ethics.

American Association of Dental Office Managers

The American Association of Dental Office Managers (AADOM) is a relatively new organization that has been created for dental office managers and practice administrators. This organization deals with specific issues related to the dental business office, and it makes special efforts to ensure that its members maintain confidentiality. More information may be found at www.dentalmanagers.com.

ETHICAL AND LEGAL CONSIDERATIONS FOR THE ADMINISTRATIVE ASSISTANT

Vigilance

Each day, the dental professional is confronted with ethical and legal decisions. The basis for each of these decisions may change as laws and societal expectations affect the delivery of dental care. As discussed previously, each member of the dental profession must constantly be attentive to the changes taking place in the laws that affect the practice of dentistry. Although the administrative assistant has contact with the clinical areas of the office, emphasis in this text is placed only on those areas that directly relate to the activities of the dental administrative assistant. Box 4-3 lists those activities that the administrative assistant may encounter that could potentially lead to litigation. The following discussion provides the administrative assistant with a practical understanding of various issues. These situations also should provoke one's critical-thinking processes to consider other situations that may be common to a dental practice.

BOX 4-3

Common Business Activities That May Lead to Potential Litigation

- Making false accusations about another person in verbal or written communication
- Providing another party or agency with confidential information without patient consent
- Entering inaccurate data on patient records
- Duplicating copyrighted material without permission
- Using unauthorized software
- Gaining illegal access to computer data
- Maliciously or deliberately damaging data in a computer
- Falsely entering data on insurance claims
- Failing to follow federal or state disease transmission or waste management regulations
- Failing to maintain accurate local, state, or federal governmental records

Assignment of Duties

As described in the section about the state dental practice act, it is the responsibility of the licensed dentist to assign or delegate specific procedures to dental auxiliaries. If a duty that is illegal within the state is assigned to the dental assistant, the dentist is liable for this illegal action. Furthermore, if a dental assistant performs a procedure that is not legally delegable to be performed by the assistant; the assistant is liable for such action.

Several factors should be considered in the areas of delegation. First, before an employee is hired, requests for appropriate documentation for certification or licensure should be made. Copies of documentation provide evidence that the person does indeed have the specified credentials. This may include transcripts, certificates of completion, or additional licenses. Second, the administrative assistant or office manager must be responsible for retaining current copies of all employee credentials on file. In some states, this may include current licenses, reports related to background checks, and cardiopulmonary resuscitation (CPR) or other certifications. Third, if the employer–employee relationship is incorrectly handled as a result of inappropriate delegation or direction, this may create tension or conflict in the office environment. An assistant may feel that, if the dentist assigns a task, it must be performed because the dentist is an authority figure. The assistant may feel that his or her job will be jeopardized if the task is not completed. There is significant risk associated with the performance of a task that is illegal or that should not have been delegated or one for which an assistant is not qualified or does not have the appropriate credentials. If a dental assistant performs an illegal act, the assistant may be subject to charges of negligence. The administrative assistant and all dental auxiliaries must be up to date concerning the scope of practice, and they must understand what can be delegated by a dentist to a particular staff member.

PRACTICE NOTE

If a task or procedure that is not legal within the state is delegated to the dental assistant, the dentist is liable for this illegal action.

CONSENT

Consent is the voluntary acceptance of or agreement with what is planned or done by another person. To examine or treat a patient without consent constitutes an unauthorized touching and makes the person committing the act guilty of battery. Battery is contact with someone that may result in bodily harm or offensive touching. Informed consent for the delivery of dental care can occur via two different mechanisms: implied consent and express consent.

PRACTICE NOTE

Consent is the voluntary acceptance of or agreement with what is planned or done by another person.

Informed Consent

Informed consent is a concept that has evolved for decades in courts and legislatures to assist patients with determining the care that they find acceptable. It has resulted in more disclosure on the part of the provider to allow the patient to make an informed decision. The basis for the concept of informed consent is that every adult of sound mind has the right to determine what can and cannot be done with his or her body. For that person to make a proper judgment, he or she must be given appropriate information by the healthcare provider. The patient must be given enough information about the proposed treatment, in understandable language, to make an intelligent decision as to whether to proceed with the treatment. Moreover, the patient must have ample opportunity to ask questions and have them answered.

In general, courts and legislatures have defined specific elements that describe informed consent. These elements state that consent must be given freely; treatment and diagnosis must be described in understandable language; risks, benefits, and estimates of the success of treatment must be described; the prognosis if no treatment is given and alternative treatment plans must be explained; and the patient must be given the opportunity to ask questions and have them answered.

It is important to remember that, if these conditions are not met, the courts may conclude that the patient did not consent to the procedure and therefore the dentist may be liable for actions such as battery or negligence (depending on the individual state). Failure to obtain informed consent may be considered negligent, because the dentist did not meet his or her duty to get the consent.

For consent to be legally valid, it must be informed and given freely, and the patient must be an adult of sound mind. Patients under the influence of alcohol, drugs, or severe stress may not have sufficient mental capacity to grant permission for treatment. When a dentist treats a minor, only the parent or guardian of the minor may grant consent. This excludes grandparents, caregivers, and siblings. However, parents may authorize another party to grant consent for treatment during the parents' absence. Such authorization must be signed and provided to the dental office before treatment consent is obtained. In some situations, the minor being treated may have divorced parents. It is important to determine if one or both biologic parents must provide consent for dental treatment to occur.

An emancipated minor is someone who has not reached the age of majority but who, as a result of certain circumstances, can provide consent himself or herself. An emancipated minor may be married or in the military; alternatively, due to personal circumstances, he or she is not relying on a parent for financial support. An example of this would be a young woman who has children of her own, who does not live with her parents, and who receives no financial support from her parents. In all consent situations, for adults and emancipated minors, a variety of consent forms are available and should be used before any and all invasive procedures.

Specialty practices such as endodontics and oral surgery have forms designed specifically for their disciplines. Informed consent is also important for care that is provided in a general practice. Figure 4-2 shows an example of a consent form for a general practice. These forms must be signed, dated, and retained in the patient record. It is not recommended to have the patient sign an informed consent form that gives the provider permission to "perform any and all procedures." This violates the intent of the concept of informed consent as well as the patient's right to have adequate and appropriate information when making a decision about a specific recommendation or treatment option.

Express Consent

Express consent is achieved either orally or in writing. When a dentist prepares a treatment plan, writes it down, and presents the patient with a copy to sign after providing a description that incorporates the elements of informed consent, this is express consent. A dentist may also verbally describe the treatment plan, and the patient may verbally agree to it.

Implied Consent

Other agreements that flow automatically from the relationship between the patient and the dental professional fall under the category of implied consent. Implied consent is based on the actions of the patient and the provider.

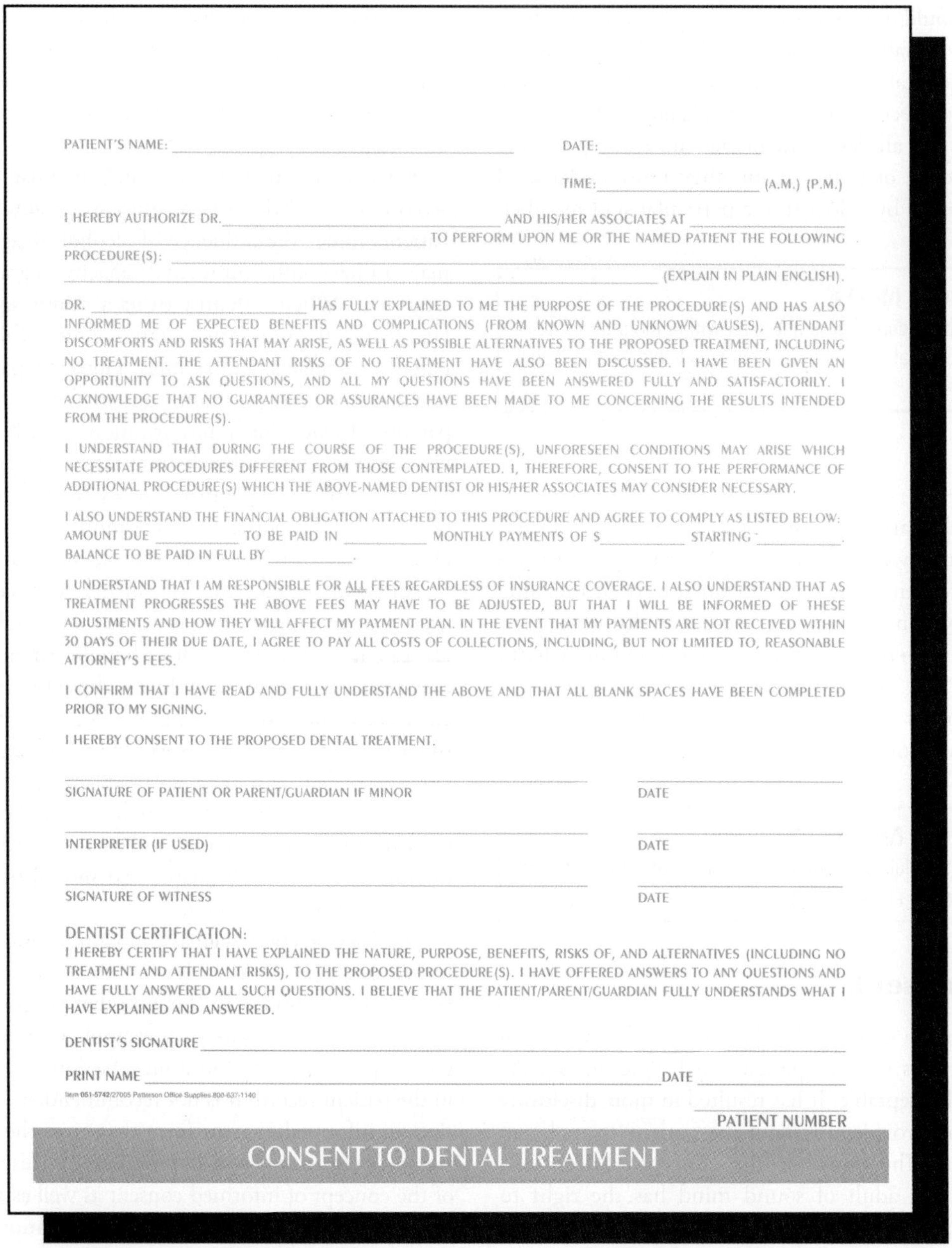

PATIENT'S NAME: ______________________ DATE: ______________

TIME: ______________ (A.M.) (P.M.)

I HEREBY AUTHORIZE DR. ______________________ AND HIS/HER ASSOCIATES AT ______________________ TO PERFORM UPON ME OR THE NAMED PATIENT THE FOLLOWING PROCEDURE(S): ______________________ (EXPLAIN IN PLAIN ENGLISH).

DR. ______________ HAS FULLY EXPLAINED TO ME THE PURPOSE OF THE PROCEDURE(S) AND HAS ALSO INFORMED ME OF EXPECTED BENEFITS AND COMPLICATIONS (FROM KNOWN AND UNKNOWN CAUSES), ATTENDANT DISCOMFORTS AND RISKS THAT MAY ARISE, AS WELL AS POSSIBLE ALTERNATIVES TO THE PROPOSED TREATMENT, INCLUDING NO TREATMENT. THE ATTENDANT RISKS OF NO TREATMENT HAVE ALSO BEEN DISCUSSED. I HAVE BEEN GIVEN AN OPPORTUNITY TO ASK QUESTIONS, AND ALL MY QUESTIONS HAVE BEEN ANSWERED FULLY AND SATISFACTORILY. I ACKNOWLEDGE THAT NO GUARANTEES OR ASSURANCES HAVE BEEN MADE TO ME CONCERNING THE RESULTS INTENDED FROM THE PROCEDURE(S).

I UNDERSTAND THAT DURING THE COURSE OF THE PROCEDURE(S), UNFORESEEN CONDITIONS MAY ARISE WHICH NECESSITATE PROCEDURES DIFFERENT FROM THOSE CONTEMPLATED. I, THEREFORE, CONSENT TO THE PERFORMANCE OF ADDITIONAL PROCEDURE(S) WHICH THE ABOVE-NAMED DENTIST OR HIS/HER ASSOCIATES MAY CONSIDER NECESSARY.

I ALSO UNDERSTAND THE FINANCIAL OBLIGATION ATTACHED TO THIS PROCEDURE AND AGREE TO COMPLY AS LISTED BELOW: AMOUNT DUE __________ TO BE PAID IN __________ MONTHLY PAYMENTS OF $__________ STARTING __________. BALANCE TO BE PAID IN FULL BY __________.

I UNDERSTAND THAT I AM RESPONSIBLE FOR <u>ALL</u> FEES REGARDLESS OF INSURANCE COVERAGE. I ALSO UNDERSTAND THAT AS TREATMENT PROGRESSES THE ABOVE FEES MAY HAVE TO BE ADJUSTED, BUT THAT I WILL BE INFORMED OF THESE ADJUSTMENTS AND HOW THEY WILL AFFECT MY PAYMENT PLAN. IN THE EVENT THAT MY PAYMENTS ARE NOT RECEIVED WITHIN 30 DAYS OF THEIR DUE DATE, I AGREE TO PAY ALL COSTS OF COLLECTIONS, INCLUDING, BUT NOT LIMITED TO, REASONABLE ATTORNEY'S FEES.

I CONFIRM THAT I HAVE READ AND FULLY UNDERSTAND THE ABOVE AND THAT ALL BLANK SPACES HAVE BEEN COMPLETED PRIOR TO MY SIGNING.

I HEREBY CONSENT TO THE PROPOSED DENTAL TREATMENT.

______________________ ______________
SIGNATURE OF PATIENT OR PARENT/GUARDIAN IF MINOR DATE

______________________ ______________
INTERPRETER (IF USED) DATE

______________________ ______________
SIGNATURE OF WITNESS DATE

DENTIST CERTIFICATION:
I HEREBY CERTIFY THAT I HAVE EXPLAINED THE NATURE, PURPOSE, BENEFITS, RISKS OF, AND ALTERNATIVES (INCLUDING NO TREATMENT AND ATTENDANT RISKS), TO THE PROPOSED PROCEDURE(S). I HAVE OFFERED ANSWERS TO ANY QUESTIONS AND HAVE FULLY ANSWERED ALL SUCH QUESTIONS. I BELIEVE THAT THE PATIENT/PARENT/GUARDIAN FULLY UNDERSTANDS WHAT I HAVE EXPLAINED AND ANSWERED.

DENTIST'S SIGNATURE ______________________

PRINT NAME ______________________ DATE ______________

Item 051-5742/27005 Patterson Office Supplies 800-637-1140

____
PATIENT NUMBER

CONSENT TO DENTAL TREATMENT

FIGURE 4-2 Informed consent form. (Courtesy Patterson Office Supplies, Champaign, IL.)

Both implied and express consent trigger responsibilities for both parties: those that the dentist owes to the patient and those that the patient owes to the dentist. Accepting a patient for treatment indicates that the dentist agrees to accept certain responsibilities for that patient's dental care. Likewise, if a patient agrees to accept treatment by the dentist, it is considered that the patient assumes certain responsibilities. Boxes 4-4 and 4-5 list implied responsibilities for each of these parties.

Informed Refusal

A patient may decline a recommended procedure or a referral recommendation from a dentist. Examples include the refusal of radiographs, periodontal care, fluoride treatments, or referral to a specialist or physician. An office should document this refusal for recommended care in writing. The informed refusal process parallels the principles found in informed consent. An informed refusal form should include the specific recommended procedures, the potential risks (to both oral and general health) of declining the procedure, and an opportunity for the patient to ask and have their questions answered. The dentist, the patient, and a witness such as the administrative assistant should sign the form, and the date should be recorded. If an allegation of negligence occurs, the informed refusal may assist in the defense of the dentist. Not all courts recognize informed refusal. However, documentation is helpful for defending allegations of negligence.

BOX 4-4

Implied Duties Owed by the Dentist to the Patient

- Use reasonable care in the provision of services as measured against acceptable standards set by other practitioners with similar training in a similar community.
- Be properly licensed and registered, and meet all other legal requirements to engage in the practice of dentistry.
- Obtain an accurate health (medical and dental) history of the patient before a diagnosis is made and treatment is begun.
- Employ competent personnel and provide for their proper supervision.
- Maintain a level of knowledge in keeping with current advances in the profession.
- Use methods that are acceptable to at least a respectable minority of similar practitioners in the community.
- Refrain from performing procedures that are not evidence-based or experimental
- Obtain informed consent from the patient before instituting an examination or treatment.
- Refrain from abandoning the patient, and ensure that care is available in emergency situations.
- Charge a reasonable fee (by community standards) for services.
- Refrain from exceeding the scope of practice authorized by your license or permitting those acting under your direction to engage in unlawful acts.
- Keep the patient informed of his or her progress.
- Refrain from undertaking any procedure for which you are not qualified.
- Complete care in a timely manner.
- Keep accurate records of the treatment rendered to the patient.
- Maintain confidentiality of the patient's information.
- Inform the patient of any untoward occurrences during the course of treatment.
- Make appropriate referrals, and request necessary consultations.
- Comply with all laws that regulate the practice of dentistry.
- Practice in a manner that is consistent with the codes of ethics of the profession.
- Use universal precautions during the treatment of all patients.

BOX 4-5

Implied Duties Owed by the Patient to the Dentist

- Cooperate in the care by following homecare or other reasonable instructions, taking prescribed medications, and showing up for recall visits.
- Keep appointments, and notify the office of cancellations or appointment delays.
- Provide honest answers to questions asked on the history form and by the dentist and office personnel.
- Notify the office staff or the dentist of any change in health status.
- Pay a reasonable fee for the service if no fee is agreed on verbally or in writing.
- Remit the fee for services within a reasonable time.

MANAGED CARE

Some patients may pay for their dental care from their own funds, whereas other patients may have dental insurance. Dental insurance is designed to pay, depending on the service provided, a portion of the total cost of dental care received. There are several different types of individual, family, and group dental insurance plans. There are three general categories of insurance: 1) indemnity, which is usually called *dental insurance,* allows you to see any dentist you choose who has agreed to accept the plan and the coverage offered; 2) preferred provider organizations (PPOs) and network dental plans; and 3) dental health managed organizations (DHMOs) in which patients are assigned or select a dentist network member or an in-network dental office and use the dental benefits in that network. There are also some states that fund dental care through a state-supported insurance program that allows certain populations, such as children on social services, to obtain care. A dental staff member who is responsible for collecting fees should be familiar with the plans that are accepted in a particular dental office. An insurance carrier may require specific paperwork and documentation before dental care can be provided, or an insurance company may require the patient to pay the dental office for services and then the patient will submit a form for reimbursement. In other situations, the dental office directly bills the insurance company to collect payment.

Dental insurance may cover the total costs of some procedures (e.g., all preventive care, including sealants, fluoride treatments, and prophylaxis) and only a percentage of restorative care. If the administrator has questions about a patient's coverage or about the documentation that an insurance carrier requires, then he or she should contact the insurance company. If an office does accept dental insurance, an administrator should be careful that they never agree to do something that would be considered insurance fraud. For example, if there is a family in which both spouses have dental insurance, only one insurance company should be billed for care that is provided to a particular family member. In some situations, a staff person may be asked to commit insurance fraud by billing for a procedure that was not provided, being asked to alter an insurance submission form by changing the date of when the treatment was provided, or adding on extra fees or costs. Insurance companies can audit dental records and detect if fraud has occurred, and this can carry criminal penalties.

Managed care refers to a cost-containment system of healthcare insurance that may direct the use of health benefits by restricting the type, level, and frequency of treatment; limiting access to care to certain entities or practitioners; and basing the level of reimbursement for services on a capitation or other risk basis. Limitations imposed by managed care companies are generally directed at payment for services, but the policies may also limit the actual services received by a patient.

In this way, managed care systems raise several legal and ethical issues for the dentist and other healthcare professionals. Patients may ask dentists to render only the treatment that is covered by the insurance plan rather than the necessary treatment based on the patient's needs. Insurance companies are profit driven and may not sufficiently consider the health-care professional's responsibilities. Capitated plans can cause an ethical dilemma for a dentist when, for example, a dentist is paid for patient care whether or not it is provided, because it is obvious that it is not in the dentist's short-term economic interest to provide that care. If certain care is not reimbursed, a patient may decline needed treatment because of financial concerns. For the patient's interest to be protected, the dentist must be relied on to adhere to both legal and ethical principles.

RISK MANAGEMENT PROGRAMS

A dental professional teaches preventive concepts to patients with a firm conviction that such practice will prevent the progression of current disease or eliminate the potential for future oral health disease or problems. This concept can be applied to the prevention or reduction of risk of malpractice claims. Most dental societies, organizations, and institutions are taking an active role in providing seminars and programs in risk management. The dental administrative assistant can play an important role in encouraging participation in such seminars as well as in documenting staff participation. In addition, there may be online resources or webinars that can be viewed to educate and inform all dental teams about their ethical and legal obligations. Lifelong learning and education are critical to reducing risks that may harm the patient, the provider, or the office's reputation.

Risk management programs primarily highlight examples of activities in which dentists were found liable. These examples provide a starting point for educating dentists and their staff regarding specific strategies to avoid exposing themselves to such liability. Often these programs accomplish this goal by reviewing case studies and describing situations in which a plaintiff (i.e., a patient) was successful in a lawsuit against a dentist. Risk management programs help the dental professional to identify, analyze, and manage risky behaviors in the dental office. A commitment to risk management applies to all members of the dental team.

Risk management programs generally include information about operating safety, product safety, quality assurance, and waste disposal. Operating safety programs emphasize methods of functioning in an environment that ensures the safety of the patient, the staff, and the visitors. Programs about product safety update the dental team with regard to the use of current materials, equipment, and methods of evaluation; they also address the storage and maintenance of these products. Quality assurance programs provide information about evaluating all systems used in the provision of care of a patient. Waste disposal programs provide the most current information about disposing of medical and dental waste. Risk management programs can also provide suggestions about appropriate communication and record-keeping strategies to protect all members of the dental team. In addition, risk management may address compliance issues, such as Occupational Safety and Health Administration (OSHA) and Health Insurance Portability and Accountability Act of 1996 (HIPAA) obligations. Risk management education in combination with competent practice assists with reducing the potential for allegations of malpractice leading to litigation.

ABANDONMENT

Abandonment is defined as the severance of a professional relationship with a patient who is still in need of dental care and proper transfers or referrals. Although this legal concept primarily affects the dentist, the administrative assistant should be aware of its existence and assist the dentist with following the appropriate steps to terminate a dentist/patient relationship.

A dentist/patient relationship can end for a number of reasons. The dentist may decide to retire, become ill, or choose to sell the practice. A dentist may also seek to end a relationship with a patient because the patient is uncooperative, fails to return for appointments, or owes a balance. In some instances, all of the treatment for the patient is up to date. In other instances, the treatment plan has not been completed, and more dental care is needed. If the relationship is going to be terminated, a letter should be sent to the patient. The contents of the letter should indicate the date that the relationship will end, which is usually 30 to 60 days from the time that the letter is written. The dental office should offer to provide only emergency care during that time period. The patient should be encouraged to seek another provider to have their oral health needs addressed and preventive services provided. The letter should clearly state that, if the patient needs a referral in the same geographic area, he or she may contact the local dental society (include the name, address, and phone number of the dental society). Finally, the office should offer to forward copies of the patient's dental records after the patient has signed a release and provided a forwarding address. The letter should indicate that there will be a reasonable fee charged for the duplication of appropriate records; it should be noted that some states have guidelines as to what a dental office can charge a patient for duplication of dental records. A copy of the letter and the returned receipt should be retained in the patient record. It would be prudent for the dentist to have a written policy regarding this issue. The policy should be posted or otherwise communicated to all patients so that there are no surprises and so that liability is mitigated when a patient receives such a letter. Similarly, if an office is sold to another provider, many regulations may require the dental office to notify patients about the transfer of their records to a new dental practice owner. In addition, patients must also be informed that they have the option not to have their records transferred to a new owner. If a patient notified an office that they would like their records forwarded to another provider, the administrative assistant should honor that request. In both situations (i.e., termination of the dentist/patient relationship or sale of the dental practice), the administrative assistant plays an important role. It may be the administrative assistant's responsibility to draft the letters to the patients, to maintain copies in the patient's chart, and to inform the dentist of the results of the communication with the patient.

The administrative assistant should also ensure that the transfer of information meets federal and state law requirements for patient records, including privacy requirements. Dental records are considered medical records, and state laws may dictate specific guidelines. In addition, the privacy of patient information must be protected as outlined by HIPAA. Information about HIPAA can be found at www.hhs.gov/ocr/privacy/index.html.

The administrative assistant should be cautious about talking with patients after a letter to terminate the relationship has been forwarded. Frequently a patient will call the office and seek an additional explanation or attempt to negotiate a return to the office. If a decision is made to terminate a patient, the office should not waver in its decision and only repeat the objective information found in the letter. For example, if the dentist chose to terminate the patient because the patient was uncooperative in care that is the only reason that should be provided, without any further explanation. Additional explanation is unnecessary, because it may provide the patient with information that could be misinterpreted and lead to patient accusations of discrimination or defamation.

FRAUD

Fraud is a deception that is deliberately practiced to secure unfair or unlawful gain. One of the most common practices of fraud is in the obtaining of fees through third-party payments by misrepresentation.

An example of a fraudulent action occurs when a patient has insurance coverage from July 1 of the past year until June 30 of the current year, after which time the patient would no longer receive this benefit. The patient had maximum benefit coverage of $1200 for the year and to date had only used $450 of the benefit. Toward the end of June, it was determined that the patient needed a fixed bridge. The patient was informed of the fee for the bridge. The patient was further informed that, after June 30, the services would not be covered and that she would be responsible for payment. The patient argued that it was the responsibility of the dentist to alter the date on the claim form so that it appeared she received all of the treatment prior to her dental insurance coverage ending. She implied that, if the dentist altered the record, she would remain a "paying" patient.

It is fraud to change the date on the claim form to indicate that the bridge was inserted before June 30 when indeed the bridge would not be inserted until mid July. Although efforts might be made to complete the case prior to the deadline, a better solution is to provide an explanation to the patient that she is asking you to commit fraud. In addition, the patient should understand that fraud is a criminal activity as well as one that insurance companies may identify during an audit of a dental practice. Some patients will accept the explanation; others may be disappointed and choose not to have any additional care provided.

Another example of a fraudulent act occurs when a patient's dental fee is covered by two insurance carriers that require the coordination of benefits. The claim forms are processed. A check is received from the primary carrier for the correct amount of money. However, when a check is received from the secondary carrier, the amount is in excess of the fee, and it appears the secondary carrier has paid the same amount as a primary carrier. Consequently, there is extra payment received. The assistant records the payment as it should have been on the patient's financial record but enters the entire check into the deposit, which leaves an excess of funds in the account. The administrative assistant is obligated to immediately inform the insurance carrier after the check in excess of the correct payment is received. It is possible to enter the check into a deposit, but then a check for the amount of overpayment must be written and returned to the insurance carrier with the appropriate explanation concerning overpayment error. The return of the overpayment should be documented in the appropriate financial record section of the patient's chart or file.

RECORDS MANAGEMENT

Nothing can be more valuable for defending against potential litigation than clear and concise records. The maintenance of such records is a vital responsibility of the administrative assistant. As discussed in other areas of this text, the importance of including complete and thorough information in a patient's record cannot be overemphasized. The individual responsible for documentation should record the exact date, the type of treatment provided, the materials used, any complications, and special notations about the treatment as well as any untoward incidents. An untoward incident is an event, incident, occurrence, or accident that could have or did lead to unintended harm, loss, or damage to a patient, visitor, or member of the staff. In addition, patient comments, questions, and reactions must be recorded in an objective manner. If a patient makes a statement about his or her dental care, such as saying something about being dissatisfied with the color of the teeth in a denture that he or she has received, it should be clear in the record that such a comment was made. For example, this could be recorded as follows: "Patient stated, 'I think the color of my teeth is too bright.'" This records the patient's reaction so that it is clear what was said and by whom. Signatures of the treating operators and, if appropriate, the recorder or reporter should be included. Good documentation results in a good defense if there are allegations in the future. Individuals in a dental operatory cannot always remember specifically what was asked or stated. Documenting patient comments in the chart provides a record of the interaction between the patient and the provider or a member of the dentist's staff.

Any irregularities or unusual incidents occurring between patients and providers or patients and employees should be documented. Such documentation may include narratives of an event, such as an accidental needlestick. These incidents require a report that includes the name of the employee, the name of the patient being treated, and the date and time of the injury.

In addition, what events occurred after the needlestick should also be included. Other incidents that may warrant documentation include unusual behavior on the part of a patient toward a staff member and how the issue was addressed or resolved.

DEFAMATION OF CHARACTER

Defamation of character is the communication of false information to a third party about a person that results in injury to that person's reputation. Such communication can be verbal (slander) or written (libel). The false statement could be about a person's product, business, profession, or title to property. A dental professional should make statements about a patient or other professional only as they relate to the rendering of dental care and only to other dental care providers involved in that care.

NEGLIGENCE

Negligence is an act of omission (neglecting to do something that a reasonably prudent person would do) or commission (doing something that a reasonably prudent person would not do). To prove negligence, it is necessary to prove that there has been a breach of duty owed, including deviation from the standard of care. In a dental negligence case, it is often necessary to provide expert testimony. To prove negligence, the plaintiff must show that there is an obligation to provide care according to a specified standard; that there was failure to meet that standard; that the failure to meet the standard led to injury; and that there was in fact an actual injury to the patient.

Although most often this action involves direct patient care, indirect patient care can also be a basis for finding negligence. Therefore, by the way of example, the administrative assistant who may be assigned to such tasks as sterilization or other supportive clinical tasks should be aware that negligence can occur as a result of activities that do not involve direct contact with the patient.

The Health Care Quality Improvement Act of 1986 authorized the creation by the federal government of a National Practitioner Data Bank (NPDB) as a central repository to collect and release information about professional competence and conduct. The repository includes information about paid malpractice claims and adverse reports of healthcare licensees. In most states, when a dentist is found negligent, the adverse act is reported to the NPDB. The administrative assistant may review this act and research the NPDB at www.npdb-hipdb.com.

INVASION OF PRIVACY

Invasion of privacy is a tort that refers to a number of wrongs involving the use of otherwise private information. Federal regulations such as HIPAA were created to protect patient privacy by providing specific guidelines concerning dental records. In the dental field, tort may involve the publishing or otherwise making known or using information related to the private life or affairs of a person without that person's approval or permission, prying into private affairs, or appropriating the plaintiff's identity for commercial use.

When an insurance company employee contacts an administrative assistant to clarify information about a patient on a claim form, the potential for invasion of privacy is present. For example, the insurance company asks for the verification of data from the patient's chart. They may request specific information, such as date of birth of a child patient or the father's name. The administrative assistant offers to fax this information to the insurance company. To save time, the assistant simply transfers a copy of the entire patient record, including information that should not have been shared about a communicable disease. This action has now placed the patient record in a setting not requested and not otherwise authorized by the patient. Thus, the patient's privacy has been violated.

The administrative assistant should have requested that the incomplete form be returned to the dental office or that a written request for information clarification be made by the insurance company. Only the information requested should have been provided, and it should have been reviewed to be certain that the information was part of the claim form that the patient had signed. In addition, if information is forwarded via a fax machine or scanned using a computer, the administrative assistant should make sure that the area where the information is being forwarded is secure. Often a cover sheet will be placed on a fax to indicate that the information is confidential and should not be shared so that the entity receiving the information is reminded about the requirement to keep such information confidential.

Another potential invasion of privacy situation could occur when an administrative assistant is having difficulty collecting a payment for services rendered in a dental office. The patient had failed to make payment on an account of $3000 for the past 12 months. During a private conversation about the account, the patient informed the administrative assistant that her business was about to enter bankruptcy and that her spouse had just been diagnosed with schizophrenia and was recovering from a serious alcohol dependency. During a discussion with a friend who worked in a local business, the assistant shared the story about the patient, who was a well-known member of the community. Disparaging remarks and personal information about the patient were passed on to the listener. The patient became aware that her circumstances had been discussed, and the source of information was traced to the assistant.

To prevent this situation, all staff must recognize that any information that a patient provides to the dental staff remains confidential within the office. No information about a patient should be shared outside of the office. If specific information is required for insurance purposes, for example, permission must be sought from the patient. When a patient requests a transfer of the records of his or her dental treatment, a signed authorization for transfer should be completed by the patient. The administrative assistant once again must adhere to HIPAA regulations.

GOOD SAMARITAN LAW

During the last two to three decades, every state in the United States has passed some form of legislation that grants immunity for acts performed by a person who renders care in an emergency situation. This concept, called the *Good Samaritan law,* was considered necessary to create an incentive for healthcare providers to provide medical assistance to the injured in cases of automobile accidents or other disasters without the fear of possible litigation. This law is intended for individuals who do not seek compensation but rather are solely interested in providing care to the injured in a caring, safe manner, with no intent to do bodily harm. This law does not provide protection for a negligent healthcare provider who is being compensated for services.

AMERICANS WITH DISABILITIES ACT

In 1990, the federal government enacted legislation to ensure that persons with some degree of disability are not discriminated against. The Americans with Disabilities Act (AwDA)—not to be confused with the American Dental Association (ADA)—affects the dental office in the area of prohibitions against employment discrimination and by requiring facilities be accessible to physically and mentally compromised patients. In 2008, the ADA Amendments Act (ADAAA) was passed to broaden the definition of disability and provide clear guidelines as to who is eligible within the Act. The law provides guidelines to protect patients from discrimination and requires dental offices to modify their facilities or make other accommodations to allow access to dental care. For example, the office must have doorways that will allow a patient in a wheelchair the ability to enter a building by using a ramp and having a door that opens and is wide enough to allow the patient to enter. The law also outlines legal protections so that an applicant, who can perform the functions of a particular job, will not be discriminated against because of their disability. Similarly, the law protects employees from being fired if they have a disability and may require the office to make reasonable accommodations so that an employee can adequately fulfill their job responsibilities.

Box 4-6 shows a list of titles that describe the provisions of the AwDA. This federal mandate is aimed at the elimination of discrimination against individuals with disabilities, and it includes clearly defines enforceable standards. Attention should be given to Title III and Title V, because they specifically relate to the dental office. It is important for the office manager to obtain a copy of this act for the office and to routinely update the office policies as required. The address for the Office of Americans with Disabilities is available at www.usdoj.gov/crt/ada/adahom1.htm.

COMPUTER SECURITY

The administrative assistant may be exposed to potential activities that could cause illegal or unethical activity while using a computer. Computer security refers to safeguards that are implemented to prevent and detect unauthorized access or deliberate damage to a computer system and data. A computer crime is the use of a computer to commit an illegal act.

In a dental office, the most common activity that would violate computer integrity is software theft or piracy. Some people make an illegal copy of a program, a CD, or a DVD instead of paying for an authorized copy. Software theft is a violation of copyright law, and it is a crime. For large users, such as dental schools and other healthcare institutions, most software companies provide a site license and discounts for multiple copies.

Although most dental offices use personal computers rather than a mainframe, the potential for gaining unauthorized access to data can still exist. If a dental assistant inadvertently gains access to unauthorized or confidential data on a computer, that

BOX 4-6

Provisions of the Americans with Disabilities Act

Title I	Protects the rights of people with disabilities to employment; defines disability, describes who is covered and who is not covered by the act, defines qualified individuals, and covers the obligations of employers to hire people with disabilities
Title II Part A	Extends protections given to people with disabilities under Section 504 of the Rehabilitation Act of 1973 to state and local governments
Title II Part B	Covers access by people with disabilities to public transportation
Title III	Requires that public accommodations operated by private entities do not discriminate against persons with disabilities; addresses access by people with disabilities to public accommodations (e.g., restaurants, shops, malls), commercial facilities, private agencies that offer examinations or courses related to licensing or certification, and transportation provided by private agencies
Title IV	Prohibits discrimination against disabled individuals in the area of communication, especially hearing-impaired and speech-impaired individuals; Title IV is enforced by the Federal Communications Commission (FCC)
Title V	Contains miscellaneous provisions regarding the continued viability of other state or federal laws that provide disabled persons with equal or greater rights than the act; specifically, this section prohibits state or local governments from discriminating against individuals with disabilities

person should exit the file that includes this data and report to the appropriate supervisor that a confidential file was accidentally compromised. However, making changes in a confidential file without authorized permission constitutes an unethical and possibly illegal act. Refer to the HIPAA standards in Chapter 7 to ensure information integrity.

MAKING ETHICAL DECISIONS

The administrative assistant has many factors to consider when fulfilling routine duties in the dental business office. During all activities, consider the ethical issues that apply to all tasks being performed. Routinely review the steps listed in Box 4-7 in making ethical decisions.

BOX 4-7

An Ethical Decision Making Model

1. Specifically identify the ethical issue or dilemma. Dilemmas occur when a practitioner is caught between competing obligations and has to weigh two or more options to resolve the situation.
2. Gather and review important facts or information pertinent to the situation.
3. List alternatives that could be used to resolve the problem
4. Evaluate each alternatives using ethical principles, codes, laws and regulations to determine the best alternative.
5. Make a decision choosing the best alternative that is ethically and legally appropriate.
6. Act on the decision.

LEARNING ACTIVITIES

1. Explain the two types of informed consent (implied and express) that apply to the delivery of dental care.
2. Describe the four elements that are necessary to prove that a dental provider has committed negligence.
3. Identify 12 steps that should be followed when making ethical decisions.
4. Identify 12 implied duties that a dentist owes a patient.
5. List five inappropriate or incorrect business office activities that could lead to potential litigation.

Please refer to the student workbook for additional learning activities.

BIBLIOGRAPHY

American Dental Association: *ADA principles of ethics and code of professional conduct (revised)*, Chicago, 2012, American Dental Association.

Dental Assisting National Board: *State fact booklet*, Chicago, 2014, Dental Assisting National Board.

D'Cruz L: *Legal aspects of general dentist practice*, St Louis, 2006, Mosby.

Davison JA: *Legal and ethical considerations for dental hygienists and assistants*, St Louis, 2000, Mosby.

Zarkowski P, Aksu MN: *Employment Law.* In Dunning, DG and Lange, BM, editors: *Dental Practice Transition*, Ames, IA, 2009, Wiley-Blackwell.

Zarkowski P: *Ethical and Legal Concepts.* In Darby, M and Bushee E, editors: *Comprehensive Review of Dental Hygiene*, ed 7, St Louis, 2011, C.V. Mosby.

Zarkowski P: *Legal and Ethical Decision Making in Dental Hygiene.* In Darby, M And Walsh, M, editors: *Dental Hygiene Theory and Practice*, St Louis, 1995, ed 2, 2003, ed 3, 2010, ed 4, 2014, Saunders.

RECOMMENDED WEBSITES

www.danb.org.

State-Specific Dental Assistant Information

www.usdoj.gov/crt/ada/adahom1.html.

www.ada.org.

http://www.danb.org/Meet-State-Requirements/State-Publications.aspx.

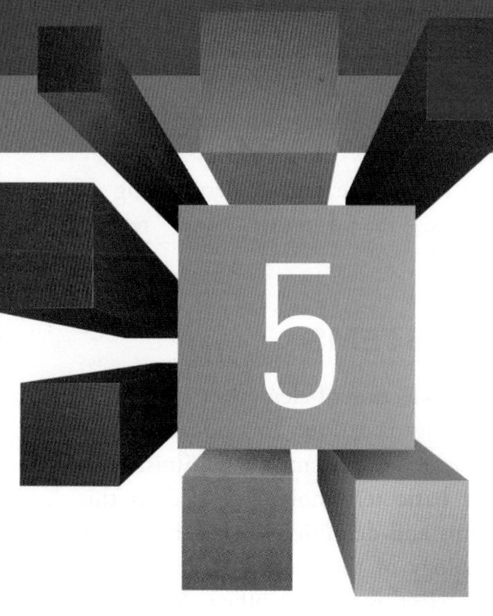

5 Business Office Technology

http://evolve.elsevier.com/Finkbeiner/practice

LEARNING OUTCOMES

1. Define the key terms in this chapter.
2. Discuss how the digital age has impacted dentistry and why implementing a change to a computer system is important to all staff members.
3. Describe the elements of information systems.
4. Explain the four operations of a computer.
5. Explain how digital technology can be used to increase profitability and the purpose of a feasibility study.
6. Understand the various general and specific task software or apps available.
7. Discuss integrated apps and list the guidelines to follow when selecting apps.

KEY TERMS

App This term is short for *application.* Apps are programs that are designed to make users more productive or to assist them with personal tasks.

Byte The basic unit of measurement of information storage in computer science, which is made up of eight bits that are grouped together as a unit. A byte provides enough different combinations of 0s and 1s to represent 256 individual characters.

Central processing unit (CPU) The electronic component of a computer's motherboard that interprets and carries out the basic instructions that operate the computer.

Computing device An electronic device that operates under the control of instructions stored in its own memory that can accept data, process the data according to specified rules, produce results, and store the results for future use.

Data A collection of unprocessed items, which can include text, numbers, images, audio, and video.

Database A structured collection of records or data that is stored in a computer system. The structure is achieved by organizing the data according to a database model.

Digital literacy This concept involves having a current knowledge and understanding of computers, mobile devices, the Internet, and related technologies.

Digital office A term used to describe the increasing use of computer-based information technology in office work.

Electronic spreadsheet Application software that allows the user to organize data in rows and columns and to perform calculations using this data.

Feasibility study An analysis of business practices that is one of the most reliable ways to determine what types of updates the computing devices in the practice require and whether new digital technologies are needed.

Hardware The electric, electronic, and mechanical components contained in a computing device.

Information system A collection of elements that provide accurate, timely, and useful information.

Intelligent printer The laser printer that shapes characters through the use of light (laser beams). An intelligent printer is able to collate, stack, and place images on both sides of the paper.

Internet A worldwide collection of networks that connects millions of businesses, government agencies, educational institutions, and individuals.

Mobile device A hand-held computing device that is usually Internet capable. These include smartphones, digital cameras, portable media players, and e-book readers.

Software
A series of instructions that tells a computer what to do and how to do it.

NOTE: Please refer to Box 5-3 for additional technology-related terms and their accompanying images.

The Digital Age has affected modern dentistry, and it helps the dentist and the dental staff to be more productive and remain on the cutting edge. Digital technology in the office involves the application of computers and associated electronic equipment to prepare and distribute information. Indeed, the computer has made an impact on the profession of dentistry, and it is used routinely in the clinical and business applications of the office. The dental staff should expect their duties as well as the way they work to change from time to time. The need for high productivity and quality performance means that all dental health care workers must be willing to change work methods and adapt to modern digital changes.

Few businesses today can avoid the explosion in the need for more information and technology. The prudent selection of digital technology equipment is a major component of dental office productivity and efficiency. There are millions of digital devices in all types of offices in the United States, and the numbers are growing. In fact, office automation using the Internet has been called the "primary way to do business in a high-tech world." Some form of computer usage is now present in more than 90% of dental offices in North America. The digital office is a workplace in which sophisticated computers and other electronic equipment carry out many of the office's routine tasks and provide more options for gathering, processing, displaying, and storing information. Some applications of digital technology in the business office are outlined in Box 5-1.

The digital revolution that led to the information age has had a profound effect on the business office. The use of digital office technology in the dental business office allows the staff to be more organized and efficient. It can help to automate routine office tasks, improve cash flow, and increase accuracy. Today a patient in a general practice can have a radiograph digitally processed and transferred to the oral surgeon before the patient even leaves the general dentist's office. This concept can be likened to the application of four-handed dentistry in the clinical setting, because both result in improved patient care, increased productivity, and a reduction of stress on the dental staff. Because technology changes, you must keep up with the changes to remain digitally literate. Digital literacy involves having a current knowledge and understanding of computers, mobile devices, the Internet, and related technologies.

INFORMATION SYSTEMS

An information system is a collection of elements that provide accurate, timely, and useful information. To understand the procedure for using an information system, the administrative assistant must understand basic terminology related to this concept. A glossary of terms and definitions helps the novice to understand the terminology of the modern digital office, and it can be useful when selecting current office equipment. Box 5-2 contains a detailed list of basic increments of storage for an information system.

Figure 5-1 depicts the five elements that make up the information system:

1. Computers or hardware (the equipment)
2. Apps or software (programs)
3. Data
4. Personnel
5. Procedures

Computers and Other Hardware

Hardware is the information system's physical equipment. The central piece of hardware in the information system is the computer (Figure 5-2). A computing device collects data, processes the data arithmetically and logically, produces output as a result of the processing, and stores the result for future use. This device could take the form of a smartphone, a tablet, a notebook, a hand-held device, a headset, a laptop, a card reader, a digital pen, or even a desktop computer.

Other digital technologies prevalent in the business office today include telephone systems with the capacity for voicemail or paging, voice headsets, facsimile (fax) machines, copy machines, calculators, dental imagers, scanners, and digital cameras (Box 5-3). The notebook, laptop, or tablet computer

BOX 5-1

Business Office Apps

- Electronic charting
- Computerized scheduling
- Online office procedure manuals
- Addition of progress notes to online records
- Automated insurance claims
- Purchase of supplies from online supply warehouses
- Telemarketing with websites
- Communicating to staff and patients with texts, tweets, or e-mails
- Enrollment in online college courses
- Provision of a means for continuing education
- Allowance for "virtual group practices" in which solo practitioners share one set of records
- Consultation with experts from all over the world

BOX 5-2

Increments of Storage for Information Systems

Storage Term	Approximate Number of Bytes
Kilobyte (KB)	1 thousand
Megabyte (MB)	1 million
Gigabyte (GB)	1 billion
Terabyte (TB)	1 trillion
Petabyte (PB)	1 quadrillion
Exabyte (EB)	1 quintillion
Zettabyte (ZB)	1 sextillion
Yottabyte (YB)	1 septillion

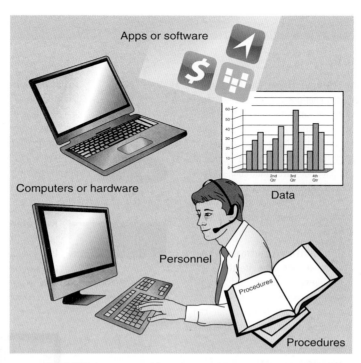

FIGURE 5-1 The five elements of an information system.

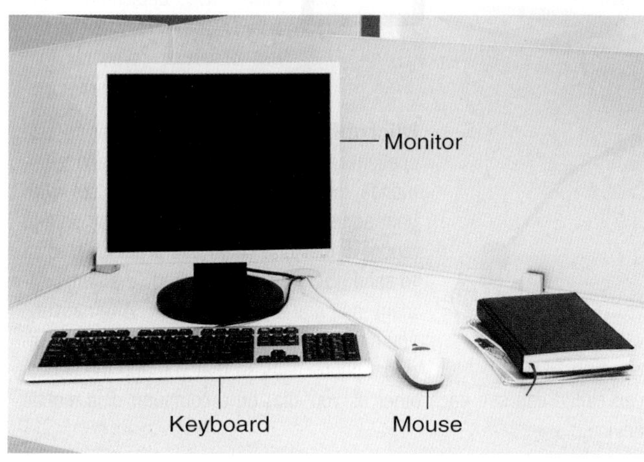

FIGURE 5-2 Components of a microcomputer. (Copyright © 2014 Tereh, BigStock.com.)

with a wireless network is becoming popular with dentists as they seek to work from room to room or to conduct office business outside of the office. Digital technology can help enhance productivity and customer service within a dental practice in the following ways:

- Digital voicemail allows both incoming and outgoing telephone messages to be recorded and processed.
- Pagers carried by members of the office staff allow them to be signaled when needed.
- Digital voice equipment records voice sounds as input for a voice-activated system; for later transcription; for referral letters; for recording information for a patient's clinical record; or for recording research reports, minutes of a staff meeting, or the summary of a conference.
- Fax machines send and receive documents or other graphic images over the telephone systems or the Internet.
- Copy machines reproduce letters, pages from magazines and books, charts and drawings, financial reports, clinical records, and statements from patients' ledger cards. (Box 5-4 lists several features of copiers.)
- Calculators found in computer software or those purchased separately are a great help to assistants with many routine duties that require mathematical skills. Many other calculators are inexpensive enough to be sold at department and discount stores and also at office machine dealers. The price of a calculator is not determined entirely by its number of functions, although this is an important factor. The types of components and materials used to produce the machine also affect the price (Box 5-5).
- Digital cameras and intraoral cameras allow images to become part of the patient record. Data are stored, and a hard copy of the intraoral condition can be printed. Cosmetic imagers are capable of displaying proposed changes that will result from specific treatment.
- Scanners input text or graphical data directly into computer storage. Any of these devices may be directly connected to the computer system to provide a centralized source of information. Chapter 10 includes detailed descriptions of telecommunications systems and techniques.
- Laptop, notebook, and tablet computers enable the dentist and staff to go from room to room or to work outside of the office at meetings or conferences while remaining in contact with the office via e-mail or the Internet.

BOX 5-3

Selected Technology Terms

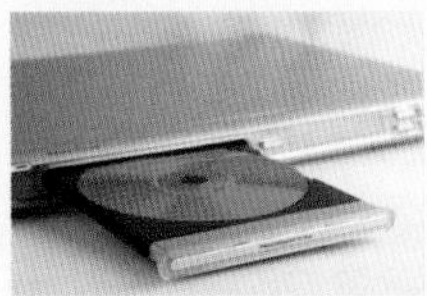

Storage device: There are three main types of consumer-grade computer storage: internal, external, and network attached. Internal storage is generally a hard drive or a solid-state drive (SSD) that hosts your computer's operating systems and programs. External storage comes mostly in the form of external drives that connect to a computer via a peripheral port, such as a USB flash drive, a memory card, or an optical drive (CD or DVD). Finally, network attached storage (NAS) solutions are those that connect to a switch or a router to provide storage space and services to the entire network.

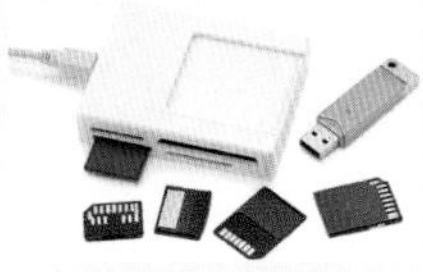

Card reader/writer: A card reader/writer is useful for transferring data directly to and from a removable flash memory card, such as the ones used in a camera or a music player. Make sure that the card reader/writer can read from and write to the flash memory cards that are used.

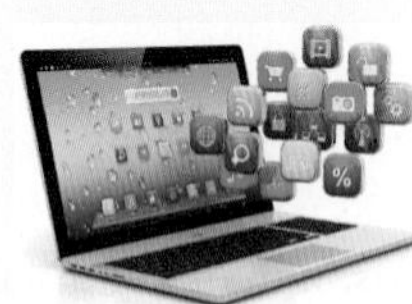

Cloud storage: Cloud storage is an Internet service that provides offsite storage to computer users. Cloud storage companies can provide storage for patient records, radiographs, or other professional documents. This can create a backup or duplicate version in case the original is lost, damaged, or destroyed.

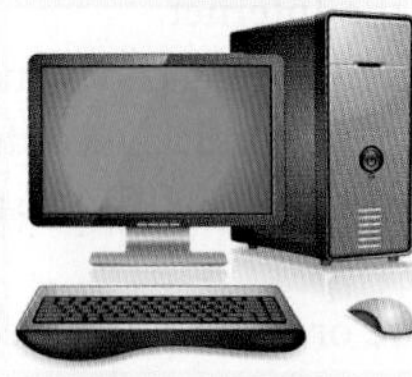

Desktop computer: A desktop computer is a personal computer designed to be in a stationary location, where all of its components fit on or under a desk. Minimal configuration would include a screen, a keyboard, and a mouse with a tower. Sometimes the processing circuitry of the tower is contained in the screen, thereby eliminating the tower.

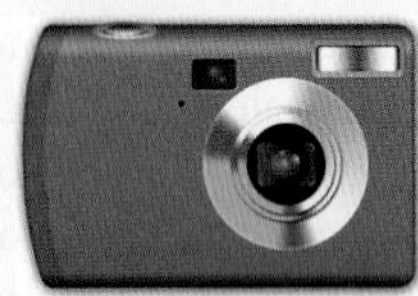

Digital camera: For the dental office, an inexpensive point-and-shoot digital camera should be considered. These are small enough to carry around, they usually operate automatically in terms of lighting and focus, and they contain storage cards for storing photographs. All of these features may also be built into smartphones or other mobile devices.

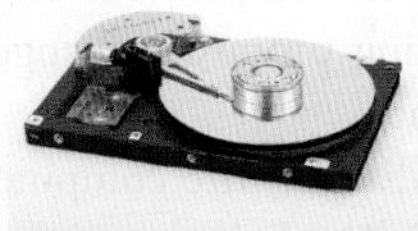

Hard disk: A hard disk is a storage device that contains one or more inflexible circular platters that use magnetic particles to store data, instructions, and information. Desktop and laptop computers often contain at least one hard disk that is mounted inside the computer's case; this is called a *fixed disk* because this hard disk is not portable. External hard disks are separate, portable, freestanding hard disks that either attach with a cable or are wireless. Hard disks today have capacities that are measured in gigabytes and terabytes.

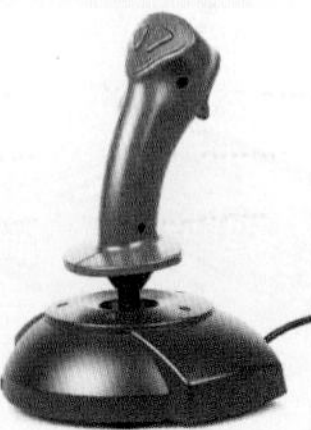

Joystick/wheel: If a computer is used to play games, then a joystick or wheel should be purchased. These devices—especially the more expensive ones—provide for realistic game play with force feedback, programmable buttons, and specialized levers and wheels. These might be useful for patient education apps in which the joystick can be used to allow the patient to navigate through a virtual tour of the mouth.

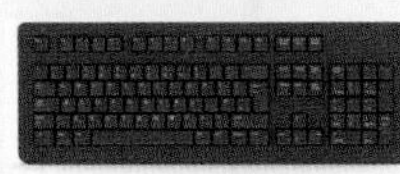

Keyboard: The keyboard is one of the more important devices used to communicate with the computer. For this reason, make sure that the keyboard purchased has 101 to 105 keys, that it is comfortable and easy to use, and that it has a USB connection. A wireless keyboard should be considered, especially if there is a small desk area.

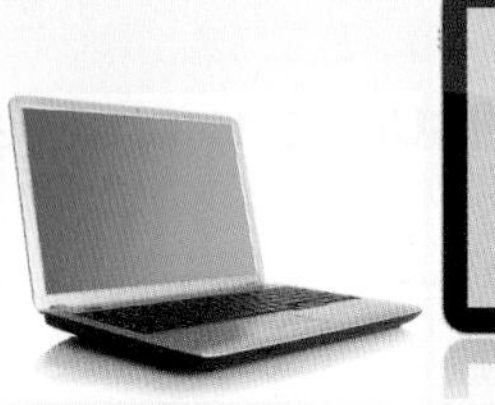

Laptop, notebook, or tablet computer: These are portable personal computers that are designed to fit on a user's lap. Sometimes they may have detachable keyboards, or they may involve the use of virtual keyboards that can be found on the screen.

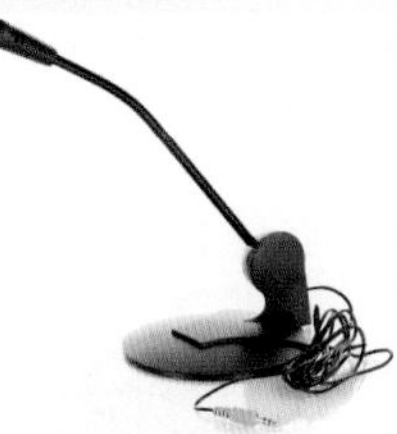

Microphone: To record audio or to use speech recognition to enter text and commands, purchase a close-talk headset with gain adjustment support or a desktop plug-in model. Either one could use a person's voice to send a text message, schedule an appointment, and dial a phone number. Alternatively, you may opt for video calling instead of traditional phone calls so that you and the person you called can see each other as you chat on a computer or a mobile device.

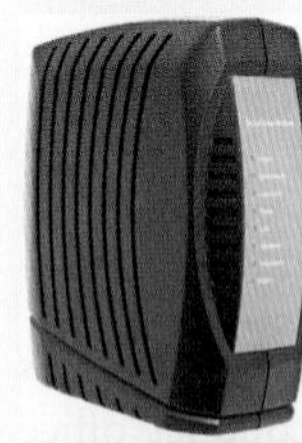

Modem: Most computers come with modems to connect them with the Internet or with a wireless network. Some modems also have fax capabilities. The modem chosen should be rated at 56 kbp.

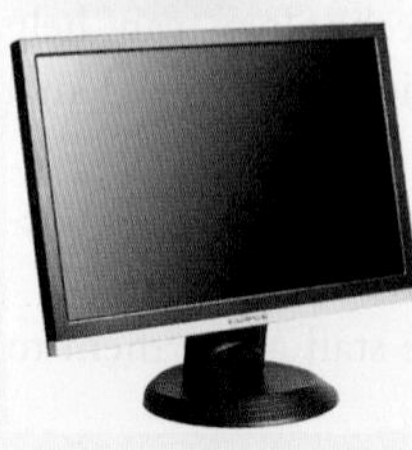

Monitor: The monitor is the screen on which documents are viewed, e-mail messages are read, and pictures are observed. A screen with a minimum size of 17 inches is recommended, but, if you are planning to use the computer for graphic design or game playing, a 19- or 21-inch monitor should be chosen. An LCD

BOX 5-3—cont'd

Selected Technology Terms

flat-panel monitor should be considered, especially if space is an issue. A touch-screen monitor may be used in some areas; this allows the user to interact by touching areas of the screen without using the mouse. Mobile computers and devices typically integrate the display into their same physical case and support touch-screen input.

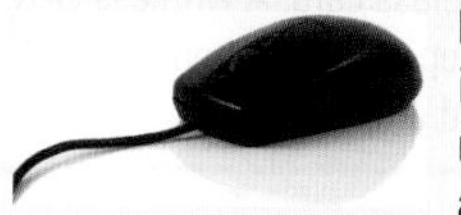

Mouse or pointing device: The mouse is used constantly with the computer. For this reason, spend a few extra dollars, if necessary, and purchase a mouse with an optical sensor and a USB connection. The optical sensor replaces the need for a mouse ball, which means that a mouse pad is not needed. For a personal computer (PC), make sure that the mouse has a wheel, which acts as a third button in addition to the top two buttons on the left and right. An ergonomic design is also important, because the hand is on the mouse most of the time when using the computer. A wireless mouse should be considered to eliminate the cord and to allow the assistant work at short distances from the computer. A pointing device is an input device that allows a user to control a small symbol on the screen; this is typically used with laptops or tablets.

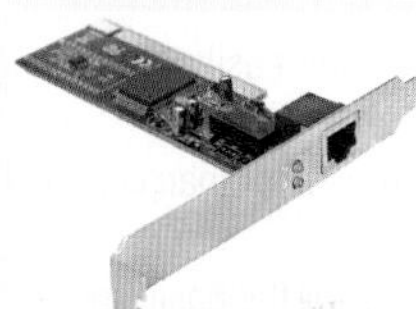

Network card: If planning to connect to a network or use broadband (cable or DSL) to connect to the Internet, then purchase a network card. Broadband connections require a 10/100 PCI Ethernet network card.

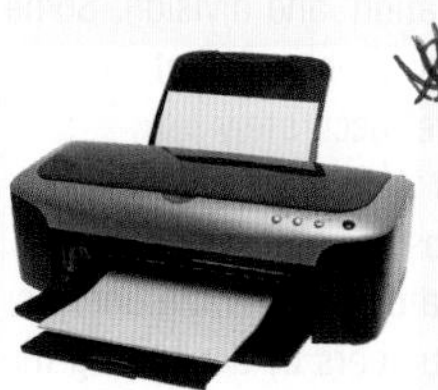

Printer: The two basic printer choices are ink jet and laser. Color ink jet printers cost from $50 to $300, on average, whereas laser printers cost from $300 to $2000. In general, the cheaper the printer, the lower the resolution and speed and the more often the ink cartridge or toner must be changed. Laser printers print faster and with a higher quality than an ink jet printer, and their toner generally costs less. If color is desired, then go with a high-end ink jet printer to ensure the quality of the printing. The duty cycle (i.e., the number of pages that will be printed each month) also should be a determining factor. If the duty cycle is on the low end (i.e., hundreds of pages per month), then stay with a high-end ink jet printer rather than purchasing a laser printer. If planning to print photographs taken with a digital camera, then purchase a photo printer. A photo printer is a dye-sublimation printer or an ink jet printer with higher resolution and features that allow for the printing of quality photographs. Most printers support wireless connectivity.

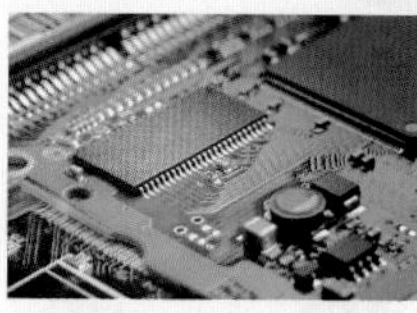

Processor: To select the right processor, first determine your needs. Determine the amount of power that you have with your current processor, and then research current processors. Another thing to consider when updating processors is considering that what used to be done with a desktop model may now be accomplished with a tablet or laptop or even with a hand-held mobile device.

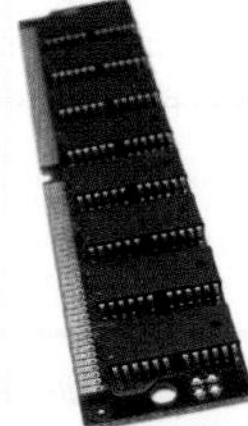

RAM: Random access memory (RAM) plays a vital role in the speed of the computer. Make sure that the computer purchased has at least 1 GB of RAM. If there is extra money to invest in the computer, consider increasing the amount of RAM. The extra money spent for RAM will be well spent.

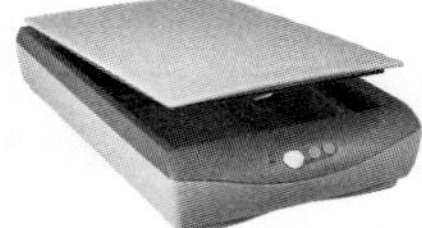

Scanner: The most popular scanner purchased with a computer today is the flatbed scanner that can attach to the computer either with a cable or wirelessly. When evaluating a flatbed scanner, check the color depth and resolution. Some scanners are duplex scanners, which means that they can scan both sides of a document.

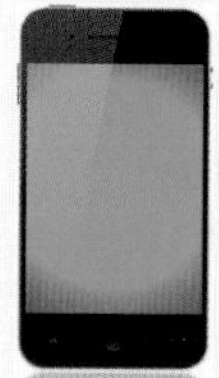

Smartphone: A smartphone is an Internet-capable phone that usually includes a calendar, an appointment book, an address book, a calculator, a notepad, games, and several other apps. Smartphones typically communicate wirelessly with other devices or computers.

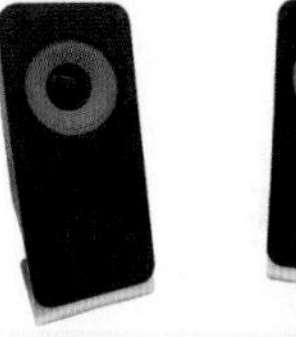

Speakers: Speakers allow you to hear audio in the form of music, voice, or other sounds. Most personal computers and mobile devices have small internal speakers, or you can attach earbuds or headphones for personalized listening. Purchasing a good sound card, quality speakers, and a separate subwoofer that amplifies the bass frequencies of the speakers can turn the computer into a premium stereo system.

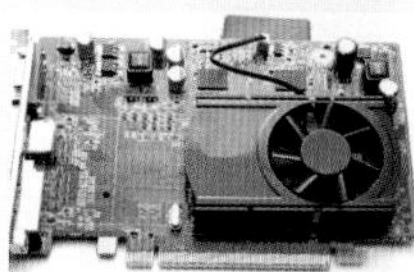

Video graphics card: Most standard video cards satisfy the monitor display needs of home and small office users. If the purchaser is a game player or a graphic designer, a higher-quality video card can be selected. The higher refresh rate will further enhance the display of games, graphics, and movies.

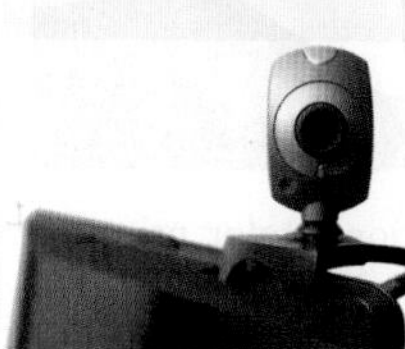

PC video camera: A PC video or web cam is a small camera that can be used to capture and display live video (in some cases with sound), primarily on the Internet. A PC video camera can also be used to capture, edit, and share videos and still photos. The camera sits on the monitor or desk. These functions can also be found on a smartphone.

Continued

BOX 5-3—cont'd

Selected Technology Terms

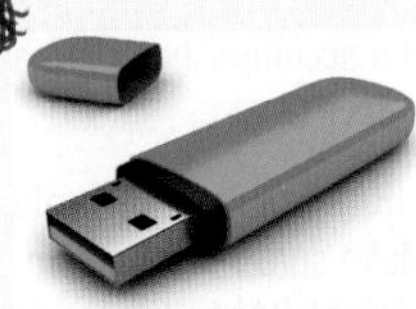

USB flash (jump) drive: If different computers are used and if access to the same data and information is needed, then this portable miniature storage device that can fit on a key chain is ideal. USB flash drive capacities vary from 128 MB to 4 GB.

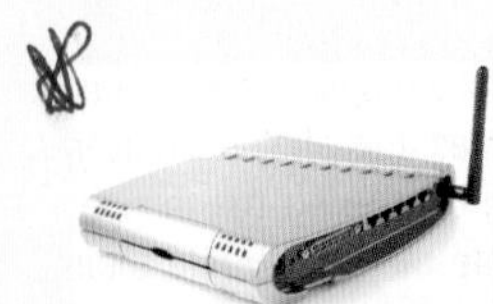

Wireless LAN access point: A wireless local area network (LAN) access point allows for the networking of several computers so that they can share files and access the Internet through a single cable modem or DSL connection. Each device connected requires a wireless card. A wireless LAN access point can offer a range of operation of up to several hundred feet, so be sure that the device has a high-powered antenna.

Data from Shelly GB, Cashman TJ, Vermaat ME: *Discovering computers: Fundamentals edition*, Boston, 2004, Course Technology.

BOX 5-4

Features to Consider When Selecting or Using Copiers

- Style of copier: tabletop size or standalone floor model
- Volume of work to be done: low, mid, or high volume
- Quality of copy desired: clear and sharp
- Selection of paper size for reports, ledger cards, and letters
- Ability to reproduce from a colored original or colored ink
- Speed and output: number of copies per minute
- Ability to make copies on regular office forms and paper
- Availability of outside copying business or other specialized copying services to handle a large volume of documents (e.g., a new office policy manual)

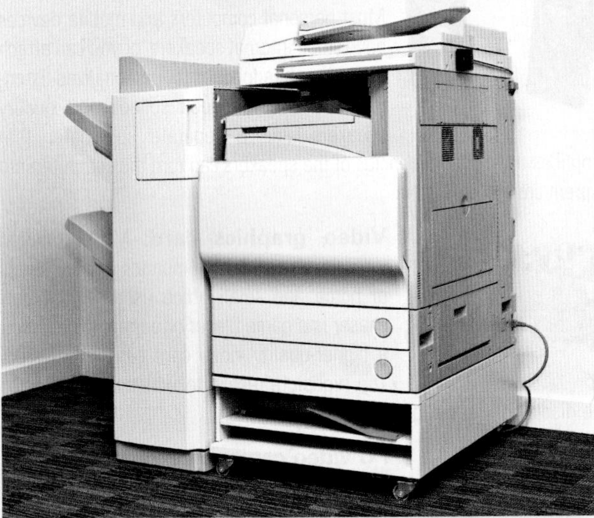

Multitask machine that performs four functions: color printing, scanning, plain-paper faxing, and copying. (Copyright © 2014 Markus, BigStock.com.)

BOX 5-5

Features to Consider When Selecting a Calculator

- Type of display
- Printing capabilities
- Quality of keyboard
- Type of batteries: For portable models, are they easily obtained? Are they throwaway or rechargeable?
- Durability of components and materials: Factors other than cost will influence the selection of a calculator.
- Ease of operation: The calculator should allow for the basic computations of addition, subtraction, multiplication, and division. Some machines can solve difficult trigonometry problems that only an accomplished mathematician could answer accurately.
- Decimal functions: A fixed decimal restricts the number of decimals; a floating decimal puts no restriction on the position of the decimal point.
- Repeat and constant operations: This feature allows the operator to add or subtract a series of identical numbers by depressing the *add* or *subtract* function key repeatedly.
- Memory register: Figures can be added to or subtracted from and are available until the register is cleared.

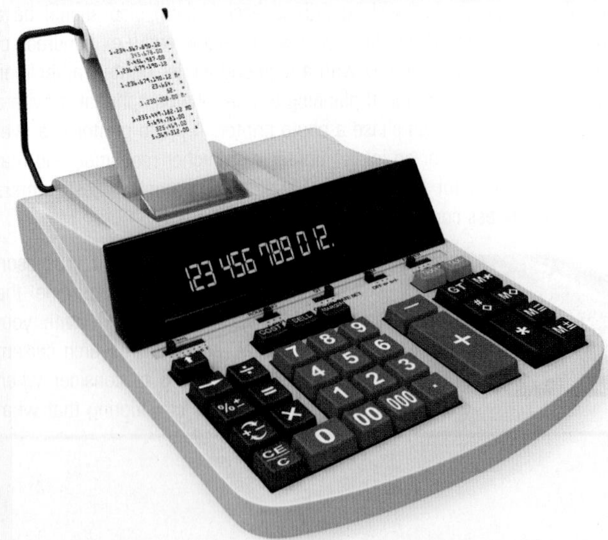

Calculator. (Copyright © 2014 Nerthuz, BigStock.com.)

A mobile device is a computing device that is small enough to be held in your hand. Because of their reduced size, the screens on mobile devices are small, often between 3 and 5 inches. Some mobile devices are Internet capable, which means that they can wirelessly connect to the Internet. You can often exchange information between the Internet and a mobile device or between a computer or network and a mobile device. Popular types of mobile devices are smartphones, digital cameras, portable media players, and e-book readers.

Apps and Software

The computer system is directed by a series of instructions called a *computer program* or a software *application,* which directs the sequence of operations that the computing system is to perform. Apps in the dental office may include software specifically designed for dental practice management as well as general-purpose software such as word processors, spreadsheets, and database systems. Apps may be provided with the computer system, or they may be purchased as individual or bundled packages. A typical desktop window is shown in Figure 5-3.

Data

The term *data* refers to the facts or figures that the information system needs to produce accurate and timely information. Data are the raw material of the information system, and they are manipulated or processed by the computer to produce the finished product or the information needed. For example, the administrative assistant enters data such as treatment rendered. In addition, the fees and payments on a financial record are calculated. The finished product can result in a statement or an insurance claim form. If the data are incorrect, the resulting information will be incorrect. Remember, "garbage in, garbage out." The amount of storage offered by a *byte* is roughly equivalent to one character of text. For example, typing the letters *a*, *b*, and *c* requires three bytes of storage. Data is measured in the storage terms shown in Box 5-2.

Personnel

For some larger computer installations, properly trained information processing personnel are required to operate and maintain the information system or network. However, in most dental practices, the administrative assistant is responsible for the accuracy of both the input and output of the information system as well as the system's setup and maintenance. When an information system is installed in an office, most system vendors provide a training session for the staff. Alternatively, they may provide a social media site for self-training or for building a community of users. As updated versions are released, notifications about system improvements are posted. Most software suppliers offer ongoing telephone helplines or Internet-based support options on a monthly or yearly basis.

Procedures

Procedures are the written versions of policies that help to maintain the information system efficiently. Specialized manuals can be assembled, or these procedures may be included in the office procedures manual described in Chapter 2.

PRACTICE NOTE

If any of the elements of the information system—the computing device, the apps, the data, the personnel, or the procedures—are missing or flawed, the entire system may be affected.

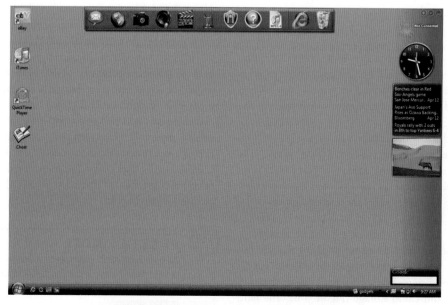

FIGURE 5-3 Parts of a typical desktop window.

OPERATIONS AND THE INFORMATION SYSTEM

Information Processing Cycle

Regardless of the computing device that is selected for business office use, such a device is capable of performing four general operations known as the *information processing cycle*. These four operations are (1) input, (2) process, (3) output, and (4) storage. By using these four processes, the computing device will process the data into information.

Parts of a Computing Device

Input Device

The most common means of entering information and instructions into a computer is the keyboard (Figures 5-4 and 5-5). Special keys may include a numeric keypad, cursor control keys, and function keys. In addition to the keyboard, there are a host of other data-collection devices, including the mouse or trackball, touch screens, graphic input devices, scanners, and voice input devices. These devices may input data directly, without any keystrokes. The trend today is to eliminate keystrokes whenever possible, thereby increasing the accuracy of the data.

Processor

The processor is the controlling unit of the computing system that contains the electronic circuitry needed to manipulate data. This unit is known as the central processing unit (CPU; see Figure 5-4), and it directs and controls all of the computer's activities. As the data are accepted from the input device, they are processed by the apps. The apps contain a series of instructions that direct the computer to perform a sequence of tasks. The number of apps and the amount of data that can be stored in the processing unit depends on the size of the main memory of the system. The memory capacity of computers varies, but each computer has a fixed amount.

Output Device

The printer and the screen are the two most commonly used output devices (see Figure 5-4). If a paper copy (hard copy) is needed, the computer will be directed to print a copy. When no permanent record is needed, the output is displayed on the screen (soft copy).

A laser printer, which is often called an *intelligent printer*, shapes characters through the use of light (laser beams). The intelligent printer is able to collate, stack, and place images on both sides of the paper. The cost of these printers has decreased, so they now produce multiple copies more economically.

Storage Media

Storage media are used to store data and programs that are not being processed on the computer. Types of storage media include hard disks, solid-state drives, USB flash drives, memory cards, optical drives, and cloud storage (Figure 5-6). The hard disk is a rigid metal disk coated with magnetic material that makes it suitable for recording and storing data. Solid-state drives typically use flash memory; they are found on some desktops, laptops, and tablets. USB flash drives are portable storage devices that you plug into a USB port on a computer or a mobile device. Memory cards are removable flash memory devices that you insert and remove from slots in a computer, a mobile device, or a card reader. The optical compact disk system uses a laser to burn microscopic holes on the surface of a hard plastic disk. The most popular optical disk formats used for data storage are the recordable compact disk (CD-R/DVD-R) and the rewritable compact disk (CD-RW/DVD-RW). Cloud storage is an Internet-based service that provides storage options to computer users. Types of services provided by cloud storage providers vary from the storage of specific types of files (e.g., photographs, radiographs, patient records) to the backing up of entire systems in case the original is lost, damaged, or destroyed.

Networks and Telecommunication

Most computing devices today are not standalone systems; rather, they are connected together to form a network. Networks can be classified as local area networks (LANs), which connect computing devices in an office, a building, or several nearby buildings, or as wide area networks (WANs), which link computers and other devices across a city, a region, or even the world as the Internet does. How the devices connect to the network is called the *telecommunications pipeline*, which includes analog dial-up service, cable, digital subscriber line (DSL), microwave, radio, or satellite. The first three involve physical connections, and the last three use wireless technology.

PROFITABILITY OF THE INFORMATION SYSTEM

All of the high-tech equipment available today will not make the private dental office, clinic, or dental laboratory more efficient if proper procedures are not followed before investing in the information system. Before the office acquires new equipment or updates equipment of any kind, the needs of the office should be identified (Box 5-6). The major categories of equipment that should be considered include computing devices dedicated to such tasks as word processing, records management, insurance management, and accounting; scanners, copying machines; calculators; and voice processing equipment. Other specific types of equipment used to handle mail and telephone systems are discussed within the content of specific chapters of this book.

PRACTICE NOTE

All of the high-tech equipment available today will not make the private dental office, clinic, or dental laboratory more efficient if proper procedures are not followed before investing in the information system.

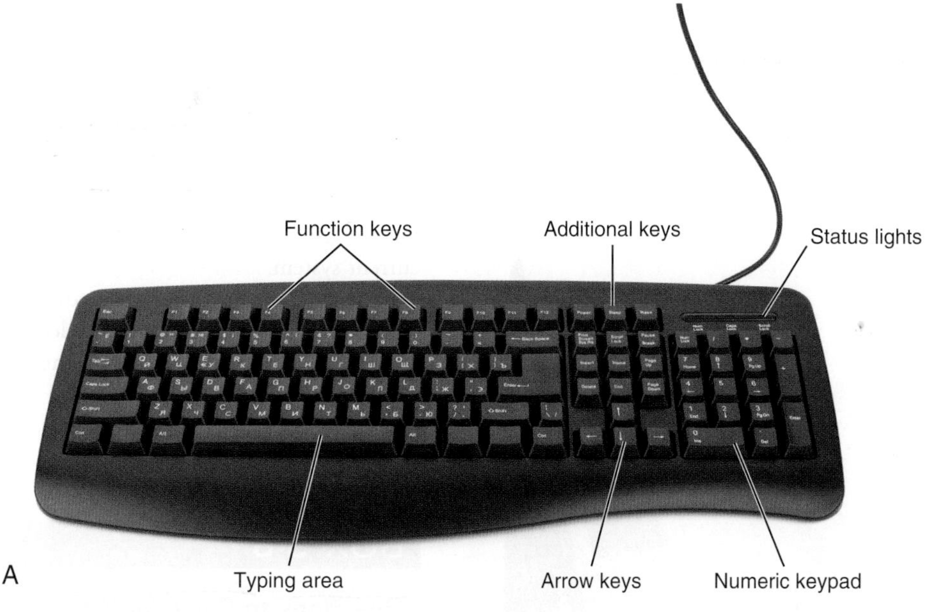

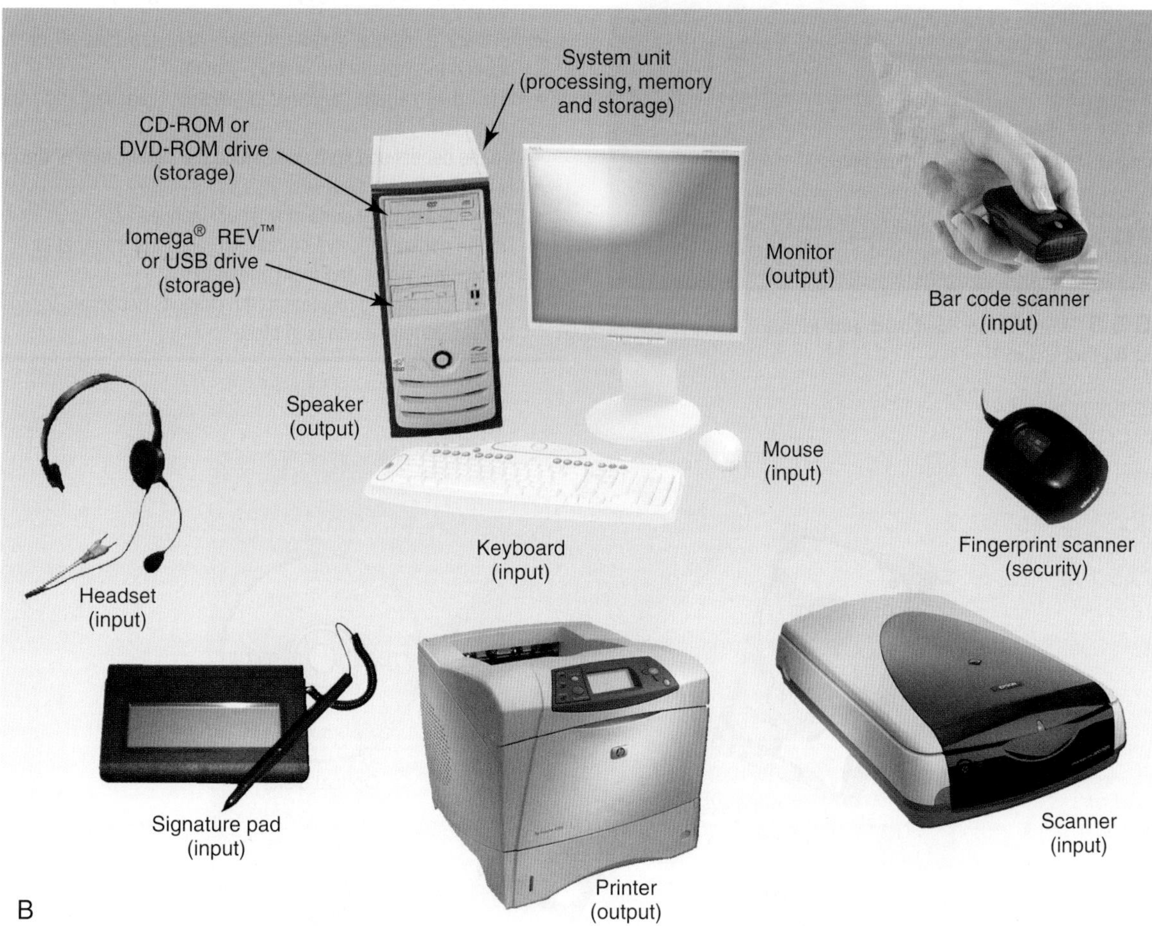

FIGURE 5-4 **A,** Computer keyboard. **B,** Computer system. (**A,** Copyright © 2014 Digitalr, BigStock.com. **B,** Courtesy Patterson Office Supplies, Champaign, IL.)

A feasibility study is one of the most reliable ways to determine what types of updates to the computer system are needed and whether new technologies are needed. This study can be conducted within the office by a vendor (usually an equipment manufacturer), an organization, or a qualified individual (e.g., the administrative assistant). A feasibility study must involve everyone who will use the system as well as other support staff. Some factors to consider when doing the feasibility study include the following: (1) the type and size of the practice, (2) the cost, (3) any changes in the practice since the initial computer purchase, (4) the abilities of the staff, and (5) training requirements. Investing in a new computer is unwise if it will only be used as a billing machine or if it will not improve the current system.

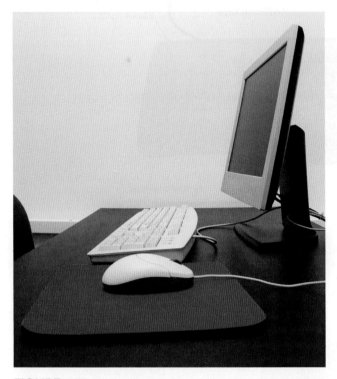

FIGURE 5-5 Workstation: keyboard and monitor. (Copyright © 2014 Drx, BigStock.com.)

After the need for a new or modified system has been established, it will be time to begin selecting the equipment and software modifications, setting up the procedures for using the equipment, training personnel, and entering or transferring data from one system to another.

BOX 5-6

Questions to Consider When Preparing to Automate or Modify an Existing System

- Is there a manual system in place that provides all of the data needed to evaluate the practice monthly?
- Has the current automated system reached its maximum potential?
- Do the dentist and staff understand the significance of the change?
- Is the staff organized?
- Does the work get done in a timely manner?
- Do the patients receive current and accurate information?
- Is the staff stable and team oriented?
- Is the staff willing to adapt to the changes necessary to modify the current system, if one is in place?

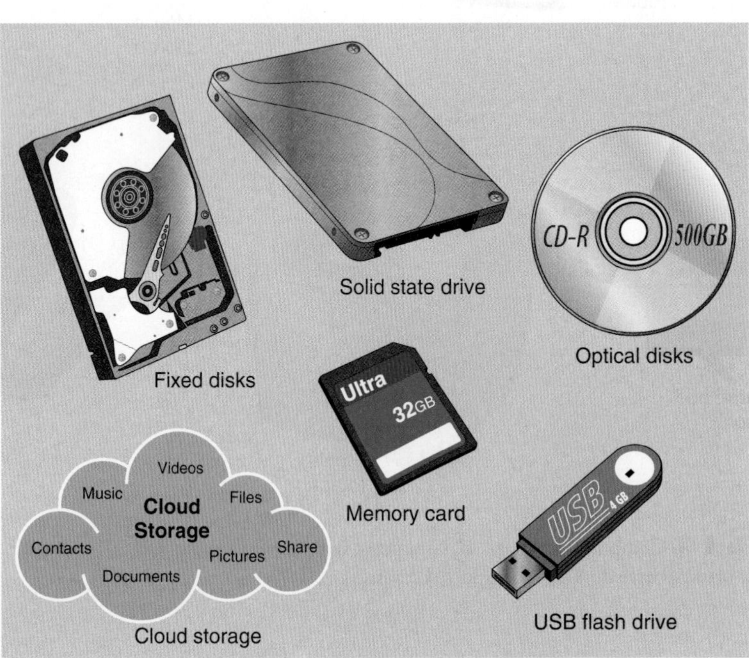

FIGURE 5-6 Different types of storage media.

APP (APPLICATION) AND SOFTWARE SELECTION

The first part of this chapter can be used as a guide for selecting the computing devices of the information system for the office needs, with the help of equipment manufacturers. The next task is the selection of the apps or software. Software is the computer programs that are written to meet specific user needs. Remember that some software companies sell both hardware and software. This is good, because the company is aware of the requirements of the software and can enable the user to select the appropriate hardware to support the chosen apps or software.

Selecting the apps and software that will perform the tasks specific to a particular office is important. Apps and software are available to perform general tasks; these include programs for word processing, spreadsheets, database management, graphics, and desktop publishing. Practice management apps and software are available to support all of the previously mentioned tasks, and they can also perform specific tasks for dental offices, including those related to account reports, patient reports, patient history, transactions, prescription history, insurance claim processing, appointment scheduling, treatment planning, summary reports, billing and aging receivables, referral tracking, income analysis, recall, and inventory management. Figures 5-7 through 5-20 include illustrations of some of the various screens that can be accessed with a commonly used software system, including the following:

- The *patient information screen* (Figure 5-7) includes comprehensive patient information.
- The *patient accounts screen* (Figure 5-8) includes accounts receivable information. A variety of payment and remittance information is found on this screen, including the minimum monthly payment, the date of the last statement, the current account balance, and any outstanding insurance or budget plan balances.
- The *patient master report* (Figure 5-9) can be filtered or sorted with the use of different criteria, such as patient zip codes, birthdays, phone numbers, insurance coverage, and more.
- The *prescription window* (Figure 5-10) lists the patient's medication history.
- The *transaction entry screen* (Figure 5-11) is a window within the American Dental Association (ADA) window that shows the ADA codes for completed treatments.
- The *claim transaction window* (Figure 5-12) is the portion of the practice management software that handles claims processing. It tracks all open claims, shows what was submitted with each claim, and allows for the electronic submission of claims.
- The *treatment plan screen* (Figure 5-13) enables the production of a treatment plan for the patient and tracks all of the planned treatment to completion.
- The *daily appointment screen* (Figure 5-14) indicates the schedule for various treatment rooms.
- The *schedule versus goal screen* allows for the viewing of a provider's scheduled appointments versus the goals for each day (Figure 5-15).
- The *family recall* feature (Figure 5-16) can pull up everyone in a specific family and identify their examination due dates.
- The *tickler file* (Figure 5-17) is provided in the appointment section of the program to collect and store information about patients who have missed, canceled, or broken appointments. It allows for the easy tracking of patients who need to be contacted to reschedule.
- *Clinical charting* (Figure 5-18) can be done in the treatment room with the use of a graphic format. Charting can be done

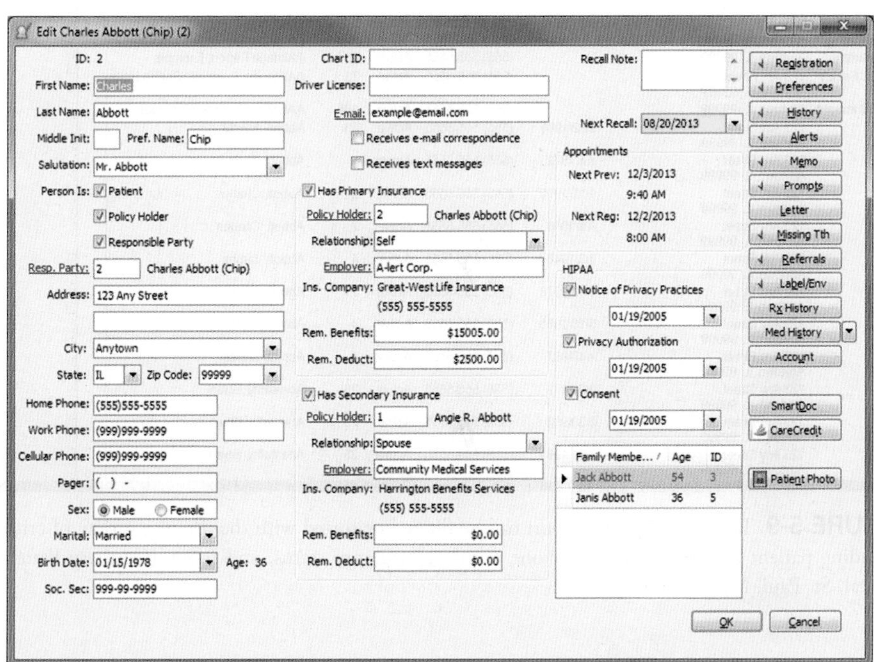

FIGURE 5-7 Patient information screen. (Courtesy Patterson Dental, St. Paul, MN.)

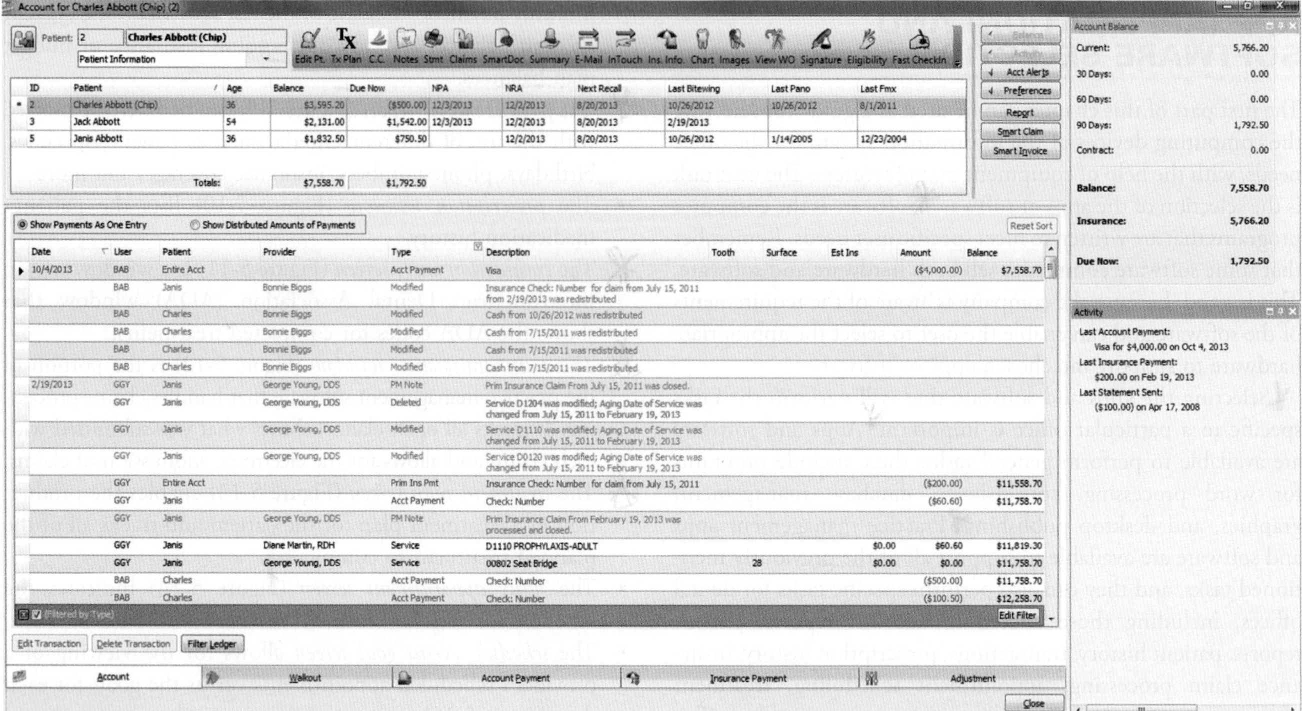

FIGURE 5-8 Patient accounts screen. (Courtesy Patterson Dental, St. Paul, MN.)

TIME 12:21 PM PTC & Associates DATE 9/17/2014

PATIENT MASTER

Patient		Address	Birthdate	Home Phone	Status	Responsible Party	
195	AA3D Image, Ortho	Anytown, IL 99999		(555) 555-5555	Active	195	AA3D Image, Ortho
137	AAImage Report, Example	Anytown, IL 99999		(555) 555-5555	Active	137	AAImage Report, Example
73	AAImages, Cosmetic Smiles I	123 Any Street Anytown, IL 99999		(555) 555-5555	Active	73	AAImages, Cosmetic Smiles Libra
166	AAImages, Schick 33 Images	Anytown, IL 99999		(555) 555-5555	Active	166	AAImages, Schick 33 Images
63	Abbott, Angela	123 Any Street Anytown, IL 99999	11/2/1980	(555) 555-5555	Active	63	Abbott, Angela
1	Abbott, Angie R	123 Any Street Anytown, IL 99999	6/8/1972	(555) 555-5555	Active	1	Abbott, Angie R
2	Abbott, Charles	123 Any Street Anytown, IL 99999	1/15/1978	(555) 555-5555	Active	2	Abbott, Charles
3	Abbott, Jack	123 Any Street Anytown, IL 99999	8/8/1960	(555) 555-5555	Active	2	Abbott, Charles
4	Abbott, James	123 Any Street Anytown, IL 99999	3/3/1948	(555) 555-5555	Active	4	Abbott, James
5	Abbott, Janis	123 Any Street Anytown, IL 99999	1/19/1978	(555) 555-5555	Active	2	Abbott, Charles
19	Abbott, Madison G	123 Any Street Anytown, IL 99999	5/18/1985	(555) 555-5555	Active	4	Abbott, James
20	Abbott, Mark	123 Any Street Anytown, IL 99999	4/4/1987	(555) 555-5555	Active	4	Abbott, James
27	Abernathy, Betsy	123 Any Street Anytown, IL 99999	9/9/1972	(555) 555-5555	Active	25	Abernathy, Bryan
25	Abernathy, Bryan	123 Any Street Anytown, IL 99999	3/3/1963	(555) 555-5555	Active	25	Abernathy, Bryan
72	Abernathy, Bryan A	123 Any Street Anytown, IL 99999	7/21/1988	(555) 555-5555	Active	25	Abernathy, Bryan

FIGURE 5-9 The patient master report can be filtered or sorted with the use of a variety of criteria, including patient zip code, birthday, phone number, insurance status, and more. (Courtesy Patterson Dental, St. Paul, MN.)

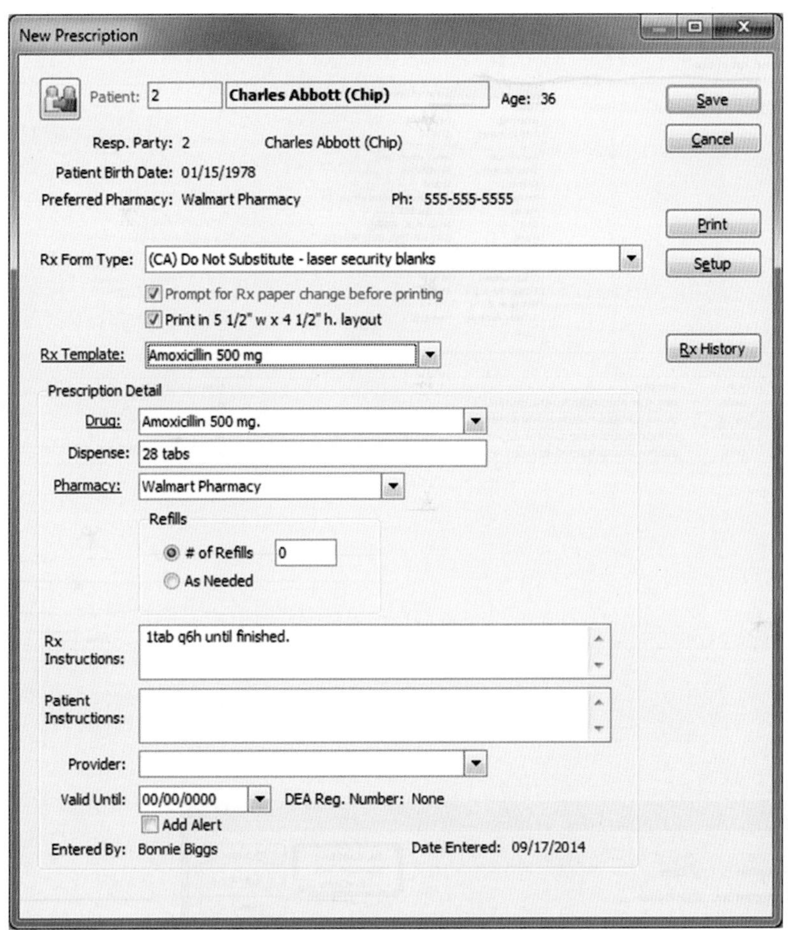

FIGURE 5-10 Prescription window. (Courtesy Patterson Dental, St. Paul, MN.)

Report Preview
File View Background

TIME 12:24 PM PTC & Associates DATE 09/17/2014

SERVICE CODES MASTER

Service Code	ADA Code	Display Abbr	Description	Service Type	Standard Fee	Time Units	Generate Recall	Status
D0120	D0120	PEXAM	PERIODIC ORAL EVALUATION	PREVENTIVE	$50.00	1	Yes	Active
D0140	D0140	LEXAM	LIMITED ORAL EVALUATION-PROBLEM	DIAGNOSTIC	$42.00	1	No	Active
D0145	D0145	D0145	ORAL EVAL PT UNDER 3/PRIM CAREGIV	DIAGNOSTIC	$0.00	1	No	Active
D0150	D0150	CEXAM	COMPREHENSIVE ORAL EVALUATION	DIAGNOSTIC	$50.00	1	No	Active
D0160	D0160	DEXAM	DETAILED & EXTENS ORAL EVAL-PRB F	DIAGNOSTIC	$25.00	1	No	Active
D0170	D0170		RE-EVAL. - LIMITED, PROBLEM FOCUSE	DIAGNOSTIC	$40.00	1	No	Active
D0180	D0180	PRExm	COMPREHENSIVE PERIODONTAL EVAL	DIAGNOSTIC	$45.00	1	No	Active
D0190	D0190	D0190	SCREENING OF A PATIENT	DIAGNOSTIC	$0.00	1	No	Active
D0191	D0191	D0191	ASSESSMENT OF A PATIENT	DIAGNOSTIC	$0.00	1	No	Active
D0210	D0210	FMX	INTRAORAL-COMPLETE (INCL. BITEWIN	DIAGNOSTIC	$85.00	1	No	Active
D0220	D0220	PAX	INTRAORAL-PERIAPICAL FIRST FILM	DIAGNOSTIC	$20.00	1	No	Active
D0230	D0230	PAX	INTRAORAL-PERIAPICAL-EACH ADDITIO	DIAGNOSTIC	$15.00	1	No	Active
D0240	D0240	OCCX	INTRAORAL-OCCLUSAL FILM	DIAGNOSTIC	$20.00	1	No	Active
D0250	D0250	EOXRA	EXTRAORAL-FIRST FILM	DIAGNOSTIC	$20.00	1	No	Active
D0260	D0260	00260	EXTRAORAL-EACH ADDITIONAL FILM	DIAGNOSTIC	$20.00	1	No	Active

Page 1 of 17

FIGURE 5-11 Service codes listed with the American Dental Association. (Courtesy Patterson Dental, St. Paul, MN.)

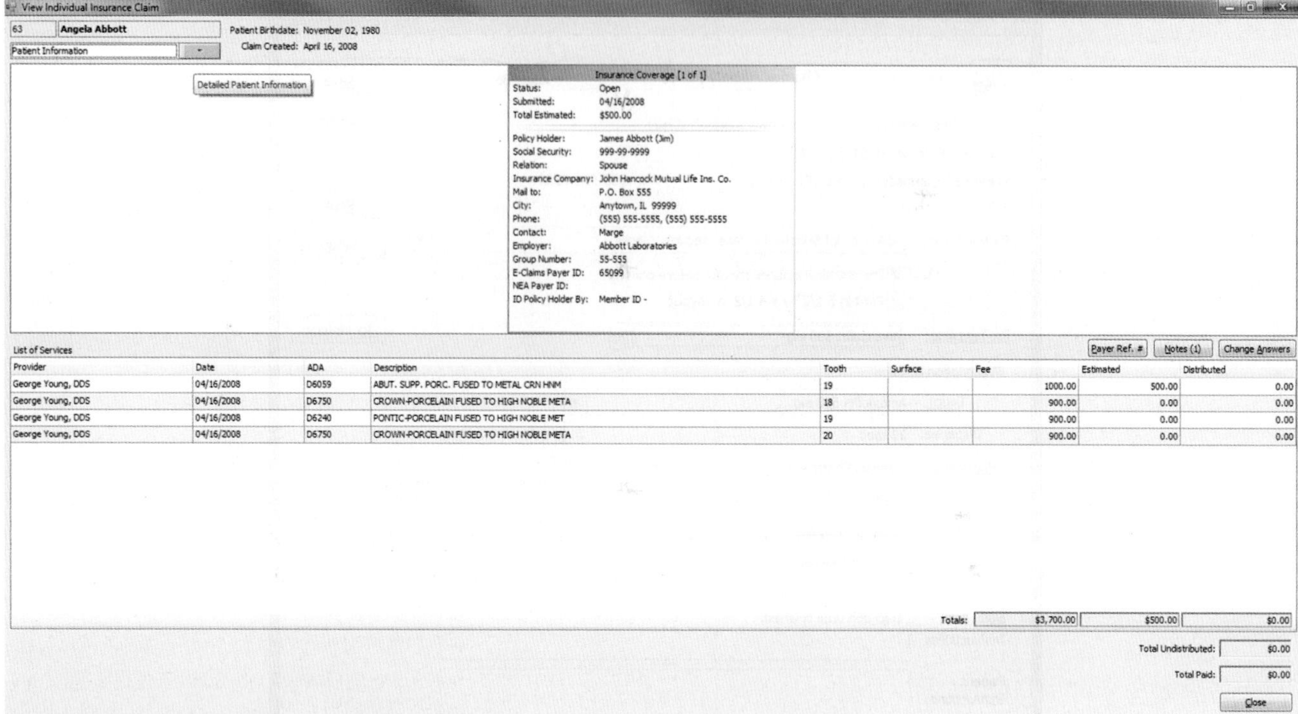

A

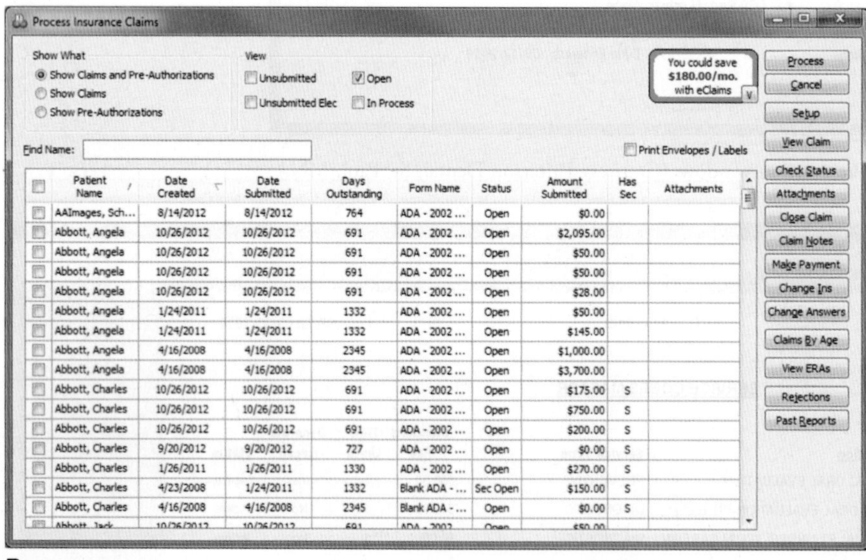

B

FIGURE 5-12 Claim transaction window. **A,** Claims view. **B,** Process in claim. (Courtesy Patterson Dental, St. Paul, MN.)

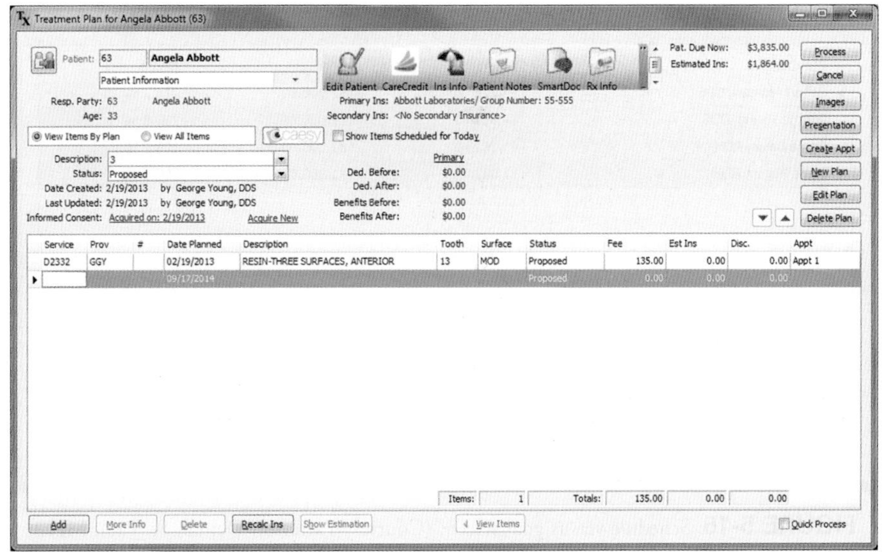

FIGURE 5-13 Treatment plan screen. (Courtesy Patterson Dental, St. Paul, MN.)

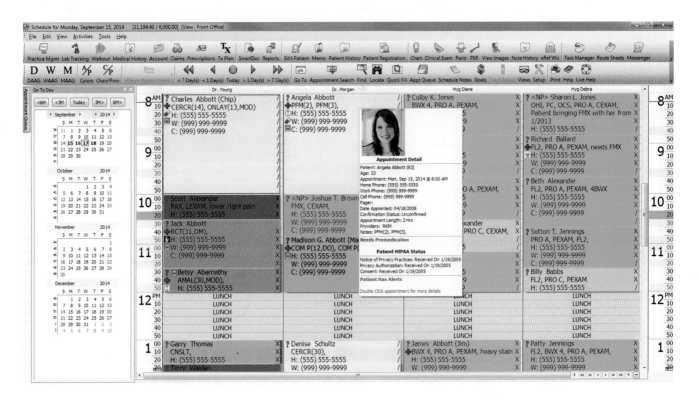

FIGURE 5-14 Daily appointment screen. (Courtesy Patterson Dental, St. Paul, MN.)

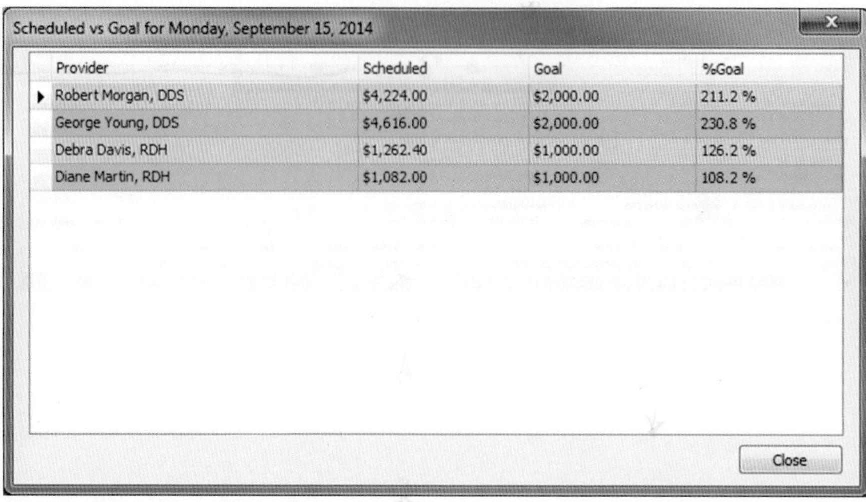

Scheduled vs Goal for Monday, September 15, 2014

Provider	Scheduled	Goal	%Goal
Robert Morgan, DDS	$4,224.00	$2,000.00	211.2 %
George Young, DDS	$4,616.00	$2,000.00	230.8 %
Debra Davis, RDH	$1,262.40	$1,000.00	126.2 %
Diane Martin, RDH	$1,082.00	$1,000.00	108.2 %

Close

FIGURE 5-15 Schedule versus goal screen. (Courtesy Patterson Dental, St. Paul, MN.)

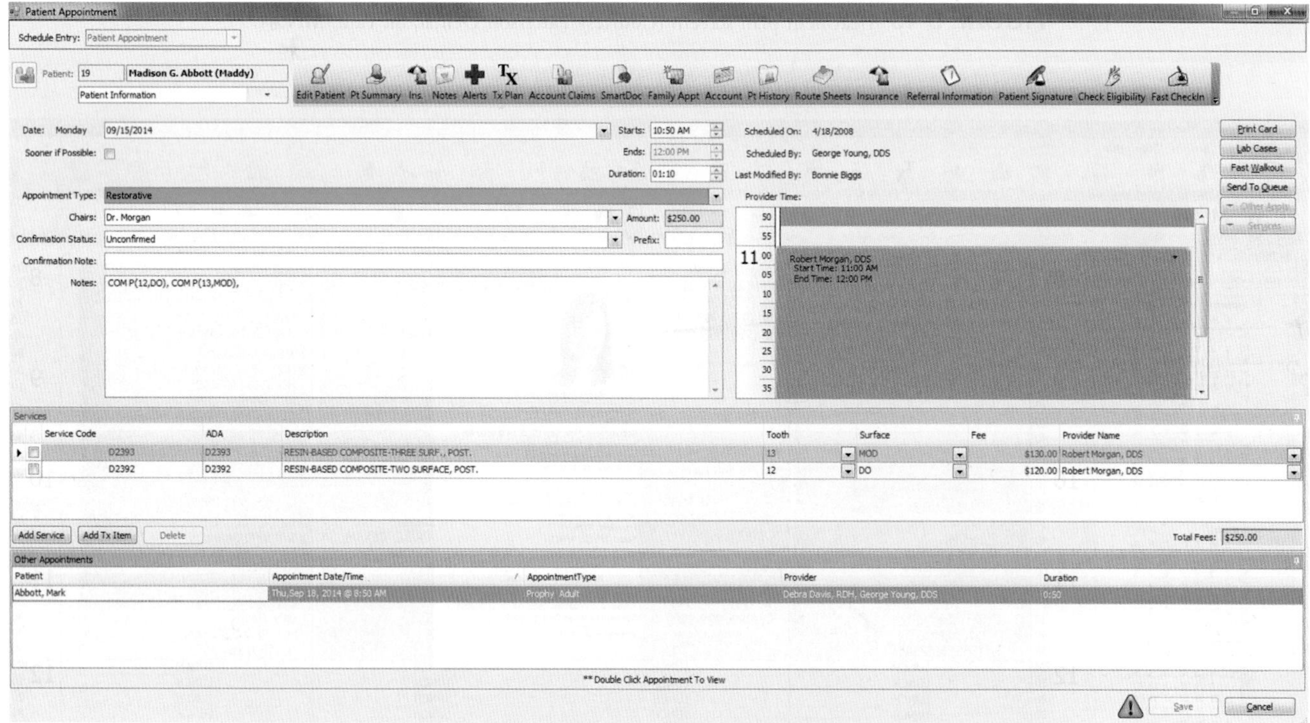

A

Family Appointment

Schedule Appointments for an Entire Family

Patient: 19 Madison G. Abbott (Maddy)

Patient Information

Site: PTC & Associates

Schedule	Patient	Next Recall	Frequency	Provider	Appointment Type	Duration
	James . Abbott	3/21/2013	6	Diane Martin, RDH	Prophy Adult	00:50
	Madison G. Abbott	2/15/2013	6	Debra Davis, RDH	Prophy Adult	00:50
	Mark . Abbott	7/27/2011	6	Debra Davis, RDH	Prophy Adult	00:50

Mark All

Clear All

Save Close

B

FIGURE 5-16 Family recall. **A,** Future dates of family member appointments. **B,** Next recall dates of each person in a family group.

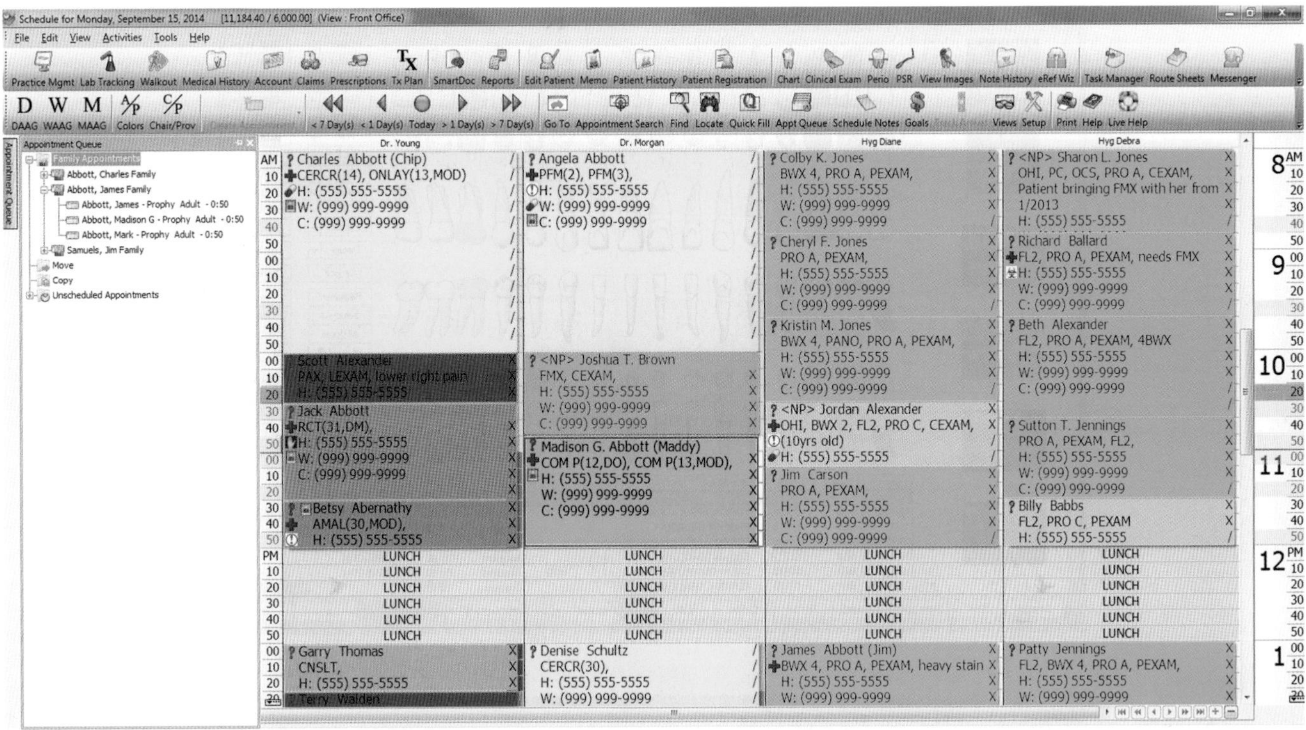

C

FIGURE 5-16, cont'd C, Appointment query screen for a family. (Courtesy Patterson Dental, St. Paul, MN.)

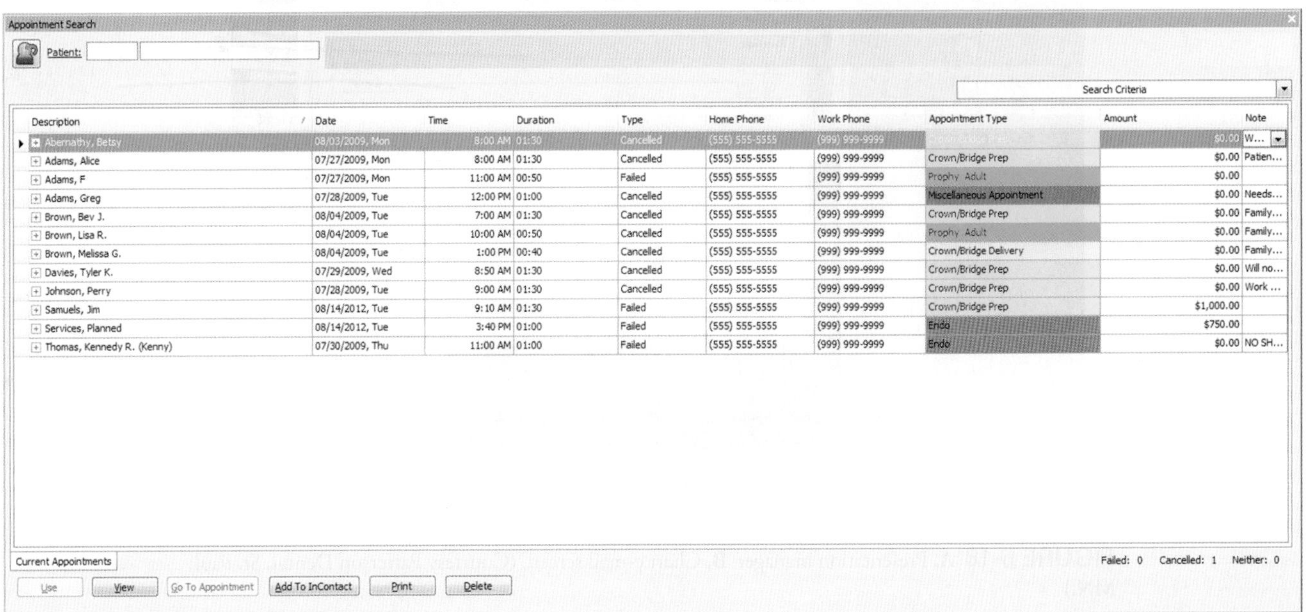

Appointment Search

Description	Date	Time	Duration	Type	Home Phone	Work Phone	Appointment Type	Amount	Note
Abernathy, Betsy	08/03/2009, Mon	8:00 AM	01:30	Cancelled	(555) 555-5555	(999) 999-9999		$0.00	W...
Adams, Alice	07/27/2009, Mon	8:00 AM	01:30	Cancelled	(555) 555-5555	(999) 999-9999	Crown/Bridge Prep	$0.00	Patien...
Adams, F	07/27/2009, Mon	11:00 AM	00:50	Failed	(555) 555-5555	(999) 999-9999	Prophy Adult	$0.00	
Adams, Greg	07/28/2009, Tue	12:00 PM	01:00	Cancelled	(555) 555-5555	(999) 999-9999	Miscellaneous Appointment	$0.00	Needs...
Brown, Bev J.	08/04/2009, Tue	7:00 AM	01:30	Cancelled	(555) 555-5555	(999) 999-9999	Crown/Bridge Prep	$0.00	Family...
Brown, Lisa R.	08/04/2009, Tue	10:00 AM	00:50	Cancelled	(555) 555-5555	(999) 999-9999	Prophy Adult	$0.00	Family...
Brown, Melissa G.	08/04/2009, Tue	1:00 PM	00:40	Cancelled	(555) 555-5555	(999) 999-9999	Crown/Bridge Delivery	$0.00	Family...
Davies, Tyler K.	07/29/2009, Wed	8:50 AM	01:30	Cancelled	(555) 555-5555	(999) 999-9999	Crown/Bridge Prep	$0.00	Will no...
Johnson, Perry	07/28/2009, Tue	9:00 AM	01:30	Cancelled	(555) 555-5555	(999) 999-9999	Crown/Bridge Prep	$0.00	Work ...
Samuels, Jim	08/14/2012, Tue	9:10 AM	01:30	Failed	(555) 555-5555	(999) 999-9999	Crown/Bridge Prep	$1,000.00	
Services, Planned	08/14/2012, Tue	3:40 PM	01:00	Failed	(555) 555-5555	(999) 999-9999	Endo	$750.00	
Thomas, Kennedy R. (Kenny)	07/30/2009, Thu	11:00 AM	01:00	Failed	(555) 555-5555	(999) 999-9999	Endo	$0.00	NO SH...

Current Appointments — Failed: 0 Cancelled: 1 Neither: 0

Use | View | Go To Appointment | Add To InContact | Print | Delete

FIGURE 5-17 Tickler file. (Courtesy Patterson Dental, St. Paul, MN.)

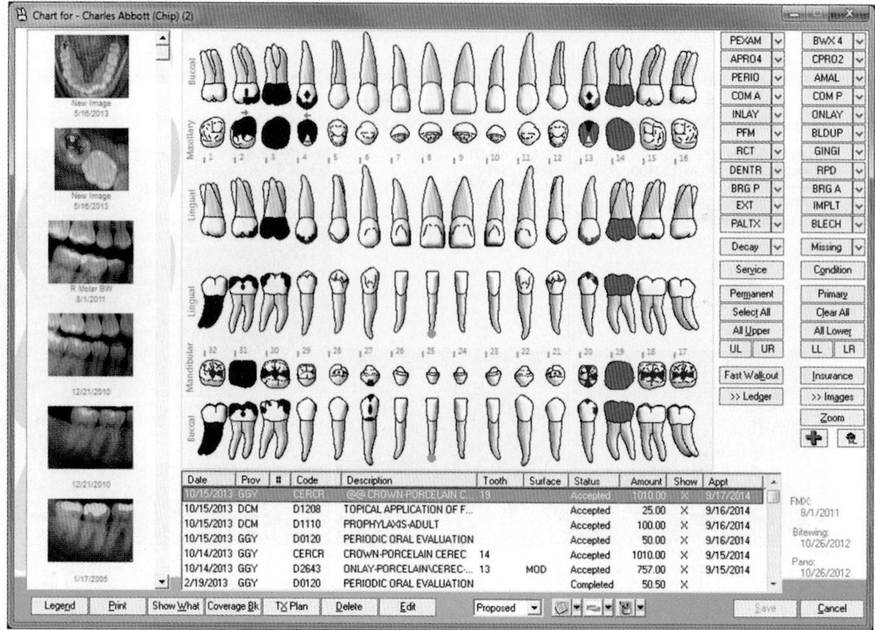

A

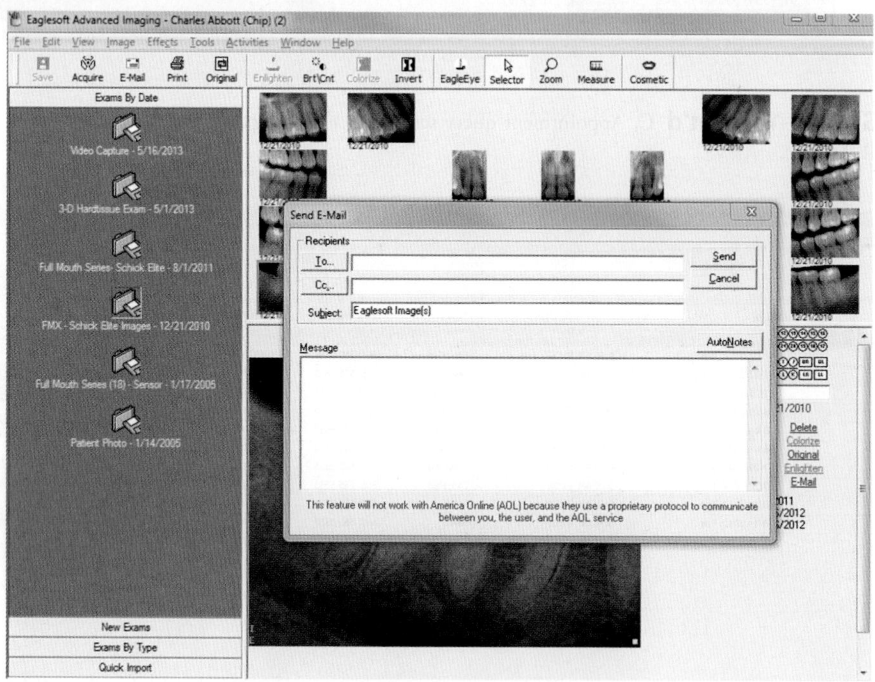

B

FIGURE 5-18 **A,** Presentation manager. **B,** Chart e-mail screen. (Courtesy Patterson Dental, St. Paul, MN.)

TIME 2:01 PM | PTC & Associates | DATE 9/17/2014

DAY SHEET
From EOD: Oct 08, 13 (10/08/13) To EOD: Oct 08, 13 (10/08/13)

Type	Production	Collections	Adjustments	A.R. Impact
Services:	$7,593.27	---	---	$7,593.27
Deleted Services	$0.00	---	---	$0.00
Taxes:	$0.00	---	---	$0.00
Deleted Taxes	$0.00	---	---	$0.00
Discounts:	$0.00	---	---	$0.00
Deleted Discounts	$0.00	---	---	$0.00
Returned Checks:	$0.00	$0.00	$0.00	$0.00
Returned Check Service Charges	$0.00	$0.00	$0.00	$0.00
Debit Adjustments	$0.00	$0.00	$0.00	$0.00
Finance Charges	$0.00	$0.00	$0.00	$0.00
Billing Charge:	$0.00	$0.00	$0.00	$0.00
Deleted Debit:	$0.00	$0.00	$0.00	$0.00
Cash Payments	---	$0.00	---	$0.00
Check Payments	---	$1,560.50	---	($1,560.50)
Other Payments	---	$2,511.42	---	($2,511.42)
Credit Adjustments	$0.00	$0.00	$0.00	$0.00
Deleted Credits	$0.00	$0.00	$0.00	$0.00
Write Offs:	$0.00	$0.00	$0.00	$0.00
Totals:	$7,593.27	$4,071.92	$0.00	

Beginning A.R.	$86,202.38
Change in A.R.	$3,521.35
Ending A.R.	$89,723.73

System Summary For Activity From EOD: Oct 08, 13 (10/08/13) To EOD: Oct 08, 13 (10/08/13)

Total Payment:	$4,071.92	Less Trans Pmts:	$4,071.92*	Total Productior	$7,593.27
Total Walkouts	$7,593.27**	Less Est. Ins:	$3,040.22****	Total Collection:	$4,071.92
Payments Made On Walkout	$3,571.92			Collection Rati	53.63%
Walkout Collection Rati	47.04%***		117.49%*****		
Patients Seen	9			Patients Seen	9
Total Productior	$7,593.27			Total Collection:	$4,071.92
Avg. Production Per Visi	$843.70			Avg. Collection Per Visi	$581.70

* Total of Payments made today less those from prior days that were deleted & recreated today due to transferring patients with history.
** Total of Services + Taxes - Discounts from the above totals less any service amounts that were both entered and deleted within this per
*** Total of Payments Made On Walkouts divided by Total Walkouts within this pe
**** Total Walkouts less any estimated insurance calculated on those walkouts. This amount does not change when the claims these are on are cl
***** Total of Payments Made On Walkouts divided by Total Walkouts less estimated insurance within this pe

FIGURE 5-19 Summary of activities. (Courtesy Patterson Dental, St. Paul, MN.)

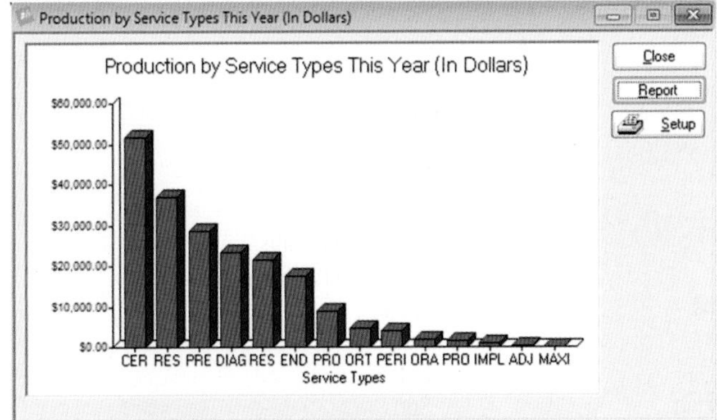

FIGURE 5-20 Provider report of actual production by service. (Courtesy Patterson Dental, St. Paul, MN.)

in a basic format, or it may include complex charts for periodontics and other specialty areas. Radiographs from the patient's chart can even be e-mailed to another dentist for evaluation.

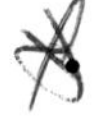

The *day sheet report* (Figure 5-19) summarizes practice activity for a period of time.

- *Annual graphic reports* are generated to illustrate categorical treatment production (Figure 5-20).

The appropriate selection of an app or software package is extremely important. For the software to be effective, the computer functions must be applicable to the specific dental practice. Stored data and information must be usable and easily accessible. The required applications should be presented to the vendor rather than asking the vendor what the dental practice should do. To be more specific, take a routine accounts receivable task and have the vendor explain how it would be processed with that company's equipment and software. Inquire how different procedures (e.g., billing, payments, appointment notification) can be combined. Another option is starting with basic software packages, such as insurance estimating and billing, appointment tracking, treatment planning, marketing, and payroll. It is strongly recommended that an office make sure that the app or software can provide all that they will need going forward. If an office will someday want to use digital radiography, it is very important that the app or software have that option available when the office needs it.

The preceding text illustrates a sampling of dental apps and software programs, all of which help to improve cash flow and increase productivity. The list goes on, however. The word processing function is also invaluable to the dental practice, and it can be integrated with the information system to improve communication with patients. When a computer is used to produce welcome letters, treatment letters, and special greetings, it can be a very effective marketing tool.

When word processing software is used on the computer, the document is prepared electronically, and it is easy to edit a document by making changes in the text. Text can be corrected by using the backspace or delete key. Words, sentences, paragraphs, or pages may be added or deleted from a document. Text can be moved from one section to another. The document is formatted according to individual specifications. For example, margins, type style, double or single spacing, underlining, boldface or italics, and page length are determined by the user. When the document is finalized and all corrections made, the document can be printed. More than one copy can be made, and each copy is an original. These documents are stored in the computer's memory, and they can be used again as is or edited and brought up to date.

Many word processing packages include other features, such as spell checking, grammar checking, and a thesaurus. Some spell-checking software enables you to add words that are common to your specific dental practice.

Word processing software can be a very productive tool for the dental practice and should be selected wisely. Box 5-7 lists common features of word processing apps and software packages.

An electronic spreadsheet app or software package allows the user to organize numeric data in a worksheet or table format. The user enters the data into the formula that has been typed in specific rows and columns, which are known as *cells*. As the data are entered into the proper cells, electronic calculations are performed automatically. Daily postings and updates can be made very easily. An electronic spreadsheet's ability to recalculate data makes this an invaluable tool for business office management.

A graphics app or software package allows the user to create graphs from numeric data; this is sometimes part of the spreadsheet software package. The most common forms of graphics are pie charts, line charts, and bar charts (see Figure 5-20). Graphs are good management tools for reviewing information and helping to communicate information more effectively. A popular graph is used in periodontal charting. In Figure 5-21 is an example of an automated periodontal probe system that records, stores, and prints the data in a readable form for the dentist or hygienist to review with the patient. When using graphics in a presentation, select the type of graph that is most appropriate for your purpose. Do not try to present too much information; use few words, be consistent, and keep the graphics simple.

INTEGRATED APPLICATIONS

Today most dental apps and software packages integrate electronic spreadsheets and word processing capabilities into the software. As stated previously, choosing the right software for the specific need of the dental practice can be difficult. The information in Box 5-8 should help with the making of this decision. The selection process for the computing device and the appropriate apps or software requires a great deal of thought

BOX 5-7

Common Features of Word Processors

Insert
- Insert character(s)
- Insert word(s)
- Insert line(s)
- Insert document(s)
- Insert graphics
- Insert pictures

Delete
- Delete character(s)
- Delete word(s)
- Delete sentence(s)
- Delete paragraph(s)
- Delete page(s)
- Delete entire document

Keyboard and Screen Control Printing
- Cursor movement
- Page up and down
- Word wrap
- Upper- and lower-case display
- Function keys
- Control keys
- Status line
- Line
- Column

Format
- Top and bottom margins
- Left and right margins
- Tab stops
- Single and double spacing

Move
- Move sentence(s)
- Move paragraph(s)
- Move blocks

Search and Replace
- Search to specific text
- Search and replace word
- Search and replace character strings

Tools
- Spelling and grammar
- Thesaurus
- Track changes
- Merge documents
- Letters and mailings
- Table
- Insert
- Delete
- Sort
- Printing
- Print columns
- Subscripts
- Superscripts
- Underline
- Boldface
- Headers
- Footers
- Page numbering
- Document title

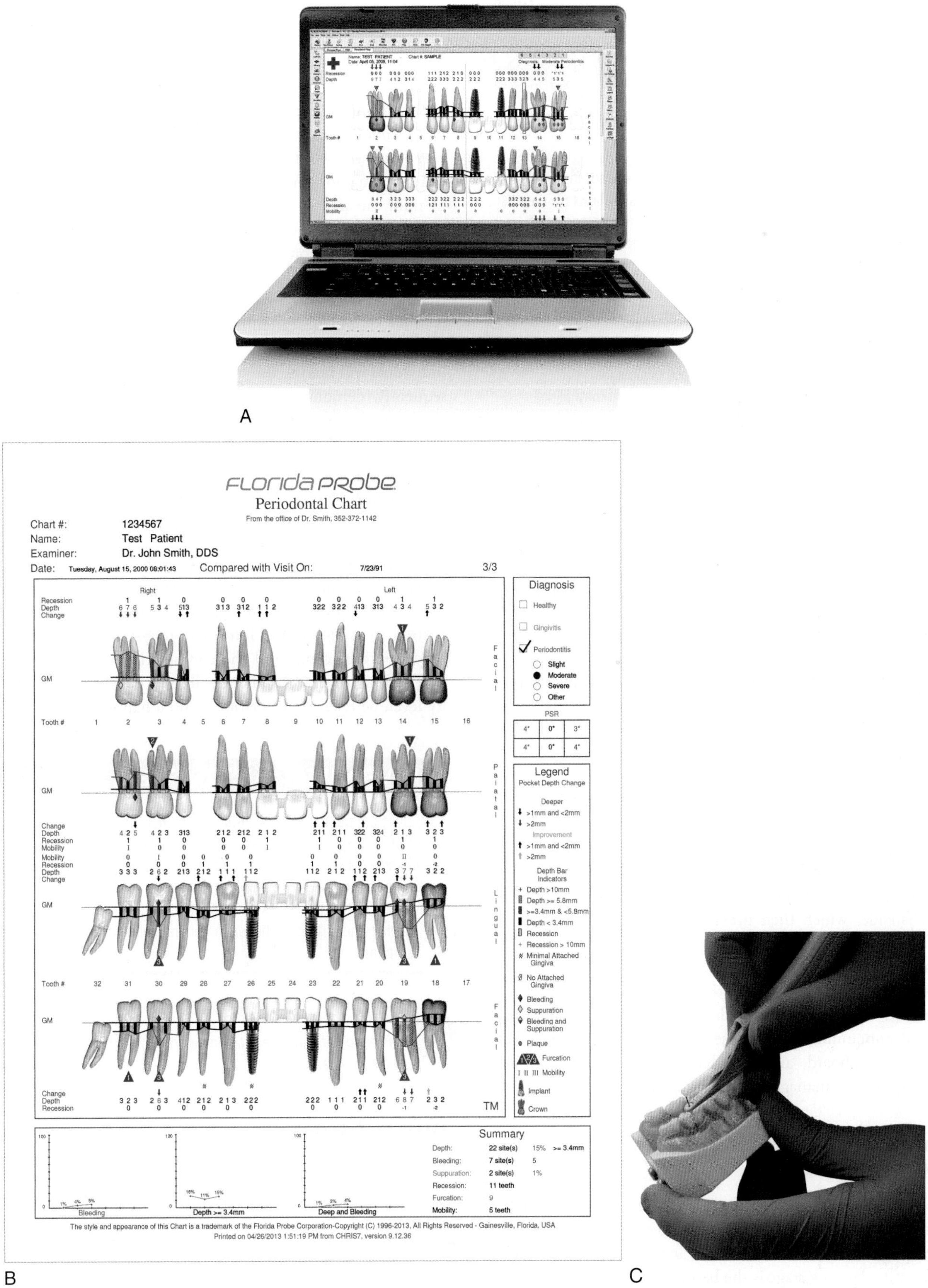

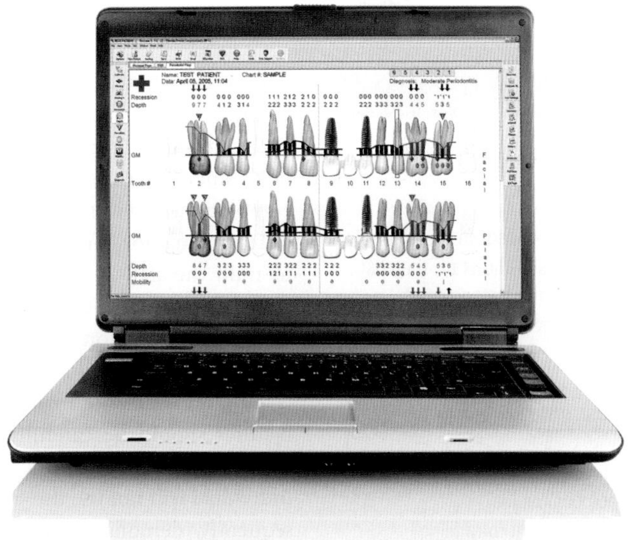

A

FLORIDA PROBE

Periodontal Chart

From the office of Dr. Smith, 352-372-1142

Chart #: 1234567
Name: Test Patient
Examiner: Dr. John Smith, DDS
Date: Tuesday, August 15, 2000 08:01:43 Compared with Visit On: 7/23/91 3/3

Right Left

Recession
Depth
Change

GM

Tooth # 1 2 3 4 5 6 7 8 9 10 11 12 13 14 15 16

Change
Depth
Recession
Mobility

Tooth # 32 31 30 29 28 27 26 25 24 23 22 21 20 19 18 17

Change
Depth
Recession

TM

Diagnosis
Healthy
Gingivitis
Periodontitis
Slight
Moderate
Severe
Other

PSR

4*	0*	3*
4*	0*	4*

Legend
Pocket Depth Change
Deeper
>1mm and <2mm
>2mm
Improvement
>1mm and <2mm
>2mm
Depth Bar Indicators
Depth >10mm
Depth >= 5.8mm
>=3.4mm & <5.8mm
Depth < 3.4mm
Recession
Recession > 10mm
Minimal Attached Gingiva
No Attached Gingiva
Bleeding
Suppuration
Bleeding and Suppuration
Plaque
Furcation
I II III Mobility
Implant
Crown

Bleeding Depth >= 3.4mm Deep and Bleeding

Summary

Depth:	22 site(s)	15%	>= 3.4mm
Bleeding:	7 site(s)	5	
Suppuration:	2 site(s)	1%	
Recession:	11 teeth		
Furcation:	9		
Mobility:	5 teeth		

Printed on 04/26/2013 1:51:19 PM from CHRIS7, version 9.12.36

B

C

FIGURE 5-21 **A,** The Florida Probe Periodontal Exam and Charting System provides highly accurate and repeatable periodontal measurements with superior charting capabilities. The system requires only a single operator, and it records, stores, and prints the examination automatically. **B,** Samples of the periodontal charts automatically produced by the Florida Probe system. **C,** Objective measurements of pocket depth and gingival recession from the cementoenamel junctions are ensured by the probe's constant 15 g of pressure. (Courtesy The Florida Probe, Inc, Gainesville, FL.)

BOX 5-8

Guidelines for Choosing the Right Apps and Software Programs

1. Determine the needs of the dental practice based on the type of practice, the size of the practice, the abilities of the staff, the cost, and the training required for the doctor and the support staff.
2. Select a vendor who is reputable and who provides fast and efficient support when there are questions.
   - Ask about other dental practices that use the system.
   - How many systems has the vendor installed within the geographic area?
   - Are the insurance forms that are processed through the system accepted by participating insurance companies?
   - Does the system provide for electronic claim form filing?
3. Determine what the software does. Does it process insurance claims, improve billing, improve practice management, improve office efficiency and auditing, track delinquent accounts, compute monthly finance charges, or aid in communications as a marketing device?
4. Identify what type of backup system is available in case of computer failure.
5. Establish how security is managed.
6. Determine the type of training available from the vendor. Systems with tutorial software are also available. Some software makes use of online instruction for the learner.

and time so that the selection can be made carefully. Everyone will have to live with the decision that is made.

Clinical Records Applications

Although it may appear that the bulk of record management is generated only in the business office, one cannot overlook the computer as a communication tool between the treatment room and the business office. A variety of charting systems allows a clinical assistant to enter data directly on a keyboard at chairside, which then provides a printout in the business office. An example of this system is shown in the periodontal examination and charting system in Figure 5-21. Systems are available for patient history taking, general and specialty charting, and treatment completed. Such a system also eliminates record contamination, because barrier covers may be placed over the keyboard, and the chances of disease transmission through record management are thus decreased.

Establishing Procedures for Computerization

There are times in the office when it is necessary to modify or change an existing system. Resistance to change can be expected if employees are not made aware of and involved in the change. The early planning stage is the best time to begin communicating with other staff members; their cooperation and support will be gained if they are made aware of the new system's advantages. The staff needs to know that the workload may need to be modified during the update or change and that the workload will be distributed to more than one individual so that it is lessened.

Establishing procedures is necessary to make sure that work flows smoothly through the entire process, from origination to completion. It will probably be necessary to update the procedures manual for computing tasks and then hold staff meetings to train the staff in the use of the new hardware or software, depending on the changes being made. A manual provides detailed information about how various tasks are completed and by whom as well as the purpose of each task.

App and software manuals that are provided by the manufacturer should be carefully evaluated. If the documentation and instructions are difficult to follow and understand, the individual will not use the system properly and efficiently. Consequently, demonstrations and regular staff meetings help to resolve any confusion or conflict that may arise with the use of the new system.

SUMMARY OF TECHNOLOGY IN THE BUSINESS OFFICE

A digital system's primary advantage is the accuracy and quality of its end product. However, without proper management and usage, the system becomes a costly investment with poor returns. A well-planned information system helps make the office more efficient, and the combination of an experienced staff and high-tech equipment will result in a higher productivity level, better patient relations, and a happier staff.

LEARNING ACTIVITIES

1. Describe the importance of an information system to dentistry.
2. List and explain the operations that computing devices can perform.
3. Describe how a feasibility study helps to determine the need for automation.
4. Describe computer apps and software.
5. Explain the difference between general and specific-task apps and software.

Please refer to the student workbook for additional learning activities.

BIBLIOGRAPHY

Fulton-Calkins PJ, Rankin DS, Shumack KA: *The administrative professional*, ed 14, Mason, OH, 2011, Thomson South-Western.

Vermaat ME, Sebok SL, Freund SM: *Discovering computers—technology on a world of computers, mobile devices, and the Internet*, Boston, MA, 2014, Course Technology, Cengage Learning.

RECOMMENDED WEBSITES

www.floridaprobe.com.
www.pattersondental.com.
www.dentistryiq.com.

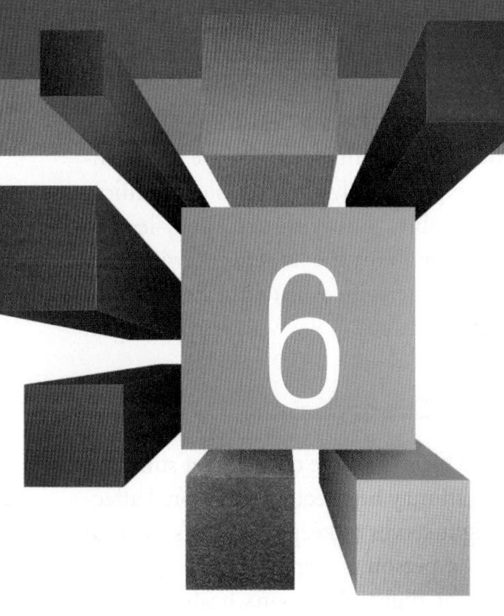

6 Office Design and Equipment Placement

 http://evolve.elsevier.com/Finkbeiner/practice

LEARNING OUTCOMES

1. Define the key terms in this chapter.
2. Describe the physical environmental factors that should be considered when designing a dental office, including:
   - Discuss the impact of the Americans with Disabilities Act on a dental practice.
   - Describe seasonal affective disorder (SAD).
   - Discuss factors to be considered when designing the reception room.
   - Discuss the importance of a business office work triangle.
   - Discuss other considerations in the design of the business office work space.
3. Provide suggestions for workstation organization and the importance of time and motion principles in a dental office.
4. Discuss the importance of body positioning and ergonomics when designing a dental office.
5. Discuss the various office supplies needed for a dental office.

KEY TERMS

Classifications of motion Classifications that refer to the amount of energy it takes to perform various tasks.

Ergonomics The science that studies the relationship between people and their work environments.

Reception room The gateway to the dental office; the reception area provides the patient's first impression of the dentist.

Time and motion A concept that refers to the amount of time and the extent of motion it takes to perform a given task.

At some point during a dental professional's career, it is likely that he or she will be asked to help design, remodel, or improve the efficiency of the dental business office. These responsibilities demand an understanding of the principles of motion economy and the placement of office equipment to create an environment in which a person can work smarter rather than harder.

In the past, more emphasis was placed on the design of the dental treatment rooms than the design of the business office. However, planning of the business office workspace is equally important. This area should be ergonomically designed so that the business staff can perform its tasks with the greatest efficiency. Ergonomics is the science that studies the relationship between people and their work environments. Interrelated physical and psychologic factors are involved in the creation of a stress-free work environment. By understanding the abilities that people have and their work patterns, it is possible to design work environments that conform to the abilities and work needs of the employee. The appropriate use of ergonomics can make the worker more productive and efficient, and it can reduce work-related discomfort and injuries.

PRACTICE NOTE
Ergonomics is the study of the effects of the work environment on health and well-being.

PHYSICAL ENVIRONMENT

Physiologic factors include color, lighting, acoustics, heating and air conditioning, space, and furniture and equipment. Color plays a major role in how a patient perceives a practice and in the staff's health, productivity, and morale. An attractive, cheerful, and efficient office inspires confidence in the staff and comfort in the patient. A drab, dirty, or untidy office can create an attitude of doubt or mistrust. Light and dark colors can be effectively used and may vary according to geographic location.

Some decorators work with dark colors for walls and then use lighter accent colors to downplay the dark base color. Designers today use a variety of color palettes to enhance an office and make it warm and comfortable for both patients and staff. Dental offices no longer need to present a stark, sterile image. A comfortable patient is a happier patient. Moreover, staff productivity is likely to be greater in a pleasant working environment. Many office plans are available; the one chosen should reflect the dentist's personality and satisfy the needs of both staff and patients.

PRACTICE NOTE
An attractive, cheerful, and efficient office inspires confidence in the staff and comfort in the patient.

Office Design and the Americans with Disabilities Act

For years, patients have had difficulty gaining access to dental treatment rooms as a result of poorly designed offices. The Americans with Disabilities Act of 1990 has influenced the design of dental offices with regard to patient treatment. Special attention should be directed to this act to ensure that the office design complies with state and federal guidelines. The Justice Department issues accessibility specifications for offices, but some states have even stricter standards. Accessibility features must be incorporated into building renovations, and those features must be accessible from elsewhere in the building. For example, making a lobby bathroom accessible to a wheelchair patient is not adequate if the patient cannot get to the lobby. Wider hallways enable a patient in a wheelchair to easily access treatment rooms and other areas of the office (Figure 6-1). Box 6-1 presents a list of recommendations for designing a barrier-free office.

The government estimates that the cost of incorporating accessibility features into new construction is less than 1% of construction costs. Because remodeling existing buildings usually is more costly, the requirements for them are less stringent. Currently the law requires only "reasonable modifications" that are "readily achievable," but both terms may lead to litigation. Further information about the Americans with Disabilities Act is available from the sources listed in Box 6-2, or it can be found online at www.ada.gov or www.access-board.gov.

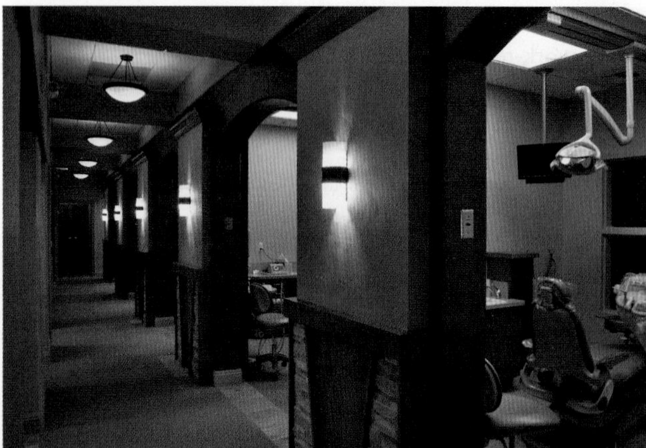

FIGURE 6-1 A hallway made wider per the specifications of the Americans with Disabilities Act enables a patient in a wheelchair to easily access the treatment rooms. (Courtesy EnviroMed Design Group, Boca Raton, FL | Austin, TX.)

Seasonal Affective Disorder

In geographic locations in which there are extremes of sunshine and darkness, patients or staff may be affected by seasonal affective disorder (SAD). Sunlight serves to keep the body's internal circadian clock in sync, so a person is alert and awake during the day and ready to sleep at night. A person's health, mood,

BOX 6-1

Design Features of a Barrier-Free Office

The following modifications used to create a barrier-free environment comply with the Americans with Disabilities Act:

- Designate handicapped parking areas.
- Install sidewalk and curb access to accommodate wheelchairs or other devices.
- Install access ramps to building and office areas.
- Widen doors and doorways to accommodate wheelchairs and other devices.
- Install raised letters and Braille on elevator controls.
- Provide visual and sound alarms.
- Install grab bars.
- Install raised toilet seats and wider stalls.
- Make paper towel dispensers accessible.
- Install paper cup dispensers at existing water fountains.
- Eliminate plush, low-density carpeting.

BOX 6-2

Sources of Information About the Americans With Disabilities Act

Office of the Americans with Disabilities Act
US Department of Justice
P.O. Box 66118
Washington, DC 20035-6738
1-800-514-0301 (voice)
1-800-514-0383 (TTY)
www.ada.gov

Architectural and Transportation Barriers Compliance Board
1111 18th Street NW, Suite 501
Washington, DC 20036
1-800-872-2253 (voice)
1-800-993-2822 (TTY)
202-272-5448 (Electronic bulletin board)
www.access-board.gov

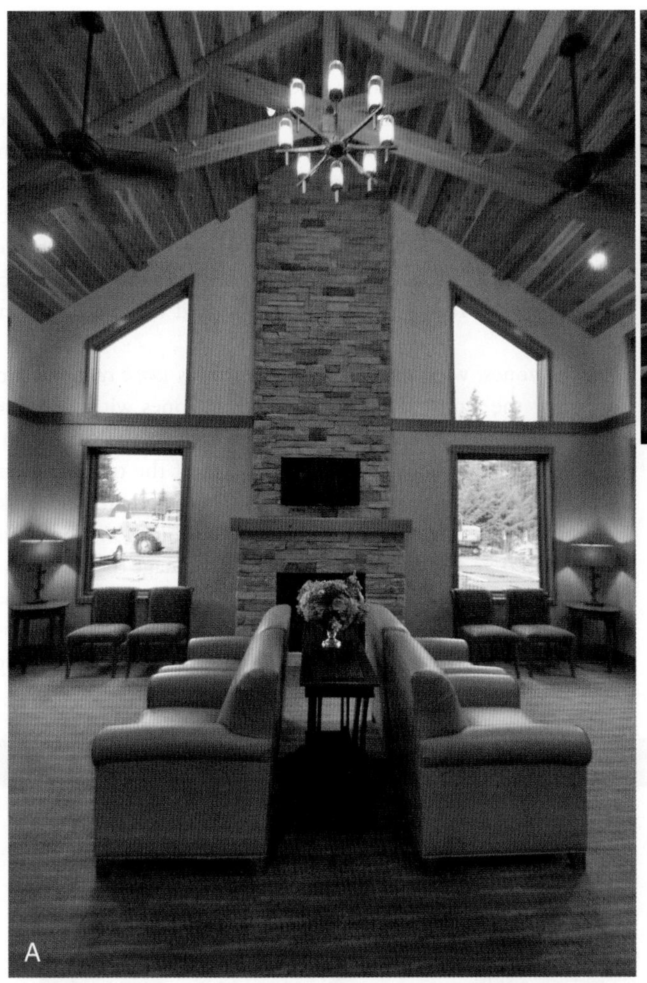

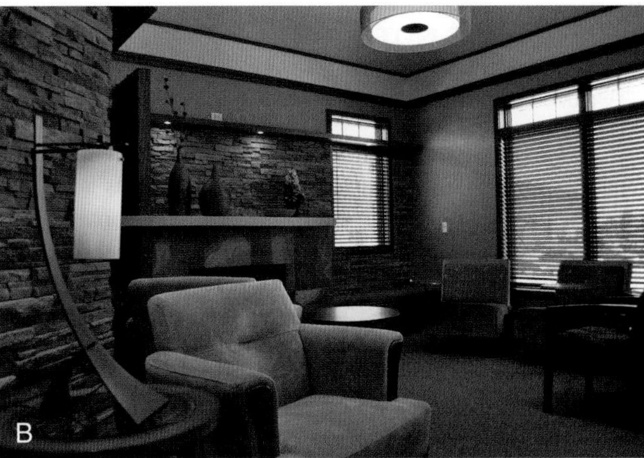

FIGURE 6-2 **A,** The reception room of a dental office reflects the theme of the practice. Open areas allow a patient personal space as well as space in which to work. **B,** A reception room with comfortable chairs provides adequate seating space (Courtesy EnviroMed Design Group, Boca Raton, Florida | Austin, Texas.)

and behavior can be affected when the quality and quantity of sunlight are lessened. A direct consequence of SAD can be winter depression or sleep disorders.

Many offices provide lighting systems to help individuals overcome SAD. If staff members are affected by SAD, it may be worth the investment in such lights to increase the health of the staff. Most of the lights are designed for the brightness needed for light therapy. With a brightness level of 10,000 lux at 18 to 24 inches, these lights have been proved to provide fast and effective light therapy at a comfortable distance. Most of these lights are easy and safe to use (i.e., they contain no harmful ultraviolet rays). It is also recommended that a person with SAD have his or her treatment room or desk placed near a window. This may not be feasible in some office designs, but it may be a factor to consider with new construction.

Design of the Reception Room

The reception room (the term *waiting room* has a negative connotation and so its use is being phased out) is the gateway to the dental office, and it provides the patient's first impression of the dentist. A warm atmosphere can be created in the reception room by furnishing a comfortable "living room" environment. The office should reflect the theme that originates in the reception room (Figure 6-2).

Patients should be able to check in with the administrative assistant at the desk as soon as they arrive. For privacy, patients should have access to a restroom off of the reception room, and appropriate signs should direct them to this area.

Seating in the reception room varies from office to office, depending on individual practice styles. A general rule is to provide two seats for each dental chair in a general practice. High-volume practices, such as orthodontics or pediatrics, require three or four seats per dental chair, whereas an oral surgery or endodontic practice needs only one or two seats per chair.

Seating space is an important consideration. People generally do not like to have others sitting too close to them. When completing forms or other business activities, a person needs some privacy. Comfort should be the major concern when selecting furniture for this area; it needs to be sturdy but not too formal or too casual. Low, cushiony couches and armless chairs are sometimes difficult for even an agile person to get out of and even more difficult for an older adult or an arthritic patient. Figure 6-2, *B*, illustrates comfortable armchairs with sturdy bases.

PRACTICE NOTE

The reception room is the gateway to the dental office, and it provides the patient's first impression of the dentist.

Special amenities are a thoughtful gesture, such as a desk-height table with an electrical outlet that makes it convenient for businesspeople or students to bring laptop computers to use while waiting. A self-serve coffee or juice bar is a considerate gesture toward busy patients. These amenities send a message that the dentist respects patients' time and wants to make the office a friendly place to visit (Box 6-3).

Business Office Work Triangle

The design of the business office can be likened to the design of a kitchen in one's home. A kitchen design starts with the "work triangle," which keeps the three primary work centers or zones in close proximity, thereby eliminating wasted effort and time. The triangle in a kitchen is measured from the center of the sink to the center of the refrigerator to the center of the cooktop. Likewise, the design of a business office can take into consideration three main zones: the reception zone, the intraoffice communication center, and the work area zone. A good rule of thumb would be to measure the distance from the center of the reception zone to the center of the communications zone and to the center of the work zone to ensure that the perimeter of the triangle does not exceed 26 feet. This distance should be uninterrupted by traffic or cabinetry. Limiting the distances between these three zones allows the business office staff to be efficient while reducing the stress associated with walking long distances.

The zones, which may also be known as *work centers*, complement the work triangle. By planning zones within the triangle, one can ensure that different tasks can be carried out without collisions. In the reception zone of the triangle, there should be adequate space to meet and greet patients and make appointments. In the intraoffice communication zone, the administrative assistant should be able to manage the telephone; to access a computer for appointments, clinical data, financial records, or other information; and to communicate with the clinical areas. The work zone maintains space for preparing,

BOX 6-3

Keys to Creating a Comfortable Reception Room

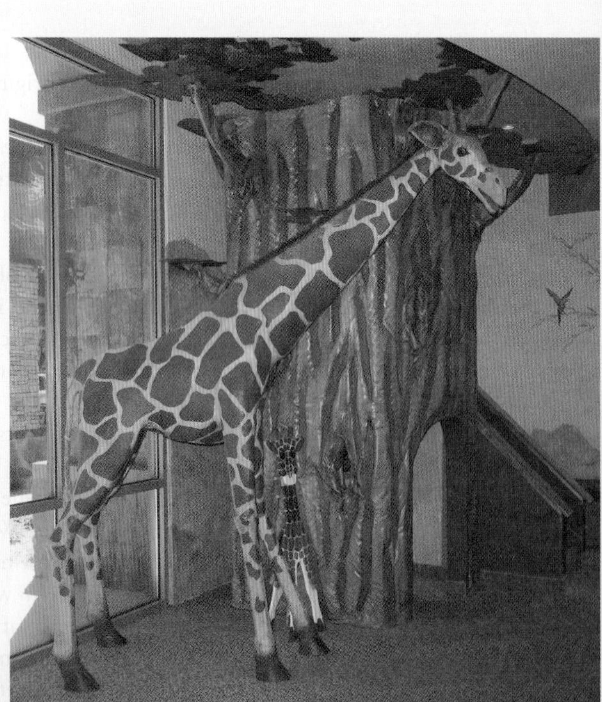

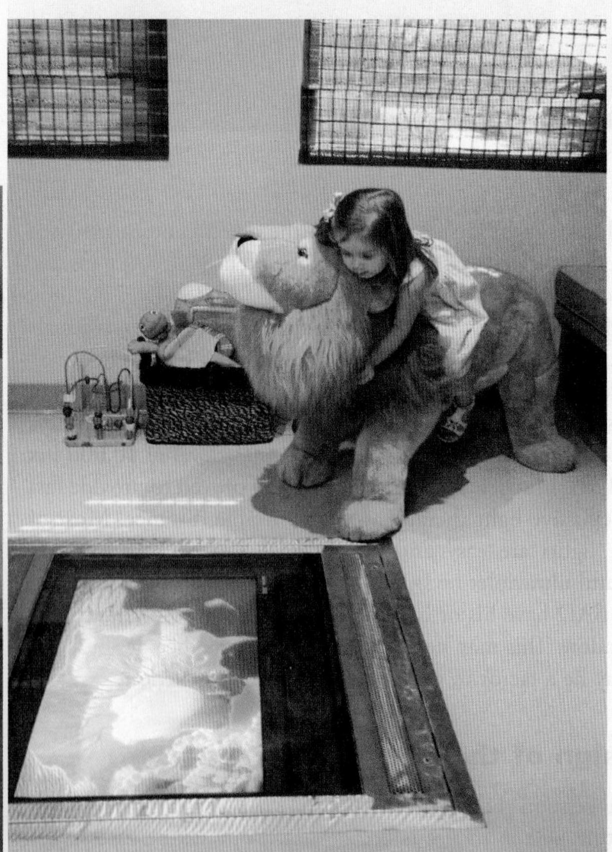

A and **B**, Children's area with alternative seating. (Courtesy of Affiliated Pediatric Dentistry and Orthodontics, Scottsdale, Arizona.)

BOX 6-3—cont'd

Keys to Creating a Comfortable Reception Room

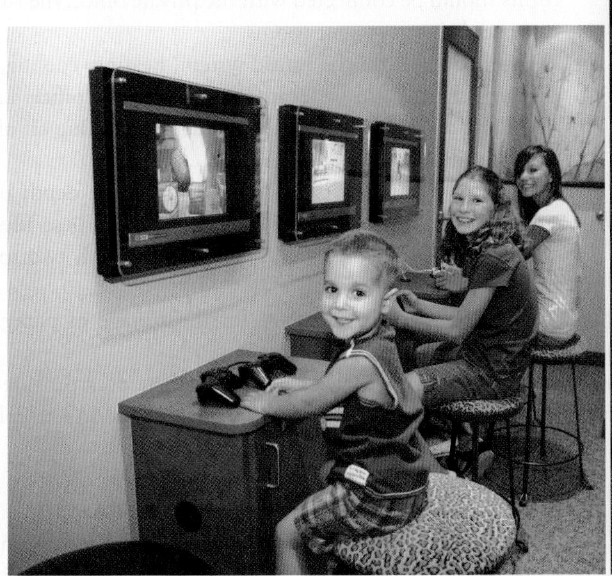

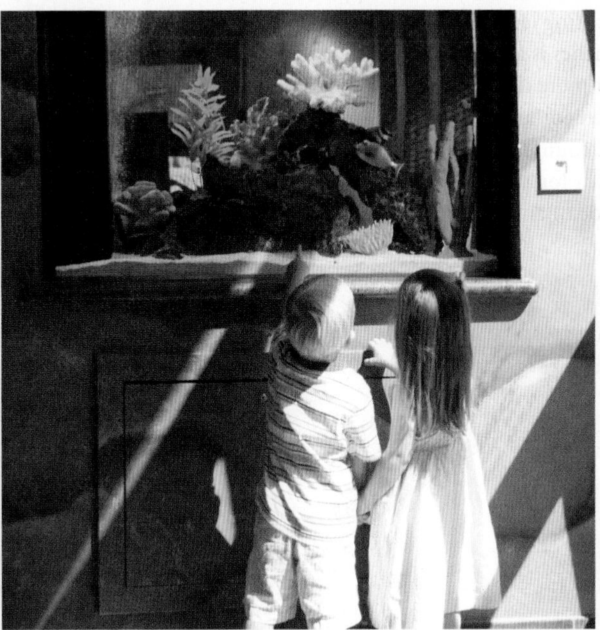

C, A video game corner provides a computer and games for children to play in the reception room. **D,** A fish tank can be entertaining to both adults and children in the reception room. (Courtesy of Affiliated Pediatric Dentistry and Orthodontics, Scottsdale, Arizona.)

- A soft warning bell or chimes should announce the patient's arrival in the reception area.
- The patient's arrival should be acknowledged immediately. A clear glass window affords privacy yet allows the administrative assistant to see all of the activity in the reception room. Today many offices are designed with open, barrier-free reception areas. Whether a window or a barrier-free opening is used, it is commonly placed 44 inches from the floor and has a size of at least 36 × 36 inches. A barrier-free environment can be created with the open concept. A desk area for physically challenged patients is positioned 27 to 29 inches from the floor.
- Coat racks should be convenient for both children and adults. A nearby bench benefits older adults, small children, and anyone putting on boots.
- Magazine racks can be placed on a wall or table for patient convenience.
- If necessary, a small children's corner can be included (see Figure 6-4, D). In many specialty offices (e.g., orthodontics, pediatric dentistry), an office theme can be created.
- The style and number of seats and tables depend on the patients' requirements. A combination of sofas and chairs also provides a comfortable seating arrangement. Chairs should be of a height and depth that afford easy seating and exiting.
- An automatic air freshener eliminates "dental" odors, and cordial "no smoking" signs can be posted at the entrance to the office and in the reception room.
- An adjoining restroom eliminates trips to the inner office.
- Wood paneling, fabric, textured wallpaper, antiques, live plants, artwork, and mirrors add warmth to the reception room and reflect the dentist's personality.
- Signs directing patients to various rooms should be large and easy for all patients to read.
- Lighting intensity and color should be adequate for the easy reading of printed materials in any part of the room.

filing, or copying records; using the fax machine; or performing other activities that require counter space or file access. Figure 6-3 illustrates an example of a work triangle.

Design of the Business Office

The business office workspace should provide a healthful and enjoyable environment that minimizes disruption and distraction. The business office should be centrally located between the reception room and the dental treatment rooms. This central location is convenient for the patient, and it allows the administrative assistant to be aware of the activities in the office. Figure 6-4 illustrates two different floor plans that make use of a central location for the business office. The first is an example of a small dental office; the second is a basic floor plan for a team concept that includes advanced functions dental staff. The factors involved in designing a business office work environment are motion economy, space planning, health issues, safety, and security. The following suggestions should also be considered:

- The administrative assistant or receptionist should be seated facing the reception room.
- Two desk heights ensure comfort and efficiency. The keyboard level should be approximately 27 inches, and the writing level should be about 29 inches (Figure 6-5). Twenty inches is an adequate depth for most working areas. A depth of more than 30 inches is excessive; it makes reaching inconvenient and reduces the amount of floor space in the office.
- A counter approximately 44 inches high provides a writing area for patients, as well as privacy for the assistant and for documents placed on the counter (see Figure 6-5).

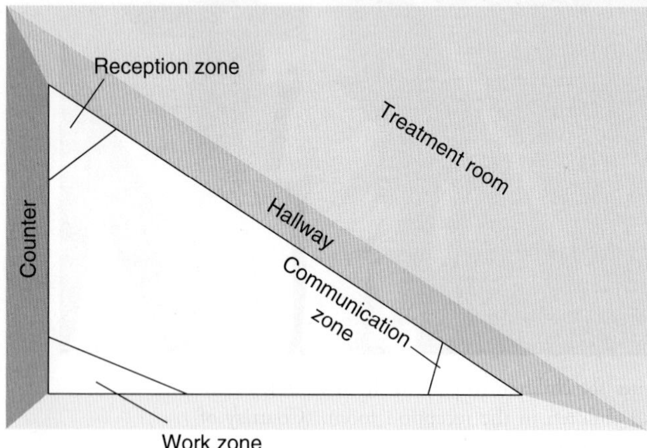

FIGURE 6-3 A business office work triangle designed to include the reception, intraoffice communication, and work zones within a 26-foot perimeter.

- The business office clock should be out of view of patients in the reception room.
- Central controls for an intercom system should be integrated with the telephone or mounted on the wall as a separate unit within easy reach of the assistant (Figure 6-6). Auxiliary units should be connected with the private office, the laboratory, and the treatment rooms.
- Master controls for the music system, heating, cooling, and lighting should also be located in the business office. Labeling these controls prevents the accidental shutting off of any of the utilities.
- Lateral or open files (see Figure 6-7) with a depth of 18 inches require less space than vertical files. These files are supplied in 30-, 36-, and 42-inch widths with two to five drawers.
- Cupboard space is necessary for the storage of paper and supplies.
- Small compartmentalized areas above the desk provide easy access to items such as appointment cards and telephone message pads.
- Telephones should be installed at each workstation and should be made hands free whenever possible.
- Desk drawers should have full suspension for maximum use.
- Inserts and dividers in drawers help with the organization of materials.
- A small area adjacent to the business office set up for private calls and conversations with patients is convenient and can be used for the completion of insurance forms.

Many of these criteria have been incorporated into the design of the business office shown in Figures 6-4 and 6-5.

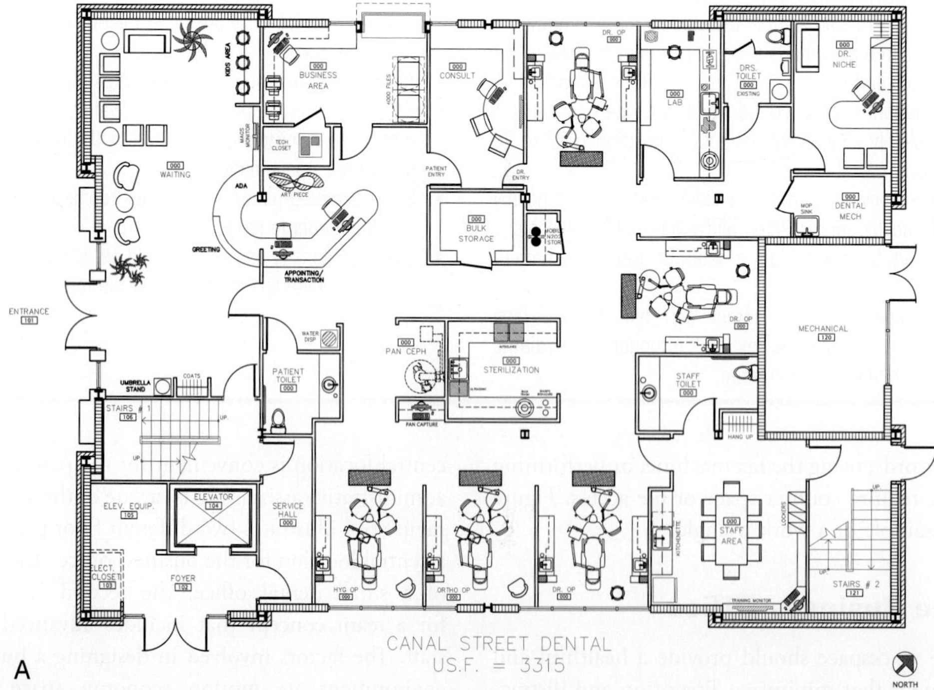

FIGURE 6-4 Sample dental office designs. **A,** A small office designed for efficiency and patient comfort includes all of the basic rooms and also provides openness.

FLOOR PLAN

1 PATIENT ENTRY
2 RECEPTION
3 TOILET ROOM
4 APPOINTMENTS
5 FRONT DESK
6 OFFICE MANAGER
7 BUSINESS AREA
8 CONSULT #1
9 CONSULT #2
10 TOILET ROOM
11 PAN-CEPH
12 OPERATORY
13 DIGITAL SCANNING
14 HYG. COORD. STAND UP
15 HYGIENE STORAGE
16 STERILIZATION
17 DOCTOR STORAGE
18 DENTAL MECHANICAL
19 CENTRAL COMPUTERS
20 CLEAN LAB
21 MESSY LAB
22 STAFF ENTRY
23 CHANGING
24 STAFF TOILET
25 STAFF LOUNGE
26 DR.'S OFFICE
27 DR.'S TOILET
28 COURTYARD
29 TRELLIS

N

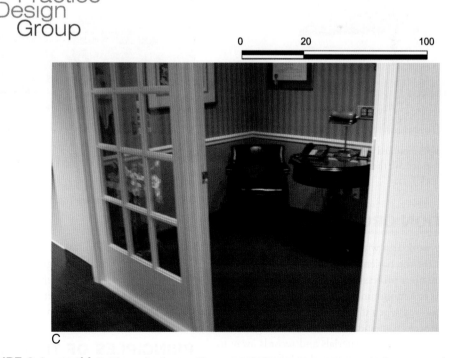

the Practice Design Group

B

0 20 100

C

FIGURE 6-4, cont'd **B,** This multi-dentist office suite includes an open concept, multiple treatment and hygiene rooms, and a larger reception area; it also provides patient privacy. **C,** A consultation room adjacent to the business office provides privacy for the patient and the dentist. (**A** and **B,** Courtesy PDGFazio Design Group, Austin, Texas. **C,** Courtesy Joseph Ellis, DDS, and Lisa Tartaglione, DDS, Grand Rapids, Michigan.)

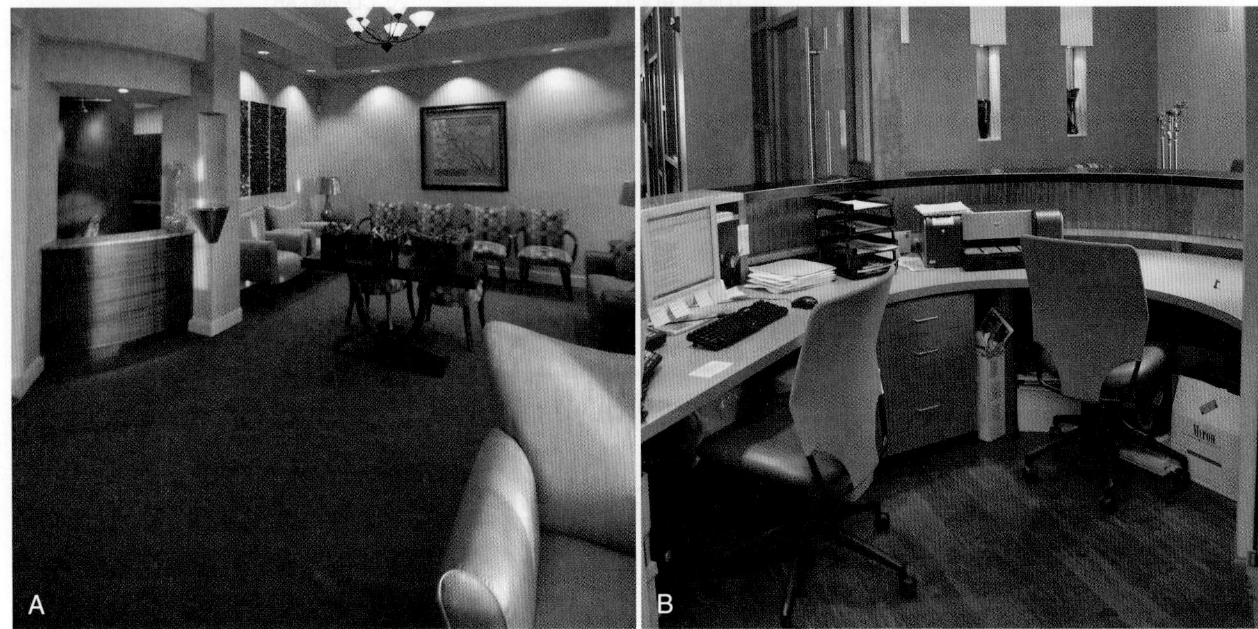

FIGURE 6-5 **A,** Counter space in the business office provides the patient with a comfortable position for performing business transactions from the reception room. **B,** The inner business office counter is working height for the staff, whereas the counter as seen from the reception room is convenient for the patient. (Courtesy EnviroMed Design Group, Boca Raton, Florida | Austin, Texas.)

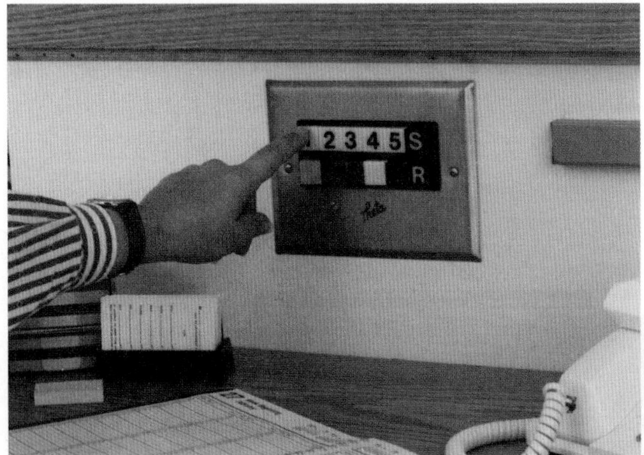

FIGURE 6-6 A wall-mounted nonverbal intercom system places controls within easy reach of the assistant. (Courtesy Theta Corp, Niagara Falls, New York.)

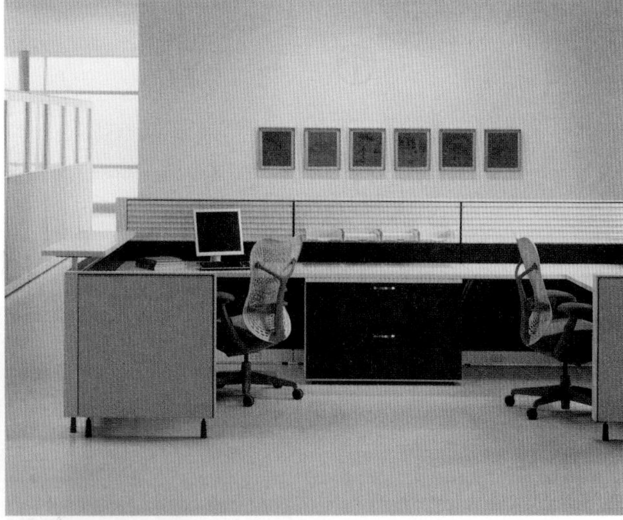

FIGURE 6-7 Lateral files require less space than vertical files. (Courtesy Herman Miller, Inc, Zeeland, Michigan.)

WORKSTATION ORGANIZATION

A neat and orderly work area within the business office creates a good impression for the patient, the staff, and other visitors to the office. Maintain a professional image in this area, and keep personal items to a minimum. Of course, the policy of the office should be followed when displaying any such items.

Keep the work area clean and neat. If outside cleaning services are used, remember to place all materials and records away to avoid loss, damage, or potential confidentiality infringement.

To help the staff submit materials to the assistant, an inbox and an outbox should be placed on the desk. Sturdy wide folders can be used to hold materials that need "To Be Faxed," "To Be Scanned," "To Be Signed," or "To Be Recorded." This type of organization will keep items from getting lost in the outbox. Keeping these materials within the work zone will ensure that they will be given appropriate attention.

PRINCIPLES OF TIME AND MOTION

When determining the placement of office equipment and supplies, the principles of time and motion should be considered.

The concept of *time and motion* refers to the amount of time and the degree of motion required to perform a given task. This principle is as important in the business office as in the dental treatment rooms. Many studies and much research have gone into minimizing the amount of time and motion it takes to perform basic chairside tasks. However, these principles have not always been applied to the dental business office. Because the dentist seldom spends time in the business office, the staff's suggestions should be considered when designing the area. Before positioning equipment and supplies, staff members should determine the most common tasks and the most routinely used materials, and they should attempt to classify the motions that are most commonly used.

During the early 1950s, researchers at the University of Alabama classified motions according to the amount of energy required to perform various chairside tasks. These classifications of motion systems (Box 6-4) can also be applied to the business office. The administrative assistant should try to use only Class I, II, and III motions, which require the least amount of energy and thus reduce stress.

To improve motion economy, it is often necessary to eliminate unnecessary steps or tasks, rearrange equipment and materials, organize procedures, simplify tasks, and evaluate outcomes. The principles of motion economy (Box 6-5) can help with the accomplishment of each of these goals, thereby reducing stress and increasing productivity in the practice.

BODY POSITIONING

Basic Principles

The administrative assistant must consider proper seating arrangements for routine daily activities. When possible, all activities should be performed in a seated position to avoid undue stress on the neck, back, and legs. A chair with a broad base, four or five casters, and a well-padded seat and back support is helpful (Figure 6-8). Improper posture while standing or sitting can lead to fatigue, which in turn affects productivity. The suggestions presented in Box 6-6 can help ensure the greatest levels of comfort and efficiency.

Figure 6-9 illustrates a proper seated posture while using a computer with a tabletop monitor. An alternative position for the computer monitor is to recess it beneath the desk as shown in Figure 6-9, *B*. The schematic drawing in Figure 6-9, *C*, illustrates the positioning of a person in an ergonomic chair when using the recessed monitor.

BOX 6-4

Classifications of Motion

Class I: Fingers-only movement
Class II: Fingers and wrist movement
Class III: Fingers, wrist, and elbow movement
Class IV: Fingers, wrist, elbow, and shoulder movement
Class V: Arm extension and twisting of the torso

BOX 6-5

Applying the Principles of Motion Economy in the Business Office

- Position materials as close to the point of use as possible.
- Use motions that require the least amount of movement.
- Minimize the number of materials to be used for a given procedure.
- Use smooth, continuous motions rather than zigzag motions.
- Organize materials in a logical sequence of use.
- Position materials and equipment in advance whenever possible.
- Use ergonomically designed stools or chairs to provide good posture and body support.
- Use body motions that require the least amount of time.
- Minimize the number of eye movements.
- Provide lighting that eliminates shadows in work areas.
- Avoid abrupt contrasts in room lighting to minimize eyestrain.
- Position computer monitors to allow for a line of sight to the screen that is within 10 to 40 degrees horizontal.
- Provide work areas that are elbow level or 1 to 2 inches lower.

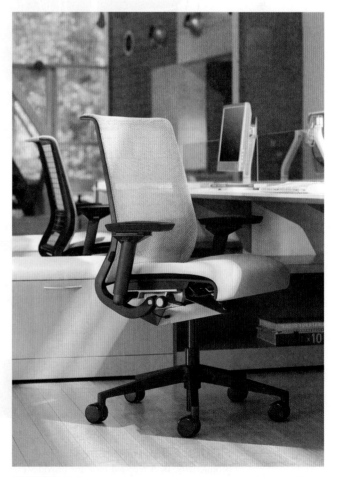

FIGURE 6-8 An ergonomically designed office chair with padded seating and proper back support promotes productivity. (Courtesy Steelcase, Inc., Grand Rapids, Michigan)

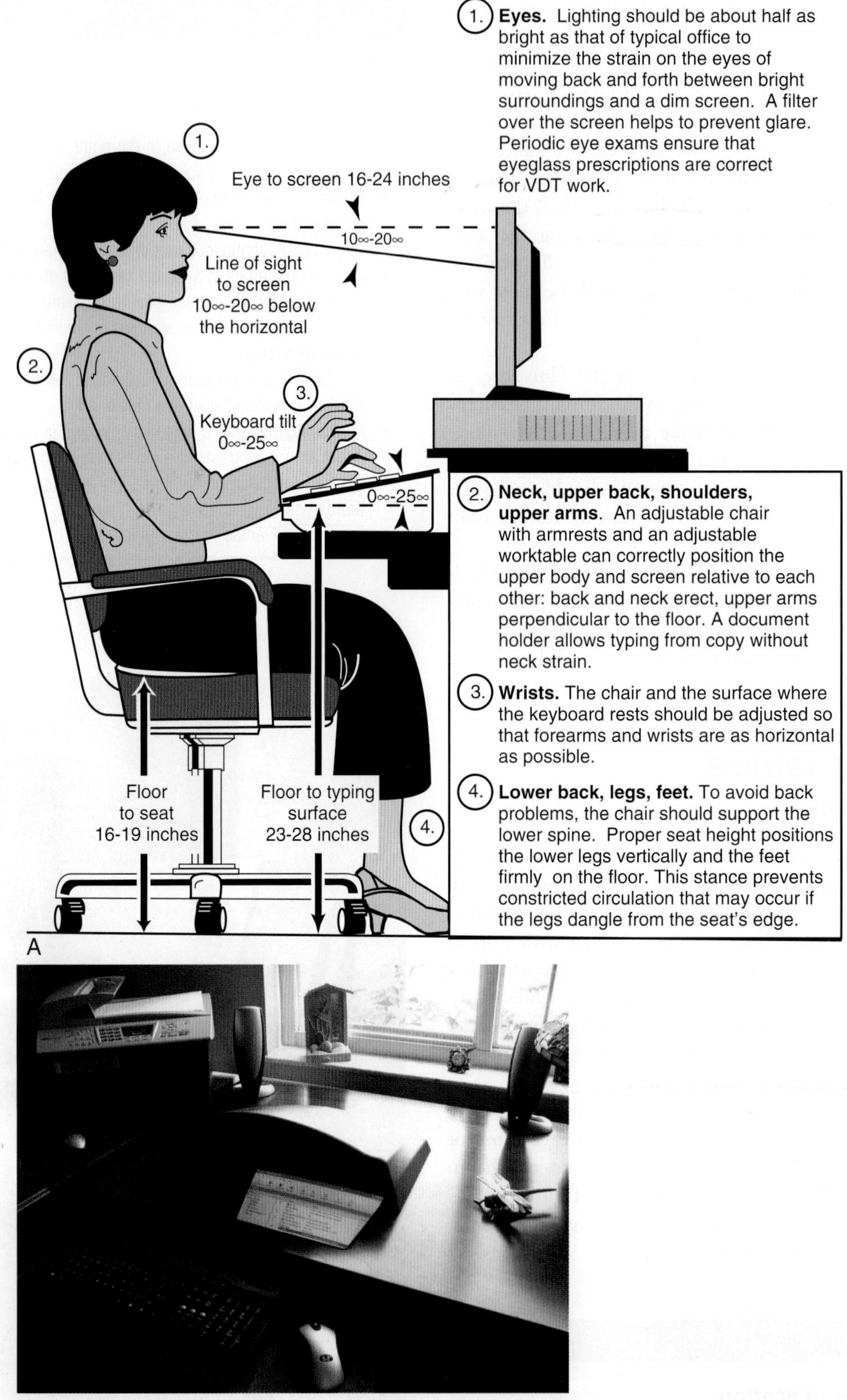

1. Eyes. Lighting should be about half as bright as that of typical office to minimize the strain on the eyes of moving back and forth between bright surroundings and a dim screen. A filter over the screen helps to prevent glare. Periodic eye exams ensure that eyeglass prescriptions are correct for VDT work.
1.
Eye to screen 16-24 inches
10∞-20∞
Line of sight to screen 10∞-20∞ below the horizontal
2.
3.
Keyboard tilt 0∞-25∞
0∞-25∞
2. Neck, upper back, shoulders, upper arms. An adjustable chair with armrests and an adjustable worktable can correctly position the upper body and screen relative to each other: back and neck erect, upper arms perpendicular to the floor. A document holder allows typing from copy without neck strain.
3. Wrists. The chair and the surface where the keyboard rests should be adjusted so that forearms and wrists are as horizontal as possible.
4. Lower back, legs, feet. To avoid back problems, the chair should support the lower spine. Proper seat height positions the lower legs vertically and the feet firmly on the floor. This stance prevents constricted circulation that may occur if the legs dangle from the seat's edge.
Floor to seat 16-19 inches
Floor to typing surface 23-28 inches
4.
A
B

FIGURE 6-9 **A,** Proper posture and positioning in relation to office equipment promotes high-level productivity. **B,** A recessed monitor provides ergonomic positioning and an increased work surface on the desk.

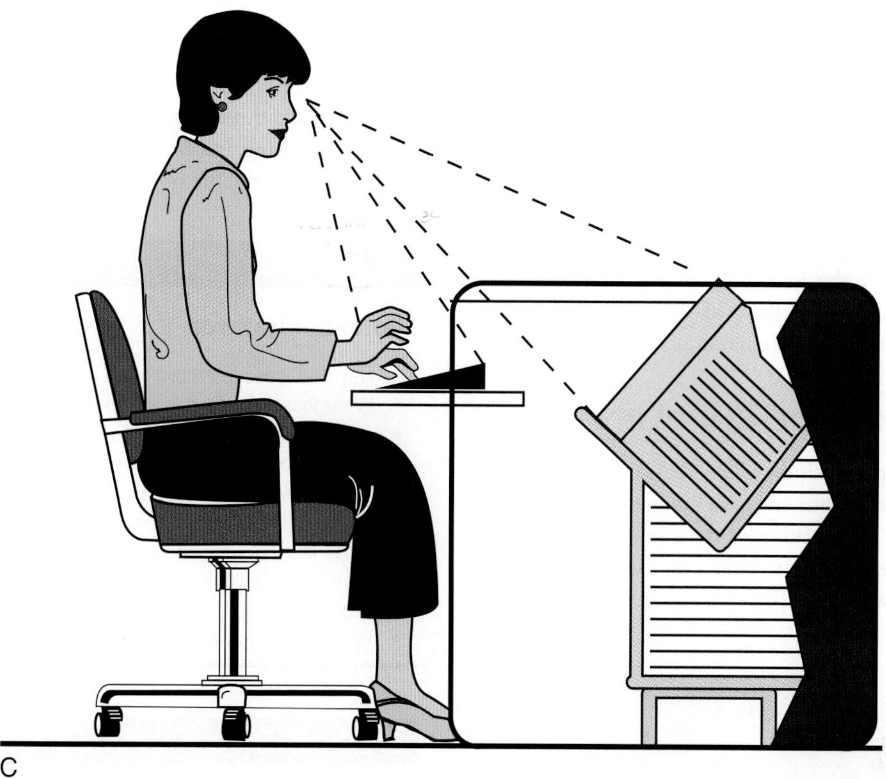

FIGURE 6-9, cont'd C, A schematic illustrates the ergonomic position of an operator using a Nova Solutions station.

BOX 6-6

Ergonomically Correct Body Positioning

- When a person is seated, the thighs should be parallel with the floor, the lower legs vertical, and the feet firmly on the floor.
- When a person is using a keyboard, the arms should be positioned so that the forearms and wrists are as horizontal as possible.
- The distance from the eyes to the computer screen should be 16 to 24 inches.
- The keyboard should tilt 0 to 25 degrees.
- The back and neck should be erect, and the upper arms should be perpendicular to the floor.
- The buttocks should be well supported by the chair seat, which should be 16 to 19 inches from the floor.

Tilt and glare are both factors to consider during monitor placement. When the recessed monitor position is used, it is necessary to follow the manufacturer's recommended position to avoid any neck problems. Two side benefits of recessed monitor placement are the elimination of the patient observing the monitor screen and additional space made available on the desktop. Persons who have used this system often wonder why they have always used the desktop monitor. For further information about this system, visit the website of Nova Solutions (www.novadesk.com). Refer to Box 6-6 for recommendations regarding desk height and foot clearance when these types of systems are used. Much of the success of an office may be attributed to its efficiency and productivity without loss or waste. Again, the goal of ergonomic body positioning should be working smarter rather than harder.

Health and Safety Issues

A variety of factors can affect the health and safety of business office personnel. For example, spending hours each day looking at a computer screen can result in eyestrain and fatigue. Repetitive keyboarding can lead to wrist discomfort and possibly to carpal tunnel syndrome, although the use of an ergonomically designed keyboard (Figure 6-10) can help reduce this stress. The following tips can help reduce fatigue and eyestrain when working at a computer:

- Make sure the screen is neither too dark nor too bright.
- If you are using the computer continuously, take a 10- to 15-minute break every 2 or 3 hours.
- Use good posture.
- Stand up every half hour.
- Periodically look away from the screen for a few minutes.
- Use an ergonomically designed mouse, such as one with a track ball.
- Use an ergonomically designed chair.
- Consider a recessed monitor system.

Safety hazards can exist in the dental business office. In 1970, the Occupational Safety and Health Act was passed to ensure that workers in the United States have safe working environments. Much has been discussed in terms of the relation of this act to the dental treatment room, but often the impact on the business area is overlooked. The Occupational Safety and Health Administration (OSHA) requires employers to provide a hazard-free work environment, which means that it is one without recognized dangers that can cause death, injury, or illness. Box 6-7 presents a list of hazards that can be found in a business office. Of course, in dental and medical offices, this list is compounded by the possibility of disease transmission (see Chapter 17). The lists in Boxes 6-7 and 6-8 can be used periodically to check for possible hazards.

SELECTING OFFICE SUPPLIES

When first setting up a business office, determining what supplies will be needed may be an overwhelming task. Many dental suppliers assist with the stocking of the clinical area, but they seldom consider the "nuts and bolts" of the business office. Box 6-9 on the following page presents a basic list of the various forms and office supplies required in a dental business office. Most office supply companies can assist you, and a variety of stationery suppliers can provide samples of stationery and forms. A walk through a favorite office supply discount store can be fascinating and fun, but only the supplies that are most needed should actually be bought.

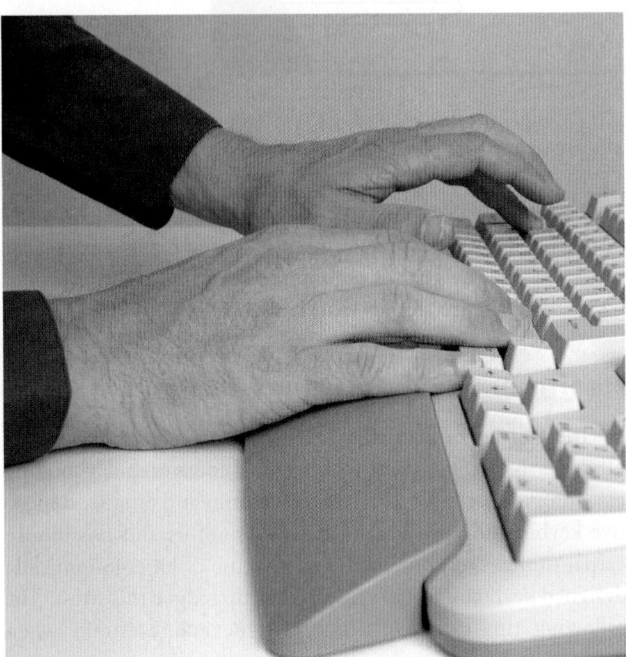

FIGURE 6-10 An ergonomic keyboard reduces overuse stress on the wrist. (Copyright © 2014 BigStock.com.)

BOX 6-7

Potential Hazards

- Frayed or loose telephone cords or electrical wires
- Wires loosely secured to the floor
- Improperly grounded wall or floor switches
- Use of improper electric current to electronic equipment
- Spilled beverages or food on the floor
- Paper cutters, knives, or spindle files
- Loose floor covering on the stairs or floor
- Wearing of jewelry that can be caught in electronic equipment (e.g., copiers)
- Open files or drawers

BOX 6-8

Hazard Checklist

The following points should be evaluated routinely to ensure that safety measures have been observed:

- Floor coverings are durable and in good repair.
- Floor surfaces in clinical areas are hard and uncarpeted.
- Antislip protection is available on smooth floor surfaces.
- Electrical equipment and cords are in safe operating condition.
- Employees have been trained in the proper operation of equipment.
- Only one drawer of a file cabinet is opened at a time.
- Office furniture has stable arms and legs and no sharp edges.
- The locations of eyewash areas are posted in laboratory and clinical areas.
- First aid kits are well stocked and readily accessible.
- "No smoking" signs are posted in visible locations.
- All guidelines for infection control from the Occupational Safety and Health Administration (OSHA) are followed and posted in visible locations.
- Hazard information is posted and available for all employees.

BOX 6-9

Basic Office Supplies

General Supplies

Ballpoint pens
Calendar and calendar holder
Clear tape with dispenser
Double-sided tape with dispenser
Erasers
Felt-tip markers
Hole puncher; one, two, and three-hole puncher
Label maker
Letter opener
Masking tape
Paper clips (small and large)

BOX 6-9

Basic Office Supplies—cont'd

Paper cutter
Paper shredder
Pen holder
Pencil sharpener
Pencil tray
Pens and pencils
Rubber bands
Rubber stamps and ink pad
Ruler
Scissors
Stapler, staples, and staple remover
Utility tray (for paper clips, pens, pencils, and other small items)
Wastebasket

Paper Supplies

Adhesive notes
Assorted envelopes (e.g., coin, large, and special mailing services envelopes)
Business cards
Copy paper (assorted sizes)
Drug reference
File folders
File folder labels
File guides
Index cards
Index tabs
Letterhead (cover and second sheets)
Letterhead and envelopes
Medical and dental dictionaries
Message reply forms
Notepads
Plain white paper
Preprinted office forms
Report covers
Ring binders
Ruled letter- and legal-size writing pads
Standard dictionary
Storage cartons
Telephone message pads
Thermal paper, if required

Appointment Management Supplies

Appointment book (optional if not computerized)
Appointment cards
Appointment schedule forms and replacement sheets for appointment book (optional if not computerized)
Work or school excuse forms

Clinical Forms (optional if not computerized)

Clinical charts with assorted forms
Colored filing labels
Consent forms
File guides
Health alert labels
Health Insurance Portability and Accountability Act (HIPAA) forms
Health questionnaire forms
Laboratory requisition forms
Occupational Safety and Health Administration (OSHA) reporting forms
Patient file envelopes and folders
Prescription pads
Referral forms
Registration forms
Safety management forms
Update forms

Financial Record Forms

Application for Employer Identification Number (SS-4)
Bank deposit slips
Bookkeeping forms (optional if not computerized)
Checkbook and replacement checks
Citizenship Eligibility Form (I-9)
Employee's Withholding Allowance Certificate Form (W-4)
Employer's quarterly tax return form (941)
Employer's annual federal unemployment tax return form (940)
Insurance claim forms
Ledger cards and forms (optional if not computerized)
Payroll forms
Statements
Transmittal of income and tax statements form (W-3)
Wage and tax statement form (W-2)

Microcomputer Supplies

CDs and DVDs
Cleaning materials
Connecting devices for USB ports
Disk cases
Disk labels
Disk mailers
Flash drives
Ink cartridges
Mouse pad
Toner cartridges

NOTE: When available, ergonomically designed supplies and materials should be purchased.

LEARNING ACTIVITIES

1. List eight suggestions for the design of a reception room.
2. Discuss 10 factors to consider when designing a business office.
3. Describe the impact of the Americans with Disabilities Act on a dental practice.
4. Describe the concept of time and motion as it applies to a dental business office.
5. Describe a system that could be used to maintain a clean and clear work area.
6. List six tips that will help reduce fatigue and eyestrain when working at a computer.

Please refer to the student workbook for additional learning activities.

BIBLIOGRAPHY

Business and Institutional Furniture Manufacturers Association International: *BIFMA ergonomics guideline*, Effingham, IL, 2008, Nova Solutions. Available at: http://www.novadesk.com/Portals/84375/docs/bifma-summary.pdf.

Fulton-Calkins PJ, Rankin DS, Shumack KA: *The administrative professional*, ed 14, Mason, OH, 2011, Thomson South-Western.

RECOMMENDED WEBSITES

www.access-board.gov
www.ada.gov
www.sad.com
www.novadesk.com

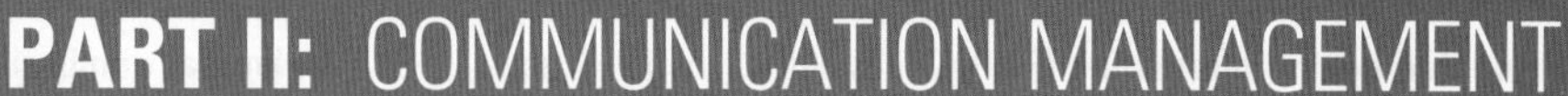

PART II: COMMUNICATION MANAGEMENT

7

Working with Dental Office Documents

Rebecca A. Nagy

 http://evolve.elsevier.com/Finkbeiner/practice

LEARNING OUTCOMES

1. Define the key terms in this chapter.
2. Discuss the records management system in a dental office and identify the various categories of records that are maintained in a dental office.
3. Discuss HIPAA and how to implement HIPAA regulations in the dental office record management system.
4. Discuss the importance of maintaining accurate clinical records, including:
   - List the components of a clinical record.
   - Discuss the purpose of certified electronic health records (EHR).
   - Explain the rules for entering data into patient records.
   - Discuss the various types of clinical data entries.
   - Explain the use of symbols and abbreviations in clinical records.
   - Describe methods of records retention and transfer.
5. Identify various types of records required by the Occupational Safety and Health Administration (OSHA) that must be maintained in a dental office.
6. Identify the various types of employee records.

KEY TERMS

Axial surface The tooth surface that runs vertically from the biting surface to the apex of a tooth.

Charting symbols A type of shorthand in the dental office that is used to enter clinical data and conditions on a graphic tooth chart in a patient's record.

Clinical abbreviations Initials or short terms used to explain a clinical condition in a patient's oral cavity.

Clinical record A collection of all information about a patient's dental treatment.

Consent form A form that is signed by the patient or by the parent or legal guardian of a pediatric patient that grants permission for the administration of an anesthetic and other specified procedures.

Electronic health record (EHR) A certified EHR is a universally standardized electronic format that makes use of compliant systems, standards, and interfaces that work together to create, manage, store, and share health information among authorized providers across multiple healthcare settings.

Fédération Dentaire Internationale (FDI) system A tooth-numbering system that assigns a two-digit number to each tooth in any quadrant. The first number indicates the quadrant in which the tooth is positioned, and the second number identifies the specific tooth.

Health history form A form on which the patient provides his or her complete health history and that is signed by the patient.

Health history update form A form that should be completed periodically to keep both the patient's health history and his or her personal information current. The patient should sign and date this form.

Health Insurance Portability and Accountability Act of 1996 (HIPAA) A federal act that protects and enhances patient rights, including requirements for ensuring the privacy and security of electronically transmitted protected health information.

Important records Records for the dental office operation that are extremely valuable but not vital. They include accounts payable and receivable, invoices, canceled checks, inventory and payroll records, and other federal regulatory records.

Information management See *records management.*

International Standards Organization (ISO) System A numbering system of teeth that can be used internationally as well as by electronic data transfer. The ISO System is based on the Federation Dentaire Internationale (FDI) System and is used in many countries.

Laboratory prescription/requisition A form that accompanies each case a dentist sends to a dental laboratory and that includes information about the case.

Nonessential records Documents that have little importance or that have value for a limited amount of time. Examples include notes regarding a task, meeting reminders, outdated announcements, and pamphlets or flyers that are no longer in use.

Occlusal surface The biting surface of a tooth.

Palmer notation system A tooth-numbering system that assigns each of the four quadrants a bracket to designate the area of the mouth in which the tooth is located.

Patient registration form A form that contains general information such as addresses and phone numbers as well as employment and insurance information. This may also be combined with a health history form.

Protected health information (PHI) This is defined by HIPAA as anything that ties a patient's name or Social Security number to that person's health, healthcare, or payment for healthcare.

Record Information in forms such as text, numbers, images, or voice that is kept for future reference.

Records management The process of establishing a logical and functional system for storing and retrieving information. This is also called *information management.*

Statute of limitations The period within which a civil suit for alleged wrongdoing may be legally filed.

Universal numbering system The most widely used tooth-numbering system. The Arabic numerals 1 through 32 are used for the permanent dentition, and the letters *A* through *T* are used for the primary dentition.

Useful records Records that include employment applications, expired insurance policies, petty cash vouchers, bank reconciliations, and general correspondence.

Vital records Essential documents that cannot be replaced, including patient clinical and financial records and the office's corporate charter and deed, mortgage, or bill of sale.

Healthcare providers, including dentists, are shifting more of their documents from paper and patient files to electronic records. In most cases, electronic records are more secure and easier for all members of the dental team to access. Offices vary with regard to their document management procedures and may use a combination of e-records and paper documents. Some dentists could easily manage with a totally paperless office, yet there are those who feel more comfortable when they have a paper record for recording documentation and reviewing history.

The business of dentistry requires a wide range of records and forms that must be scrupulously completed, maintained, and stored so that others can refer to the information later or use it to complete another task. The administrative assistant is required to maintain clinical, financial, employee, state, and federal records. Any lapses, gaps, or missed details can trigger a chain of events that negatively affect the dentist, the members of the dental team, and the patients. The administrative assistant must be very detail oriented and dedicated to maintaining all types of records that are essential to the dental practice.

OVERVIEW OF A RECORDS MANAGEMENT SYSTEM

A dental office operates on information: it is created, processed, stored, printed, and distributed in many forms to various locations and people. For the office to run smoothly and efficiently, the dental administrative assistant must establish and maintain a logical, user-friendly system for storing and retrieving information. A record is information in forms such as text, numbers, images, or voice that is kept for future reference. In a dental office, this information comes in the form of clinical, financial, radiographic, and photographic data. Records management or an information management system refers to a set of procedures used to organize, store, retrieve, remove, and dispose of records. Records have a life cycle which begins with their inception and ends with their disposition (Figure 7-1). The life cycle proceeds as follows:

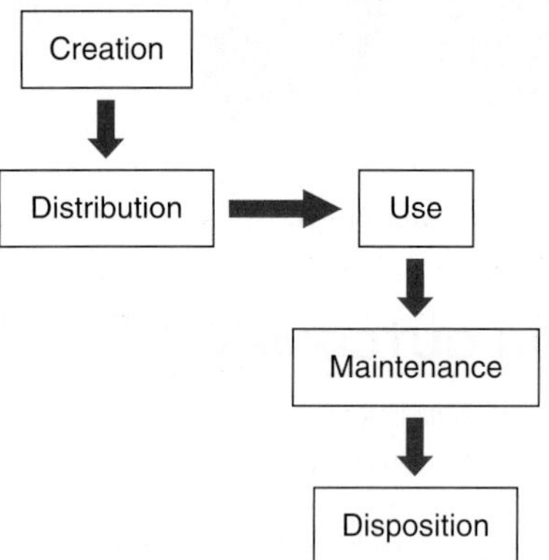

FIGURE 7-1 Life cycle of a record.

- *Creation:* This is the origination of the data. In the case of a patient record, creation begins with the completion of a patient registration form and health questionnaire. If the patient plans to continue treatment with the office, a permanent record is usually started on paper, or the information is entered into a computer. If the patient is transient (i.e., he or she will not be returning), the form for recording the data may be different from the standard form, and the record may not be stored with the active clinical charts.
- *Distribution:* The information may be distributed manually or electronically. This includes sending the patient's clinical record to the dentist for review.
- *Use:* The dentist, hygienist, or assistant records pertinent procedures, diagnoses, treatment recommendations, and miscellaneous information. These individuals refer the data to an appropriate location for further use or maintenance.

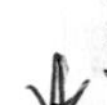

- *Maintenance:* This stage of the cycle involves determining whether the data or information should be retained. If it is to be retained, the administrative assistant must decide the best way to store it for easy retrieval and how long it should be stored. If the patient is to be seen again and become a patient of record, the clinical record is filed alphabetically either electronically or in a file folder and envelope in a protected cabinet. Some components of the record, such as notes that the dentist may have made during evaluation, may not be necessary to the treatment history and may possibly be removed and destroyed.
- *Disposition:* Clinical records are vital and must be retained for a period that is consistent with the state statute of limitations. Electronic data can be transferred to external devices or secure repositories for storage. Paper records, which have no backup, must be kept in a safe, dry area. After the legal time limit has passed, a decision can be made to either destroy the record because it no longer has value to the office, or to continue storing it as an important document.

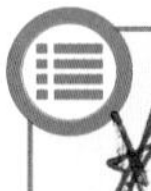

PRACTICE NOTE
Records have a life cycle that begins with creation and ends with disposition.

CATEGORIES OF RECORDS

The administrative assistant must be able to decide which records to keep, how to organize and store them, how long they legally must be retained, and when to dispose of them. In general, records can be categorized as *vital, important, useful,* or *nonessential* and as *active* or *inactive.*

Vital Records

Vital records are essential documents that cannot be replaced. These include patients' clinical and financial records and the office's corporate charter and deed, mortgage, or bill of sale. These records should be kept in a fireproof, theft-proof cabinet or safe, and copies of financial records and legal papers are often kept in a protected offsite location.

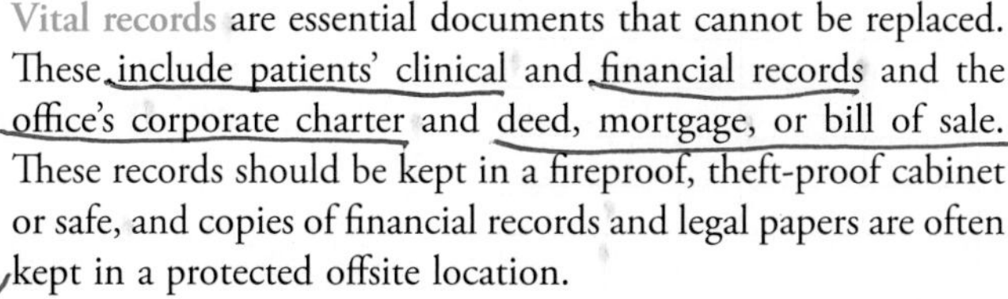

PRACTICE NOTE
Vital records are essential documents that cannot be replaced.

Important Records

Important records are extremely valuable to the operation of the office, but they are not vital. They include accounts payable and receivable, invoices, canceled checks, inventory and payroll records, and other federal regulatory records. Such records may be needed for a tax audit or if a question arises about a financial transaction. Important records generally should be retained for 5 to 7 years. Most offices keep them for about 7 years or in accordance with federal or state regulations.

Useful Records

Useful records include employment applications, expired insurance policies, petty cash vouchers, bank reconciliations, and general correspondence. This category is difficult to define, because one office may consider a document useful, whereas another might find it indispensable. These records are usually retained for 1 to 3 years. Before discarding a document, it is always wise to check with the dentist or other staff members to see if it is still needed.

Nonessential Records

Nonessential records have little importance or only have value for a limited amount of time. Examples include notes about a completed task, meeting reminders, outdated announcements, and pamphlets or flyers that are no longer in use. Common sense dictates when these materials may be discarded.

HEALTH INSURANCE PORTABILITY AND ACCOUNTABILITY ACT

The Health Insurance Portability and Accountability Act of 1996 (HIPAA), which became effective in dentistry in April 2003, has affected the business functions of the dental office in a number of ways. HIPAA laws may seem daunting at first; however, their purpose is to protect and enhance patient rights, and everyone is a patient at one time or another.

The HIPAA Privacy and Security Rules mandate federal protection for individually identifiable health information and give patients certain rights with regard to that information. Dental practices that conduct electronic transactions (e.g., claim submission, predetermination, requests for eligibility or benefit information) must comply with the federal requirements. In addition, the dental offices are required to have a business association agreement with any other company or entity with which they electronically exchange this information, such as a benefit carrier or clearinghouse.

HIPAA defines protected health information (PHI) as anything that ties a patient's name or Social Security number to that person's health, healthcare, or payment for healthcare, such as radiographs, charts, or invoices. Ensuring the privacy and security of PHI is a legal imperative, but it also protects everyone on the dental team, not just the patient. Overall, the issue of privacy is extremely important for all patient records, both paper and electronic. It is also good risk management, because it helps each dental professional to prevent potential litigation. Each person on the dental team should become familiar with state and federal privacy legislation, because individual states may have additional or more detailed requirements.

A privacy issue that affects many dental offices is the use of a sign-in sheet for patients to indicate that they have arrived for their appointment. Patient privacy must be protected, so the administrative assistant must make sure that any names on the sheet are not viewable by others. Crossing a name off of a list usually does not obliterate it completely, so tear-off labels such as those shown in Figure 7-2 are commonly used. As soon as the patient signs in, the label can be immediately removed. Other options could include a digital or computerized sign-in process.

The Administrative Simplification provisions of HIPAA require national standards for electronic healthcare transactions. All dentists who transmit or accept patients' healthcare information electronically must use these standard formats. They must also apply for and use a National Provider Identifier (NPI) in all e-transactions. Dental practices that do not have software or transmission capabilities that are compliant with the standards are able to send their data to a healthcare clearinghouse. The clearinghouse verifies the accuracy of the information, "translates" it into the legally required formats, and then transmits it to the benefit carrier or other target entity. Paper transactions are not subject to HIPAA's Administrative Simplification Statute and Rules. The most affected area in the dental office is

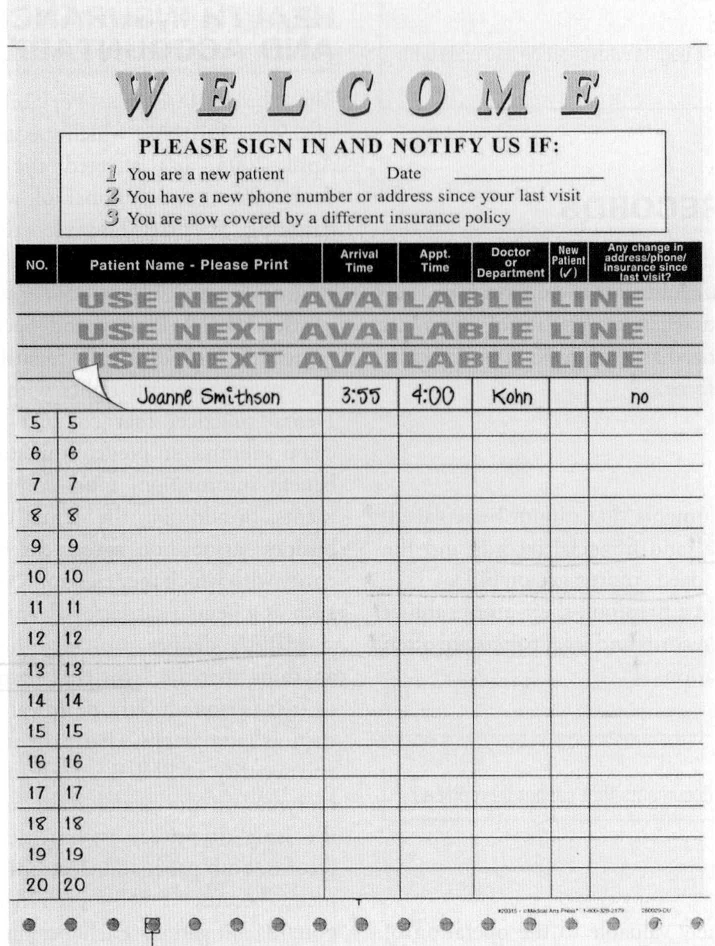

WELCOME

PLEASE SIGN IN AND NOTIFY US IF:

1 You are a new patient Date ____________

2 You have a new phone number or address since your last visit

3 You are now covered by a different insurance policy

NO.	Patient Name - Please Print	Arrival Time	Appt. Time	Doctor or Department	New Patient (✓)	Any change in address/phone/ insurance since last visit?
	USE NEXT AVAILABLE LINE					
	USE NEXT AVAILABLE LINE					
	USE NEXT AVAILABLE LINE					
	Joanne Smithson	3:55	4:00	Kohn		no
5	5					
6	6					
7	7					
8	8					
9	9					
10	10					
11	11					
12	12					
13	13					
14	14					
15	15					
16	16					
17	17					
18	18					
19	19					
20	20					

FIGURE 7-2 Sign-in form with removable lines. (Courtesy Medical Arts Press, Brooklyn Park, MN.)

the area of transmission of dental claim forms, which is reviewed in Chapter 14.

The American Dental Association (ADA) and most state dental associations have done an excellent job of providing members with the necessary tools for the implementation of HIPAA. The ADA and state dental associations as well as many dental office stationers provide a HIPAA Security Tool Kit such as the one shown in Figure 7-3. This kit contains most of the forms needed for privacy practices, including the following:

- The Notice of Privacy Practices form (Figure 7-4) presents information that the dental professional is required to give patients regarding the office's privacy practices. This form may need to be changed to reflect the dental practice's particular privacy policies or stricter state laws. The name of the practice may be on the notice, and it must be given to each patient at the date of the first service. In addition, the notice may be posted in a clear and prominent location in the office that is visible to any patient seeking service. Boxes 7-1 and 7-2 provide checklists for managing the privacy and security of patient records.

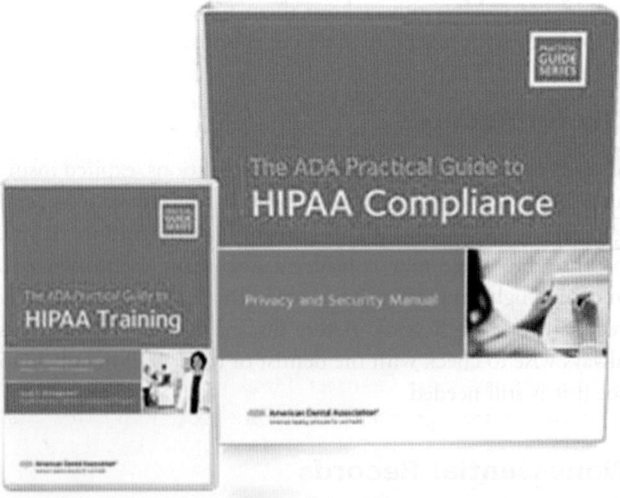

FIGURE 7-3 HIPAA security kit. (Courtesy American Dental Association, Chicago, IL.)

NOTICE OF PRIVACY PRACTICES

THIS NOTICE DESCRIBES HOW MEDICAL INFORMATION ABOUT YOU MAY BE USED AND DISCLOSED AND HOW YOU CAN GET ACCESS TO THIS INFORMATION. PLEASE REVIEW IT CAREFULLY.

This practice is required, by law, to maintain the privacy and confidentiality of your protected health information and to provide our patients with notice of our legal duties and privacy practices with respect to your protected health information.

Disclosure of Your Health Care Information

Treatment
We may disclose your health care information to other health care professionals within our practice for the purpose of treatment, payment or health care operations. (example)

> *"On occasion, it may be necessary to seek consultation regarding your condition from other health care providers associated with this practice."*

> *"It is our policy to provide a substitute health care provider, authorized by this practice, to provide assessment and/or treatment to our patients, without advanced notice, in the event of your primary health care provider's absence due to vacation, sickness, or other emergency situation."*

Payment
We may disclose your health information to your insurance provider for the purpose of payment or health care operations. (example)

> *"As a courtesy to our patients, we will submit an itemized billing statement to your insurance carrier for the purpose of payment to this practice for health care services rendered. If you pay for your health care services personally, we will, as a courtesy, provide an itemized billing to your insurance carrier for the purpose of reimbursement to you. The billing statement contains medical information, including diagnosis, date of injury or condition, and codes which describe the health care services received."*

Workers' Compensation
We may disclose your health information as necessary to comply with State Workers' Compensation Laws.

Emergencies
We may disclose your health information to notify or assist in notifying a family member, or another person responsible for your care, about your medical condition or in the event of an emergency or of your death.

Public Health
As required by law, we may disclose your health information to public health authorities for purposes related to: preventing or controlling disease, injury or disability, reporting child abuse or neglect, reporting domestic violence, reporting to the Food and Drug Administration problems with products and reactions to medications, and reporting disease or infection exposure.

Page 1

ITEM 066-6305/18252 © JULY2003

FIGURE 7-4 Notice of Privacy Practices form. (Courtesy Patterson Office Supplies, Champaign, IL.)

- Acknowledgement of Receipt of Notice of Privacy Practices (Figure 7-5) is the form the patient signs to acknowledge that he or she has received a copy of the Notice of Privacy Practices. If the patient refuses to sign the form, the administrative assistant can indicate that an attempt was made to have the patient sign in the in-office section of the form. The patient may also opt to sign a separate refusal form that may then be placed in the record.
- Business Associate Contract Terms is a contract form that ensures the integrity and confidentiality of PHI that a business associate may create or receive for or from the dental practice (Figure 7-6).

Other forms, such as the Health Information Access-Response/Delay, Complaint, and Staff Review of Policies and Procedures forms, are available in the ADA manual or from the state dental society. To ensure that records are maintained for patients, a preprinted chart label can provide information about important HIPAA information for paper patient files (Figure 7-7, *A* and *B*) or notations made in the patient computerized record.

CLINICAL RECORDS

Patient records generally fall into two categories: clinical and financial. Clinical records are reviewed in this chapter, and financial records are discussed in Chapter 15. A recall system can be considered a type of clinical record, but it is maintained separately; see Chapter 12 for a discussion of this system.

The clinical record is a collection of all of the information about a patient's dental treatment. In many practices, the clinical record is referred to as the *patient's chart;* these terms are often interchangeable. Although each patient's clinical record is used during dental treatment, updating and

BOX 7-1

HIPAA Privacy Checklist

The purpose of the HIPAA Privacy Rules is to safeguard the privacy of patients' confidential health information.

Develop:
- A written privacy policy and procedures*
- A notice of privacy practices (This must be posted.)*
- An acknowledgement of the receipt of the notice of privacy practices (Patients must sign this form.)*

Designate:
- A privacy officer to oversee enforcement of the privacy procedures
- A contact person to receive complaints and answer questions

Evaluate:
- Relationships with business associates, such as consultants, technology/computer support personnel, accountants, and other business/service people or companies who have access to your patients' protected health information (Sign business associates agreements with individuals or companies that meet necessary criteria.)*

Provide:
- Employee training regarding the provisions of the HIPAA Privacy Rules*

Document:
- All employee training and any violations of the privacy policies by employees

*An excellent resource for templates for these items is the American Dental Association's HIPAA Privacy Kit, available at www.ada.org or from a dental stationery supply house.

Modified from Mary Govoni, CDA, RDA, RDH, MBA, Clinical Dynamics, Okemos, MI (www.marygovoni.com).

BOX 7-2

HIPAA Security Checklist

The purpose of the HIPAA Security Rules is to safeguard the confidentiality and integrity of electronic data regarding patients and their protected health information.

Develop:
- A written security policy and procedures*

Designate:
- A security officer to oversee enforcement of the security procedures and protocols

Evaluate:
- Security risks that may allow unauthorized access to electronic data
- Methods used to back up and store electronic data

Provide:
- Employee training regarding the provisions of the HIPAA Security Rules*
- Access control measures (unique passwords) for all employees who access electronic data

Document:
- All employee training and any violations of the privacy policies by employees
- Periodic system audit reviews (Audit trail reports to check for unauthorized access to electronic data.)

*An excellent resource for templates for these items is the American Dental Association's HIPAA Privacy Kit, available at www.ada.org or from a dental stationery supply house.

Modified from Mary Govoni, CDA, RDA, RDH, MBA, Clinical Dynamics, Okemos, MI (www.marygovoni.com).

maintaining this record is the administrative assistant's responsibility. The successful maintenance of clinical records requires cooperation and efficiency from each member of the dental office team.

Accurate clinical records are vital for several reasons:

1. Clinical records are a narrative of the patient's care and services. They contain a detailed history and outline future treatment options.
2. In a malpractice suit, the dental record is legally admissible as evidence. It can be used for or against the dentist.
3. Dental consultants representing third-party benefit carriers may review the clinical chart and other parts of the clinical record to determine whether services have been rendered adequately or if a proposed treatment is necessary.
4. The record acts as verification of treatment rendered for Internal Revenue Service (IRS) purposes.
5. Components of the clinical records are vital in forensic odontology, which is the field of dentistry concerned with the identification of individuals on the basis of dental evidence.

Components of a Clinical Record

A patient's clinical record commonly includes the following:
- A file envelope or folder (for paper records)
- Patient registration
- Health history and updates
- HIPAA acknowledgment
- Clinical chart
- Treatment record/progress notes
- Dental diagnosis, treatment plan, and treatment estimates
- Medication history and prescriptions
- Laboratory requisitions
- Consent forms
- Consultation and referral reports
- Letters
- Postal receipts
- Radiographs
- Copies of laboratory tests

Bulkier materials such as diagnostic models are generally stored in an area other than the business office. A cross-reference in the patient record makes these materials easier to locate.

ACKNOWLEDGEMENT OF RECEIPT OF NOTICE

As required by the Privacy Regulations, I hereby acknowledge that I have received a current copy of this practice's "NOTICE OF PRIVACY PRACTICES", revision date ________________.

As required by the Privacy Regulations, ________________________________ from
Name of Staff Member
this practice has explained the "NOTICE OF PRIVACY PRACTICES" to my satisfaction.

As required by the Privacy Regulations, I am aware that this practice has included a provision that it reserves the right to change the terms of its notice and to make the new notice provisions effective for all protected health information that it maintains.

Requests:

☐ I wish to file a "Request for Restriction" of my Protected Health Information.

☐ I wish to file a "Request for Alternative Communications" of my Protected Health Information.

☐ I wish to object to the following in the "Notice of Privacy Practices":

____

____

I understand that this office may change their Notice of Privacy Practices and is not required to honor the terms of the original/previous version(s).

________________________ Signature ________________ Date

________________________ Print Name

(OFFICE USE ONLY)

Signed form received by: ________________________ Date: ________________

Good faith effort to obtain receipt: (Describe) ________________________

____

____

 ITEM 066-6289/18243 © JULY2003

FIGURE 7-5 Acknowledgement of Receipt of Notice of privacy practices. (Courtesy Patterson Office Supplies, Champaign, IL.)

Although the dentist chooses the components and mode of the clinical record, staff members' input is valuable to ensure that all of the information needed to manage the business systems is collected accurately and efficiently. Most offices use computerized systems for at least part of the administration process, but they may keep paper documents for some data. The practicality and need for paper documents continues to decline as the capability and scope of dental software provide secure, user-friendly functions and storage for all types of clinical records.

Electronic Health Records

Legislation and mandates from the federal government are key drivers of the movement for all healthcare providers to use electronic health records (EHRs) in a universally standardized format. The ultimate goal of the EHR system is to enable the sharing of health information among authorized providers across multiple healthcare settings. Under this system, healthcare providers would be required to use certified healthcare record technology that has been approved by specifically designated federal agencies as using compliant systems, standards, and interfaces that work together to create, manage, store, and share information. Although the terms *electronic medical records* (EMR) and *electronic dental records* (EDR) are also used, EHR is generally used to indicate certified technology systems.

Patient File Envelope or Folder for Paper Records

Most dental practices use an 8½ × 11-inch file envelope or folder to contain clinical paper documents. Records of

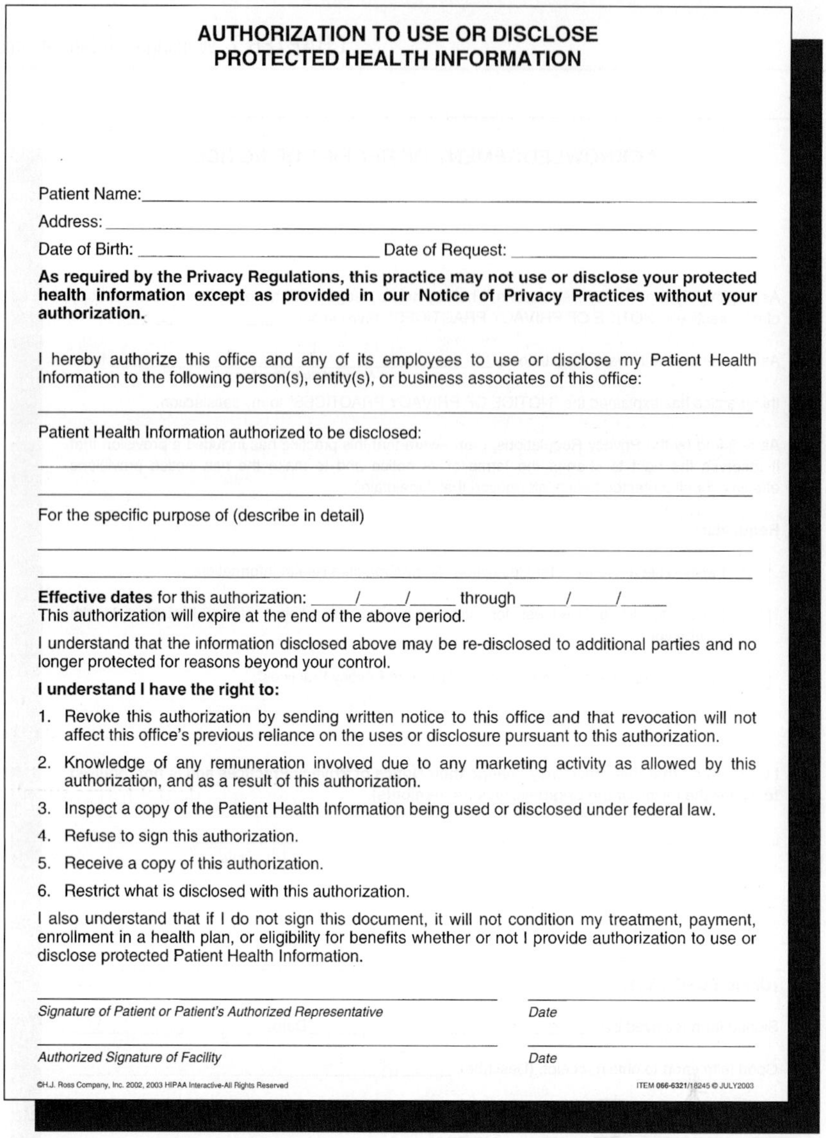

AUTHORIZATION TO USE OR DISCLOSE PROTECTED HEALTH INFORMATION

Patient Name:______________________________

Address:______________________________

Date of Birth: ________________ Date of Request: ________________

As required by the Privacy Regulations, this practice may not use or disclose your protected health information except as provided in our Notice of Privacy Practices without your authorization.

I hereby authorize this office and any of its employees to use or disclose my Patient Health Information to the following person(s), entity(s), or business associates of this office:

____

Patient Health Information authorized to be disclosed:

____

____

For the specific purpose of (describe in detail)

____

____

Effective dates for this authorization: _____/_____/_____ through _____/_____/_____
This authorization will expire at the end of the above period.

I understand that the information disclosed above may be re-disclosed to additional parties and no longer protected for reasons beyond your control.

I understand I have the right to:

1. Revoke this authorization by sending written notice to this office and that revocation will not affect this office's previous reliance on the uses or disclosure pursuant to this authorization.
2. Knowledge of any remuneration involved due to any marketing activity as allowed by this authorization, and as a result of this authorization.
3. Inspect a copy of the Patient Health Information being used or disclosed under federal law.
4. Refuse to sign this authorization.
5. Receive a copy of this authorization.
6. Restrict what is disclosed with this authorization.

I also understand that if I do not sign this document, it will not condition my treatment, payment, enrollment in a health plan, or eligibility for benefits whether or not I provide authorization to use or disclose protected Patient Health Information.

______________________________ ________________
Signature of Patient or Patient's Authorized Representative *Date*

______________________________ ________________
Authorized Signature of Facility *Date*

 ITEM 066-6321/18245 © JULY2003

FIGURE 7-6 Preprinted HIPAA Record of Disclosures forms for patient charts. (Courtesy Patterson Office Supplies, Champaign, IL.)

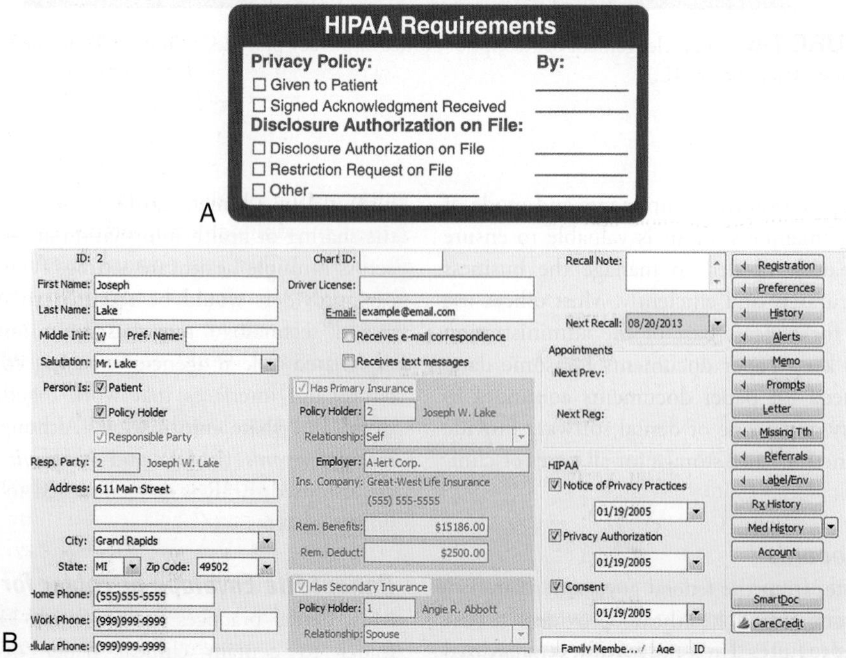

HIPAA Requirements

Privacy Policy: **By:**
☐ Given to Patient ________
☐ Signed Acknowledgment Received ________
Disclosure Authorization on File:
☐ Disclosure Authorization on File ________
☐ Restriction Request on File ________
☐ Other ____________ ________

A

ID: 2
First Name: Joseph
Last Name: Lake
Middle Init: W Pref. Name:
Salutation: Mr. Lake
Person Is: ☑ Patient
☑ Policy Holder
☑ Responsible Party
Resp. Party: 2 Joseph W. Lake
Address: 611 Main Street
City: Grand Rapids
State: MI Zip Code: 49502
Home Phone: (555)555-5555
Work Phone: (999)999-9999
Cellular Phone: (999)999-9999

Chart ID:
Driver License:
E-mail: example@email.com
☐ Receives e-mail correspondence
☐ Receives text messages
☑ Has Primary Insurance
Policy Holder: 2 Joseph W. Lake
Relationship: Self
Employer: A-lert Corp.
Ins. Company: Great-West Life Insurance (555) 555-5555
Rem. Benefits: $15186.00
Rem. Deduct: $2500.00
☑ Has Secondary Insurance
Policy Holder: 1 Angie R. Abbott
Relationship: Spouse

Recall Note:
Next Recall: 08/20/2013
Appointments
Next Prev:
Next Reg:
HIPAA
☑ Notice of Privacy Practices 01/19/2005
☑ Privacy Authorization 01/19/2005
☑ Consent 01/19/2005
Family Membe... / Age ID

Registration
Preferences
History
Alerts
Memo
Prompts
Letter
Missing Tth
Referrals
Label/Env
Rx History
Med History
Account
SmartDoc
CareCredit

B

FIGURE 7-7 **A**, Preprinted label for patient's chart to affirm that HIPAA requirements are met. **B**, Notation on an electronic record stating that the patient has completed the HIPAA information form. (Courtesy Patterson Office Supplies, Champaign, IL.)

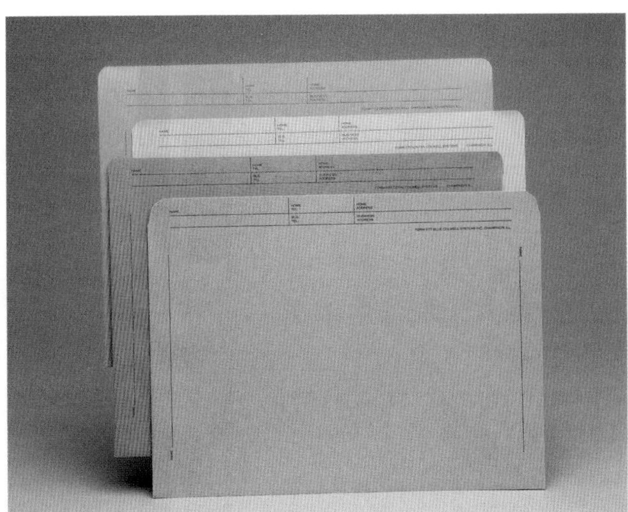

FIGURE 7-8 Patient file envelopes. (Courtesy Patterson Office Supplies, Champaign, IL.)

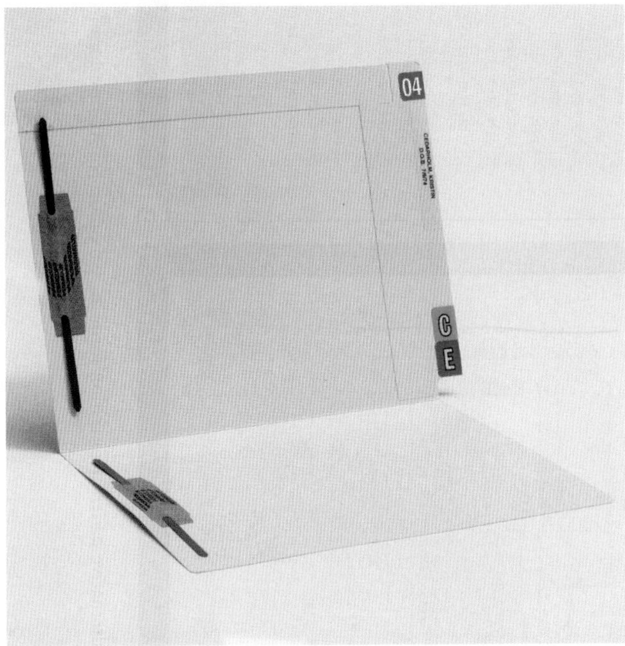

FIGURE 7-9 File folder with two two-hole fasteners. (Courtesy Patterson Office Supplies, Champaign, IL.)

treatment for transient or one-time patients may be kept together in one folder or file location. File envelopes may be plain or color-coded. They are supplied in a preprinted format with spaces for patient information, including the patient's name, address, and telephone number (Figure 7-8). This type of envelope is widely used, and it satisfies the needs of many practices.

Another very common type of storage for paper records is an end-tab file folder with one or two two-hole fasteners (Figure 7-9). This type of folder requires the use of vertical-style records. The folders generally have a reinforced tab for easy label placement. They are also precut for the quick insertion of a two-hole file fastener. Options include folders with pockets and diagonal cuts, expandable folders, and polyvinyl pockets to hold small materials such as radiographs and CDs.

Whether folders or envelopes are used, some form of color-coding is necessary to make sorting, storing, and retrieval easier. Color-coding can be done as an alphabetical system, or, in a group practice, it can be used to categorize by dentist. In addition to a label with the patient's name, either an alpha or numeric label system can be used to sort the records. Year aging labels can be used to identify inactive patient records that may need to be purged from the active storage system.

Patient Registration and Health History Forms

Although they are often combined, these two forms contain two different types of data. The information gathered on these forms should be retained in the patient's paper file or by scanning the completed form into a computer. Generic paper forms are available from dental forms suppliers. Custom forms can be designed by most companies at an additional cost to address the special needs of a specific office. Electronic versions of these forms are also available.

Some forms address privacy issues with questions such as, "May we leave a message on your answering machine at the phone number you have given?" or "May we contact you at a cell phone number or text message you?" Most supply companies provide patient forms in English and Spanish versions for use in various areas of the country. Many offices with Spanish-speaking patients have both versions available.

The **patient registration form** contains general information such as addresses, telephone numbers, and e-mail address as well as employment and insurance information (Figure 7-10). This form enables the staff members to become better acquainted with the patient, and it can provide information for third-party payments and credit checks. Make sure that no nicknames are used and that all data are accurate, because this information is used later to complete insurance forms. Incomplete information on this form can complicate account collection later. In addition, many offices use a breakdown of benefits form to gather and organize detailed benefit coverage from the patient's insurance carrier (Figure 7-11). Keep patients' records current by asking if there have been any changes in their personal, work, or insurance information at each visit (Figure 7-12).

Each patient should fill out a **health history form** (Figure 7-13) and then date and sign it. If the dentist prefers to ask these questions in person, the patient should verify the answers recorded and then sign the form. The health history form for a child should be completed by a parent or legal guardian, not by the child or a babysitter (Figure 7-14).

The patient's history should be reviewed when the person returns for treatment if several months have elapsed since the

A

Welcome

Thank you for selecting our dental healthcare team! We will strive to provide you with the best possible dental care. To help us meet all your dental healthcare needs, please fill out this form completely in ink. If you have any questions or need assistance, please ask us - we will be happy to help.

Patient # ____
SS#/SIN ____

Patient Information (CONFIDENTIAL)

Date ____
Name ____ Birthdate ____ Home Phone ____
Address ____ City ____ State/Prov. ____ Zip/P.C. ____
Email ____ Cell Phone ____
Check Appropriate Box: ☐ Minor ☐ Single ☐ Married ☐ Divorced ☐ Widowed ☐ Separated
If Student, Name of School/College ____ City ____ State/Prov. ____ ☐ Full Time ☐ Part Time
Patient or Parent/Guardian's Employer ____ Work Phone ____
Business Address ____ City ____ State/Prov. ____ Zip/P.C. ____
Spouse or Parent/Guardian's Name ____ Employer ____ Work Phone ____
Whom may we thank for referring you? ____
Person to contact in case of emergency ____ Phone ____

Responsible Party

Name of Person Responsible for this Account ____ Relationship to Patient ____
Address ____ Home Phone ____
Email ____ Cell Phone ____
Driver's License# ____ Birthdate ____ Financial Institution ____
Employer ____ Work Phone ____ SS#/SIN ____
Is this person currently a patient in our office? ☐ Yes ☐ No
For your convenience, we offer the following methods of payment. Please check the option you prefer. Payment in full at each appointment.
☐ Cash ☐ Personal Check Credit Card ☐ VISA ☐ MasterCard ☐ I wish to discuss the office's payment policy.

Insurance Information

Name of Insured ____ Relationship to Patient ____
Birthdate ____ SS#/SIN ____ Date Employed ____
Name of Employer ____ Union or Local # ____ Work Phone ____
Address of Employer ____ City ____ State/Prov. ____ Zip/P.C. ____
Insurance Company ____ Group # ____ Policy/ID # ____
Ins. Co. Address ____ City ____ State/Prov. ____ Zip/P.C. ____
How much is your deductible? ____ How much have you used? ____ Max. annual benefit ____

DO YOU HAVE ANY ADDITIONAL INSURANCE? ☐ Yes ☐ No IF YES, COMPLETE THE FOLLOWING:

Name of Insured ____ Relationship to Patient ____
Birthdate ____ SS#/SIN ____ Date Employed ____
Name of Employer ____ Union or Local # ____ Work Phone ____
Address of Employer ____ City ____ State/Prov. ____ Zip/P.C. ____
Insurance Company ____ Group # ____ Policy/ID # ____
Ins. Co. Address ____ City ____ State/Prov. ____ Zip/P.C. ____
How much is your deductible? ____ How much have you used? ____ Max. annual benefit ____

Over Please

B

PATIENT INFORMATION (CONFIDENTIAL)

NAME ____ FIRST ____ MI ____ LAST ____ DATE ____
ADDRESS ____ CITY ____ STATE/PROV. ____ ZIP/P.C. ____
E-MAIL ____ CELL PHONE ____ HOME PHONE ____
SS#/SIN ____ BIRTHDATE ____
CHECK APPROPRIATE BOX: ☐ MINOR ☐ SINGLE ☐ MARRIED ☐ DIVORCED ☐ WIDOWED ☐ SEPARATED
IF COLLEGE STUDENT, F.T. / P.T., NAME OF SCHOOL ____ CITY ____ STATE/PROV. ____
PATIENT'S OR PARENT'S/GUARDIAN'S EMPLOYER ____ WORK PHONE ____
BUSINESS ADDRESS ____ CITY ____ STATE/PROV. ____ ZIP/P.C. ____
SPOUSE OR PARENT'S/GUARDIAN'S NAME ____ EMPLOYER ____ WORK PHONE ____
WHOM MAY WE THANK FOR REFERRING YOU? ____
PERSON TO CONTACT IN CASE OF AN EMERGENCY ____ PHONE ____

RESPONSIBLE PARTY

NAME OF PERSON RESPONSIBLE FOR THIS ACCOUNT ____ RELATIONSHIP TO PATIENT ____
ADDRESS ____ HOME PHONE ____
DRIVER'S LICENSE # ____ BIRTHDATE ____ SS#/SIN ____
EMPLOYER ____ WORK PHONE ____
IS THIS PERSON CURRENTLY A PATIENT IN OUR OFFICE? ☐ YES ☐ NO

INSURANCE INFORMATION

NAME OF INSURED ____ RELATIONSHIP TO PATIENT ____
BIRTHDATE ____ SS#/SIN ____ DATE EMPLOYED ____
NAME OF EMPLOYER ____ UNION OR LOCAL # ____ WORK PHONE ____
EMPLOYER ADDRESS ____ CITY ____ STATE/PROV. ____ ZIP/P.C. ____
INSURANCE CO. ____ TEL. # ____ GRP # ____ POLICY / I.D. # ____
INS. CO. ADDRESS ____ CITY ____ STATE/PROV. ____ ZIP/P.C. ____
HOW MUCH IS YOUR DEDUCTIBLE? ____ HOW MUCH HAVE YOU USED? ____ MAX ANNUAL BENEFIT? ____

DO YOU HAVE ANY ADDITIONAL INSURANCE? ☐ YES ☐ NO IF YES, COMPLETE THE FOLLOWING:

NAME OF INSURED ____ RELATIONSHIP TO PATIENT ____
BIRTHDATE ____ SS#/SIN ____ DATE EMPLOYED ____
NAME OF EMPLOYER ____ UNION OR LOCAL # ____ WORK PHONE ____
EMPLOYER ADDRESS ____ CITY ____ STATE/PROV. ____ ZIP/P.C. ____
INSURANCE CO. ____ TEL. # ____ GRP # ____ POLICY / I.D. # ____
INS. CO. ADDRESS ____ CITY ____ STATE/PROV. ____ ZIP/P.C. ____
HOW MUCH IS YOUR DEDUCTIBLE? ____ HOW MUCH HAVE YOU USED? ____ MAX ANNUAL BENEFIT? ____

X ____
SIGNATURE OF PATIENT OR PARENT/GUARDIAN IF MINOR ____ PATIENT NUMBER ____

REGISTRATION

FIGURE 7-10 **A,** Front of an alternative patient registration form. **B,** Common registration form. (Courtesy Patterson Office Supplies, Champaign, IL.)

INSURANCE BREAKDOWN FORM

Subscriber Name_____________________________ SS or ID#__________________ DOB____________

Employer____

Patient Name_____________________________ DOB____________ Relation to Subscriber________

Ins. Co. Name____ Elec. Payor ID#_______________

Address____

Phone #______________________ Group #_____________________

Spoke to_____________________ Date____________ By____________________

Effective______________________ Calendar or Benefit Year_____________to______________

Deductible: Indiv. $_______ Family $_______ Yearly Max $_______ Ded on Preventive? YES NO

Preventive covered at_____% Basic covered at_____% Major covered at_____%

Includes____________________________________ Includes____________________________________

Includes____________________________________

Is there a waiting period for: Basic work? YES NO satisfied_____ Major work? YES NO satisfied_____

FMX every_____yrs Is patient eligible now? YES NO Pts. last FMX or Pano_____ Pano addition to FMX? YES NO

Prophylaxis _____time(s) in_____ Exams_____time(s) in_____ Bitewings_____ time(s) in_____

Limitations_______________________________________

Does the patient have any history of perio treatment (4341)? YES NO When_____ Frequency_____time(s) in_____

Is 4910 (perio prophy) covered? YES NO Frequency_____time(s) in_____ Limitations____________________________________

Is there sealant coverage (1351)? YES NO A_____% Limitations____

Are posterior composites covered (2385)? YES NO Limitations____

Are onlays covered (2642)? YES NO At_____% Limitations____

Are inlays covered (2610)? YES NO At_____% Limitations____

Are build-ups covered (2950)? YES NO At_____% Limitations____

Are crowns paid at? PREP SEAT EITHER

Replacement clause: crowns and bridges_____yrs. partials and dentures_____yrs.

Orthodontic coverage? YES NO At_____% Separate ded $_____ Lifetime Max $_____ Age limit_____yrs.

Are nightguards covered (9940)? YES NO At_____% Limitations____

Are prior extractions covered (missing tooth clause)? YES NO Limitations____

Annual benefits used-to-date $________ Year___________

Has the individual deductible been met? YES NO Family deductible? YES NO

FIGURE 7-11 Insurance benefit breakdown form. (Courtesy Patterson Office Supplies, Champaign, IL)

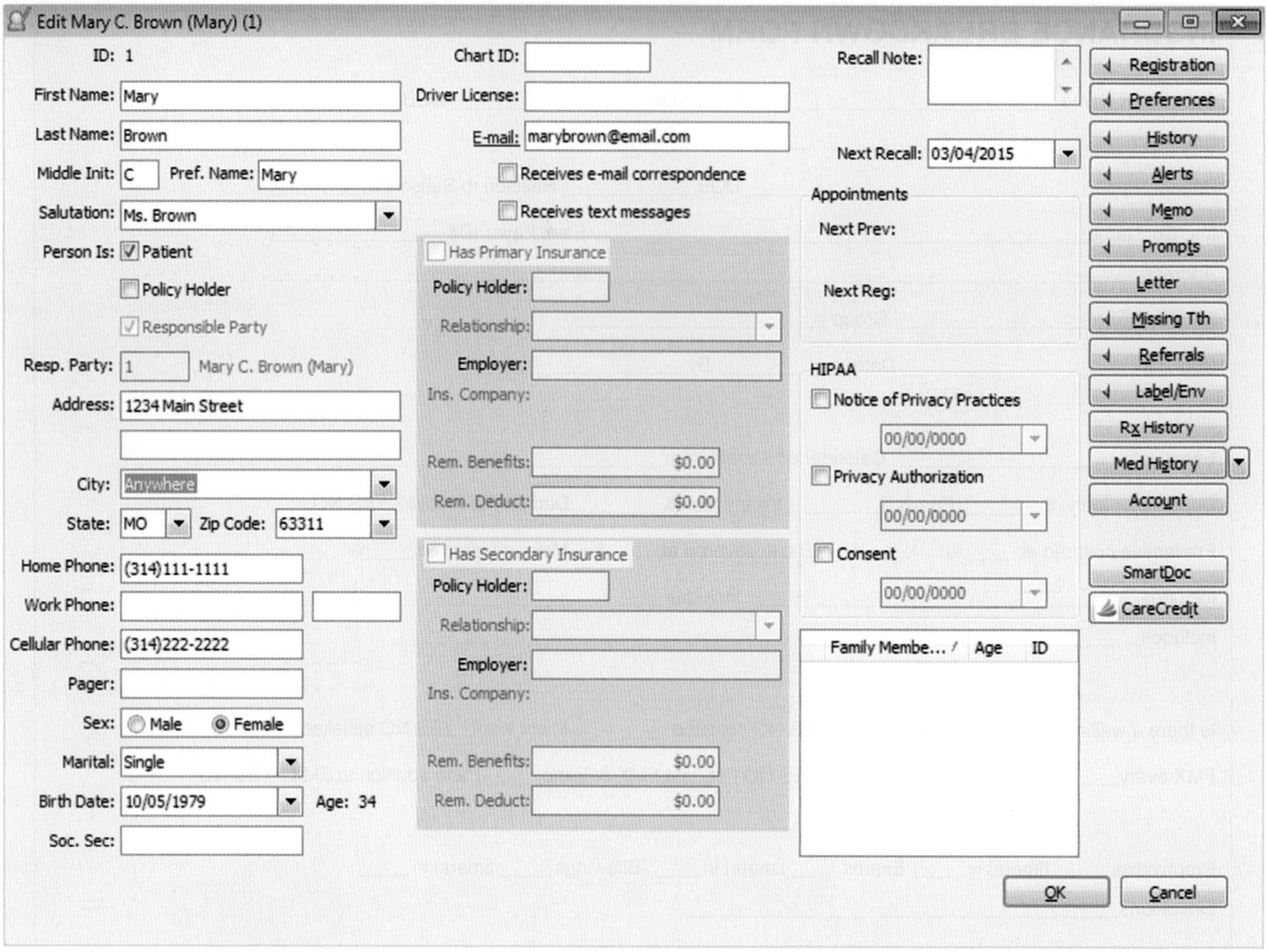

FIGURE 7-12 Screenshot of patient information software page. (Courtesy Patterson Office Supplies, Champaign, IL)

last visit. Depending on the dental office's policy and the length of time since the patient was seen, the administrative assistant may have the patient fill out a complete health history form or a shorter **health history update form** (Figure 7-15). The patient should sign and date this form.

Many types of patient registration and health history forms are available in print and electronic formats. The forms can be filled out by the patient when he or she presents for an appointment; they can be mailed or e-mailed so that the patient can complete the forms and bring them in; or they can be posted to the dental office's website and filled out online. Regardless of the format used, it is important to remember that a current and accurate health history serves as a preventive measure during patient treatment and as a defense in malpractice suits.

When a patient is filling out the forms in the office, certain conditions need to be present:

- Provide the patient with a comfortable location with relative privacy.
- If using a paper form, put it on a clipboard with a ballpoint pen (not a pencil) attached.
- Do not ask the questions in a public area of the business office. This can compromise the patient's right to privacy if his or her answers are overheard by other people. If the office has new patients complete these forms when they present for their appointment, ask them to arrive 15 minutes early.
- Make sure that a parent or legal guardian completes the forms for a child.
- Keep the information absolutely confidential. The patient record is not for public review and should not become a feature of lunchtime gossip.
- Review the forms to ensure that they have been completed and signed. Patients may avoid questions that they do not understand or do not want to answer. If the patient says, "I don't think this question has anything to do with my teeth," explain how the answer relates to their dental care. If the question cannot be justified, it should not be on the form.

A person's privacy is protected by law, and questions that may be considered discriminatory or in violation of a patient's rights must be avoided. Consequently, the administrative assistant must be aware of the state laws that protect a person's rights and recommend changes to the form that accommodate these

Health History Form

ADA American Dental Association www.ada.org

E-mail: Today's Date:

As required by law, our office adheres to written policies and procedures to protect the privacy of information about you that we create, receive or maintain. Your answers are for our records only and will be kept confidential subject to applicable laws. Please note that you will be asked some questions about your responses to this questionnaire and there may be additional questions concerning your health. This information is vital to allow us to provide appropriate care for you. This office does not use this information to discriminate.

Name: Last First Middle | Home Phone: Include area code ( ) | Business/Cell Phone: Include area code ( )

Address: Mailing address | City: | State: | Zip:

Occupation: | Height: | Weight: | Date of birth: | Sex: M F

SS# or Patient ID: | Emergency Contact: | Relationship: | Home Phone: ( ) | Cell Phone: ( ) Include area codes

If you are completing this form for another person, what is your relationship to that person?

Your Name Relationship

Do you have any of the following diseases or problems: *(Check DK if you Don't Know the answer to the question)* Yes No DK

- Active Tuberculosis ☐ ☐ ☐
- Persistent cough greater than a 3 week duration ☐ ☐ ☐
- Cough that produces blood ☐ ☐ ☐
- Been exposed to anyone with tuberculosis ☐ ☐ ☐

If you answer yes to any of the 4 items above, please stop and return this form to the receptionist.

Dental Information *For the following questions, please mark (X) your responses to the following questions.*

Yes No DK

- Do your gums bleed when you brush or floss? ☐ ☐ ☐
- Are your teeth sensitive to cold, hot, sweets or pressure? ☐ ☐ ☐
- Does food or floss catch between your teeth? ☐ ☐ ☐
- Is your mouth dry? ☐ ☐ ☐
- Have you had any periodontal (gum) treatments? ☐ ☐ ☐
- Have you ever had orthodontic (braces) treatment? ☐ ☐ ☐
- Have you had any problems associated with previous dental treatment? ☐ ☐ ☐
- Is your home water supply fluoridated? ☐ ☐ ☐
- Do you drink bottled or filtered water? ☐ ☐ ☐
- If yes, how often? Circle one: DAILY / WEEKLY / OCCASIONALLY
- Are you currently experiencing dental pain or discomfort? ☐ ☐ ☐
- Do you have earaches or neck pains? ☐ ☐ ☐
- Do you have any clicking, popping or discomfort in the jaw? ☐ ☐ ☐
- Do you brux or grind your teeth? ☐ ☐ ☐
- Do you have sores or ulcers in your mouth? ☐ ☐ ☐
- Do you wear dentures or partials? ☐ ☐ ☐
- Do you participate in active recreational activities? ☐ ☐ ☐
- Have you ever had a serious injury to your head or mouth? ☐ ☐ ☐

Date of your last dental exam:

What was done at that time?

Date of last dental x-rays:

What is the reason for your dental visit today?

How do you feel about your smile?

Medical Information *Please mark (X) your response to indicate if you have or have not had any of the following diseases or problems.*

Yes No DK

- Are you now under the care of a physician? ☐ ☐ ☐
- Physician Name: Phone: Include area code ( )
- Address/City/State/Zip:
- Are you in good health? ☐ ☐ ☐
- Has there been any change in your general health within the past year? ☐ ☐ ☐
- If yes, what condition is being treated?
- Date of last physical exam:
- Have you had a serious illness, operation or been hospitalized in the past 5 years? ☐ ☐ ☐
- If yes, what was the illness or problem?
- Are you taking or have you recently taken any prescription or over the counter medicine(s)? ☐ ☐ ☐
- If so, please list all, including vitamins, natural or herbal preparations and/or diet supplements:

Medical Information *Please mark (X) your response to indicate if you have or have not had any of the following diseases or problems.*

(Check DK if you Don't Know the answer to the question) Yes No DK

- Do you wear contact lenses? ☐ ☐ ☐
- **Joint Replacement.** Have you had an orthopedic total joint (hip, knee, elbow, finger) replacement? ☐ ☐ ☐ Date: ______ If yes, have you had any complications? ______
- Are you taking or scheduled to begin taking either of the medications, alendronate (Fosamax®) or risedronate (Actonel®) for osteoporosis or Paget's disease? ☐ ☐ ☐
- Since 2001, were you treated or are you presently scheduled to begin treatment with the intravenous bisphosphonates (Aredia® or Zometa®) for bone pain, hypercalcemia or skeletal complications resulting from Paget's disease, multiple myeloma or metastatic cancer? ☐ ☐ ☐ Date Treatment began:
- Do you use controlled substances (drugs)? ☐ ☐ ☐
- Do you use tobacco (smoking, snuff, chew, bidis)? ☐ ☐ ☐ If so, how interested are you in stopping? (Circle one) VERY / SOMEWHAT / NOT INTERESTED
- Do you drink alcoholic beverages? ☐ ☐ ☐ If yes, how much alcohol did you drink in the last 24 hours? ______ If yes, how much do you typically drink in a week? ______

WOMEN ONLY Are you:

- Pregnant? ☐ ☐ ☐
- Number of weeks: ______
- Taking birth control pills or hormonal replacement? ☐ ☐ ☐
- Nursing? ☐ ☐ ☐

Allergies - Are you allergic to or have you had a reaction to: To all **yes** responses, specify type of reaction. Yes No DK

- Local anesthetics ☐ ☐ ☐
- Aspirin ☐ ☐ ☐
- Penicillin or other antibiotics ☐ ☐ ☐
- Barbiturates, sedatives, or sleeping pills ☐ ☐ ☐
- Sulfa drugs ☐ ☐ ☐
- Codeine or other narcotics ☐ ☐ ☐
- Metals ☐ ☐ ☐
- Latex (rubber) ☐ ☐ ☐
- Iodine ☐ ☐ ☐
- Hay fever/seasonal ☐ ☐ ☐
- Animals ☐ ☐ ☐
- Food ☐ ☐ ☐
- Other ☐ ☐ ☐

Please mark (X) your response to indicate if you have or have not had any of the following diseases or problems. Yes No DK

- Artificial (prosthetic) heart valve ☐ ☐ ☐
- Previous infective endocarditis ☐ ☐ ☐
- Damaged valves in transplanted heart ☐ ☐ ☐
- Congenital heart disease (CHD)
  - Unrepaired, cyanotic CHD ☐ ☐ ☐
  - Repaired (completely) in last 6 months ☐ ☐ ☐
  - Repaired CHD with residual defects ☐ ☐ ☐

Except for the conditions listed above, antibiotic prophylaxis is no longer recommended for any other form of CHD.

- Cardiovascular disease ☐ ☐ ☐
- Angina ☐ ☐ ☐
- Arteriosclerosis ☐ ☐ ☐
- Congestive heart failure ☐ ☐ ☐
- Damaged heart valves ☐ ☐ ☐
- Heart attack ☐ ☐ ☐
- Heart murmur ☐ ☐ ☐
- Low blood pressure ☐ ☐ ☐
- High blood pressure ☐ ☐ ☐
- Other congenital heart defects ☐ ☐ ☐
- Mitral valve prolapse ☐ ☐ ☐
- Pacemaker ☐ ☐ ☐
- Rheumatic fever ☐ ☐ ☐
- Rheumatic heart disease ☐ ☐ ☐
- Abnormal bleeding ☐ ☐ ☐
- Anemia ☐ ☐ ☐
- Blood transfusion ☐ ☐ ☐ If yes, date: ______
- Hemophilia ☐ ☐ ☐
- AIDS or HIV infection ☐ ☐ ☐
- Arthritis ☐ ☐ ☐
- Autoimmune disease ☐ ☐ ☐
- Rheumatoid arthritis ☐ ☐ ☐
- Systemic lupus erythematosus ☐ ☐ ☐
- Asthma ☐ ☐ ☐
- Bronchitis ☐ ☐ ☐
- Emphysema ☐ ☐ ☐
- Sinus trouble ☐ ☐ ☐
- Tuberculosis ☐ ☐ ☐
- Cancer/Chemotherapy/Radiation Treatment ☐ ☐ ☐
- Chest pain upon exertion ☐ ☐ ☐
- Chronic pain ☐ ☐ ☐
- Diabetes Type I or II ☐ ☐ ☐
- Eating disorder ☐ ☐ ☐
- Malnutrition ☐ ☐ ☐
- Gastrointestinal disease ☐ ☐ ☐
- G.E. Reflux/persistent heartburn ☐ ☐ ☐
- Ulcers ☐ ☐ ☐
- Thyroid problems ☐ ☐ ☐
- Stroke ☐ ☐ ☐
- Glaucoma ☐ ☐ ☐
- Hepatitis, jaundice or liver disease ☐ ☐ ☐
- Epilepsy ☐ ☐ ☐
- Fainting spells or seizures ☐ ☐ ☐
- Neurological disorders ☐ ☐ ☐ If yes, specify: ______
- Sleep disorder ☐ ☐ ☐
- Mental health disorders ☐ ☐ ☐ Specify: ______
- Recurrent Infections ☐ ☐ ☐ Type of infection: ______
- Kidney problems ☐ ☐ ☐
- Night sweats ☐ ☐ ☐
- Osteoporosis ☐ ☐ ☐
- Persistent swollen glands in neck ☐ ☐ ☐
- Severe headaches/migraines ☐ ☐ ☐
- Severe or rapid weight loss ☐ ☐ ☐
- Sexually transmitted disease ☐ ☐ ☐
- Excessive urination ☐ ☐ ☐

Has a physician or previous dentist recommended that you take antibiotics prior to your dental treatment? ☐ ☐ ☐

Name of physician or dentist making recommendation: Phone:

Do you have any disease, condition, or problem not listed above that you think I should know about? ☐ ☐ ☐
Please explain:

NOTE: Both Doctor and patient are encouraged to discuss any and all relevant patient health issues prior to treatment.
I certify that I have read and understand the above and that the information given on this form is accurate. I understand the importance of a truthful health history and that my dentist and his/her staff will rely on this information for treating me. I acknowledge that my questions, if any, about inquiries set forth above have been answered to my satisfaction. I will not hold my dentist, or any other member of his/her staff, responsible for any action they take or do not take because of errors or omissions that I may have made in the completion of this form.

Signature of Patient/Legal Guardian: Date:

FOR COMPLETION BY DENTIST

Comments:

FIGURE 7-13 ADA Health History Form. (Courtesy American Dental Association, Chicago, IL)

WELCOME

Your Child
Child's Name ______
Nickname ______ Sex ______
Birthdate ______ Age ______
SS# / SIN ______
School ______ Grade ______
Child's Home Address ______
City ______ State/Prov. ______ Zip/P.C. ______
Phone ______

Responsible Party
Name ______
Relationship ______
Address ______
City ______ State/Prov. ______ Zip/P.C. ______
Email ______
Phone ______ SS#/SIN ______
DL# ______

Who is responsible for making appointments?
Name ______ Best time to call ______
Home Phone ______ Cell Phone ______ Time ______ Day ______
Work Phone ______ Ext. ______

Mother ☐ Stepmother ☐ Guardian
Name ______
Home Phone ______ Cell Phone ______
Work Phone ______ Ext. ______
Email ______
Employer ______
Occupation ______
SS#/SIN ______ D.O.B. ______
DL # ______
Marital Status ☐ Single ☐ Married ☐ Divorced ☐ Widowed ☐ Separated

Father ☐ Stepfather ☐ Guardian
Name ______
Home Phone ______ Cell Phone ______
Work Phone ______ Ext. ______
Email ______
Employer ______
Occupation ______
SS#/SIN ______ D.O.B. ______
DL # ______
Marital Status ☐ Single ☐ Married ☐ Divorced ☐ Widowed ☐ Separated

Primary Insurance
Insured's Name ______
Relationship ______
Birthdate ______ SS#/SIN ______
Employer ______ Date Employed ______
Occupation ______
Insurance Company ______
Group # ______ Employee # ______
Ins. Co. address ______ State/ ______ Zip/ ______
City ______ Prov. ______ P.C. ______

Additional Insurance
Insured's Name ______
Relationship ______
Birthdate ______ SS#/SIN ______
Employer ______ Date Employed ______
Occupation ______
Insurance Company ______
Group # ______ Employee # ______
Ins. Co. address ______ State/ ______ Zip/ ______
City ______ Prov. ______ P.C. ______

Financial Arrangements
For your convenience, we offer the following methods of payment. Please check the option which you prefer.
Payment in full at each appointment. ☐ Cash ☐ Personal Check Credit Card ☐ Visa ☐ MC ☐ Discover ☐ AMEX
☐ I wish to discuss the office's payment policy.

designs by lee

Dental & Health History **CONFIDENTIAL** Patient ID # ______

Your child's overall health as well as any medications which your child takes could have an important interrelationship with the dental care your child receives. Please answer each of the following questions completely.

How often does your child brush? ______ How often does your child floss? ______
Is your child's water fluoridated? ☐ Yes ☐ No Does your child take fluoride supplements? ☐ Yes ☐ No
Does your child:
Suck thumb/finger ☐ Yes ☐ No Grind teeth ☐ Yes ☐ No
Suck/Bite lip ☐ Yes ☐ No Clench jaws ☐ Yes ☐ No
Bite/Chew nails ☐ Yes ☐ No Gag easily ☐ Yes ☐ No
Chew hard objects (pencils, etc.) ☐ Yes ☐ No Tonsils/Adenoids removed ____ age ☐ Yes ☐ No
Speech Problem ☐ Yes ☐ No
Previous dentist ______ Address ______
Date of last dental visit? ______
Has your child had difficulty with previous dental visits? ☐ Yes ☐ No
Child's physician ______ Address ______
Phone # ______
Previous Hospitalizations/Surgeries/Serious Illnesses? ______ When? ______

Is your child currently taking medications? ☐ Yes ☐ No (if yes, please list)
Has your child ever taken FenPhen/Redux? ☐ Yes ☐ No
Does your child have a history of allergies/sensitivities/adverse reactions to any drugs or medications (penicillin, Novocain, etc.)? ☐ Yes ☐ No (if yes please describe) ______
Does your child have a history of allergies to any other substances (latex, environmental, etc.)? ☐ Yes ☐ No

Has your child ever had any of the following:
Asthma ☐ Yes ☐ No
Cancer ☐ Yes ☐ No
Hepatitis ☐ Yes ☐ No
HIV/AIDS ☐ Yes ☐ No
Hemophilia ☐ Yes ☐ No
A persistent cough or throat clearing not associated with a known illness (lasting more than 3 weeks) ☐ Yes ☐ No
Abnormal Bleeding ☐ Yes ☐ No
Acid Reflux ☐ Yes ☐ No
Stomach, liver or kidney problems ☐ Yes ☐ No
Handicaps/Disabilities ☐ Yes ☐ No
Tuberculosis ☐ Yes ☐ No
Diabetes ☐ Yes ☐ No
Rheumatic Fever ☐ Yes ☐ No
Congenital Heart Defect ☐ Yes ☐ No
Heart Murmur ☐ Yes ☐ No
Convulsions/Epilepsy ☐ Yes ☐ No
Osteoporosis ☐ Yes ☐ No
Hearing Impairment ☐ Yes ☐ No
Handicap/Disabilities ☐ Yes ☐ No

Please explain any medical problem that your child has: ______

Authorization & Release
I understand that providing incorrect information can be dangerous and it is my responsibility to inform the office of any changes in the child's medical status. I also authorize the staff to perform the necessary services the child may need.
I also authorize the release of any information including the diagnosis and the records of treatment or examination rendered, to third party payers and/or other health practitioners. I authorize and request my insurance company to pay directly to the Dentist or Dentist's group insurance benefits otherwise payable to me. I understand that my insurance carrier may pay less than the actual bill for services. I agree to be responsible for payment of all services rendered on my behalf or my dependents.

Signature of patient (or parent/guardian if minor) ______ Date ______
Dentist Review

Signature of Dentist ______ Date ______

028-9926/41000 PATTERSON OFFICE SUPPLIES 800.637.1140

FIGURE 7-14 Registration and health history form for children. (Courtesy Patterson Office Supplies, Champaign, IL.)

PATIENT'S NAME ____________ DATE OF BIRTH ____________

DATE	I HAVE REVIEWED THE ATTACHED HEALTH HISTORY. MY HEALTH AND MEDICATIONS HAVE CHANGED AS FOLLOWS (IF NO CHANGE, WRITE "NO CHANGE")	DENTIST'S SIGNATURE	PATIENT'S OR GUARDIAN'S SIGNATURE

ITEM 07-0515783/27004 COLWELL 1.800.637.1140

PATIENT NUMBER

HEALTH HISTORY UPDATE

A

Medical History Update

Patient Name____________ Birthdate___/___/___ Patient Number____________

I have reviewed the attached MEDICAL HISTORY. My (or the patient's) health and medications have changed as follows (if no change, write "No Change"):

Signature of Patient (or Guardian) Date

Update reviewed by Dr.____________

I have reviewed the attached MEDICAL HISTORY. My (or the patient's) health and medications have changed as follows (if no change, write "No Change"):

Signature of Patient (or Guardian) Date

Update reviewed by Dr.____________

I have reviewed the attached MEDICAL HISTORY. My (or the patient's) health and medications have changed as follows (if no change, write "No Change"):

Signature of Patient (or Guardian) Date

Update reviewed by Dr.____________

I have reviewed the attached MEDICAL HISTORY. My (or the patient's) health and medications have changed as follows (if no change, write "No Change"):

Signature of Patient (or Guardian) Date

Update reviewed by Dr.____________

16803/051-1113

B

FIGURE 7-15 Common health history update forms. (Courtesy Patterson Office Supplies, Champaign, IL.)

rights. Local and state dental associations monitor legislation that affects dentists and keep members informed. As legal changes occur, most suppliers update their forms for compliance.

Clinical Chart

A wide selection of dental charts is available for both general and specialty practices, but both electronic and paper formats have several basic points in common: patient identification (name, date of birth), a tooth chart diagram (permanent, deciduous, or a combination of both), and an area for clinical notes. Clinical notes may include general oral condition, the state of the gingival tissue, temporomandibular joint issues, and the dates of the placement of fixed or removable prosthetics. Most supply companies offer a special service for dentists who want to design their own paper charts; however, the customization of software products is generally unavailable or cost prohibitive.

Most paper charts are 8½ × 11 inches in size, made of heavy paper stock, and printed on both sides (Figure 7-16). One side of the record contains a tooth chart, an overview of the patient's health history, and general oral information or clinical notes. Some forms are designed to allow for the recording of periodontal measurements on the tooth chart, or the dentist or hygienist may use a separate form for periodontal charting (Figure 7-17).

The layout and design of clinical records may vary in different software systems, but these generally include the same information as the paper chart, which often involves a feature for recording periodontal measurements (Figure 7-18).

Treatment Record/Progress Notes

The reverse side of the paper clinical chart or a separate treatment sheet may be used for entering the services rendered and the associated fees. Progress notes can be included here or documented on a different sheet. Computer software systems generally have modules for entering services and fees and for recording notes. The administrative assistant enters the date, services, and fees into the patient's financial record where payments and balances are maintained.

Dental Diagnosis, Treatment Plan, and Estimate

This form includes the dentist's diagnosis and the treatment plan recommended for the patient (Figure 7-19). In many cases, the patient can select options in the treatment plan. After the consultation has been completed and treatment has been accepted by the patient, the form may be signed by the person responsible for the account. Often a clause is included to explain that the fee quoted is an estimate and that unforeseen circumstances may affect the final fee for the service.

Consultation and Referral Report

In some cases, the dentist refers a patient to another dentist for examination, evaluation, and diagnosis. The form shown in Figure 7-20 includes information about the patient, the reason for the referral, and an anticipated treatment plan. This form is sent to the referring dentist, with a copy being sent to the patient as well. The consultant enters an evaluation and recommendation on the form and returns it to the dentist.

Medication History and Prescriptions

Having a history and current list of all medications taken by a patient helps to prevent the prescription of drugs that could lead to unsafe interactions or that may negatively affect a chronic health condition. As in a medical practice, medications are prescribed for a dental patient on a paper prescription form (Figure 7-21, *A* and *B*) or through a qualified electronic prescribing system. E-prescription systems must be certified EHR technology; these can be stand-alone modules or part of a complete EHR system. With e-prescribing, dentists can route prescriptions electronically to the patient's preferred pharmacy in addition to reviewing the patient's medication history and insurance information. Some states require specific formats for prescription forms, and virtually all states authorize e-prescribing for the majority of prescription drugs (noncontrolled substances). If a patient elects to use a mail-order prescription service, prescriptions can usually be submitted on paper, via fax, or through an electronic portal.

Laboratory Requisitions

Many states require that a prescription or **laboratory requisition** form (Figure 7-22) accompany each case that a dentist sends to a dental laboratory. This blueprint improves communication between the dentist and the laboratory technician and helps eliminate illegal dental practices, thereby protecting the patient.

Consent Form

A **consent form** is commonly used in dentistry as a preventive measure against malpractice suits. The form, which is signed by the patient or by the parent or legal guardian of a pediatric patient, grants permission for the administration of anesthetic and other specified procedures. It is impossible to have a consent form for every phase of treatment, and it is unrealistic to believe that a general consent form that covers every possible procedure would be upheld in court. Therefore, a written summary of the treatment plan as agreed upon by the patient and dentist and that is dated and signed by both parties is a more acceptable format for such consent. Chapter 4 reviews the use of various types of consent forms in the dental office (see Figure 4-2).

Refusal of Treatment

There may be a time in the dental practice when a patient refuses to undergo recommended treatment for a condition that presents potential risks. To ensure that litigation does not ensue, the dentist should have the patient sign a refusal of treatment form (Figure 7-23) that includes the nature of the treatment, alternative treatments, treatment risks, and risks if no treatment is rendered.

Letters

Copies of all written communications sent to or concerning a patient should become part of the patient's clinical record.

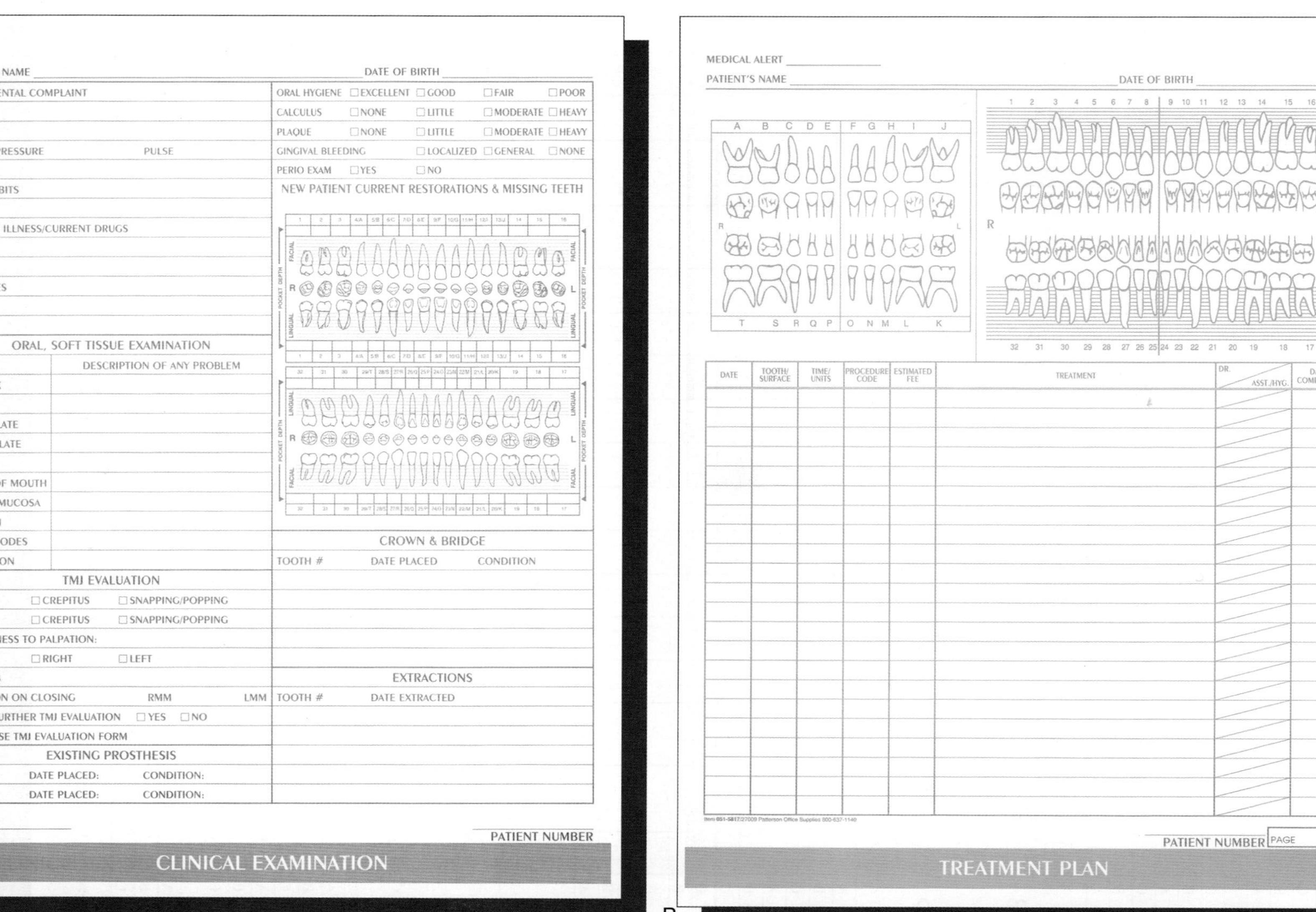
A

PATIENT'S NAME ______ DATE OF BIRTH ______

CHIEF DENTAL COMPLAINT	ORAL HYGIENE ☐EXCELLENT ☐GOOD ☐FAIR ☐POOR
	CALCULUS ☐NONE ☐LITTLE ☐MODERATE ☐HEAVY
	PLAQUE ☐NONE ☐LITTLE ☐MODERATE ☐HEAVY
BLOOD PRESSURE PULSE	GINGIVAL BLEEDING ☐LOCALIZED ☐GENERAL ☐NONE
	PERIO EXAM ☐YES ☐NO
ORAL HABITS	NEW PATIENT CURRENT RESTORATIONS & MISSING TEETH
EXISTING ILLNESS/CURRENT DRUGS	
ALLERGIES	

ORAL, SOFT TISSUE EXAMINATION

AREA	DESCRIPTION OF ANY PROBLEM
PHARYNX	
TONSILS	
SOFT PALATE	
HARD PALATE	
TONGUE	
FLOOR OF MOUTH	
BUCCAL MUCOSA	
LIPS SKIN	
LYMPH NODES	
OCCLUSION	

CROWN & BRIDGE

TOOTH #	DATE PLACED	CONDITION

TMJ EVALUATION

RIGHT ☐CREPITUS ☐SNAPPING/POPPING
LEFT ☐CREPITUS ☐SNAPPING/POPPING
TENDERNESS TO PALPATION:
TMJ ☐RIGHT ☐LEFT
MUSCLES
DEVIATION ON CLOSING RMM LMM
NEEDS FURTHER TMJ EVALUATION ☐YES ☐NO
IF YES, USE TMJ EVALUATION FORM

EXTRACTIONS

TOOTH #	DATE EXTRACTED

EXISTING PROSTHESIS

MAX. DATE PLACED: CONDITION:
MIN. DATE PLACED: CONDITION:

DATE ______ PATIENT NUMBER ______

CLINICAL EXAMINATION

B

MEDICAL ALERT ______
PATIENT'S NAME ______ DATE OF BIRTH ______

DATE	TOOTH/ SURFACE	TIME/ UNITS	PROCEDURE CODE	ESTIMATED FEE	TREATMENT	DR. / ASST./HYG.	DATE COMPLETED

PATIENT NUMBER PAGE

TREATMENT PLAN

FIGURE 7-16 **A,** Adult clinical chart (general practice). **B,** Treatment plan that may accompany a clinical chart. (Courtesy Patterson Office Supplies, Champaign, IL.)

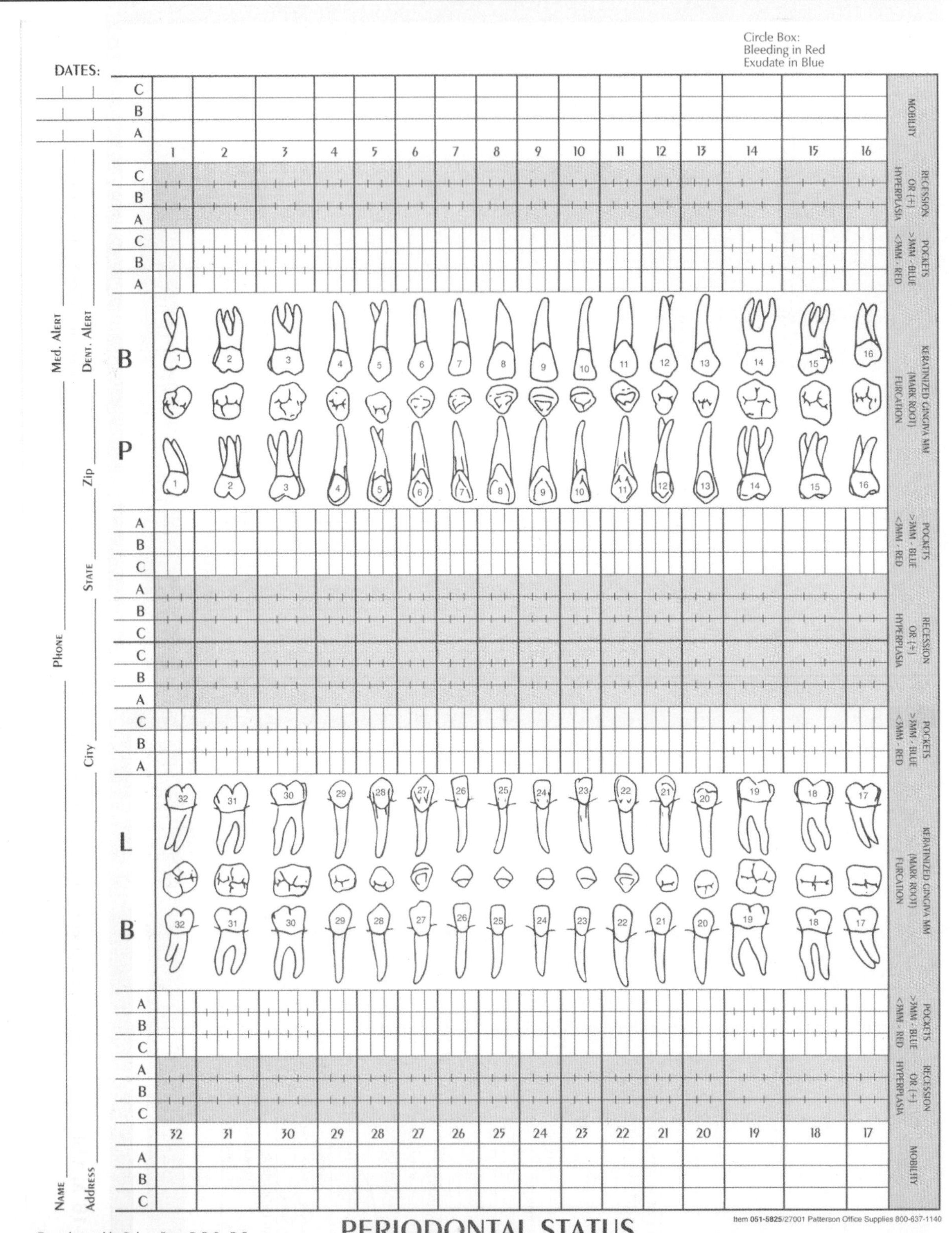

Circle Box:
Bleeding in Red
Exudate in Blue

DATES:

Med. Alert
Dent. Alert
Zip
State
Phone
City
Name
Address

	1	2	3	4	5	6	7	8	9	10	11	12	13	14	15	16	
C, B, A																	MOBILITY
C, B, A																	RECESSION OR (+) HYPERPLASIA
C, B, A																	POCKETS >3MM - BLUE <3MM - RED
B	1	2	3	4	5	6	7	8	9	10	11	12	13	14	15	16	KERATINIZED GINGIVA MM (MARK ROOT) FURCATION
P	1	2	3	4	5	6	7	8	9	10	11	12	13	14	15	16	
A, B, C																	POCKETS >3MM - BLUE <3MM - RED
A, B, C																	RECESSION OR (+) HYPERPLASIA

	32	31	30	29	28	27	26	25	24	23	22	21	20	19	18	17	
C, B, A																	RECESSION OR (+) HYPERPLASIA
C, B, A																	POCKETS >3MM - BLUE <3MM - RED
L	32	31	30	29	28	27	26	25	24	23	22	21	20	19	18	17	KERATINIZED GINGIVA MM (MARK ROOT) FURCATION
B	32	31	30	29	28	27	26	25	24	23	22	21	20	19	18	17	
A, B, C																	POCKETS >3MM - BLUE <3MM - RED
A, B, C																	RECESSION OR (+) HYPERPLASIA
A, B, C																	MOBILITY

Form designed by Robert Ryan, D.D.S., P.C.

PERIODONTAL STATUS

Item 051-5825/27001 Patterson Office Supplies 800-637-1140

FIGURE 7-17 Periodontal specialty clinical chart, front. (Courtesy Patterson Office Supplies, Champaign, IL.)

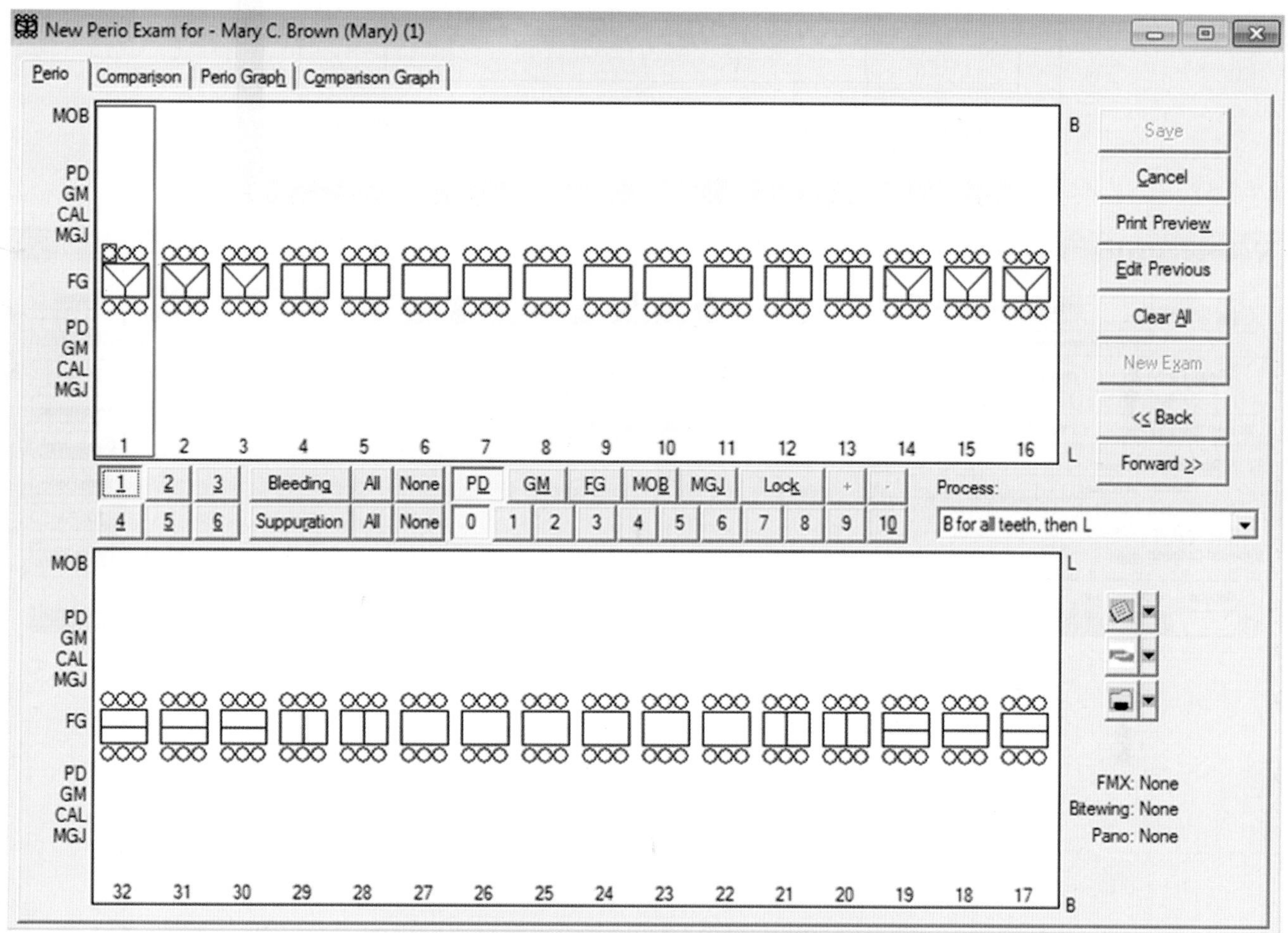

FIGURE 7-18 Screenshot of tooth chart software page.

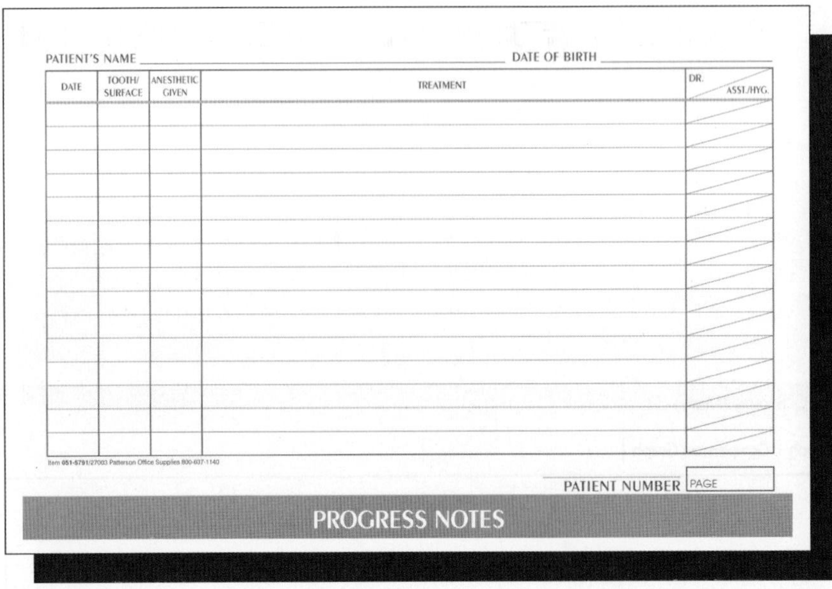

PATIENT'S NAME ______ DATE OF BIRTH ______

DATE	TOOTH/ SURFACE	ANESTHETIC GIVEN	TREATMENT	DR. / ASST./HYG.

PATIENT NUMBER ______ PAGE

PROGRESS NOTES

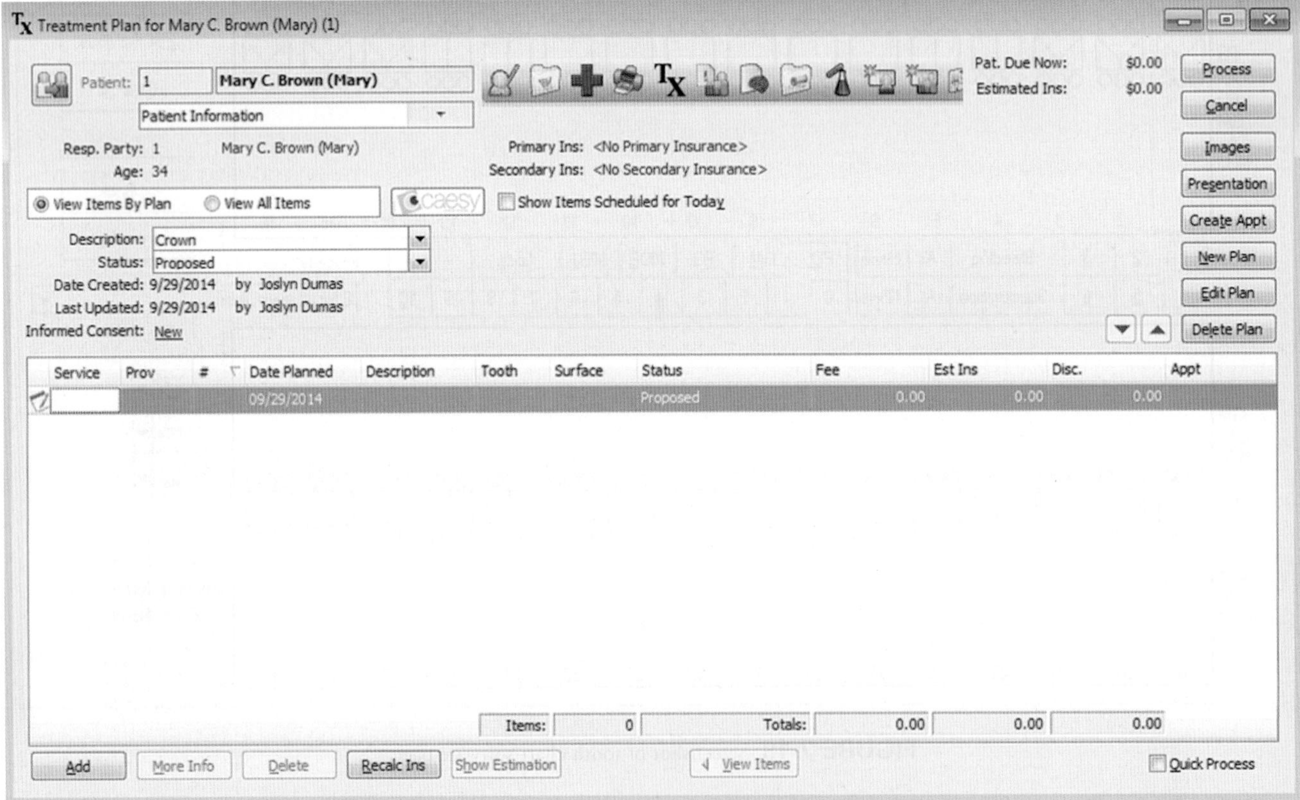

FIGURE 7-19 A clinical chart for recording treatment data and a screenshot of a treatment plan estimate. (Courtesy Patterson Office Supplies, Champaign, IL.)

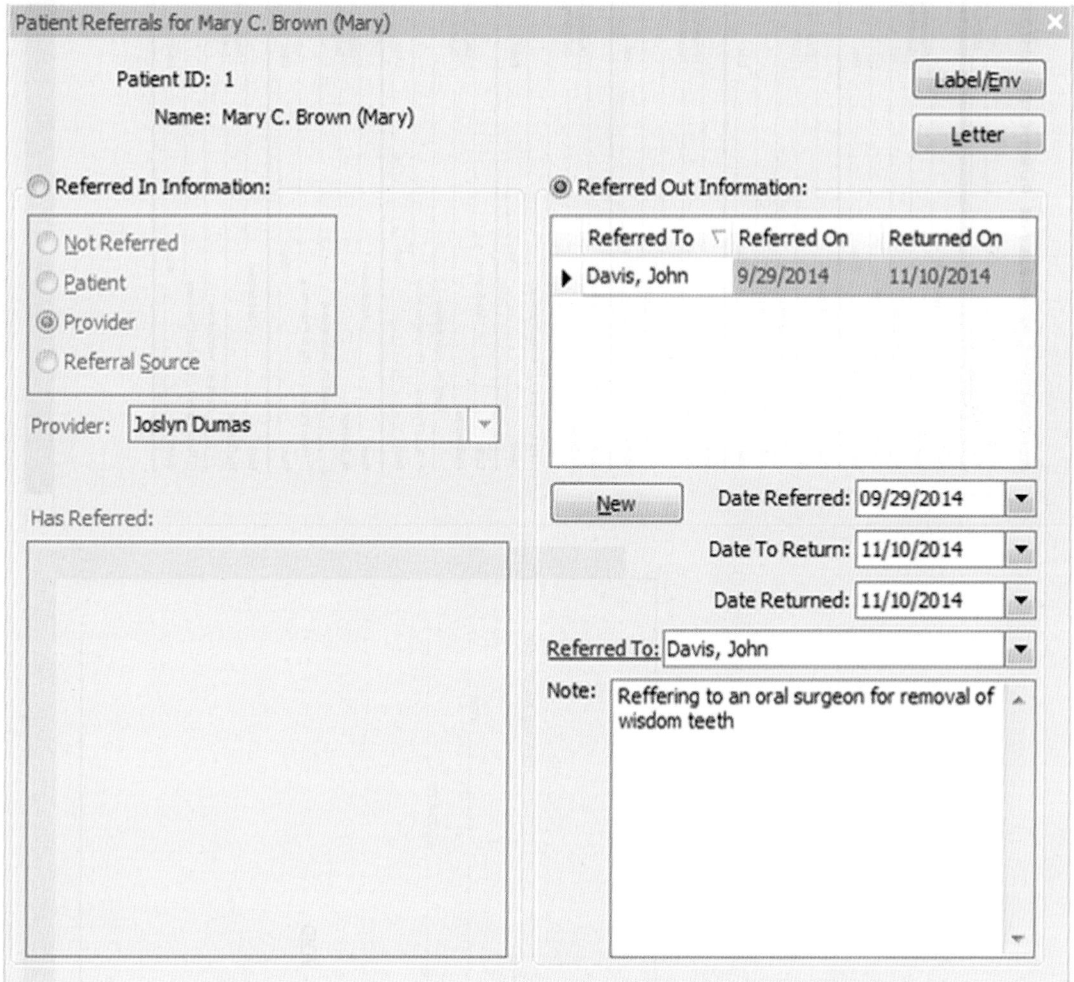

FIGURE 7-20 Screenshot of patient treatment record software page.

A

JOSEPH W. LAKE, D.D.S.
611 Main Street, S.E.
Grand Rapids, MI 49502

Telephone 616-101-9575 DEA Reg. No. 0000000

NAME ______ AGE ______

ADDRESS ______ DATE ______

℞

SAMPLE - VOID

☐ Label

Refill ____ Times

B

Rx/MEDICATION HISTORY

NAME ______ AGE ____ DATE ______ ACCT# ______
ALLERGIES ______ MEDICAL ALERT ______

Date ______ Medication ______
Rx/Dosage ______ ☐ Dispense as Written ☐ Substitute Permitted Qty ______ Freq ______
______ Refill (s), Instructions ______
☐ Rx to Patient / ☐ Rx to Pharmacy ______
Start: ______ Stop: ______ Disc: ______ Initials ______

Date ______ Medication ______
Rx/Dosage ______ ☐ Dispense as Written ☐ Substitute Permitted Qty ______ Freq ______
______ Refill (s), Instructions ______
☐ Rx to Patient / ☐ Rx to Pharmacy ______
Start: ______ Stop: ______ Disc: ______ Initials ______

Date ______ Medication ______
Rx/Dosage ______ ☐ Dispense as Written ☐ Substitute Permitted Qty ______ Freq ______
______ Refill (s), Instructions ______
☐ Rx to Patient / ☐ Rx to Pharmacy ______
Start: ______ Stop: ______ Disc: ______ Initials ______

Date ______ Medication ______
Rx/Dosage ______ ☐ Dispense as Written ☐ Substitute Permitted Qty ______ Freq ______
______ Refill (s), Instructions ______
☐ Rx to Patient / ☐ Rx to Pharmacy ______
Start: ______ Stop: ______ Disc: ______ Initials ______

Date ______ Medication ______
Rx/Dosage ______ ☐ Dispense as Written ☐ Substitute Permitted Qty ______ Freq ______
______ Refill (s), Instructions ______
☐ Rx to Patient / ☐ Rx to Pharmacy ______
Start: ______ Stop: ______ Disc: ______ Initials ______

Date ______ Medication ______
Rx/Dosage ______ ☐ Dispense as Written ☐ Substitute Permitted Qty ______ Freq ______
______ Refill (s), Instructions ______
☐ Rx to Patient / ☐ Rx to Pharmacy ______
Start: ______ Stop: ______ Disc: ______ Initials ______

Date ______ Medication ______
Rx/Dosage ______ ☐ Dispense as Written ☐ Substitute Permitted Qty ______ Freq ______
______ Refill (s), Instructions ______
☐ Rx to Patient / ☐ Rx to Pharmacy ______
Start: ______ Stop: ______ Disc: ______ Initials ______

FIGURE 7-21 A, Prescription form. **B,** Custom medication history form. (Courtesy Patterson Office Supplies, Champaign, IL.)

WARD | a dti company

1068 Charles H. Orndorf Drive • Brighton, MI • 48116 • P 810 534 9273 • F 810 534 9278

Crown and Bridge Rx

RX DATE _____

CASE # _____

DATE WANTED TIME

DOCTOR INFORMATION
Name _____
Address _____
Telephone _____

PATIENT INFORMATION
Name _____
Sex _____ Age _____
O Diagnostic wax up O Pearltemps[TM] (provisionals)
O Call me (before proceeding with case)

Rx

HAVE YOU INCLUDED THE FOLLOWING?
O Impression
O Bite
O Opposing
O Shade
O Pre-op model
O Photos
O Model of temps
O Bite stick
O Face bow

PLEASE SEND
O Prescription forms
O Plastic bags
O Case boxes

RETURN FOR
O Die Trim
O Metal try-in
O Finish
O Evaluation
O Wax check
O Bisque bake try-in

IF INSUFFICIENT ROOM
O Reduce and mark
O Metal occlusion
O Reduction coping
O Please call

IF CASE WILL NOT DRAW
O Make reduction copings
O Please call

O Surgical Stent

SHADE _____ STUMP _____

AMOUNT OF TRANSLUCENCY
O Light O Medium O Heavy

VALUE
O Bright O Medium O Low

MIDLINE SHIFT
R _____ MM L _____ MM
_____ MM
Length of centrals from cervical margin
O Close Diastema

CIRCLE TEETH NUMBERS
1 2 3 4 5 6 7 8 9 10 11 12 13 14 15 16
32 31 30 29 28 27 26 25 24 23 22 21 20 19 18 17

OCCLUSAL STAINING
O None
O Light
O Medium
O Dark
O Hypo-calcification
O Shade tab enclosed

MOLD OF CROWN DESIRED
O Follow study model
O Match existing
O Make ideal

SURFACE ANATOMY
O Smooth
O Textured
O Mamelon development
O Match existing

METAL
O High noble O Noble

OCCLUSION
O Metal O Porcelain

LATERAL EXCURSION
O Cuspid guidance O Group function

PONTIC DESIGN
O Harmony O Ovate O Ridge Lap
O Cone O Hygienic

PONTIC TISSUE RELIEF
O Yes mm deep _____ O No _____

LABIAL MARGIN
O Fine metal collar on tooth # _____ O Show no metal standard on # _____
O Show no metal 360° on tooth # _____ O Porcelain Butt Margin on tooth # _____

CONTACTS
O Broad O Normal O Point

OCCLUSAL CLEARANCE
O Positive Contact O Cusp Fossa O Out of Occlusion O Foil Relief

Doctor's Signature _____ License # _____

White - Lab Copy Yellow - Lab Copy Blue - Doctor's Copy

A

FIGURE 7-22 **A,** Example of a laboratory prescription/requisition form for a crown and bridge.

Continued

Doctor ____ Patient ____
Address ____ Age ____ Sex ____
City ____ St ____ Zip ____
Phone ____
Date Sent: ____
Try in Date: ____
Finish Date: ____

Please send:
☐ RX Forms ☐ Mailing Boxes ☐ Other____

PARTIALS AND DENTURES (Please ✓)

CASE DESIGN
☐ Full Upper ☐ Partial Upper
☐ Full Lower ☐ Partial Lower
☐ Cusil Denture ☐ Jump Denture
☐ Other____
☐ Reline ☐ Repair
☐ Custom Tray ☐ Surgical Tray
☐ Bite Block ☐ Post Dam
☐ Relief ☐ Altered Cast
☐ Please exclude identification
☐ Please mark denture for ID purposes as: ____

FACIAL CHARACTERISTICS
☐ Square ☐ Dominant rt side
☐ Square Tapering ☐ Dominant lft side
☐ Tapering ☐ Diastema
☐ Ovoid

MATERIALS
Anterior Teeth: ☐ Porc ☐ Plastic
Shade ____ Mold ____
Posterior Teeth: ☐ Porc ☐ Plastic
Shade ____ Mold ____
☐ Economy Acrylic ☐ Cast Chrome
☐ Regular Acrylic ☐ Temporary
☐ Personalized Acrylic ☐ Flipper
Vinyl ____ Soft liner ____

ADDITIONAL INSTRUCTIONS

DESIGN CASE
UPPER — RIGHT, LEFT (teeth 1–16)
LOWER — LEFT, RIGHT (teeth 17–32)
CHARACTERIZATION

FORM 9410

CROWN AND BRIDGE (Please ✓)

MATERIALS
☐ Porcelain to Metal
☐ High Noble (yellow)
☐ Noble (white)
☐ Base - N.P.
☐ All Porcelain
☐ Composite
☐ Other ____
☐ All Metal
☐ High Noble (yellow)
☐ Noble (yellow)
☐ Economy (yellow)
☐ Noble (white)
☐ Base - N.P. (yellow)
☐ Base - N.P. (white)

CASE DESIGN
☐ Full Crown ☐ Facing
☐ ¾ Crown ☐ Porc Butt Margin
☐ Inlay ☐ Other ____
☐ Onlay ☐ ____
☐ Full Ridge ☐ Partial Ridge ☐ No Ridge ☐ Point Contact ☐ No Contact

Ridge Relief: ☐ None ☐ Slight ☐ Medium ☐ Heavy
Contact ☐ Mesial ☐ Distal
No Contact ☐ Mesial ☐ Distal
Occlusal tight:
OK to trim? ☐ Yes ☐ No

METAL DESIGN (Please ✓)
(A) (B) (C) (D) (E) (F) (G) (H) (J) (K) (L) (M) (N)

ADDITIONAL INSTRUCTIONS

DOCTOR PLEASE RETAIN DUPLICATE COPY

Signature ____
License Number ____ State ____

Thank You!

B

FIGURE 7-22, cont'd B, Laboratory prescription form with provisions for dentures, crowns, and bridges. (Courtesy Patterson Office Supplies, Champaign, IL.)

REFUSAL OF PERIODONTAL TREATMENT

I have been advised and understand on this date that I have periodontal disease that may cause gum and bone inflammation or loss, and that it can lead to loss of my teeth. The severity of my condition today is slight/moderate/advanced. I have been informed that I have pocket depths as follows:

Depth	*Tooth Number(s)*
3-5 mm	______________
6-7 mm	______________
8+ mm	______________

Various treatment options for this condition have been explained to me, including gum surgery, replacement, extraction, as well as my right to refuse treatment. I have had the opportunity to read this form and ask questions, and my questions have been answered to my satisfaction. I am electing to refuse treatment and agree to release and hold harmless this office and the undersigned dentist from any liability for any adverse effects of my decision.

Signature of Patient/
Parent or Guardian ______________

Print Name ______________ Date ______________

Interpreter (if used) Signature ______________

Print Name ______________ Date ______________

Witness Signature ______________

Print Name ______________ Date ______________

Dentist Certification:
I hereby certify that I have explained the nature, purpose, benefits, risks of, and alternatives (including no treatment and attendant risks), to the proposed procedures. I have offered answers to any questions and have fully answered all such questions. I believe that the patient/parent/guardian fully understands what I have explained and answered.

Dentist's Signature ______________

Print Name ______________ Date ______________

REFUSAL OF PERIODONTAL TREATMENT

Item 051-3713/9085 Patterson Office Supplies 800-637-1140

FIGURE 7-23 Refusal of Periodontal Treatment form. (Courtesy Patterson Office Supplies, Champaign, IL.)

These are valuable for future dealings with the patient, and they could also become evidence in a malpractice suit.

Postal Receipts

Radiographs or other records transferred to another dentist via the US Postal Service should be sent by certified mail with a return receipt requested. The receipt verifies that the films were mailed and by whom the package was received.

Radiographic Films

A patient's radiographic films should be labeled with the patient's full name, the date of the exposure, the number and type of films, and the dentist's name. If radiographs are copied and mailed or transmitted to another practitioner, the name and date of transfer should be noted in the clinical chart. In addition, a signed release request from the patient must be retained in the patient's record.

Test Results

Dated copies of test results are kept in the patient's clinical record. These could include allergy testing and caries or periodontal risk evaluations (Figure 7-24).

Entering Data on a Clinical Chart

Several types of data are entered in the various components of a patient's record, including the charting of existing conditions, which is done with a variety of symbols and codes; the recording of treatment procedures and codes; treatment plans; and discussions with the patient about recommended treatment. Medical warnings are also noted and can be called out with warning flags as shown in Figure 7-25. Some paper clinical charts provide space on the back of the form for handwritten notes, or they may be entered by the dentist or the assistant

ADA American Dental Association®
America's leading advocate for oral health

Caries Risk Assessment Form (Age >6)

Patient Name:				
Birth Date:		Date:		
Age:		Initials:		
		Low Risk	Moderate Risk	High Risk
Contributing Conditions		Check or Circle the conditions that apply		
I.	**Fluoride Exposure** (through drinking water, supplements, professional applications, toothpaste)	☐Yes	☐No	
II.	**Sugary Foods or Drinks** (including juice, carbonated or non-carbonated soft drinks, energy drinks, medicinal syrups)	Primarily at mealtimes ☐		Frequent or prolonged between meal exposures/day ☐
III.	**Caries Experience of Mother, Caregiver and/or other Siblings** (for patients ages 6-14)	No carious lesions in last 24 months ☐	Carious lesions in last 7-23 months ☐	Carious lesions in last 6 months ☐
IV.	**Dental Home**: established patient of record, receiving regular dental care in a dental office	☐Yes	☐No	
General Health Conditions		Check or Circle the conditions that apply		
I.	**Special Health Care Needs** (developmental, physical, medical or mental disabilities that prevent or limit performance of adequate oral health care by themselves or caregivers)	☐No	Yes (over age 14) ☐	Yes (ages 6-14) ☐
II.	**Chemo/Radiation Therapy**	☐No		☐Yes
III.	**Eating Disorders**	☐No	☐Yes	
IV.	**Medications that Reduce Salivary Flow**	☐No	☐Yes	
V.	**Drug/Alcohol Abuse**	☐No	☐Yes	
Clinical Conditions		Check or Circle the conditions that apply		
I.	**Cavitated or Non-Cavitated** (incipient) **Carious Lesions or Restorations** (visually or radiographically evident)	No new carious lesions or restorations in last 36 months ☐	1 or 2 new carious lesions or restorations in last 36 months ☐	3 or more carious lesions or restorations in last 36 months ☐
II.	**Teeth Missing Due to Caries in past 36 months**	☐No		☐Yes
III.	**Visible Plaque**	☐No	☐Yes	
IV.	**Unusual Tooth Morphology** that compromises oral hygiene	☐No	☐Yes	
V.	**Interproximal Restorations - 1 or more**	☐No	☐Yes	
VI.	**Exposed Root Surfaces** Present	☐No	☐Yes	
VII.	**Restorations with Overhangs** and/or **Open Margins; Open Contacts** with Food Impaction	☐No	☐Yes	
VIII.	**Dental/Orthodontic Appliances** (fixed or removable)	☐No	☐Yes	
IX.	**Severe Dry Mouth (Xerostomia)**	☐No		☐Yes

Overall assessment of dental caries risk: ☐ Low ☐ Moderate ☐ High

Patient Instructions:

ADA American Dental Association®
America's leading advocate for oral health

Caries Risk Assessment Form (Age >6)

Circle or check the boxes of the conditions that apply. Low Risk = only conditions in "Low Risk" column present; Moderate Risk = only conditions in "Low" and/or "Moderate Risk" columns present; High Risk = one or more conditions in the "High Risk" column present.

The clinical judgment of the dentist may justify a change of the patient's risk level (increased or decreased) based on review of this form and other pertinent information. For example, missing teeth may not be regarded as high risk for a follow up patient; or other risk factors not listed may be present.

The assessment cannot address every aspect of a patient's health, and should not be used as a replacement for the dentist's inquiry and judgment. Additional or more focused assessment may be appropriate for patients with specific health concerns. As with other forms, this assessment may be only a starting point for evaluating the patient's health status.

This is a tool provided for the use of ADA members. It is based on the opinion of experts who utilized the most up-to-date scientific information available. The ADA plans to periodically update this tool based on: 1) member feedback regarding its usefulness, and; 2) advances in science. ADA member-users are encouraged to share their opinions regarding this tool with the Council on Dental Practice.

FIGURE 7-24 ADA Caries Risk Assessment Form.

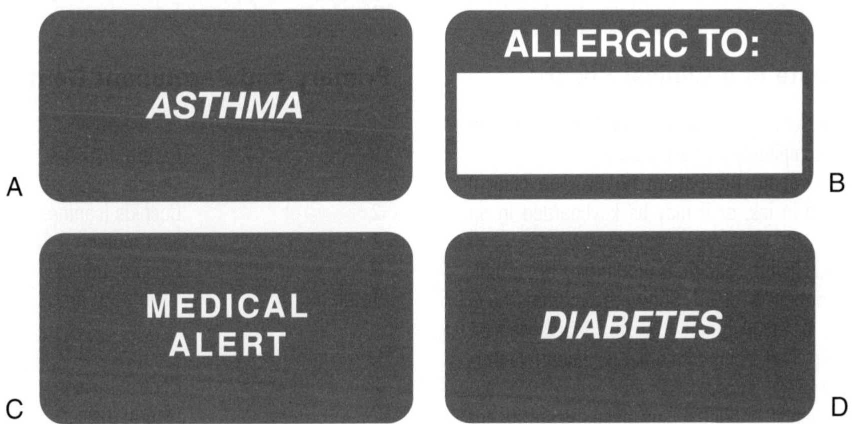

FIGURE 7-25 Medical warning flags used in a patient record.

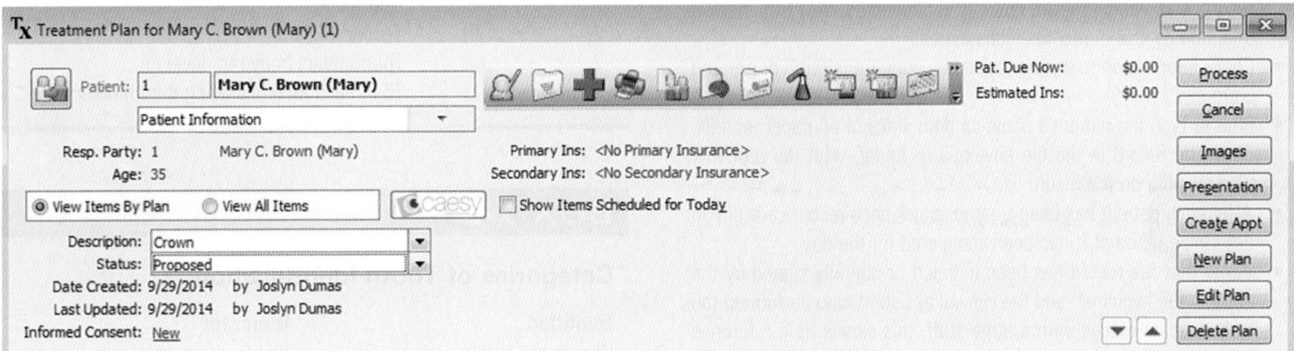

FIGURE 7-26 Screenshot of a data entry page for a patient treatment record.

into a computer terminal or tablet. All data entered in a patient's clinical chart as well as progress notes should be dated, accurate, comprehensive, and initialed or digitally verified by the treating dentist, hygienist, and assistant (Figure 7-26). One of the major concerns during legal proceedings is incomplete data on a patient record. All interactions (including nonactions, such a patient declining or delaying treatment) should be recorded in the clinical record. Failure to document any activity completely and accurately may prove costly in a lawsuit. Box 7-3 lists several rules for entering data, beginning with the creation of the record.

Types of Clinical Data Entries

Entering information on the patient's clinical chart or progress notes involves the use of tooth-numbering systems, abbreviations, and symbols. The administrative assistant must understand each of these systems as well as the basic descriptions of the oral cavity. For example, there are two arches: the maxilla or maxillary arch (upper jaw) and the mandible or mandibular arch (lower jaw). There are four quadrants: maxillary right and left and mandibular right and left. There are six segments: the maxillary and mandibular right and left posterior segments, which include the molars and the premolars (bicuspids), and the two anterior segments, which include all anterior teeth on the right and left in both arches, from canine (cuspid) to canine (cuspid).

PRACTICE NOTE

The failure to document any activity completely and accurately may prove costly in a lawsuit.

Tooth Nomenclature

The administrative assistant should be able to identify the names and numbers of the teeth in both the primary and permanent dentition (see Box 7-4). Mixed dentition (a combination of primary and permanent teeth) usually exists from approximately 6 to 12 years of age. For example, a child may have lost the primary central incisors, and the first permanent molars may have erupted; however, the primary first and second molars are still firmly in place. Mixed dentition occasionally occurs in an adult when a primary tooth is retained as a result of a missing or misaligned permanent tooth.

Teeth present a good appearance and provide support for other structures. They also aid in swallowing, mastication, digestion, and the production of speech and phonetics. The primary

BOX 7-3

Rules for Entering Data in a Clinical Record

- Transfer the information from the registration and health history form to the dental chart completely and accurately.
- Enter general information about the patient neatly. The clinical record must be completed in ink, or it may be keyboarded in an electronic record.
- Make sure that any serious health conditions or allergies are prominently displayed in the patient's record. Software programs have fields for warning flags, or small brightly colored labels can be placed inside the patient's chart along with other confidential information (see Figure 7-25.)
- The clinical assistant, hygienist, or dentist may make the entries for services rendered in the clinical record. Data can be entered on a barrier-protected keyboard in the treatment room or on a keyboard outside of the treatment room. Both methods provide a neater record, and, when they are properly implemented, they can improve infection control in records management.
- Check information to ensure that it has been transferred or entered correctly.
- Print or type the patient's name on both sides of all paper records. Place the record in the file envelope or folder, with the patient's name visible on the record.
- After each patient has been treated, check each record carefully to determine whether it has been completed for the day.
- Verify that the record has been initialed or digitally signed by the dentist, the hygienist, and the clinical assistant who performed the treatment. In offices with a large staff, this serves as a reference for follow up; it may be needed in case of a lawsuit.
- Ensure that all codes and charting techniques are consistent with the system used in the office. A list of these codes and symbols should be available to all staff members, and it should be posted in each treatment room or be available in a dropdown screen on the computer.
- Never make a derogatory remark about a patient in the record that could prove damaging in a lawsuit.

BOX 7-4

Primary and Permanent Dentition

Primary Dentition

2	Central incisors
2	Lateral incisors
2	Cuspids (canines)
2	First molars
2	Second molars
Total:	10 in each arch

Permanent Dentition

2	Central incisors
2	Lateral incisors
2	Cuspids (canines)
2	First premolars
2	Second premolars
2	First molars
2	Second molars
2	Third molars (may not develop)
Total:	16 in each arch (including third molars)

BOX 7-5

Categories of Tooth Identification

Dentition	Quadrant
Primary	Right
Permanent	Left
Arch	**Specific Tooth**
Maxillary	First premolar, central incisor,
Mandibular	and so on

dentition creates the framework for the eruption of a healthy permanent dentition. Premature loss of the primary teeth can be directly related to future dental disease or other dental anomalies. Likewise, the loss of a single permanent tooth can be the start of serious dental impairment if it is not replaced. The administrative assistant plays an important role in patient education. He or she is responsible for teaching patients about how to retain healthy teeth and a healthy mouth for a lifetime. To be an effective team member, the administrative assistant must understand and be able to communicate to patients the reasons for maintaining dental health and why this is intrinsic to good overall health.

A qualified clinical assistant understands the correct identification of a tooth in the oral cavity and the sequence of terms used to identify it. Confusion in the order of identification can cause many communication problems and administrative issues. The correct sequence of identification most commonly used is as follows: the dentition, the arch, the quadrant, and the specific tooth (see Box 7-5). For example, when describing a patient's complaint, the problem tooth should be defined as the permanent maxillary right first molar.

Tooth-Numbering Systems

Every dental office makes use of a specific numbering system to chart the patient's oral cavity or to refer to dental treatment to be performed. There are several numbering systems, and the dentist and staff choose which one is used in the office. The objective of a numbering system is to identify each tooth numerically or alphabetically. This number or letter provides an abbreviated form of tooth reference, and it helps with consistent records management. The three most common numbering systems are the Universal Numbering System, the Palmer Notation System, and the Fédération Dentaire Internationale (FDI) system.

Universal/National Numbering System. The most popular numbering system is the universal/national numbering system. It uses the Arabic numerals from 1 through 32 for the permanent dentition and the letters *A* through *T* for the primary dentition.

The universal system begins numbering the permanent teeth with the most posterior tooth in the maxillary right quadrant; this is the third molar, and it is assigned as tooth #1. Numbering

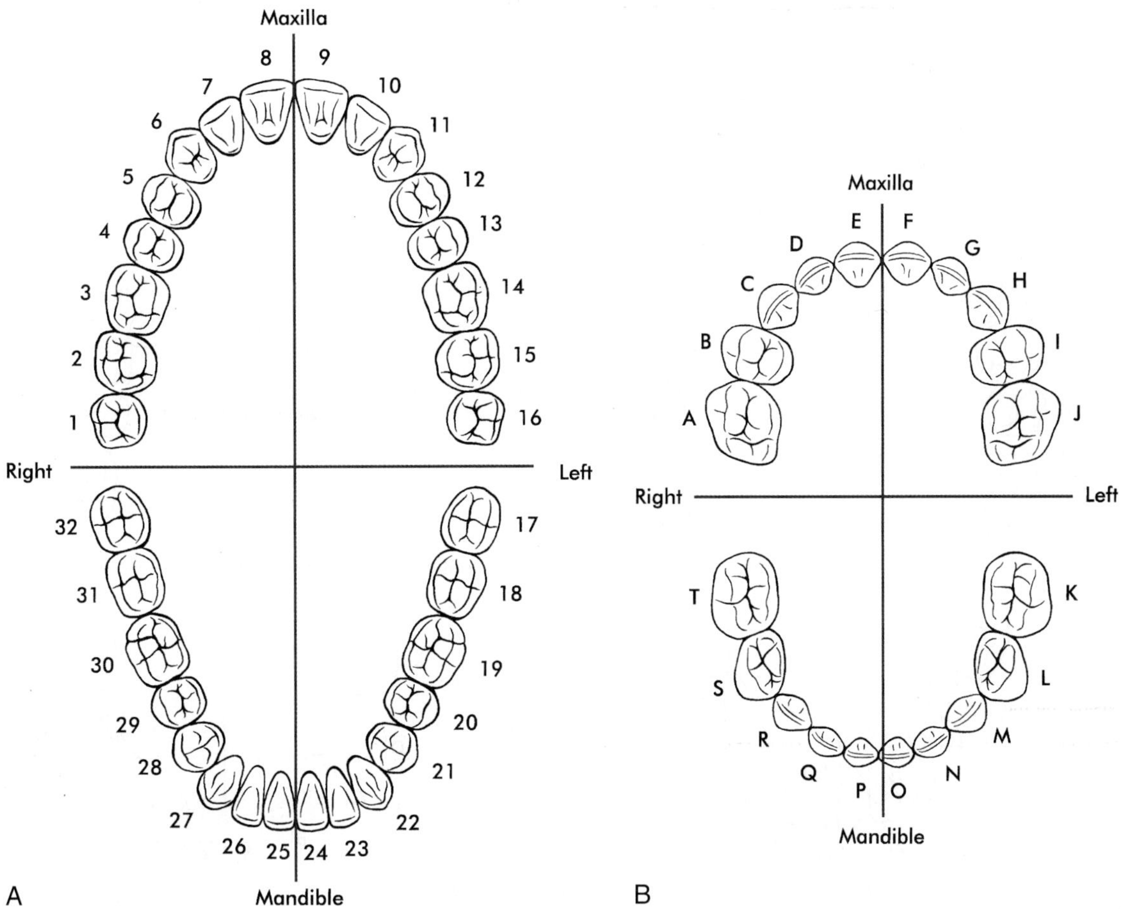

FIGURE 7-27 Universal numbering system. **A,** Permanent dentition. **B,** Primary dentition.

for the primary dentition begins with #A for the primary maxillary right second molar. The numbering continues toward the anterior midline to the right central incisor, which is tooth #8 of the permanent dentition and tooth #E of the primary dentition. The numbering continues to the maxillary left quadrant, from the midline to the most posterior tooth, which is #16 of the permanent dentition and #J of the primary dentition. The numbering drops to the mandibular left quadrant to permanent tooth #17 or primary tooth #K and then across the arch to the mandibular right most posterior tooth, tooth #32 or #T (Figure 7-27).

Palmer Notation System. The Palmer notation system assigns each of the four quadrants a bracket to designate the area of the mouth in which the tooth is found. In Figure 7-28, *A*, the left side of the chart represents the patient's right side, and the right side of the chart represents the patient's left side. It might be depicted as follows:

Maxillary right	Maxillary left
Mandibular right	Mandibular left

Each permanent tooth in the individual quadrants is assigned a number from 1 through 8, with #1 beginning at the midline and increasing to #8 distally. This may be written as follows:

Maxillary right central incisor #1⌋
Maxillary left central incisor ⌊#1
Mandibular right central incisor #1⌉
Mandibular left central incisor ⌈#1

The direction of the bracket indicates the arch, and the number within the bracket indicates the tooth, as follows:

Maxillary right third molar #8⌋
Maxillary left second molar ⌊#7
Mandibular right first premolar #4⌉
Mandibular left lateral incisor ⌈#2

For the primary dentition, brackets are used to assign a quadrant, but the teeth are designated by the letters *A* through *E*. *A* specifies the central incisors, and *E* specifies the second molars (Figure 7-28, *B*).

International Standards Organizational System/ Fédération Dentaire Internationale System. To create a numbering system that could be used internationally as well as by electronic data transfer, the World Health Organization accepted the International Standards Organization (ISO) System for teeth. In 1996, the ADA accepted the ISO system, in addition to the Universal/National System. The ISO system is based on the

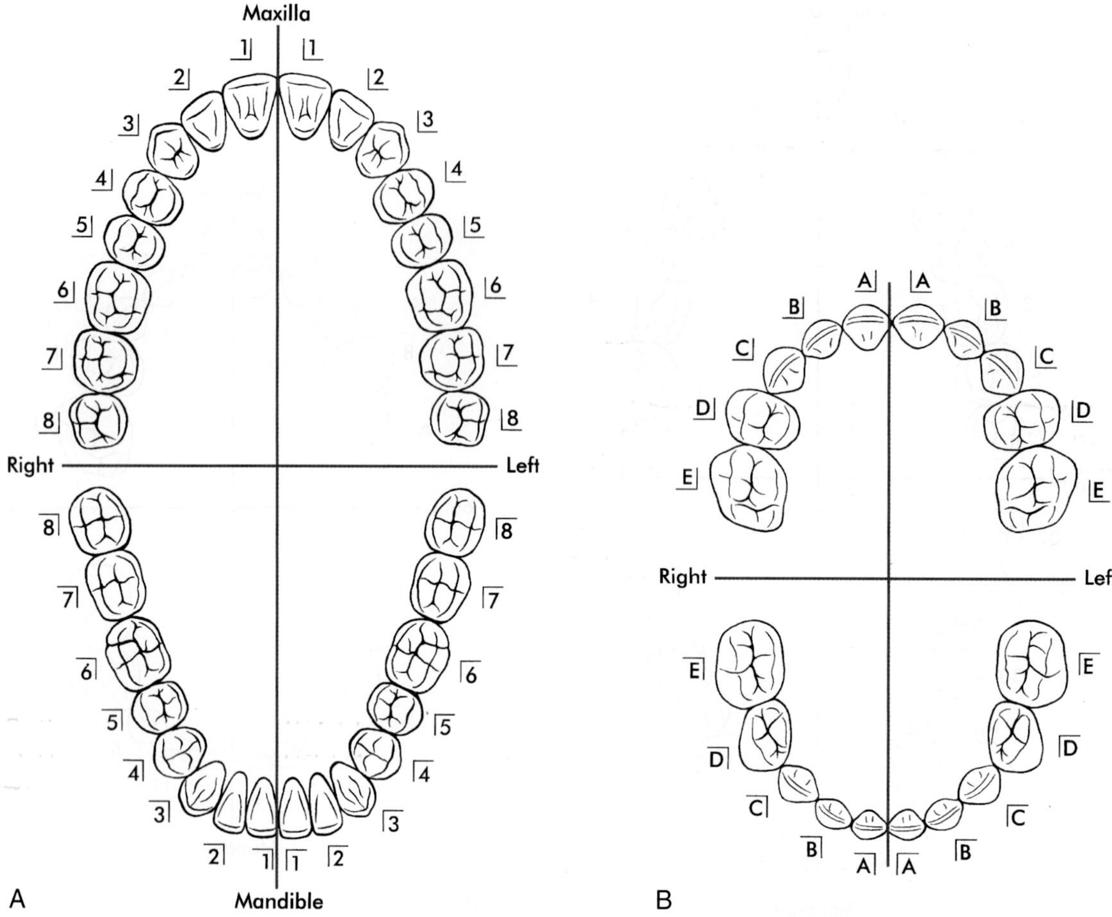

FIGURE 7-28 Palmer notation numbering system. **A,** Permanent dentition. **B,** Primary dentition.

Fédération Dentaire Internationale (FDI) System and is used in many countries.

The ISO/FDI system (Figure 7-29) assigns a two-digit number to each tooth in each quadrant. The first number indicates the quadrant in which the tooth is positioned, and the second number identifies the specific tooth. The numbers 1 through 4 are assigned to the quadrants of the permanent dentition, and the numbers 5 through 8 are assigned to the quadrants of the primary dentition.

Number	Quadrant
1	Permanent maxillary right
2	Permanent maxillary left
3	Permanent mandibular left
4	Permanent mandibular right
5	Primary maxillary right
6	Primary maxillary left
7	Primary mandibular left
8	Primary mandibular right

The second number identifies the specific tooth in the arch. The numbers 1 through 8 are assigned to the permanent dentition and 1 through 5 to the primary dentition, starting at the midline and moving posteriorly. Tooth #1 in all arches indicates a central incisor, and then the numbering proceeds to the last tooth in the quadrant. The two assigned numbers are read separately, with the first digit signifying the quadrant and the second digit identifying the tooth. Some examples are as follows:

Permanent maxillary right central incisor: #11 (number one-one)

Permanent maxillary left central incisor: #21 (number two-one)

Permanent mandibular left central incisor: #31 (number three-one)

Permanent mandibular right central incisor: #41 (number four-one)

The primary dentition is handled in the same manner. However, because there are only five teeth per quadrant, the numbers would range from 1 through 5 for each tooth and 5 through 8 for the quadrants. Therefore, the primary maxillary right first molar is #54 (number five-four), and the primary mandibular left lateral incisor is #72 (number seven-two).

Tooth Surfaces

During routine charting procedures, the clinical assistant uses a set of alpha codes for tooth surface annotation. The use of

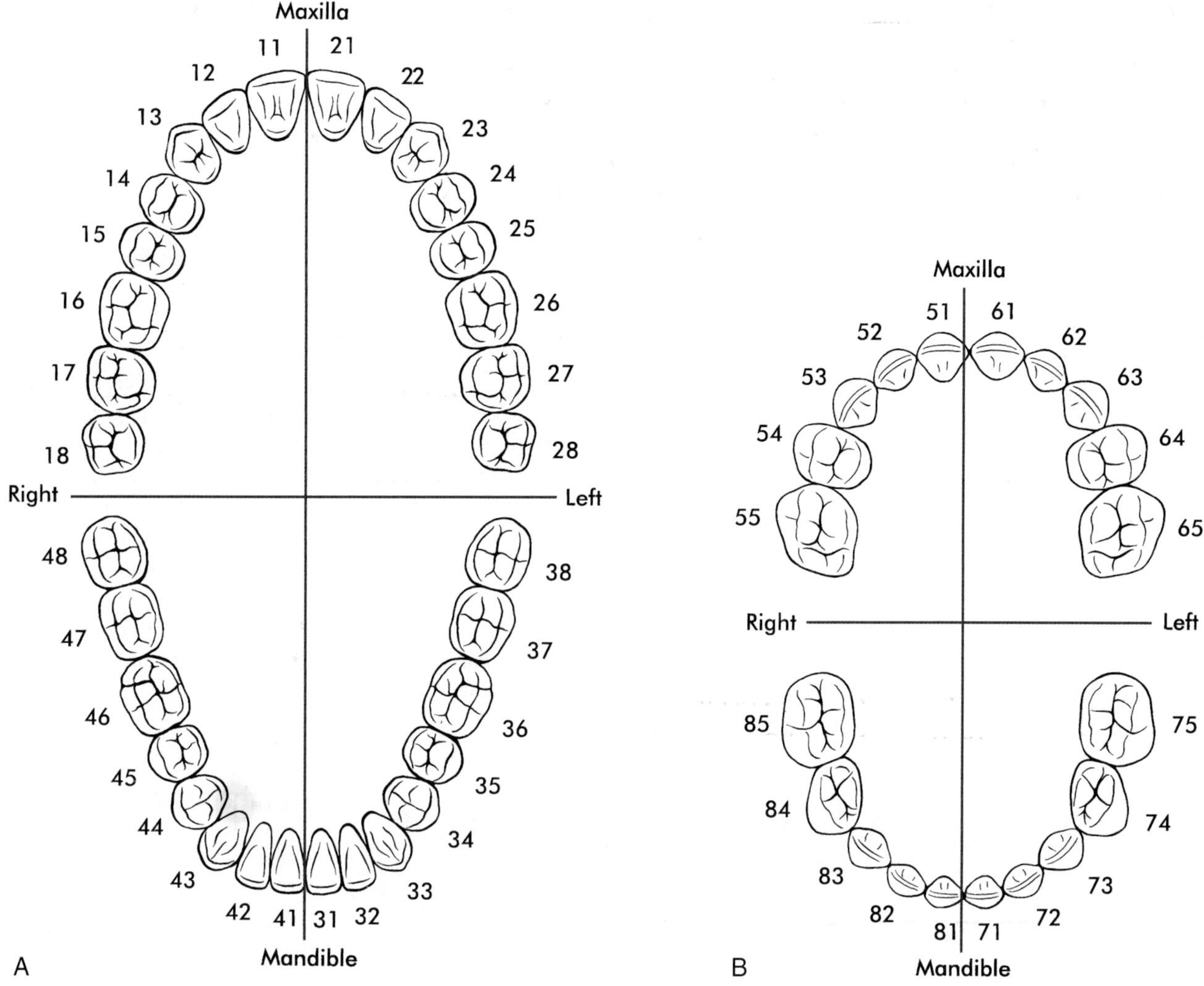

FIGURE 7-29 ISO/Fédération Dentaire Internationale (FDI) system. **A,** Permanent dentition. **B,** Primary dentition.

tooth nomenclature and surface annotation makes it easy to identify an area of a specific tooth in which there may be dental decay, a fracture, or a restoration. The administrative assistant must be familiar with this terminology to complete insurance forms and to consult with other staff about patient treatment.

All crowns of the teeth are divided into surfaces, which are identified by their position in relation to the oral cavity. For example, the surfaces nearest the lips are referred to as the *labial* or *facial surfaces.* The posterior teeth (the premolars and molars) have five surfaces. The anterior teeth (the incisors and canines) have four surfaces plus a ridge. Both anterior and posterior teeth have four axial surfaces. The axial surface runs vertically from the biting surface to the apex of a tooth. The posterior teeth have one additional surface, the occlusal surface, which is the horizontal surface that runs perpendicular to the other axial surfaces.

The surfaces of the teeth not only have names, but they are also identified by letters or numbers. This surface annotation is used to simplify charting notations and for all insurance reports. The letter or number is commonly placed as a superscript (above the print line) next to the tooth number. For example, when using the universal numbering system to describe a procedure involving the mesial surface of the permanent maxillary left first molar, the assistant would write "#14^{M}" or "#14^{1}." The surfaces of the teeth are indicated as follows (Figure 7-30):

- The *mesial surface* (M or 1) is the axial surface closest to the midline of the mouth.
- The *distal surface* (D or 2) lies directly opposite the mesial surface and is the axial surface farthest from the midline.
- The *facial surface* (F or 3) faces the cheek and lips or the exterior of the mouth.
- The *labial surface* (LA or 3) is the same as the facial surface, but it is found facing only the lips on the anterior teeth. This letter combination is not used frequently, because it requires an extra space in data entry; the designation for the facial surface (F) is used more often.
- The *buccal surface* (B or 3) is the same as the facial surface, but it is found on posterior teeth only, facing the cheeks.
- The *lingual surface* (L or 4) is the surface closest to the tongue.

- The *occlusal surface* (O or 5) is found only on posterior teeth on a vertical plane; this refers to the biting surface of the teeth.
- The *incisal ridge* (or *edge* or *surface*) (I or 5) is found only on anterior teeth that have a biting edge.

The *proximal areas* or *surfaces* are where two teeth abut or face each other. Most teeth have two proximal surfaces: the mesial and the distal proximal surfaces; however, for the third molars, only the mesial surface may be considered a proximal surface. *Interproximal* denotes the area between two proximal teeth. For example, a carious lesion on the proximal surface is called *interproximal decay.*

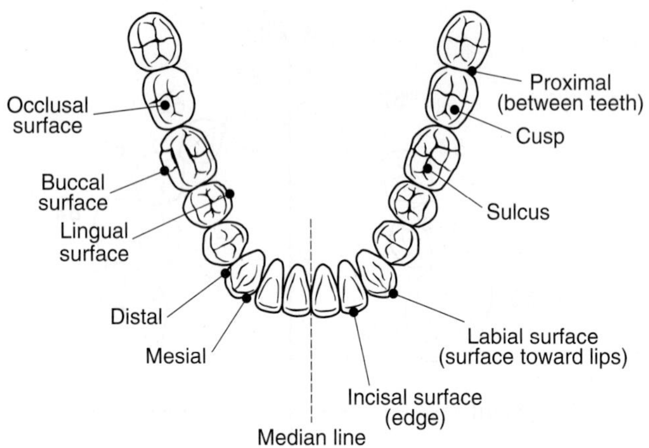

FIGURE 7-30 Tooth surface annotation.

When more than one surface is involved (e.g., mesial, occlusal, and distal), the surface annotations are placed in order from mesial to distal: for example, "#19^{MOD}" rather than "#19^{DOM}" or "#19^{ODM}." This standardization provides for uniform communication among dental professionals.

Charting Symbols and Abbreviations

Charting symbols are a form of shorthand used in the dental office to create a visual representation on a paper or electronic anatomical diagram that shows conditions in and around the patient's teeth (Figure 7-31). The dentist can use this information for diagnosis and treatment planning, or the administrative assistant can quickly identify conditions in the patient's mouth without reading through a lengthy description. Figure 7-32 presents a variety of symbols that are commonly used in a dental office. Clinical abbreviations are short versions of or initials for common clinical terminology. Table 7-1 contains a detailed list of commonly used abbreviations.

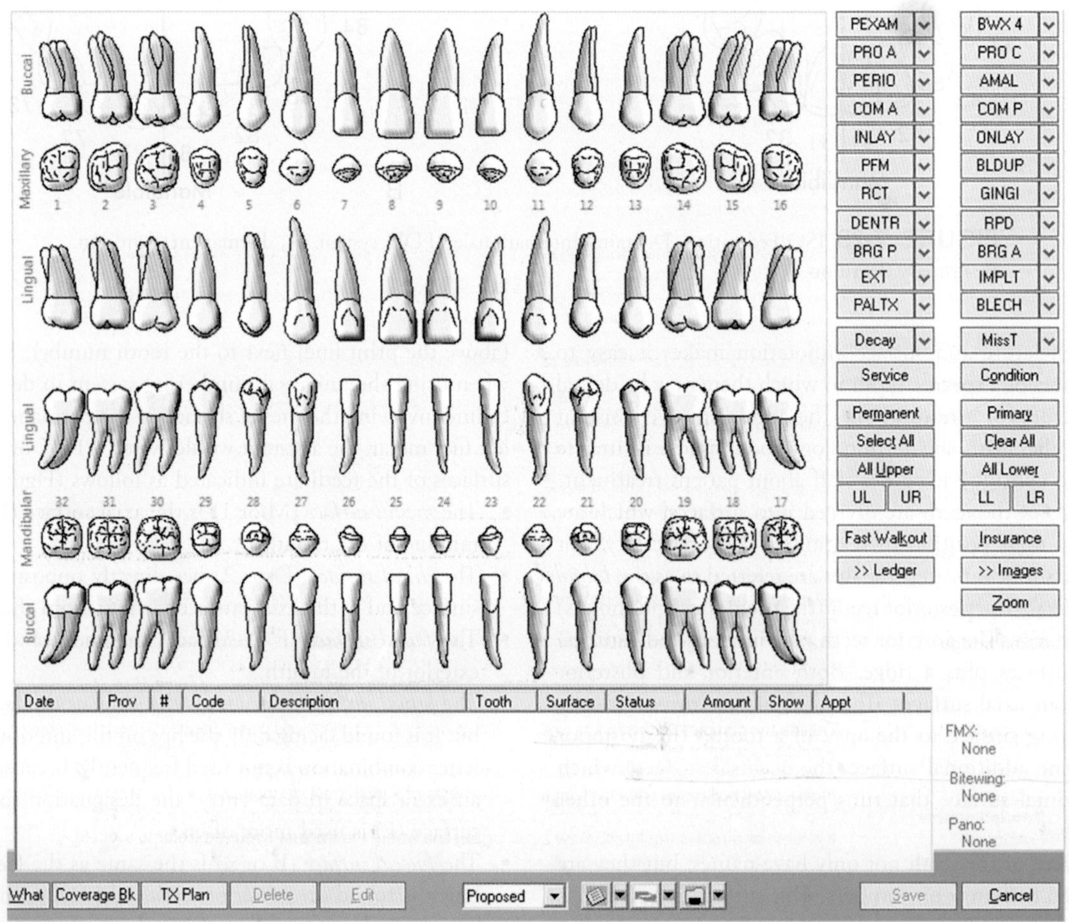

FIGURE 7-31 Screenshot of a tooth charting software page.

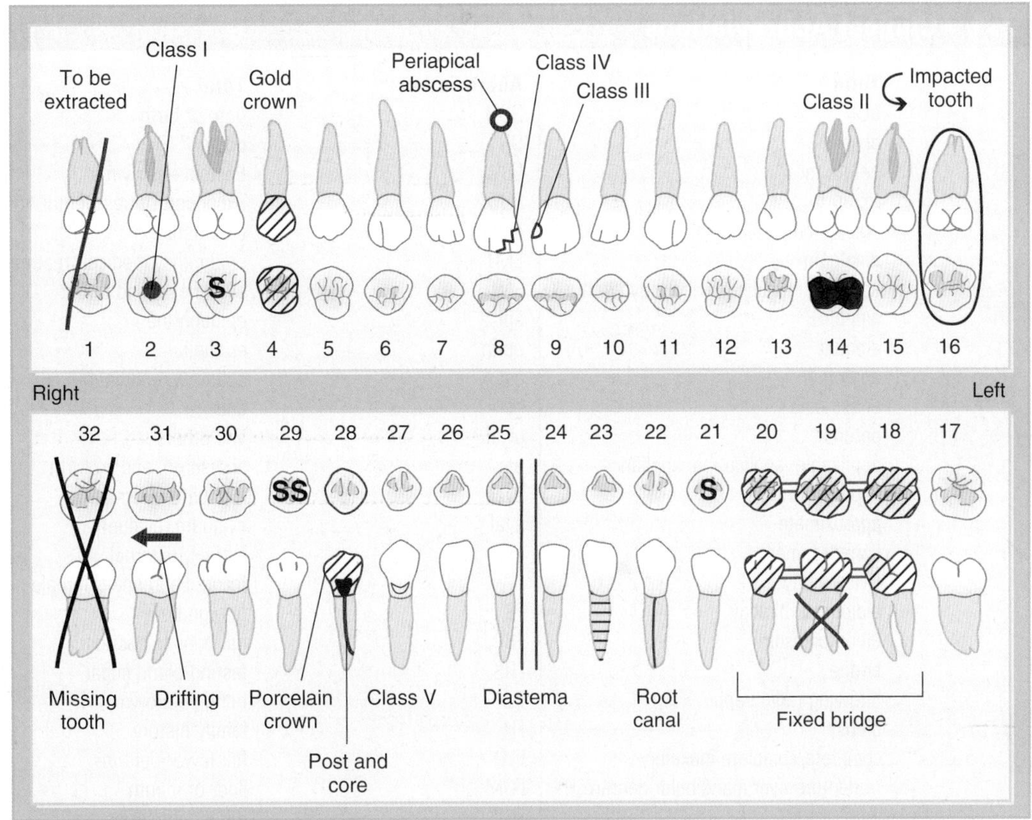

Charting Symbol	Description
Amalgam	Outline the surfaces that are involved (refer to teeth 2 and 14).
Composite	Outline the surfaces involved (refer to teeth 9 and 27).
Porcelain fused to metal (PFM)	Outline the tooth and draw diagonal lines on the occlusal or lingual surface where metal appears (refer to tooth 28).
Gold	Outline the crown of the tooth and place diagonal lines (refer to tooth 4).
Sealant	Place an "S" on the occlusal surface (refer to teeth 3 and 21).
Stainless steel crown	Outline crown of tooth and place "SS" on occlusal surface (refer to tooth 29).
To be extracted	Draw a red diagonal line through the tooth. An alternative method is to draw two red parallel lines through the tooth (refer to tooth 1).
Missing tooth	Draw a black or blue "X" through the tooth. It does not matter if the tooth was extracted or it never erupted, just as long as the tooth is not visible in the mouth. If a quadrant, or arch, is edentulous, make one "X" over all teeth (refer to tooth 32).
Impacted or unerupted	Draw a red circle around the whole tooth, including the root (refer to tooth 16).
Decay	Depending on the caries classification, outline and color the area for amalgam (refer to tooth 2), or outline the area for composite (refer to tooth 9).
Recurrent decay	Outline the existing restoration in red to indicate decay in the area (refer to tooth 14).
Root canal	Draw a line through the center of each root involved (refer to tooth 22).
Periapical abscess	Draw a red circle at the apex of the root to indicate infection (refer to tooth 8).
Post and core	Draw a line through the root that requires a post; then continue the line into the gingival one third of the crown, making a triangle shape (refer to tooth 6).
Rotated tooth	If a tooth has rotated in its position, indicate the direction the tooth has turned by placing a red arrow to the side of the tooth (refer to tooth 15).
Diastema	When there is more space than normal between two teeth, draw two red vertical lines between the areas (refer to teeth 24 and 25).
Fixed bridge	Draw an "X" through the roots of the missing tooth or teeth involved. Then draw a line to connect each of the teeth that make up the bridge. The type of material used to make the bridge will determine whether you outline the crown for porcelain, use diagonal lines for gold, or use a combination of the two (refer to teeth 18-20).
Full crown	Outline the complete crown if it is to be a porcelain crown, or outline and place diagonal lines if it will be a gold crown (refer to tooth 4).
Drifting	Place a red arrow pointing in the direction a tooth is drifting (refer to tooth 31).
Implant	In red, draw horizontal lines through the root or roots of a tooth (refer to tooth 23).
Bonded veneer	Veneers cover only the facial aspect of a tooth. Outline the facial portion only (refer to tooth 26).
Fractured tooth or root	If a tooth or a root is fractured, draw a red zigzag line where the fracture occurred (refer to tooth 8).

FIGURE 7-32 A variety of symbols used in charting.

TABLE 7-1 Clinical Abbreviations

Abbreviation	Term
@	at
abc	abscess
ac	before meals
ad	to, up to
adj	adjustment
a, ag, am	amalgam
AIDS	acquired immunodeficiency syndrome
amp	ampule
amt	amount
anat	anatomy
Anes/anest	anesthesia
ant	anterior
appl	applicable, application, appliance
appt	appointment
approx	approximate
BF	bone fragment
bid	twice a day
bio	biological, biology
BP	blood pressure
Br	bridge
BW	bitewing radiograph
Bx	biopsy
C/C	complete/complete maxillary denture over mandibular denture
$\bar{c}$	with
C	composite
calc	calculus
caps	capsules
cav	cavity
CC	chief complaint
cc	cubic centimeter
CDA	Certified Dental Assistant
Cer	ceramic
CHF	congestive heart failure
cm	centimeter
CM	cast metal
comp	compound, composite
conc	concentrate
Cond	condition
Cont	continue
Cr	crown
CSX	complete series x-rays
cur	curettage
CV	cardiovascular
CVA	cerebrovascular accident
D	distal
DV	devitalized
dbl	double
DDS	Doctor of Dental Surgery/Science
DEF	defective
DH	Dental Hygienist, dental hygiene
Dx	diagnosis
DM	diagnostic models
DMD	Doctor of Dental Medicine
DMF	decayed, missing, and filled
DO	disto-occlusal
DOB	date of birth
DR	doctor
EBV	Epstein–Barr virus
EDDA	Expanded Duties Dental Assistant
emerg	emergency
EMT	emergency medical treatment
ENT	ears, nose, and throat
epi	epinephrine
epith	epithelial
est	estimate, estimation
et	and
et al	and others
etc	and so on, and so forth
evac	evacuate, evacuation
eval	evaluate, evaluation
ext	extract, external
F	facial, Fahrenheit, female
FB	foreign body
FBI	full bony impaction
FBS	fasting blood sugar
FGC	full gold crown
FH	family history
FLD	full lower denture
FOM	floor of mouth
FMS	full mouth series
FMX	full mouth radiographs
FR or frac	fracture
FOM	full range of motion
frag	fragment
freq	frequent, frequency
FUD	full upper denture
G	gold
GI	gold inlay
ging	gingiva, gingivectomy
GP	general practitioner
H_2O	water
H_2O_2	hydrogen peroxide
HAV	hepatitis A virus
HBP	high blood pressure
HBV	hepatitis B virus
HCV	hepatitis C virus
HIV	human immunodeficiency virus
Hdpc	handpiece
hosp	hospital
hr	hour
hs	hour of sleep
ht	height
Hx	history
I&D	incision and drainage
IM	intramuscular
IMP/imp	impacted/impression
inc	incisal, incisive, incise
inf	infected, inferior, infusion
inj	injection, injury
Inop	inoperable, inoperative
Irreg	irregular

TABLE 7-1 Clinical Abbreviations—cont'd

Abbreviation	Term	Abbreviation	Term
IV	intravenous	PDR	physicians' desk reference
L	lingual	Ped	pediatrics
LA	labial, lower anterior	PFM	porcelain fused to metal
lab	laboratory	PLD	partial lower denture
lac	laceration	PMT, PMTx	periodontal maintenance therapy
lat	lateral	PO, postop	postoperative; orally, by mouth
lig	ligament	Pre-op	Preoperative
ling	lingual	prep	preparation, prepare for treatment
liq	liquid	prn	as needed
LLQ, LL	lower left quadrant/lower left	Prog	prognosis
LN	lymph node	Pro, Proph	prophylaxis
LRQ, LR	lower right quadrant/lower right	PSA	posterior superior alveolar
Lt, L	left	PSR	periodontal screening and recording
M, mes	mesial	pt	patient
mand	mandibular, mandible	Px, PX, prog	prognosis
max	maximum, maxillary	q	every
MDR	minimum daily requirement	qd	every day
med	medicine, medical	qh	every hour
mg, m	milligram	q2h	every 2 hours
micro	microscopic	q4h	every 4 hours
ML	midline/mesio-lingual	qid	4 times a day
MM	mucous membrane	quad	quadrant
mm	millimeter	qn	every night
MO	mesio-occlusal	R	respiration
mo	month	RPD	removable partial denture
MOD	mesio-occluso-distal	Rx, RX	prescribed/prescription
MRI	magnetic resonance imaging	rad	radiograph
MSA	middle superior alveolar	RC	root canal
MS	multiple sclerosis	RCT, RCTx	root canal treatment
MVP	mitral valve prolapse	RDA	Registered Dental Assistant
NA	not applicable	RDH	Registered Dental Hygienist
N_2O	nitrous oxide	Rec	recession
narc	narcotic	Re-eval	re-evaluation, re-evaluate
nc	no change, no charge	Ref	refer
NCP	not clinically present	reg	regular
nec	necessary	req	requisition
neg	negative	resp	respiration
nonrep	nonrepetitive	RHD	rheumatic heart disease
norm	normal	ROA	received on account
NPO	nothing by mouth	$\overline{S}$	without
O_2	oxygen	SBE	subacute bacterial endocarditis
occ, occl	occlusal		
OH	oral hygiene	Sig	instructions on label
OHI	oral hygiene instructions	SOB	short of breath
Opp	opposite	sol	solution
OS	oral surgery	Stat	immediately
OTC	over the counter	STI	soft tissue impaction
P	pulse	stim	stimulate, stimulator
P/P	partial over (maxillary) over partial (mandibular)	strep	streptococcus pyogenes
		surg	surgery, surgeon
PA	periapical radiograph	Sx	symptom
Palp	palpitation	T	temperature
Pan/pano	panoramic oral examination	tab	tablet
Path	pathology	TAT	tetanus antitoxin
PBI	partial bony impaction	TB	tuberculosis
PD	periodontal debridement	TBI	toothbrush instructions

Continued

TABLE 7-1 Clinical Abbreviations—cont'd

Abbreviation	Term	Abbreviation	Term
temp	temperature	VD	venereal disease
tid	three times a day	vss	vital signs stable
TLC	tender loving care	wh	white
TMD	temporomandibular dysfunction	Wnd	wound
TMJ	temporomandibular joint	WNL	within normal limits
TPR	temperature, pulse, respiration	wt	weight
Tx	treatment	X	times (e.g., 4×); x-ray
U, u	unit	y/o	years old
unk	unknown	YOB	year of birth
UL/ULQ	upper left quadrant	Yr	year
URI	upper respiratory infection	↑	increase
UR/URQ	upper right quadrant	↓	decrease

Records Retention

The minimum retention period for a patient's record should be consistent with the statute of limitations within the state. The statute of limitations, which is the period within which a civil suit for alleged wrongdoing may be legally filed, varies from state to state. The average minimum amount of time for the retention of a patient's records is approximately 6 years after the performance of the last treatment, but the dentist may decide to retain some or all records longer than that. Chapter 8 offers suggestions for longer-term storage.

Records Transfer

Requests for the transfer of records are made for many reasons, including the following: (1) the patient wants to change dentists; (2) the patient is moving out of the area; (3) the dentist wants to consult with another dentist; and (4) the patient has been referred to another dentist.

Care must be taken when completing a request for the transfer of a patient's records. By law, any information regarding a patient's care and treatment is confidential and privileged. This privilege belongs to the patient, not to the dentist. Therefore, for the dentist's protection, it is prudent to obtain a written consent signed by the patient or the patient's legal representative before transferring records to anyone other than the patient. The patient's right to privacy may only be superseded by a legal action or court order directing the dentist to release specific records to a designated party, such as a lawyer, judge, or other legal representative. In general, if the following suggestions are followed, record transfer can be handled efficiently and confidentially.

PRACTICE NOTE

By law, any information about a patient's care and treatment is confidential and privileged.

The dental office's responsibilities include the following:

- Must provide accurate and complete dental records
- Cannot change dental records without maintaining the readability of the original entry and must date and record the reason for any changes
- Should obtain a signed consent form from the patient or legal guardian or the advice of legal counsel before providing copies of or allowing access to a patient's dental records to anyone other than the patient
- Must retain records in accordance with the state statute
- Must keep original records
- Can charge a reasonable clerical fee for furnishing records in accordance with local standards
- Can charge a reasonable professional fee for preparing and furnishing a narrative report for the patient
- Should require advance payment for clerical and preparation service in accordance with local standards
- Should use certified mail with return receipt requested when sending records via the US Postal Service (The receipt verifies that the materials were received.)

OCCUPATIONAL SAFETY AND HEALTH ADMINISTRATION RECORDS

Chapter 17 details the responsibilities of the administrative assistant for disease prevention. Specific records must be maintained for the Occupational Safety and Health Administration (OSHA). The *Regulatory Compliance Manual* (see Figure 17-2, *B*) developed by the ADA is an important source of samples and suggestions for developing the documents required by federal regulations.

Occupational Safety and Health Administration Records Relating to Each Employee

- Medical records
- Copies of employee hepatitis B vaccination records

- Hepatitis B declination forms
- Exposure incident forms
- Follow-up documents for exposure incidents
- OSHA training records

EMPLOYEE RECORDS

Several employee records must be maintained in the office. These must be accurate, and they must be maintained with strict confidentiality. The administrative assistant is responsible for periodically updating these records. Many of the records relate to payroll, and these are discussed in Chapter 16.

Employee records are classified into various categories, such as the following:

Employment Forms

- Applications for employment (see Chapter 18)
- Employment agreements (see Chapter 18)
- Merit evaluation forms (see Chapter 18)
- Health forms and medical records
- Federal Employment Eligibility Verification forms (Form I-9; see Figure 2-8)

Employment Tax Information Forms (see Chapter 16)

- Employer identification number
- Amounts and dates of all wage, annuity, and pension payments
- Names, addresses, Social Security numbers, and documents of employees and recipients
- Periods for which employees and recipients are paid while absent due to sickness or injury as well as the amount and weekly rate of payments made by the dentist or third-party payers
- Copies of employees' and recipients' income tax withholding allowance certificates
- Any employee copies of federal form W-2 that were returned as undeliverable
- Dates and copies of tax deposits made
- Copies of filed tax returns
- Records of fringe benefits provided, including substantiation under IRS Code Section 274 and related regulations

LEARNING ACTIVITIES

1. Describe the impact of HIPAA on a dental practice. Why is this important to patients and healthcare professionals?
2. List the various categories of records, and give examples of dental office documents that fit into each category.
3. Explain why the clinical record is a vital record in the dental office.
4. Describe the parts of a clinical record.
5. Describe the retention and transfer of clinical records in the dental office.

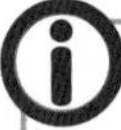

Please refer to the student workbook for additional learning activities.

BIBLIOGRAPHY

Fulton-Calkins PJ, Rankin DS, Shumack KA: *The administrative professional*, ed 14, Mason, OH, 2011, Thomson South-Western.

Matthews A: Data storage and dental healthcare, Online IQ, December 18, 2013.

Michigan Dental Association: *Disposal of dental records [member's only]*, Lansing, MI, 2008, Author. Available at: www.smilemichigan.com. Accessed November 10, 2008.

Michigan Dental Association: *Dental records access and release [member's only]*, Lansing, MI, 2008, Author. Available at: www.smilemichigan.com. Accessed November 10, 2008.

RECOMMENDED WEBSITES

www.ada.org/prof/resources/topics/hipaa/index.asp
www.hhs.gov/ocr/hipaa
www.hipaacomply.com/hipaafaq.htm
www.hipaadvisory.com
answers.hhs.gov/cgi-bin/hhs.cfg/php/enduser/std_alp.php
www.marygovoni.com
www.smilemichigan.com

8 Storage of Business Records

Kathy J. Zwieg

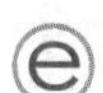 http://evolve.elsevier.com/Finkbeiner/practice

LEARNING OUTCOMES

1. Define the key terms in this chapter.
2. Discuss the importance of records management, both paper and electronic, and the benefit of keeping dental practice records readily available.
3. Describe the basic steps for preparing records for filing and the importance of cross-referencing, retrieval, and record retention.
4. Discuss the various classifications of filing systems including the basic alphabetical indexing rules.
5. Discuss the storage and care of electronic files.
6. Discuss the equipment and storage supplies necessary for both the "paperless" and paper storage of files.
7. Discuss the importance of managing workstation records effectively and list several tips for successful records management.

KEY TERMS

Alphabetical filing system A method of filing in which the arrangement of names appears in sequence from A to Z.

Card file A file that can be used to store small cards (3- × 5-inch, 4- × 6-inch, or larger) that are used for specialized systems.

Chronological filing system A method of filing by date. This system can be used within an alphabetical, geographical, subject, or numerical system by filing the most recent correspondence in the front of the file folder.

Cross-referencing This system alerts staff members that a record normally kept in a specific location has been stored elsewhere.

EDR Electronic dental record.

EHR Electronic healthcare record.

Encryption The process of encoding messages or information in such a way that only authorized parties can view it.

Geographical filing system A method of filing in which location is the important factor of reference. The principle is essentially the same as that of alphabetical filing except that it is done by territorial division (e.g., state, city, street) rather than by name.

Lateral file A file that is similar to a vertical file except that the longest side opens and the files are stored as if they were placed on a bookshelf.

Numerical filing system A method of filing that assigns a number to each new patient or account.

Open-shelf filing A method of filing that is similar to lateral filing but with no doors to close.

Password A word or string of characters used to prove one's identity or access approval to gain access to electronic records, which should be kept private for each authorized individual.

Retrieval The removal of records from files using proper "charge-out" methods.

Scanner A piece of equipment that optically scans and digitizes paper documents for inclusion in the electronic patient record.

Subject filing system A method of filing that uses an alphabetical arrangement of papers according to the subject or topic of the papers.

Tickler file A chronological method of filing that serves as a follow-up file and that contains the days of the month and the months of the year to alert the administrative assistant to perform a task.

Vertical file A file that stores records in drawers. File folders are placed on the folder's edge and arranged according to the filing method selected.

Vast amounts of information are generated in the dental office each day. The idea of a paperless office is becoming more of a reality as more certified electronic dental records (discussed in Chapter 7) become available, and the vast majority of dental offices in the United States are adapting to these technologies. To meet state and federal privacy and security standards, traditional methods of paper record storage will also need to be used for some time. In Chapter 7, disposition is identified as the final stage of a dental record, either destruction or storage. The administrative assistant is responsible for managing and maintaining records (both paper and electronic files) to meet state and federal requirements. This chapter discusses records storage. A sound understanding of records management and the indexing rules associated with records storage—whether electronic or paper—will continue to be an essential skill for the administrative assistant to possess.

A dental office produces many kinds of information, including clinical and financial records, radiographs, computer-aided design and manufacturing (CAD/CAM) models, and other diagnostic models. The inability to find a document quickly is frustrating and can often delay a decision, diagnosis, or payment. Such delays can be costly and stressful.

A record is stored information on any media created or received by the office that is evidence of its operations or that has a value that required its retention for a period of time. For example, information may be kept as follows:

- Written and recorded electronically or on paper, as in a patient's clinical or financial record
- In written form, such as employee records
- As completed written federal forms for Occupational Safety and Health Administration (OSHA) records, tax and insurance records, and accounts receivable and payable
- As an oral recording that captures the human voice and that is stored via electronic storage media
- In e-mails, spreadsheets, databases, word processing documents, or other computer software systems stored electronically
- As radiographs, videos, digital photographs, and CAD/CAM models stored electronically
- In the form of models or other replicas of a patient's oral cavity

Records are assets to the dental practice. They provide legal value by providing evidence of treatment and business transactions. Records may provide information about articles of incorporation, real estate, and contracts. Records also provide information about the day-to-day operation of the practice, historic evidence of treatment, employee data, and financial activity. Thus, the maintenance of these records becomes a major responsibility of the administrative assistant to ensure the smooth flow of the practice as well as the safety and security of the practice.

To many administrative assistants, filing is one of those dreaded routine jobs done when the administrative assistant can "get around to it" or "has the time." Although the vast implementation of electronic records in the dental office is minimizing the task of paper filing, there is still a need to understand basic filing principles for those items that do require manual organization. These principles apply to electronic records organization as well.

Dental practice records must always be readily available. Wise planning can save a tremendous amount of time and effort. The heart of any professional office is its records management system. Business office files should not be a place to *put* materials but rather a place to *find* materials. Systematic plans for storage, retrieval, transferring, protection, and retention must be established for both paper and electronic files. When planning for the office files, consider their ease of retrieval as well as their confidentiality and safety. The needs of the office, the size of the dental practice, and the space available for equipment and storage are factors that must be considered when establishing efficient systems.

PRACTICE NOTE

The heart of any professional office is its records management system.

PREPARING RECORDS FOR FILING

Basic Steps

Certain routines should be followed when preparing materials for filing: (1) set aside some time each day or every few days for filing paper records; (2) keep papers or records to be filed in a basket marked "To be filed"; and (3) file electronic records immediately in the appropriate electronic folder. Make backup copies of all electronic files as they are completed.

Before mastering the different filing systems, it is necessary to learn and understand some basic steps, which are generally done in the order of inspecting, indexing, coding, sorting, and storing:

- *Inspecting:* Review each record to determine whether it is something that must be filed. If it can be disposed of (check the retention schedule or the originator of the form), dispose of it. If it is to be retained, continue to the next step.
- *Indexing:* Determine under which caption or name an item is to be filed. Indexing is a mental process that requires the making of a decision. For example, if the record is a receipt for a payment that was just made from the dentist's checking account, the administrative assistant must decide into which file to place the receipt. If files are organized by subject, file the receipt under the subject to which it pertains (e.g., a receipt for an electric bill might be filed under "Utilities" or "Electricity"). For a patient's clinical record, use an alphabetical system, and break down the patient's name into the first, second, and third units to consider for filing. Electronic records are indexed by determining in which directory the file should be located and by following a uniform procedure for naming the files. Do not name electronic files with characters or words that do not identify the subject of the record.
- *Coding:* After the caption or title of the record has been determined, assign a code by highlighting, typing, or writing a caption on a paper record or by giving the electronic file a name. On an electronic record, this is done by creating a descriptive file name and including it on the document under the initials of the creator. If an electronic file also exists in paper form, the file name on the document allows for quick and easy retrieval. Examples of coding are shown in Figure 8-1. The clinical record is coded with the patient's name, and the electronic document is coded with the name of the originator and other important information about the document.
- *Sorting:* The records are arranged in the order in which they are to be placed in the file (e.g., if the file is alphabetical,

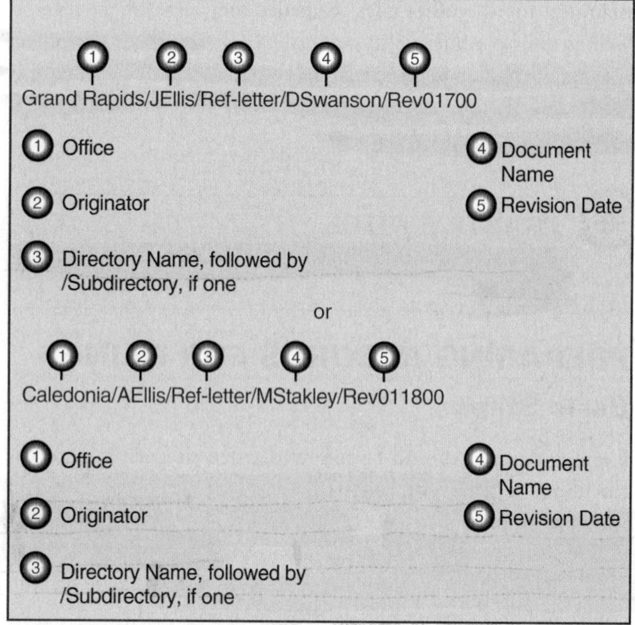

FIGURE 8-1 Electronic coding at the bottom of a document refers to the originator of the document, the directory name, the subdirectory (if used), and the document name.

put the records in alphabetical order). Electronic files are sorted as the files are saved in the correct directory. The system then sorts the files either alphabetically by file name, by date, or by any other designation made.

- *Storing*: Put any necessary paper documents in folders and records in similarly organized file drawers. Check and double-check that the documents are being filed correctly.

PRACTICE NOTE

Check and double-check that you are entering information into an electronic record correctly (e.g., confirm spelling) and that you are filing a paper document correctly.

Two other aspects of document storage—cross-referencing and retrieval—deserve special consideration:

1. Cross-referencing alerts staff members that a record normally kept in a specific location has been stored elsewhere. A cross-reference can be provided by making a copy of the record and filing it in the referenced file with a note that it is a copy, or a cross-reference sheet can be put in the file. A cross-reference sheet contains the name of the document, the date it was filed, a brief description of the subject of the record, and the places where the record can be found. This type of cross-referencing is often found in a library card catalog.

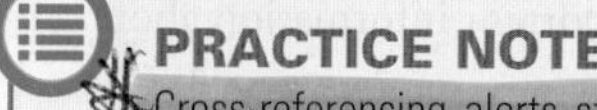

PRACTICE NOTE

Cross-referencing alerts staff members that a record normally kept in a specific location has been stored elsewhere.

2. Retrieval is the removal of records from files using proper "charge-out" methods. When an entire file folder is removed, an out-folder is put in the place of the removed folder. The out-folder has the name of the individual or department that removed the folder and the date that it was removed. Out-guides or substitution cards may be used instead of an out-folder.

Although it does not commonly happen with patient clinical charts during routine treatment, a record may need to be removed from a file and used in another location for consultation or study. In such cases, the out-folder should denote the area to which the record has been taken. Electronic filing lessens the chance for a lost record, but loss can occur when coding is done incorrectly, when names or information is misspelled, when data is entered incorrectly, and when the record is not placed in the correct electronic file.

Records Retention

It is not cost-effective to maintain unnecessary records and filing cabinets. Many records in the dental office are retained in accordance with state statutes. If the practice is large, a retention schedule may have been developed for various documents. If the office does not have a retention schedule, the administrative assistant should check with the dentist before deciding how documents should be transferred or destroyed. Check with your state dental board for state requirements. The National Archives and Records Service, a federal agency, has produced a helpful reference entitled *Guide to Record Retention Requirements;* it is available from the Superintendent of Documents, U.S. Government Printing Office, Washington, DC 20402.

The retention and destruction of files have taken on additional importance since the federal Revised Rule 26 of the Rules of Civil Procedure was approved in December 1993. This rule requires organizations to make available all relevant records that must be kept in compliance with prevailing statutes and regulations. Delay or failure to find information makes an office vulnerable to financial loss and adverse legal judgments.

As a dental practice transitions from paper to electronic records, it may not be feasible or practical to store the paper records within the practice confines. After the contents of the paper record have been transferred or scanned into the electronic record (Figure 8-2), the paper record may be boxed according to one of the five basic systems listed below and relocated to a proper storage facility. These facilities provide off-site storage and retrieval services in a safe, secure, climate-controlled environment should a paper record ever need to be reviewed. The administrative assistant is typically responsible for communicating with these businesses and arranging for the transfer of records between the dental practice and the storage location.

CLASSIFICATION OF FILING SYSTEMS

Five Basic Systems

The five basic classification systems of filing are the alphabetical system, the geographical system, the numerical system, the

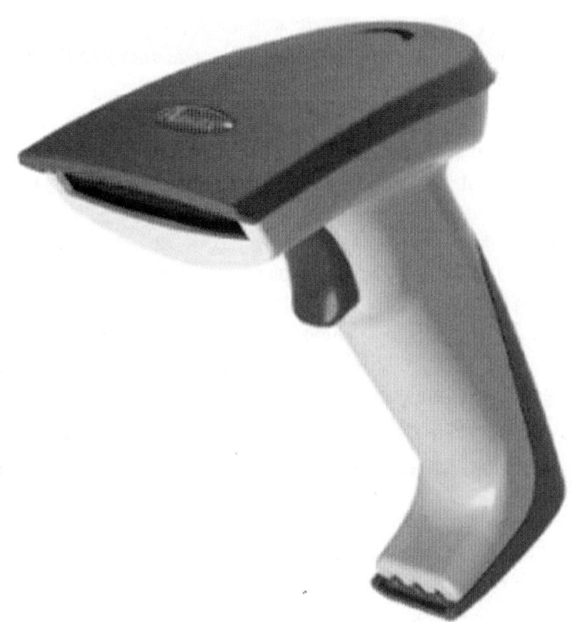

FIGURE 8-2 Electronic scanner. (Copyright © 2014 Karam Miri Photography, BigStock.com.)

subject system, and the chronological system. All of these methods except the chronological system basically apply alphabetical procedures. The method used in a dental office depends on the type of practice and the sophistication of the office's systems, but it is not uncommon to use several of these methods for various types of filing, whether electronic or paper.

PRACTICE NOTE

Delay or failure to find information makes an office vulnerable to patient dissatisfaction, financial loss, and adverse legal judgments.

Selecting the Appropriate Filing System

Alphabetical System

In an alphabetical filing system, the arrangement of names appears in sequence from A to Z. The alphabetical filing system accounts for about 90% of the filing that a person is likely to perform, and it can be applied to various captions. Standard rules exist for alphabetizing correctly. Box 8-1 illustrates alphabetical indexing rules that can be applied to a variety of situations.

Geographical Filing System

In a geographical filing system, location is the important factor of reference. The principle of geographical filing is essentially the same as alphabetical filing except that geographical filing is done by a territorial division (e.g., state, city, street) rather than by name. Coding should be done in a manner similar to that of the alphabetical system by marking the caption under which the item will be filed (see Figure 8-1).

Numerical Filing System

The numerical filing system involves a method of assigning numbers to each new patient or account. Numbers assigned are then recorded on an alphabetical card index or a computer file for future reference. Additional papers related to the same patient or account are subsequently filed according to the number originally allocated. In large clinics with access to computer centers, a numerical system can be used to great advantage, because computers handle numerical data faster than alphabetical characters.

Subject Filing System

The subject filing system is the alphabetical arrangement of papers according to the subject or topic of the papers. This system is used when it is more desirable to assemble information by topic than by name. For example, a subject file may be preferred if the dentist is involved in research or writing for publications. If a subject area is very broad, it can be broken down into smaller divisions with the use of secondary guides. This system is effective only if the administrative assistant is totally aware of the dentist's involvement in the relevant subject areas. Alternatively, it may be used for filing receipts for accounts payable.

Chronological Filing System

Basic System. The chronological filing system is a method of filing by date. It can be used within an alphabetical, geographical, subject, or numerical system by filing the most recent correspondence in the front of the file folder. This system can also be used for treatment records in a patient's clinical chart. The most current treatment data sheet would appear first, followed by past treatment records.

Tickler File. Another type of chronological classification system is a tickler file or follow-up file (Figure 8-3). The most common type of tickler file contains the days of the month and the months of the year. A manual tickler file is a card file that contains the days of each month, from 1 to 31. Items to be completed are filed in the slot of the day planned to complete the task. Time should be taken each day to review the tickler file. The tasks scheduled for a certain day should be performed on that day, or their notation should be moved to the appropriate day if the activity has been rescheduled. This can be done electronically in software that provides a calendar: simply add the task to be completed on a certain day, and then the calendar will come up for that day with the various tasks listed. A separate task card can even be created for each task that includes information specific to that task. Care should be taken to ensure that an activity is not placed on a weekend day or on a holiday when the office will be closed. The files for these days should be carefully checked in advance to ensure that the task is done before the weekend or holiday or placed in the slot of a later day. An advantage of electronic healthcare records is that information is filed automatically and may be retrieved in a variety of formats and levels of detail to be used by the administrative assistant. For example, if the practice would like to review geographic information about its patient base, it may run a

BOX 8-1

Indexing Rules for the Alphabetical System

Names of individuals are indexed by units. The last name (surname) is the key unit. This is followed by the first name (given name), which is the second unit, and then by the middle name or initial, which is the third unit. Alphabetize names by comparing the first units of the names letter by letter. Consider second units only when the first units are identical. Consider third units only if the first and second units are identical, and so on.

Name	1	2	3
Alice J. Gooding	Gooding	Alice	J.
Alice Marie Goodman	Goodman	Alice	Marie
William Grafton	Grafton	William	

If the last names are the same, consider the second indexing unit.

Name	1	2	3
Frank Martin	Martin	Frank	
George Martin	Martin	George	
George C. Martin	Martin	George	C.

If the last names are the same but vary in spelling, consider each letter.

Name	1	2	3
Joy Read	Read	Joy	
Janice Reed	Reed	Janice	
Phyllis J. Reid	Reid	Phyllis	J.

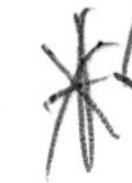

Initials are considered the same as a whole word and are filed before names beginning with the same initial. Names with no initial are filed before those with an initial (i.e., "nothing before something").

Name	1	2	3
Arthur Stone	Stone	Arthur	
C. Stone	Stone	C.	
Charles Stone	Stone	Charles	

If two people have the same name, they are indexed according to the alphabetical order of their city of residence and then by their state of residence. If two people have the same name and live in the same city, they are indexed according to the names of the streets on which they live.

Name	1	2	3
Richard Murphey (Grand Rapids)	Murphey	Richard	Grand Rapids
Richard Murphey (Grandville)	Murphey	Richard	Grandville

Surname prefixes are considered part of the last name and not as separate words. A hyphenated surname (e.g., Meyer-Schafer) is considered a single indexing unit. A compound personal name that is not hyphenated (e.g., Catherine Myers Schafer) is treated as separate indexing units.

Name	1	2	3
Connie MacDonald	MacDonald	Connie	
Connie McDonald	McDonald	Connie	
Alice Meyer-Schafer	Meyer-Schafer	Alice	
Martin O'Connor	O'Connor	Martin	
Frank M. O'Dell	O'Dell	Frank	M.
Catherine Myers Schafer	Schafer	Myers	Catherine

If the first word in a compound surname is one of the standard prefixes (e.g., "St." in "St. James"), the surname is indexed as a single unit.

Name	1	2	3
Edward St. James	Saint James	Edward	
William St. Johns	Saint Johns	William	
James E. Sutton	Sutton	James	E.

Titles and degrees are disregarded, but they may be placed in parentheses after the names.

Name	1	2	3
Professor Joseph C. Kline	Kline	Joseph	C. (Prof.)
Father Patrick O'Reilly	O'Reilly	Patrick (Fr.)	
Capt. C. J. Walters	Walters	C.	J. (Capt.)

A seniority designation is not considered an indexing unit, but it can be used as an identifying element to distinguish between identical names.

Name	1	2	3
Charles D. Flynn Jr.	Flynn	Charles	D. (Junior)
Charles D. Flynn Sr.	Flynn	Charles	D. (Senior)

Titles used without a complete name should be considered as the key indexing unit.

Name	1	2	3
Father Patrick	Father	Patrick	
Sister Mary Martha	Sister	Mary	Martha

Articles, conjunctions, and prepositions are disregarded in indexing.

Name	1	2	3
The Litton Dental Clinic	Litton	Dental	Clinic (The)

A firm or business name is indexed in the order written unless it contains an individual's name.

Name	1	2	3	4	5
The Harvey F. Andrew Dental Laboratory	Harvey	F.	Andrew	Dental	Laboratory (The)
Grand Rapids Dental Laboratory	Grand	Rapids	Dental Laboratory		
Horton Dental Ceramics	Horton	Dental	Ceramics		

BOX 8-1

Indexing Rules for the Alphabetical System—cont'd

Agencies of the federal government are indexed under United States Government and then according to department, division, subdivision, and location for adequate differentiation.

Name	1	2	3	4	5	6
Federal Bureau of Investigation	United	States	Govt. Justice	Federal Investigation	(Dept. of) (Bur. of)	
Bureau of Labor	United	States	Govt. Labor	Labor	Statistics	(Dept. of) (Bur. of)

State, county, and city governments are indexed according to location and then by department, division, or subdivision.

Name	1	2	3
Park Department, Kent County	Kent	County	Park (Dept.)
Michigan State Department of Education	Michigan	State	Education (Dept. of)
Grandville Department of Health	Grandville	City	Health (Dept.)

Numbers spelled as words in business names are filed alphabetically. Numbers written in digit form are filed before letters or words.

Name	1	2	3	4
5-Cent Copy Center	5	Cent	Copy	Center
Four Seasons Health Spa	Four	Seasons	Health	Spa
Seventh Street Photo Center	Seventh	Street	Photo	Center

- Names of schools are first indexed by the name of the city in which the school is located and then by the name of the school.
- Local banking or other institutions with branch offices are indexed as the name is written. However, if banks from several cities are involved, the first indexing unit is the city in which the bank is located, and the name of the bank follows.
- Numbers, including Roman numerals, are filed before alphabetical information. However, all Arabic numerals come before Roman numerals.
- Acronyms, abbreviations, and television and radio call letters are treated as one unit. Company names are filed as you see them.

report by zip code. Should a practice want to know more about its pediatric patients, the patient files may be searched by age. Detailed data can then be reviewed, and this may prove instrumental in furthering practice growth and development.

ELECTRONIC FILES

Storage

The storage of electronic records requires the ability to back up electronic patient records as well as word processing, database, and spreadsheet files. With more dental practices becoming paperless, the need for secure and reliable electronic storage has become more critical. First, the data need to be encrypted or coded in a secure way so that only authorized staff can view or retrieve them. Electronic records and systems should also be password-protected, with dental personnel having different levels of password access, depending on their responsibilities. For example, a clinical assistant would need access to clinical information, whereas a practice manager would likely require access to the entire system. A password is a string of characters, including letters and numbers, and is used to prove one's identity or to log in to gain access to electronic information. Passwords should be kept private for each authorized individual.

It is highly recommended to use at least two backup processes for electronic data: one maintained locally and one completely distinct and independent that is kept off-site. These processes provide regular and secure backup services that include system monitoring, alarms should an error or failure occur, testing, and full data retrievability should the need ever arise. Online backup capabilities can be practice-saving because records maintained in this way are impervious to fire, flood, theft, and other elements. These forms of storage are discussed in Chapter 5.

In most dental offices in which other electronic records such as Microsoft Word and Excel are used, files are typically stored on a hard drive. These should be backed up regularly and securely, just as an electronic healthcare or dental record (EHR or EDR) would be.

Care of Recordable Media

Recordable media includes magnetic disks, optical disks (CDs and DVDs), tape, PC cards, smart cards, and flash drives.

If a dental practice is making use of any of these devices, special attention must be paid to the storage of recordable media to prevent the damage and loss of data. Each manufacturer may recommend specific care for its products, but, in general, disks should be protected from dust, magnetic fields, extreme temperatures, liquids, and vapors. Box 8-2 presents several suggestions to ensure the safe storage of data.

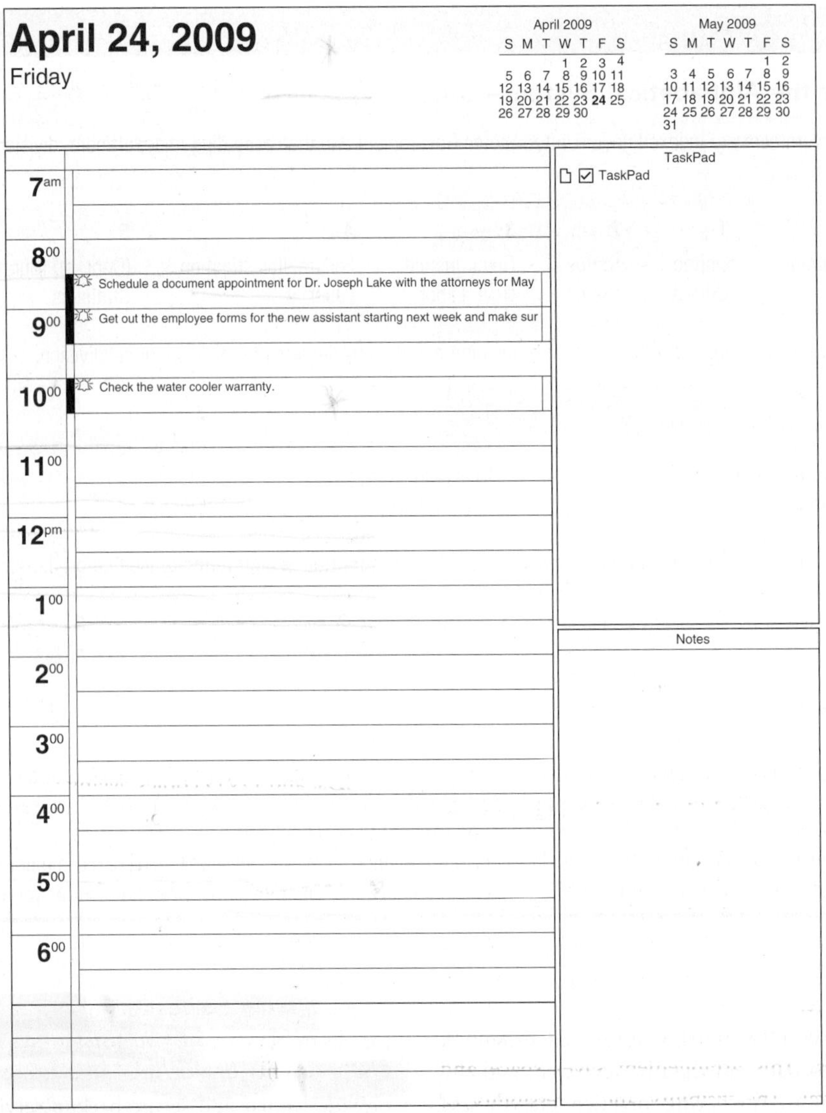
April 24, 2009
Friday
April 2009
S M T W T F S
1 2 3 4
5 6 7 8 9 10 11
12 13 14 15 16 17 18
19 20 21 22 23 24 25
26 27 28 29 30
May 2009
S M T W T F S
1 2
3 4 5 6 7 8 9
10 11 12 13 14 15 16
17 18 19 20 21 22 23
24 25 26 27 28 29 30
31
7am
8 00
Schedule a document appointment for Dr. Joseph Lake with the attorneys for May
9 00
Get out the employee forms for the new assistant starting next week and make sur
10 00
Check the water cooler warranty.
11 00
12pm
1 00
2 00
3 00
4 00
5 00
6 00
TaskPad
TaskPad
Notes

FIGURE 8-3 An electronic calendar used as a tickler file easily reminds the administrative assistant of tasks that need to be performed on a specific day.

BOX 8-2

Recordable Media Care

- Never touch the internal disk; handle disks only by the protective outer cover.
- Do not expose disks to magnetic fields, such as those produced by telephones, radio speakers, or computer screens.
- Keep media at temperatures of 50° to 140° F (10° to 60° C); avoid extreme temperatures.
- Protect media from dust and foreign particles.
- Do not expose media to water or other liquids.
- If media contain permanent information, use the write-protect system to prevent data loss. (Write-protect is a feature on a CD, DVD, or tape that prevents existing data from being written over.)

EQUIPMENT

Even in the paperless dental practice, there is still a need for office and filing equipment. On the basis of the office systems that have been chosen, the administrative assistant must determine what types of supplies and equipment are necessary to maintain the system. The equipment should be practical for day-to-day use and storage.

The term *filing equipment* refers to the actual structures that store files or records. Most manufacturers supply a variety of models in different colors with assorted features. Many practices still use vertical files, but open-shelf or lateral filing systems have become very popular as well, especially if space is limited. A vertical file stores records in drawers; file folders are placed on the folder's edge and arranged according to the filing method selected. Vertical files are available in cabinets with one to five or more drawers, and they may accommodate either an $8\frac{1}{2}$- ×

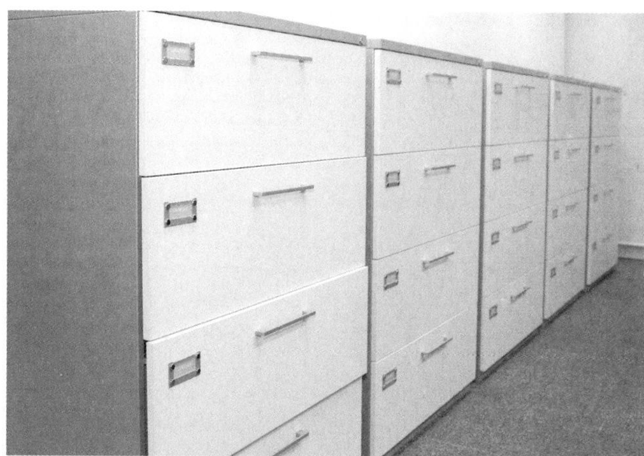

FIGURE 8-4 Lateral file. (Copyright © 2014 Karam Miri Photography, BigStock.com.)

11-inch (letter size) or 8½- × 14-inch (legal size) file. These are not the best file cabinets to use for saving space, because room is required for both the cabinet itself and the pull-out drawer space; this means that approximately double the space of the vertical cabinet is needed.

A lateral file (Figure 8-4) is similar to a vertical file, except that the longest side opens and the files are stored as if they were placed on a bookshelf. Lateral files have the added advantage of providing a countertop for reviewing files removed from the cabinet or for displaying books and other materials. Like vertical files, lateral files also are designed to accommodate letter- or legal-sized files. Less actual floor space is needed because these cabinets can store more files and require less floor and pull-out drawer space.

Open-shelf filing is the most popular filing system among modern dental practices. This arrangement saves space and speeds filing and retrieval. The visibility and accessibility of open-shelf filing have proved to be two of the many advantages of this arrangement (Figure 8-5). As compared with a closed-drawer filing system, open-shelf units hold twice as many files on half the floor space. The files give a visible sense of location and allow users to take full advantage of index guides and color-coding techniques. Misfiled information becomes less of a problem. However, because the files are open, dirt and dust may accumulate if covers are not used.

A card file can be used to store small cards (3 × 5-inch, 4 × 6-inch, or larger) that are used for specialized systems. An example of the use of the rotary or Rolodex file (Figure 8-6, *A*) is for addresses, e-mail addresses, telephone numbers, and fax numbers of dental suppliers, laboratories, and dental associates that are commonly contacted. This same information may be stored electronically in an address file (Figure 8-6, *B*).

When selecting filing equipment for a dental office, the administrative assistant should also consider a fire-protection file. As a precaution against fire destruction, vital records should be placed in the file at the end of each workday. If the dental practice is making use of these methods, these records could include the patients' ledger cards, the appointment book, copies of CDs, and DVD copies. Many dentists buy an additional file for storing valuable records away from the office.

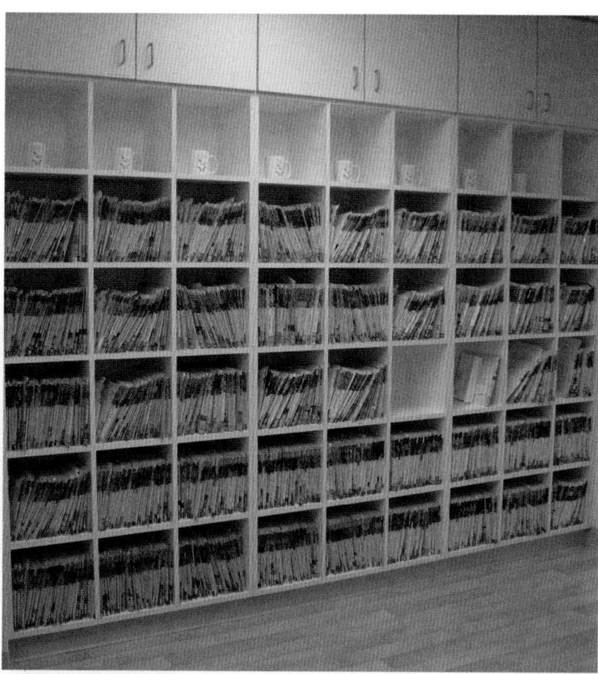

FIGURE 8-5 Open-shelf file.

STORAGE SUPPLIES

Filing supplies for paper storage include file guides, file folders, folder labels (in a variety of colors for color coding), cross-reference sheets, and out-guides.

File guides, which are usually made of heavy cardboard, divide the file drawer into separate sections. The division is indicated by a tab that extends above the guide. The guides divide the alphabet into sections, or they may show a division in a numerical sequence. The file drawer is marked on the outside to correspond with the division of the filing arrangement.

File folders are usually made of Manila paper or another heavy type of material. Folders may be obtained in a variety of cuts, which allow the tabs to be arranged in a staggered fashion. The tabs may be on the far-left side, or they may be center cut, one-third cut, or one-fifth cut.

In dental practices that use paper records, most prefer to use patient file folders or envelopes with labels that come in a variety of colors. This type of file and label guards against misplaced records (e.g., radiographs) and provides space for the patient's name, address, and telephone number. Most file folders can be labeled with gummed labels, which are available in a variety of styles (e.g., rolls of labels, peel-off labels, continuous folded strips) and colors that will make the folders easier to locate and refile (Figure 8-7). In a group practice, a different color may be used to designate the patients of each dentist. Color coding may also be used for other pertinent patient information.

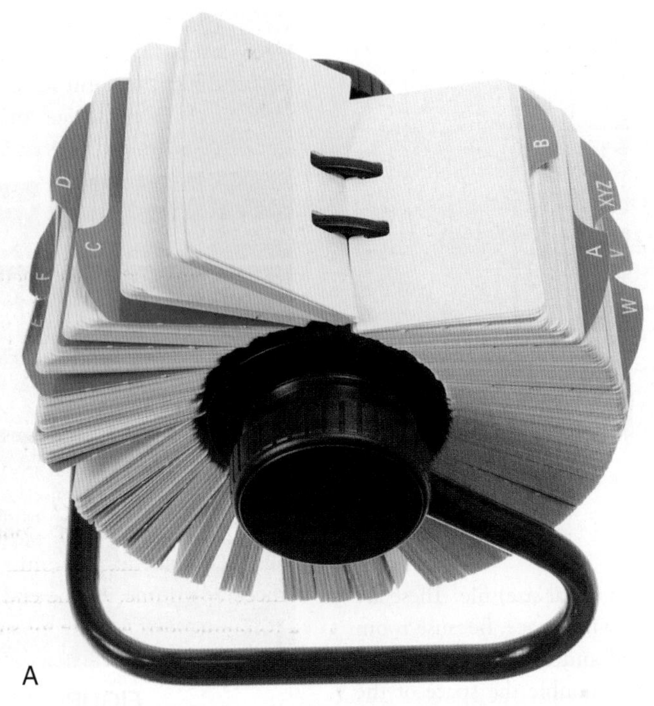

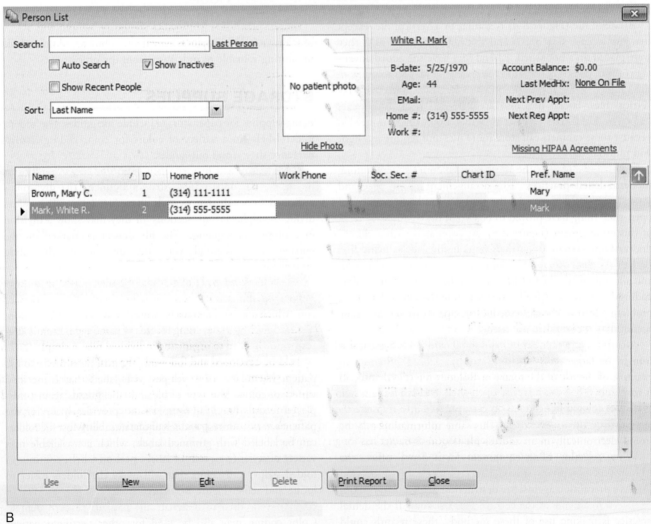

A

Person List

Search: [ ] Last Person

[ ] Auto Search [✓] Show Inactives

[ ] Show Recent People

Sort: Last Name

No patient photo

Hide Photo

White R. Mark

B-date: 5/25/1970
Age: 44
EMail:
Home #: (314) 555-5555
Work #:

Account Balance: $0.00
Last MedHx: None On File
Next Prev Appt:
Next Reg Appt:

Missing HIPAA Agreements

Name	ID	Home Phone	Work Phone	Soc. Sec. #	Chart ID	Pref. Name
Brown, Mary C.	1	(314) 111-1111				Mary
Mark, White R.	2	(314) 555-5555				Mark

Use New Edit Delete Print Report Close

B

FIGURE 8-6 **A,** Rolodex file. **B,** Electronic address file. (**A,** Copyright © 2014 Homestudio, BigStock.com. **B,** Courtesy Patterson Office Supplies, Champaign, Illinois.)

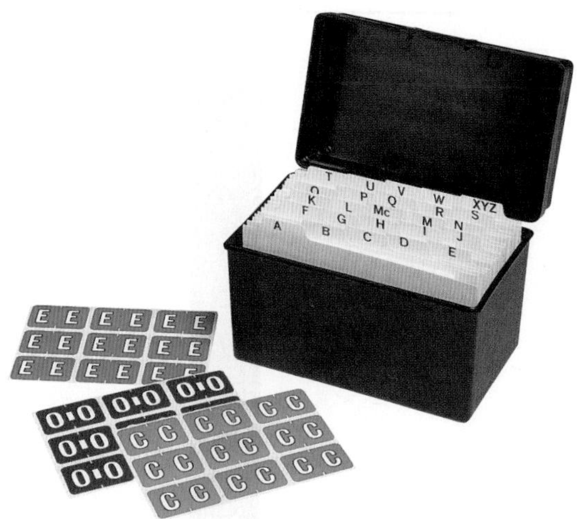

FIGURE 8-7 Label kit with assorted colored labels. (Courtesy Patterson Office Supplies, Champaign, Illinois.)

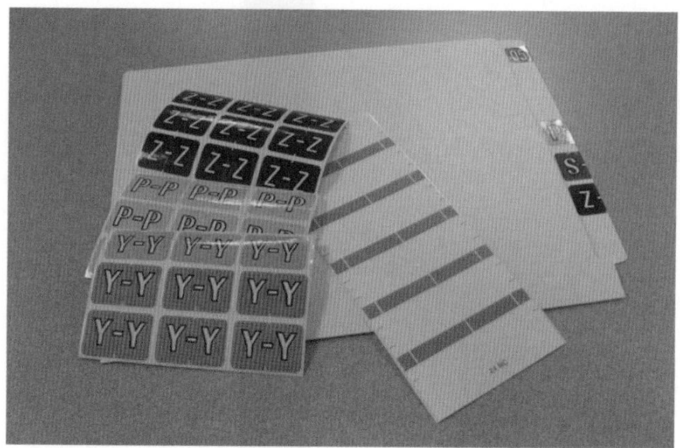

FIGURE 8-8 Patient file folders with colored filing labels.

Points to remember when making the labels include the following: (1) the labels should be keyed and printed rather than handwritten; (2) the keying should begin two or three spaces from the left edge of the label and at a uniform distance (usually one line space) from the top edge of the label; (3) the name may be keyed in all capital letters, or the first letter of each important word may be capitalized; and (4) the established format should be followed consistently.

The color coding of file folders aids in fast retrieval and refiling. Figure 8-8 shows a typical open-shelf, end-tab filing system that uses colored filing labels on each file folder to translate the alphabetical rules discussed earlier into a color-coding scheme. The assignment of color to each alphabetical character has long been recognized by efficiency experts as a time and energy saver. When patient charts are filed alphabetically and when each letter in the alphabet has a different file label color, color-block patterns begin to form in the open-shelf system that immediately direct the eye toward the proper filing areas. This virtually eliminates the misfiling that is common with non–color-coded systems. By assigning a different color to each number, large filing systems that use the numeric system can also benefit from the added efficiency of color coding.

Sometimes cross-referencing is necessary within the filing system. Cross-referencing helps the administrative assistant to locate or file the information in its proper location. For example, if a letter is to be filed by the dental clinic name rather than by the name of the individual who has written the letter, the administrative assistant may look under the individual's name and find the cross-reference sheet, which will indicate the name of the clinic (Figure 8-9).

Strong consideration should be given to an off-site online backup system that performs its services each day during the office's downtime. At the end of this chapter is an example of a recommended website for such services. Although companies that provide these services currently may not be required under law to meet the level of standards that the practice must, there are organizations that are service compliant with HIPAA requirements. These companies should be willing and able to produce a written business agreement that describes their practices and procedures.

There will also likely be a small need for the supplies necessary for electronic records management. This may include specially designed storage units for disks or tapes. These units may be small plastic or fabric containers that hold one to five CDs or DVDs, plastic or wooden desktop boxes, rotary files, or ring binders with vinyl pages that have pockets. A digital tape backup system is necessary when large amounts of data stored on hard disks must be recorded. Some of these systems store the entire contents of a hard disk on a single minicassette.

MANAGING WORKSTATION RECORDS EFFECTIVELY

Regardless of the types of records or systems used in a dental office, organization of the workstation is an absolute necessity for successful records management. Almost all assistants spend some of their workday filing records of some type. Even if filing duties are limited to organizing individual files, a simple system should be developed and followed. The goal should be to establish a system that allows for easy retrieval. Successful retrieval means being able to find a record or document when needed in a minimal amount of time. As stated previously, this type of efficiency promotes patient satisfaction, eliminates time and motion, and ultimately helps to prevent financial loss. Box 8-3 presents tips for successful records management.

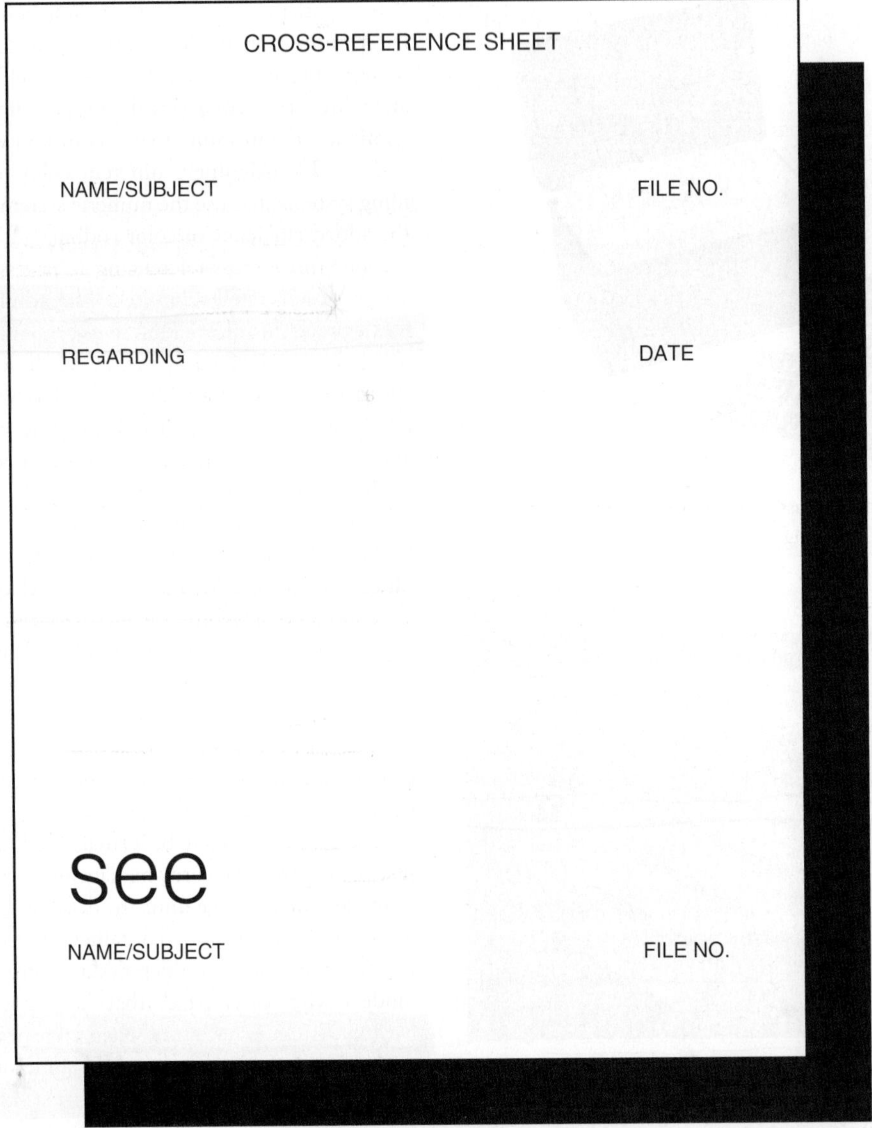
CROSS-REFERENCE SHEET

NAME/SUBJECT FILE NO.

REGARDING DATE

see

NAME/SUBJECT FILE NO.

FIGURE 8-9 Cross-reference sheet.

BOX **8-3**

Tips for Successful Records Management

Paper Records

- Organize incoming and outgoing papers in an inbox and an outbox. Use a stackable style that has three trays, and label the trays "In," "Out," and "Hold." The hold tray is for papers that do not have to be acted upon immediately.
- Use desk drawer files for forms, stationery, procedural handbooks, and other routinely used items.
- Use logbooks to record recurring events or data, such as long-distance telephone calls, petty cash, and appointment call lists.
- Keep a correspondence or chronological file, and date each folder for the year. This will provide a fingertip reference for all correspondence pertaining to a patient or a given activity. Of course, a copy of the correspondence must also be filed in the patient's paper record or scanned into his or her electronic record.
- Plan a work schedule that includes filing as part of the daily routine.
- When placing records in a folder, remove the folder from the file far enough so that the material can be placed completely in the folder and so that it does not extend over the top edge of the folder or tab.
- Be careful to place materials in the correct folder and not behind or in front of another folder.
- Do not use paper clips on filed material; it is easy for other materials to attach themselves to these clips. Staples are better if

BOX 8-3

Tips for Successful Records Management—cont'd

materials must be held together, but remove one staple before adding another.
- To avoid filing errors, designate as few people as possible to file and retrieve records.
- When searching for lost records, check letter transposition and the alternate spellings of names.
- Replace folders as they become worn out.
- Avoid overuse of the miscellaneous file.

Electronic Records
- If using portable recordable media, store the media in a file box specifically designed for that media style and according to safety and security requirements.
- Label each medium with a general classification.
- Print an index of the documents currently on the medium each time a new document is added. The index can be folded and placed in the jacket or kept in a reference notebook.
- When the media source becomes full and the same label is needed for a new disk, number the disks in consecutive order (e.g., "Letters 1," "Letters 2"). Mark each new medium with the date that it was first used.
- Store documents in electronic folders named to represent the activity that the folder represents (e.g., "Correspondence," "Recall," "Patient charts").

LEARNING ACTIVITIES

1. List four steps for preparing materials to be filed.
2. Define the five basic methods of filing.
3. Describe the use of the following filing equipment:
   a. Vertical file
   b. Open-shelf file
   c. Card file
   d. Rolodex file
   e. Tickler file
   f. Electronic file
4. Explain how color coding can be used in dental office files.
5. List six helpful hints for more efficient filing.

Please refer to the student workbook for additional learning activities.

BIBLIOGRAPHY

Fulton-Calkins PJ, Rankin DS, Shumack KA: The administrative professional, ed 14, Mason, OH, 2011, Thomson South-Western.

Vermaat ME, Sebok SL, Freund SM: Discovering computers—technology in a world of computers, mobile devices, and the Internet, Boston, 2014, Cengage Learning, Course Technology.

RECOMMENDED WEBSITES

www.ada.org.
www.amia.org.
www.drbackup.net.
www.hhs.gov.

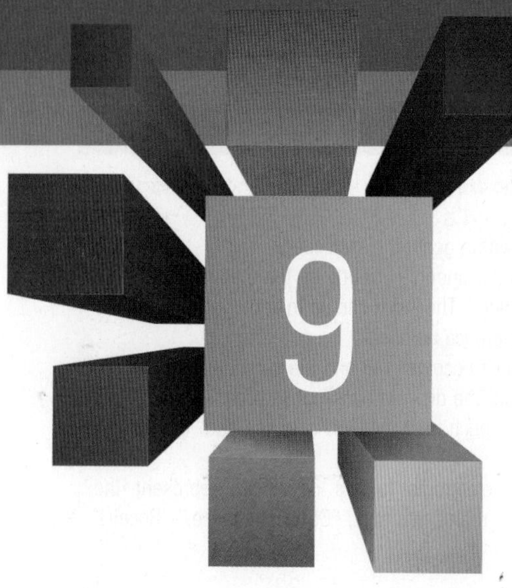

Written Communications

http://evolve.elsevier.com/Finkbeiner/practice

LEARNING OUTCOMES

1. Define the key terms in this chapter.
2. Describe the various types of written communication in a dental office.
3. Select stationery supplies.
4. Identify the characteristics of effective correspondence.
5. Identify the parts of a business letter.
6. Review rules of punctuation and capitalization and discuss ways of entering telephone numbers in a letter.
7. Describe the basic steps for preparing effective written communication and how to prepare the envelope for outgoing mail.
8. Observe ethical and legal obligations in written communication.
9. Explain the use of e-mail in the dental office and the importance of applying common business etiquette to the use of e-mail.
10. Discuss other written types of communication.
11. Discuss managing office mail including:
    - Identify the classifications of mail.
    - Identify special mail services.
    - Discuss the process for packaging laboratory cases.
    - Explain the procedure for processing incoming mail.
    - Discuss how to manage mail in the dentist's absence.

KEY TERMS

Attention line A line at the beginning of a letter that directs the letter to a particular individual or department within an organization.

Body The main portion of a letter that includes the message.

Complimentary close A courteous ending to a letter, such as "Sincerely," "Yours truly," or "Sincerely yours."

Copy notation This informs the recipient of the letter to whom additional copies were sent. Several types of notations are possible, including mail, computer copy, blind copy, postscript, and second-page headings.

Date line The line that contains the date on which the letter was keyboarded. When using printed letterhead stationery, this line usually begins two lines below the lowest line of the letterhead.

E-mail Electronic mail used to communicate within the office and with external sources.

Inside address The address that provides all information for mailing the letter and that includes the recipient's name, the name of the company (if appropriate), the street number and name, the city, and the zip code.

Interoffice memorandum Written communication within the organization or office.

Keyboarded signature The name and title of the person sending the letter or communication.

Mixed punctuation The use of punctuation within a letter. For example, a colon follows the salutation, and a comma follows the close.

Open punctuation The elimination of punctuation after the salutation and the close.

Reference initials The initials of the person who produced the letter or memo if it is different than the signature.

Salutation Formal greeting to the reader.

Subject line A statement that concisely states what the letter is about.

Today one may ask if written communication is as important in the dental office as it has been in the past. The answer is a resounding *yes.* Because e-mail is such a widely used vehicle for communicating today, the administrative assistant will probably write more than in the past. Many professionals find themselves writing their colleagues more than telephoning them.

Written communication in all of its forms remains extremely important. In addition to e-mail, the administrative assistant will use instant messaging via the Internet; he or she will also write memoranda, letters, and reports. Effective written correspondence promotes goodwill for the office, whereas ineffectively written correspondence can cost the dental office greatly in terms of unhappy patients and goodwill. This cost can include—but is not limited to—the loss of patients, profits, patient satisfaction, and goodwill.

Good business and professional writing should sound like one person talking to another person. Using an easy-to-read style makes the reader respond more positively to stated ideas. There are two ways to make writing easier. First, individual sentences and paragraphs should be easy to read so that the reader can easily skim the first paragraph or read the entire document in as short a time as possible. Second, the document should be visually pleasant, and it should include structure signposts that lead the reader through the document.

Good business and professional writing is closer to a conversation and less formal than the style of writing that has traditionally earned high marks for college essays and term papers. However, many dental professionals also use professional papers that are easy to read and that provide a good visual impact. Most people have several styles of talking that they vary instinctively, depending on the audience. This will also be the case with writing in the dental office. A letter to a dentist regarding a professional technique or a letter to a dental supplier demanding better service may be formal, whereas an e-mail to a colleague will be informal and perhaps even chatty.

Chapter 7 examined the various types of documents generated in the dental office. Now it is time to review the importance of other types of written communication in a dental practice, specifically the use of letters, forms, and newsletters. These documents are all created by the administrative assistant for a variety of reasons. This chapter discusses the creation and production of written communication, how such communication is distributed, and how incoming written communication is processed in both physical and electronic forms.

LETTERS

A variety of written documents are generated in the dental office, but none are as important as the letters that seek to enhance public relations with patients and professional colleagues. These letters should be original, and they should help to enhance the practice's professional image. Most important, the administrative assistant should be proud to mail these letters from the office.

With the use of word processing in the dental office, the dreaded task of creating an original letter each time one is needed is eliminated. Today's administrative assistant can have a supply of sample letters stored as templates in an electronic file. When necessary, the assistant can transform the sample into an original letter that is professional and that can be personalized within minutes.

The types of written communication most commonly sent from a dental office include thank you notes for the referral of patients, letters of appreciation, birthday and holiday greetings, congratulatory letters, sympathy messages, patient transfer letters or letters of consultation, recall notices, collection letters, order letters, and newsletters.

Referral Thank You Letters

The dentist should be appreciative of the confidence expressed by a patient who refers a new patient to the office and should acknowledge such a referral with a personally signed letter. In fact, some dentists include small gift cards or a lottery ticket with the thank you note. Although this letter should mention the name of the referred patient, it should never divulge any confidential information about that patient's treatment. However, if this letter is to be sent to a physician or another dentist, a reference statement may be made about the patient's diagnosis or prognosis, if this was discussed with the patient and the patient has signed the appropriate disclosure forms. Several examples of this type of thank you letter are shown in Figure 9-1. Note that the differences in content vary according to the situation.

Letters of Appreciation to Cooperative Patients

A cooperative patient is often overlooked and taken for granted. Often one thinks only of the patients who create frustration. A dentist should acknowledge a patient who is prompt for appointments, who maintains a regular payment plan, and who cooperates with prescribed homecare plans. This is a chance for the dental office staff to offer sincere compliments. When the opportunity presents itself, try writing a letter as shown in Figure 9-2, and see how appreciative patients are to receive it. A letter of appreciation should be sincere, state the purpose briefly, and be written as though conversing with the patient in person.

Birthday Letters and Holiday Greetings

Patients—especially children and older adults—like to be recognized on their birthdays. These letters should be cheerful and friendly. Figure 9-3 shows a letter that could be sent to an older adult on a special birthday. Another method of handling this form of public relations is to send a birthday card. If an email address is available, eCards could also be an option for a special birthday greeting. Many professional stationers provide appropriate greeting cards for all occasions and dental specialties (Figure 9-4).

Congratulatory Letters

Through conversations with patients and via the daily newspaper, the administrative assistant may learn about the outstanding achievements of the practice's patients. Such accomplishments should not go unnoticed by the dental office staff. A letter sent to congratulate a patient must be sent promptly. Describe how the event was discovered, and include a sincere expression of congratulations (Figure 9-5). Congratulations may also be sent for the birth of a child, a wedding, or a graduation. A greeting card or a brief letter is appropriate.

A

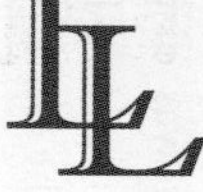

Dental Associates, PC
611 Main Street, SE
Grand Rapids, MI 49502
Phone: 616.101.9575 Fax: 616.101.9999
E-mail: office@dapc.com or Visit us at: www.Lakedental.com

Joseph W. Lake, DDS **Ashley M. Lake, DDS**

April 17, 20—

Mr. Edward Aprill
347 North Wixom
Frankfort, MI 48223

Dear Mr. Aprill:

Your expression of confidence in referring Mr. Robert Smith to my office for treatment is greatly appreciated. It is always a pleasure to welcome new patients to our practice, especially when they are referred by another satisfied patient.

It gives my staff and me a sense of satisfaction that you have been pleased with the treatment we have rendered. We will make every effort to provide Mr. Smith with the same complete and thorough dentistry we have provided you during these past five years.

Thank you again for your confidence.

Sincerely,

Joseph W. Lake, DDS

je

B

Dental Associates, PC
611 Main Street, SE
Grand Rapids, MI 49502
Phone: 616.101.9575 Fax: 616.101.9999
E-mail: office@dapc.com or Visit us at: www.Lakedental.com

Joseph W. Lake, DDS **Ashley M. Lake, DDS**

September 15, 20—

Mr. Carl Ladley
3567 Wines Drive
Wyoming, MI 49507

Dear Carl:

It was good of you to refer one of your employees, Raymone Hunchez, to me for treatment. My staff and I are always glad to be of assistance to you and your employees whenever possible.

You and your family have been valuable members of my dental practice. We hope that we will be able to provide Mr. Hunchez the same quality service that we have provided your family in the past.

Give my best regards to Mary and the boys.

Sincerely,

Ashley M. Lake, DDS

je

FIGURE 9-1 **A,** Referral thank you letter. **B,** Informal referral thank letter to a patient who is a personal friend of the dentist.

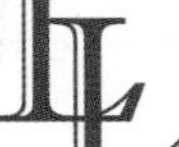

Dental Associates, PC
611 Main Street, SE
Grand Rapids, MI 49502
Phone: 616.101.9575 Fax: 616.101.9999
E-mail: office@dapc.com or Visit us at: www.Lakedental.com

Joseph W. Lake, DDS **Ashley M. Lake, DDS**

September 19, 20—

Ms. Angela Gualandi
2492 Plymouth Road
Comstock, MI 49829

Dear Ms. Gualandi:

I would like to take this opportunity to thank you for your confidence in referring your friend, Judy McKay, and her children, Debbie and Rick, to our office for treatment.

My staff and I are pleased to learn of your satisfaction. We will make every effort to justify the confidence you have shown in us during the treatment of Ms. McKay and her children.

Thank you again for your expression of confidence.

Sincerely,

Ashley M. Lake, DDS

je

C

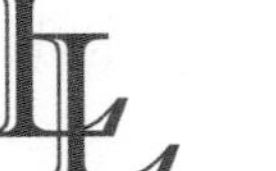

Dental Associates, PC
611 Main Street, SE
Grand Rapids, MI 49502
Phone: 616.101.9575 Fax: 616.101.9999
E-mail: office@dapc.com or Visit us at: www.Lakedental.com

Joseph W. Lake, DDS **Ashley M. Lake, DDS**

December 19, 20—

Robert W. Wells, DDS, MS
2146 Rochester Avenue
Grand Rapids, MI 49502

Dear Dr. Wells:

Mrs. Roger (Amy) Browne was in my office today for an examination. I confirmed your diagnosis of advanced periodontitis. We have set up a series of appointments for x-rays and beginning periodonatal curettage.

The prognosis is favorable and Mrs. Browne was eager to begin treatment. Thank you for this referral and the kind remarks you made to her.

Sincerely,

Joseph W. Lake, DDS

je

D

FIGURE 9-1, cont'd **C,** General referral thank you letter. **D,** Referral thank you letter to a colleague.

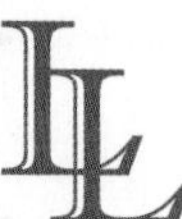

Dental Associates, PC
611 Main Street, SE
Grand Rapids, MI 49502
Phone: 616.101.9575 Fax: 616.101.9999
E-mail: office@dapc.com or Visit us at: www.Lakedental.com

Joseph W. Lake, DDS Ashley M. Lake, DDS

March 30, 20—

Mr.Ryan Hamlin
1334 Huron Road
Grandville, MI 49508

Dear Mr.Hamlin:

My staff and I would like to thank you for your cooperation during the treatment that we have just completed. A patient's cooperation and interest in his dental care is an integral part of our success.

Your cooperation in keeping your appointments, prompt payment of your account, and diligent home care has made our work much more enjoyable.

We look forward to seeing you for your oral examination in three months. We hope you continue to enjoy the wise investment you have made in your mouth.

Sincerely,

Joseph W.Lake, DDS

je

FIGURE 9-2 Letter of appreciation to a cooperative patient.

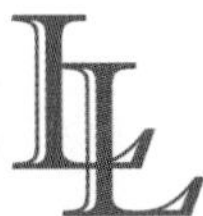

Dental Associates, PC
611 Main Street, SE
Grand Rapids, MI 49502
Phone: 616.101.9575 Fax: 616.101.9999
E-mail: office@dapc.com or Visit us at: www.Lakedental.com

Joseph W. Lake, DDS Ashley M. Lake, DDS

May 17, 20—

Mr. Joseph Divirgilius
1145 Collins Drive
Grand Rapids, MI 49502

Dear Mr. Divirgilius:

My staff and I wish to send our best wishes for a happy birthday tomorrow. We hope you will enjoy your ninety-fifth birthday and refiect on your many accomplishments.

Your longevity may be attributed to your good health and heritage, but your continued personal contributions to the community are evidence of your unselfishness. We hope your example of good citizenship will impact the youth of this city.

Again, best wishes for a happy birthday and continued good health in the future.

Sincerely,

Ashley M.Lake, DDS

je

FIGURE 9-3 Birthday letter to an older adult.

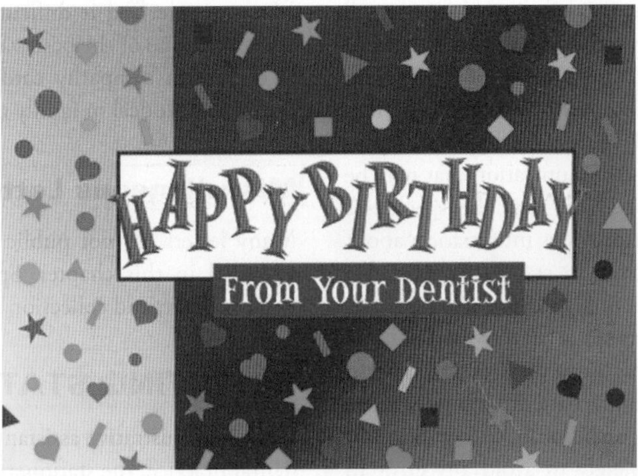

FIGURE 9-4 Birthday card. (Courtesy Patterson Office Supplies, Champaign, IL.)

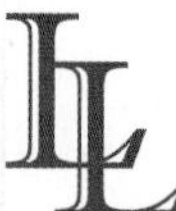

Dental Associates, PC
611 Main Street, SE
Grand Rapids, MI 49502
Phone: 616.101.9575 Fax: 616.101.9999
E-mail: office@dapc.com or Visit us at: www.Lakedental.com

Joseph W. Lake, DDS **Ashley M. Lake, DDS**

September 28, 20—

Mr.Jason Henkle
1135 Hollyhock Lane
Grand Rapids, MI 49503

Dear Mr.Henkle:

Last night the staff and I read in the *Grand Rapids News* about your promotion to Vice President of the Michigan Trust Company. We want to send our congratulations to you on this promotion.

It is a pleasure to learn of your advancement and I send my best wishes for success in this new position. I am certain this will be a challenging experience.

Again, my sincerest best wishes on your fine achievement.

Sincerely,

Ashley M.Lake, DDS

je

FIGURE 9-5 Congratulatory letter.

Referrals for Consultation or Treatment

During the treatment of a patient, it is often necessary to call upon the services of a specialist. A series of letters may be sent between the two dental offices regarding the patient's treatment. A good example of such an experience is the transfer of a patient to an orthodontist for treatment (Figure 9-6). Figure 9-7 provides examples of several forms of communication that may be used during a patient's treatment. Note that the specialist's office has used a basic format that provides information about the patient's treatment. This letter can be stored electronically, or a preprepared form can be used in a specialty office such as an orthodontics office, because there is a large patient volume and a similarity of basic treatment. Regardless of the type of form used, note that in each case the patient's name is referenced, the message is brief, and each tooth or condition is diagrammed or written out completely to avoid any error in interpretation.

Sympathy Messages

Many people find it difficult to express sympathy in a letter. Therefore, one of the best ways to handle this difficult situation is to send a sympathy card. This unexpected message often means a great deal to family members during their time of grief.

Miscellaneous Letters

Many letters are not public relations letters and thus are not included in this chapter. Specific examples of recall, broken appointment, and collection letters are discussed in Chapter 15.

SELECTING STATIONERY SUPPLIES

If the administrative assistant begins working in an established dental practice, the stationery supplies will already be available. However, he or she may have to choose business supplies if

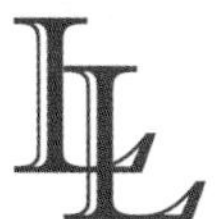

Dental Associates, PC
611 Main Street, SE
Grand Rapids, MI 49502
Phone: 616.101.9575 Fax: 616.101.9999
E-mail: office@dapc.com or Visit us at: www.Lakedental.com

Joseph W. Lake, DDS — Ashley M. Lake, DDS

September 25, 20—

Daniel R. Jacobsen, DDS, MS
2495 Packard Road SE
Grand Rapids, MI 49506

Dear Dr.Jacobsen:

I am referring Michael Moran, age 12, to you for an orthodontic evaluation. Mrs. Moran will be calling your office for an appointment. Michael appears to have a Class II malocclusion with crowding of the mandibular anterior teeth.

Enclosed you will find a complete series of radiographs that were taken on September 11, 20-- .

I will look forward to your diagnosis and assistance with this case.

Sincerely,

Joseph W.Lake, DDS

je

Enclosure: Full mouth series radiographs

FIGURE 9-6 Letter for the referral of a patient to an orthodontist.

asked to order them. Many of these supplies are listed in Chapter 6.

The office stationery (letterhead) is usually selected on the basis of simplicity, neatness, and quality. Bond paper, because of its quality, is often used. It can be made from all-cotton fiber (sometimes called *rag*), all-sulfite (a wood pulp) fiber, or any proportion of the two. High-cotton fiber bond indicates quality and prestige, and it ages without deterioration or chemical breakdown.

The following information may be used as guidelines for future stationery needs:

- A color theme for stationery items such as letterhead, envelopes, appointment cards, prescription pads, medicine envelopes, and notepads may be used. Coordinated colors (e.g., light and dark brown or blue) or contrasting tones of gray with black print are attractive combinations. Most dental stationery supply or chain office supply houses have samples of stationery stock and logo designs from which to select.
- A popular alternative to purchasing stationery is to create the letterhead with the use of appropriate computer software. A fine bond paper can be purchased. When a new letter is to be keyboarded, the letterhead is removed from the file where it is stored, the letter is prepared, and then it is printed on bond paper. This becomes less expensive and allows for more frequent changes and creativity. Clip art is available that makes it easy to create professional-looking letterhead that provides the office staff with many options. Labels with the same clip art and office information can also be created in this manner. It is important that the labels selected are compatible with the office printer.

CHARACTERISTICS OF AN EFFECTIVE LETTER

Effective letters that generate good public relations have certain common elements. Keep in mind that direct and simple writing

John G. Clinthorne, D.D.S., M.S.
H. Ludia Kim, D.M.D., M.S.
Professional Corporation
Specialists in Orthodontics
1303 Packard
Ann Arbor, Michigan 48104
(734) 761-3116

«Todays_date_in_words»

«Responsible_party_name»
«Responsible_party_address»
«Responsible_party_city_state_zip»

Dear «Responsible_party_greeting»:

Welcome to our practice! My staff and I look forward to meeting you and «Patient_first_name» on «Next_appointment_ date» at «Next_appointment_time». Be assured that «Patient_first_name possessive» first visit with us will be a pleasant and rewarding experience.

Please bring with you the enclosed information sheet as well as any insurance forms and information we may need to file with your insurance carrier.

At «Patient_first_name possessive» first visit to our office, we will proceed with an oral examination and discuss the findings with you. If a more thorough diagnosis is advisable, the following materials may be requested at an additional charge:

- Models of Teeth
- Panoramic X-ray
- Profile X-ray
- Diagnostic Photographs

After the above materials have been studied and the best course of therapy determined, the overall treatment plan will be discussed with you at a consultation appointment.

Sincerely,

John G. Clinthorne, D.D.S., M.S.
H. Ludia Kim, D.M.D., M.S.

Members American Association of **Orthodontists**

A

John G. Clinthorne, D.D.S., M.S.
H. Ludia Kim, D.M.D., M.S.
Professional Corporation
Specialists in Orthodontics
1303 Packard
Ann Arbor, Michigan 48104
(734) 761-3116

«Todays_date_in_words»

«Referring_party_name»
«Referring_party_address—line 1»
«Referring_party_address—line 2»«Referring_party_city_state_zip»

RE: «Patient_full_name» «Age: Patients_age»

Dear «Referring_party_greeting»:

DISPOSITION:
( ) Orthodontic treatment is indicated at this time and:
( ) They intend to proceed with treatment.
Records and consultation appointments have been made.
( ) They are to notify us if and when they wish to proceed.
( ) They do not intend to proceed with treatment.

( ) «Patient_first_name» has been referred to your office for:
( ) Dental examination and prophylaxis.
( ) ______________________________

( ) Orthodontic treatment may be indicated in the future and
( ) «Patient_first_name» has been placed on recall __________
( ) They prefer to call our office at a later date.

( ) Orthodontic treatment is not indicated.

REMARKS:

Members American Association of **Orthodontists**

B

FIGURE 9-7 **A,** Basic form letter from an orthodontist to welcome a new patient. Diagnosis text from the patient's record may be inserted. **B,** Basic form letter from an orthodontist to a referring dentist after examination of a patient.

John G. Clinthorne, D.D.S., M.S.
H. Ludia Kim, D.M.D., M.S.
Professional Corporation
Specialists in Orthodontics
1303 Packard
Ann Arbor, Michigan 48104
(734) 761-3116

«Todays_date_in_words»

«Responsible_party_name»
«Responsible_party_address»
«Responsible_party_city_state_zip»

Dear «Responsible_party_greeting»:

The consultation appointment to discuss «Patient_first_name possessive» orthodontic treatment is scheduled for «Next_appointment_date» at «Next_appointment_time».

We shall present to you an outline of the treatment plan and our recommendations, the estimated length of treatment, cooperation requirements, and costs. We will answer any questions you may have, as well as discuss any particular problems, that bear on the success of the treatment. Both parents are encouraged to attend to gain a thorough understanding of our services. The patient is welcome but is not required to attend.

Thank you for giving us the opportunity to be of service to you and your child. We are delighted to have «Patient_first_name» as a new patient and we look forward to a continuing relationship.

Sincerely,

John G. Clinthorne, D.D.S., M.S.
H. Ludia Kim, D.M.D., M.S.

Members American Association of **Orthodontists**

C

John G. Clinthorne, D.D.S., M.S.
H. Ludia Kim, D.M.D., M.S.
Professional Corporation
Specialists in Orthodontics
1303 Packard
Ann Arbor, Michigan 48104
(734) 761-3116

«Todays_date_in_words»

«Referring_party_name»
«Referring_party_address—line 1»
«Referring_party__city_state_zip»

Dear «Referring_party_greeting»:

I want to inform you that I have removed the fixed appliances on «Patient_full_name», age «Patients_age». The following summarizes this case to date:

TYPE OF TREATMENT:
( ) no extractions ( ) extraction of ____________
( ) partial banding ____________
( ) complete banding-duration ____________
( ) ____________

SEVERITY OF ORIGINAL PROBLEM:

Skeletal-	( ) very complex	( ) moderately complex	( ) routine
Dental-	( ) very complex	( ) moderately complex	( ) routine
Neuromuscular-	( ) very complex	( ) moderately complex	( ) routine

ORAL HYGIENE:
( ) outstanding ( ) good ( ) fair ( ) poor

COOPERATION:
( ) outstanding ( ) good ( ) fair ( ) poor

TYPE AND DURATION OF RETENTION: Approximate duration

( ) maxillary removable retainer ____________
( ) mandibular removable retainer ____________
( ) mandibular xed strap ____________
( ) ____________ ____________

THE PATIENT HAS BEEN REFERRED TO YOUR OFFICE FOR:

( ) oral prophylaxis and dental examination
( ) ____________

REMARKS:

Members American Association of **Orthodontists**

D

FIGURE 9-7, cont'd **C,** Letter to a patient confirming a consultation appointment and explaining the process. **D,** Final letter from an orthodontist to inform a referring dentist about a patient's completed treatment.

Continued

JOHN G. CLINTHORNE, D.D.S., M.S.
H. LUDIA KIM, D.M.D., M.S.

ORTHODONTICS 1303 PACKARD, ANN ARBOR, MI. 48104 734-761-3116

DR. ______ PHONE ______

NAME ______ PHONE ______

DATE ______ ______ D.D.S.

Extract Teeth Encircled

PERMANENT TEETH

UPPER

1 2 3 4 5 6 7 8 | 9 10 11 12 13 14 15 16

PATIENT'S RIGHT PATIENT'S LEFT

32 31 30 29 28 27 26 25 | 24 23 22 21 20 19 18 17

LOWER

DECIDUOUS TEETH

UPPER

A B C D E | F G H I J

PATIENT'S RIGHT PATIENT'S LEFT

T S R Q P | O N M L K

LOWER

☐ Enclosure - X-Rays
☐ Return Requested
☐ Please Keep For Your Records

If any questions ...... Please Telephone

E

FIGURE 9-7, cont'd E, Requisition used by an orthodontist to refer a patient for extraction. (Courtesy J.G. Clinthorne, DDS, and H.L. Kim, DMD, Ann Arbor, MI.)

Letterheads	**Matching Envelopes**
Standard office use: Business size $8\frac{1}{2} \times 11$ inches	No. 10 ($4\frac{1}{8} \times 9\frac{1}{2}$ inches) Same weight and fiber content as letterhead
Usually 16# or 20# bond 25% cotton fiber (rag) Executive use: Standard and Monarch size	No. 10 and No. 7 ($3\frac{7}{8} \times 7\frac{1}{2}$ inches) Same weight and fiber content as letterhead
(Monarch size: $7\frac{1}{4} \times 10$ inches) Usually 24# bond 100% cotton fiber	

is easier to read. The best word depends on context: the situation, the purpose, the audience, and the words used.

Here are some general guidelines:

- *Use words that are accurate, appropriate, and familiar.* Accurate words mean what the author is wanting to say. Appropriate words convey the attitudes that the author wants to create and fit well with the other words in the document. Familiar words are easy to read and understand.
- *Use technical terminology sparingly.* The exception to this rule is if the administrative assistant is communicating with another professional and needs to describe a condition or treatment in technical terms. However, when communicating with patients or laypersons, it is wise to use a "plain English" equivalent instead of a technical term.
- *Use active verbs most of the time.* This is common when writing for a job application or referring a patient to a

specialist. If the verb describes something that the subject is doing, the verb is active. If the verb describes something that is being done to the grammatical subject, the verb is passive.

Active: I recommend that the patient's third molar be removed.
Passive: It was recommended by me for the patient to have the third molar removed.
Active: I can expose digital radiographs.
Passive: Digital radiography is something I could do.

- *Tighten the writing.* Eliminate words that say nothing. Combine sentences to eliminate unnecessary words. Put the meaning of the sentence into the subject and the verb. Cut words if the idea is already clear from other words in the sentence. Substitute single words for wordy phrases.

Wordy: Keep this information in the patient's file for future reference.
Tighter: Keep this information for reference.
or: File this information.

Phrases beginning with *of, which,* and *that* can often be shortened.

Wordy: The issue of most importance
Tighter: The most important issue
Wordy: The estimate that is enclosed
Tighter: The enclosed estimate
Wordy: It is the case that Registered Dental Assistants are more qualified clinicians in the office.
Tighter: Registered Dental Assistants are more qualified clinicians in the office.

Combine sentences to eliminate unnecessary words. In addition to saying words, combining sentences focuses the reader's attention on key points; it makes your writing sound more sophisticated and sharpens the relationship between ideas, thus making your writing more coherent.

Wordy: I conducted a survey by telephone on Monday, April 17. I questioned 18 dental assistants, some Registered Dental Assistants, and some Certified Dental Assistants, who—according to the state directory—were all currently working. The purpose of this survey was to find out how many of them were performing advanced functions that were delegated by the state. I also wanted to find out if there were any differences in their salaries.
Tighter: On Monday, April 17, I phoned working Registered and Certified Dental Assistants to determine whether they were performing their state-delegated advanced functions and whether there was a distinction between the salaries for these two credentials.

- *Vary sentence length and structure:* A readable letter mixes sentence lengths and varies sentence structure. A really short sentence is less than 10 words long and can add punch to your letter. Really long sentences of 30 to 40 words can raise a danger flag.

A simple sentence has one main clause:

We will open a new office this month.

A compound sentence has two main clauses joined with *and, but, or,* or another conjunction. Compound sentences are used best when the ideas in the two clauses are closely related.

[Clause 1] We have hired three new dental assistants, and *[Clause 2]* they will complete their orientation next week.
[Clause 1] We hired a new intern, but *[Clause 2]* she will be unable to begin work until the end of the month.

Complex sentences have one main and one subordinate clause; they are good for showing logical relationships.

[Subordinate clause] When the new office opens, *[Main clause]* we will have an open house for local dentists and offer refreshments and door prizes.
[Subordinate clause] Because we already have a strong patient base in Livingston County, *[Main clause]* we expect that the new office will be as successful as the Ann Arbor office.

- *Use parallel structure:* Parallel structure puts words, phrases, or clauses in the same grammatical and logical form. Clarity eliminates long, meaningless words and uses language that the reader will understand. Thus, it is certain that each statement will not be misinterpreted.

Nonparallel: The position is prestigious, challenging, and also offers good money.
Parallel: The position offers prestige, challenge, and good money.
Nonparallel: The steps in the planning process include determining the objectives, an idea of who the reader is, and a list of the facts.
Parallel: Determine the objective, consider the reader, and gather the facts.

- *Put your readers in your sentences:* Use second-person pronouns *(you)* rather than third-person pronouns *(he, she, one)* or first-person pronouns *(I)* to give your writing a greater team approach. The "you" approach to letter writing requires the writer to place the reader at the center of the message.

Third person: References for patients in this office are made by our office manager, and the patient will be contacted as soon as the appointment has been confirmed with the specialist.
Second person: Once you are referred to a specialist, you will receive a confirmation of your appointment from our office manager.

PRACTICE NOTE

The "you" approach to letter writing requires the writer to place the reader at the center of the message.

In addition to considering the ideas presented here, the administrative assistant should review the basic characteristics of effective correspondence. These factors should be used as part of a review of the letter before it is sent. Remember that the letter sent from the dental office is representative of the quality of work or treatment produced in that practice and should contain the following characteristics:

- *Completeness:* Include all necessary data the reader needs to make a decision or take action.
-  *Conciseness:* State the information briefly.

BOX 9-1

Positive and Negative Words

Positive Words	Negative Words
I will	I'm sorry
Congratulations	Complaint
Concern	Difficult
Pleasure	Unpleasant
Thank you	No
Satisfactory	Can't
I can	Careless
Welcome	Error
	Inconvenient
	Disappointed

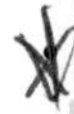
- *Confidentiality:* Release information only about the case that is relative to the contents of the letter and only after the patient has given consent to the release of specific information.

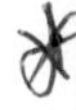
- *Courtesy:* Use good manners for good public relations. Do not make derogatory statements.

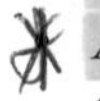
- *Accuracy:* Make sure that all of the data are correct. Check the details carefully. Use correct spelling and grammar.
- *Neatness:* Avoid smudges, tears, or wrinkles.
- *Positive language:* Use positive words that indicate helpfulness and caring (Box 9-1).
- *Orientation to reader:* Use "you"-oriented pronouns.

PARTS OF A BUSINESS LETTER

A review of the parts of a business letter and the proper placement and purpose for each part is appropriate before selecting a letter style and creating the letter. Most business letters contain the following parts:

- Date line
- Inside address (letter address)
- Salutation
- Body
- Complimentary close
- Keyboarded signature
- Reference initials
- Special notations such as attention line, subject line, or enclosures

When using most word processing software, many preformatted letter styles are available. The dates are inserted automatically, and, in most systems, the alignment and letter parts are already defined.

Date Line

The **date line** contains the date on which the letter is keyboarded. When using printed letterhead, the date usually begins two lines below the lowest line of the letterhead. (The letterhead usually takes up about 2 inches, but this may vary depending on the style and design of the letterhead.) Many times, the length of the letter determines whether the heading should be started lower on the paper; good judgment is needed. When keyboarding a personal business letter, the individual's return address is placed as the first two lines directly above the date line. The placement of the date line may be modified according to the length of the letter. When using the computer, you may view a "Print Preview" to check the appearance of the letter; necessary changes can then be made before printing. General guidelines that relate to letter length are shown in Box 9-2.

BOX 9-2

Placement of a Date Line

Letter Length	Side Margins	Top and Bottom Margins
Short (<100 words)	2 inches	3 inches
Average (101 to 200 words)	1½ inches	2 inches
Long (201 to 300 words)	1 inches	1 inches

Inside Address

The **inside address** provides all of the information for mailing the letter. The letter address should match the envelope address. When using word processing software, the envelope is often addressed from the letter address with the use of a minor key function on the computer. The information to be included is the recipient's name, the name of the company (if appropriate), the street number and name, the city, and the zip code. Three lines of space are left between the date and the first line of the letter address.

Use the titles that precede the individual's name (e.g., Mr., Mrs., Ms., Dr.), but do not use a double title (e.g., Dr. L. B. Crown, D.D.S.), because this is redundant. An official title (e.g., President) may follow the name (e.g., Ms. M. P. Colcman, President). The person's official title is often placed on the second line if it helps to balance the inside address lines. The city, state, and zip code are placed on the last line. The appropriate two-letter state postal abbreviation should be set in capital letters without a period. Leave two spaces after the abbreviation before entering the zip code.

Salutation

The **salutation** formally greets the reader. If the writer wishes the letter to be directed to an individual within a firm, it is acceptable to use an attention line. The salutation line should begin two lines below the letter address, and it should be flush with the left margin. If you are writing to an individual, the most appropriate salutation is the individual's name. For example, if the letter is addressed to Mr. Ted Monroe, the salutation would be "Dear Mr. Monroe." The salutation can be altered to be "Dear Ted" if the dentist is a close friend of the recipient. This change in formality should be recognized before the letter is keyboarded. Special situations occur when the letter is to be sent to unknown individuals or to more than one person. Suggestions for salutations to be used in common situations are shown in Box 9-3, *A*. Addresses and salutations to be used for governmental and academic officials are shown in Box 9-3, *B*.

Body of the Letter

The body of the letter contains the message. The body begins two lines after the salutation. The paragraphs within the body are single spaced, with two lines of space set between paragraphs. Paragraphs may or may not be indented, depending on the format selected. Refer to Figures 9-2 through 9-7 for the selection of the format. Many illustrations in this chapter demonstrate variations in letter format styles.

Complimentary Close

The complimentary close provides a courteous ending to the letter. It is keyboarded two lines after the last line of the body of the letter. The complimentary close is indented to the same

BOX 9-3, A

Appropriate Salutations for Various Situations

- *One person, gender unknown:* Dear M.R. Rieger
- *One person, name unknown, title known:* Dear Director of Surgical Technology
- *One woman, title unknown:* Dear Ms. Hartwig
- *Two or more women, titles known:* Dear Ms. Martin, Mrs. Leverett, and Ms. Grey
- *If all women are married:* Dear Mrs. Franks, Mrs. Johnson, and Mrs. Sullens *or* Dear Mesdames Franks, Johnson, and Sullens
- *If all women are unmarried:* Dear Miss Franks, Miss Johnson, and Miss Sullens *or* Dear Misses Franks, Johnson, and Sullens
- *If all recipients are women:* Dear Ms. Franks, Johnson, and Coady *or* Dear Mses. *or* Mss. Franks, Johnson, and Sullens
- *A woman and a man:* Dear Ms. Johnson and Mr. Ladley
- *A group or organization composed entirely of women:* Ladies or Mesdames
- *A group or organization composed entirely of men:* Gentlemen
- *A group composed of women and men:* Ladies and Gentlemen

BOX 9-3, B

Addresses and Salutations for Government and Academic Officials

The following addresses and salutations are recommended in correspondence with governmental or academic officials. In each case, the proper ways to address letters are illustrated. On the left are the addresses to use, and on the right are the appropriate salutations. When one or more examples are given, they are arranged in order of decreasing formality.

Correspondence with Government Officials

The President

Address	Salutation
The President	Dear Sir, Madam
The White House	Dear Mr. (Mrs. or Ms.) President
Washington, DC 20500	Dear Mr. President; Dear Madam President
or	
The President of the United States	
The White House	
Washington, DC 20500	

Chief Justice of the Supreme Court

Address	Salutation
The Chief Justice of the United States	Dear Sir, Madam
Washington, DC 20543	Dear Mr. or Madam Chief Justice
or	
The Honorable (full name)	
United States Supreme Court	
Washington, DC 20543	

Associate Justice of the Supreme Court

Address	Salutation
The Honorable (full name)	Dear Sir, Madam
Associate Justice of the Supreme Court	Dear Mr. or Madam Justice
Washington, DC 20543	My dear Justice (surname)
	Dear Justice (surname)

Cabinet Member

Address	Salutation
The Honorable (full name)	Dear Sir, Madam
Secretary of State	My dear Mr. or Madam Secretary
Washington, DC 20520	
or	
The Secretary of State	Dear Mr. or Madam Secretary
Washington, DC 20520	

Senator

Address	Salutation
The Honorable (full name)	Dear Sir, Madam
The United States Senate	My dear Mr. or Madam Senator
Washington, DC 20510	My dear Senator (surname)
or	Dear Senator (surname)
Senator (full name)	
The United States Senate	
Washington, DC 20510	

Representative

Address	Salutation
The Honorable (full name)	Dear Sir, Madam
The House of Representatives	My dear Representative (surname)
Washington, DC 20515	Dear Representative (surname)
or	
Representative (full name)	
The House of Representatives	
Washington, DC 20515	

BOX 9-3, B

Addresses and Salutations for Government and Academic Officials—cont'd

Chief, Director, or Commissioner of a Government Bureau

Address	Salutation
Mr., Ms., Mrs., or Miss (full name)	Dear Sir, Madam
Director of Public Information	My dear Mr., Ms., Mrs., or Miss (surname)
Department of Justice	
Washington, DC 20530	Dear Mr., Ms., Mrs., or Miss
or	
Director of Public Information	
Department of Justice	
Washington, DC 20530	

Governor

Address	Salutation
The Honorable (full name)	Dear Sir, Madam
Governor of Ohio	My dear Governor (surname)
Columbus, OH 43215	Dear Governor (surname)
or	Dear Governor
The Governor of Ohio	
Columbus, OH 43215	

State Senator

Address	Salutation
The Honorable (full name)	Dear Sir, Madam
The State Senate	My dear Senator
Columbus, OH 43215	My dear Senator (surname)
or	
Senator (full name)	Dear Senator (surname)
	My dear Mr., Ms., Mrs., or Miss (surname)
The State Senate	Dear Mr., Ms., Mrs., or Miss
Columbus, OH 43215	

State Representative

Address	Salutation
The Honorable (full name)	Dear Sir, Madam
House of Representatives	My dear Representative (surname)
Columbus, OH 43215	Dear Representative (surname)
or	My dear Mr., Ms., Mrs., or Miss (surname)
Representative (full name)	
House of Representatives	Dear Mr., Ms., Mrs., or Miss (surname)
Columbus, OH 43215	

Mayor of a City

Address	Salutation
The Honorable (full name)	My dear Sir, Madam
Mayor of the City of Ann Arbor	Dear Sir, Madam
City Hall	Dear Mr. or Madam Mayor
Ann Arbor, MI 48105	My dear Mayor (surname)
	Dear Mayor (surname)

Correspondence with Educators

President (College or University)

Address	Salutation
Dr. (full name)	My dear Sir, Madam
or	Dear Sir, Madam
(full name), Ph.D.	My dear President (surname)
President	Dear President (surname)
Ohio University	
Athens, OH 45701	

Dean of a College

Address	Salutation
Dean (full name)	My dear Sir, Madam
College of Business Administration	Dear Sir, Madam
University of Cincinnati	My dear Dean (surname)
Cincinnati, OH 45221	Dear Dean (surname)
or	
Dr. (full name)	
Dean of the College of Business Administration	
University of Cincinnati	
Cincinnati, OH 45221	

(If the individual has a doctorate degree, the salutation may be "Dear Dr. Wilson" instead of "Dear Dean Wilson.")

Professor (College or University)

Address	Salutation
(full name), Ph.D.	My dear Sir, Madam
Dr. (full name)	Dear Sir, Madam
Vanderbilt University	My dear Professor (surname)
Nashville, TN 37203	Dear Dr. (surname)

Note: Window envelopes require the date line to be placed on a line 2 inches below the top of the page.

point as the date line position if using the modified block style, or it is set flush with the left margin if using the block style. Only the first word of the complimentary close should be capitalized. The most common complimentary closes are "Very truly yours" and "Sincerely." Other acceptable closures are "Yours very truly" and "Sincerely yours."

Keyboarded Signature

The keyboarded signature appears four lines below the complimentary close. If the name and title of the individual are short, they may be placed on the same line and separated by a comma. However, if the name and title are relatively long, the name is keyboarded on the first line, and the title is placed on the second line. The comma is not placed after the name. You should attempt to make the lines as even as possible.

Reference Initials

Reference initials are the initials of the person who keyboarded the letter. They should appear in lowercase one double space after the keyboarded signature or even with the left margin. If it is policy to enter the dentist's initials in capital letters before the keyboarder's initials in lowercase, it would appear as "JWL:db" or "JWL/db."

Attention Line

You may wish to direct a letter to a particular individual or department within an organization. This can be done by using an attention line. The following example illustrates how an attention line is used if the letter has been addressed to a firm:

Apex Dental Laboratories
Attention Mr. W. W. Thomas, President

1616 W. Riverfront Street
Grand Rapids, MI 49502

The attention line indicates that the letter writer prefers that the letter be directed to a particular individual. The salutation should agree with the inside address and not with the attention line.

Subject Line

The subject line clearly states what the letter is about. For example, if writing to a patient about the office's policy regarding broken appointments, the subject line would be written as "Subject: Broken Appointments." The subject line is placed two lines after the salutation and followed by another two lines before continuing with the body of the letter. The subject line may be centered, indented like a paragraph point, or aligned with the left margin when using block style. The style of the letter will often determine the best position for the subject line. The word *Subject:* or *SUBJECT:* or the abbreviation *Re:* or *RE:* may be used, and any of these options may be underlined. Acceptable methods of using the subject line are illustrated here:

Dear Mrs. Calloway:
SUBJECT: Broken Appointments
or
Dear Mrs. Alvarez:
RE: BROKEN APPOINTMENTS
or
Dear Mrs. Alvarez:
RE: Broken Appointments

In place of a subject line, a reference number may be used. For example, in a clinical situation, the patient's registration number will appear in the same position as the subject line. It should be preceded by "Reference" or "Re":

Dear Dr. Kollasch:
Reference: No. 06920

Enclosures

It is common to transfer radiographs with a letter to another dentist when requesting a consultation. When the letter has mentioned that an item is enclosed or attached, an enclosure notation should be made. This notation is keyboarded two lines below the reference initials, and it is set even with the left margin. Two acceptable methods are as follows:

je
Enclosure
or
je
Enclosures 2

Copy Notation

When additional copies of a letter are made for distribution to various persons, reference to each recipient is commonly made in the copy notation. This informs the recipient to whom additional copies of the letter were sent. Several types of notations are possible, including mail, computer copy, blind copy, postscript, and second-page headings.

Special Mailing Notations

Notations for services such as registered mail, special delivery, or certified letters are keyboarded in all capital letters between the date and the inside address and aligned with the left margin. Other special notations, such as if a letter is considered confidential or personal, are entered in the same location.

Types of Copy Notations

With the use of word processing in the office today, copies of correspondence are stored electronically as well as filed electronically either in the patient file or in a business file folder in the office. When additional copies are made for distribution or when copies are sent electronically, it is necessary for the addressee to know this. A copy notation is keyboarded two lines below the enclosure information, if any, or it may be placed below the reference initials if there are no enclosures. When more than one person is to receive a copy, list each person on a succeeding line after indenting three spaces from the left margin. Because not all copies are computer copies, variations may be used as they apply to the various copy styles. The notation may be keyboarded as follows:

Copy to O.J. Fox, D.D.S.
or
c O.J. Fox, D.D.S. (copy)
or
cc O.J. Fox, D.D.S. (courtesy copy)
or
cc O.J. Fox, D.D.S. (courtesy copies to multiple parties)
   R.C. Campbell, D.D.S.
   M.A. Reynolds, RDA Elsevier, the above statement says that the succeeding lines should be indented three spaces from the left margin.

Blind Copy

If the person who receives the original letter does not need to know that a copy is being sent to a particular person, then a blind copy notation can be made. A copy can be sent electronically as a "bcc" (blind carbon copy), which is an available option line under the "To" line. The original copy could be printed from the computer, and the notation will then be keyboarded on the copy 1 inch from the top at the left margin, as in the following example:

bcc Barbara Rice

Postscript

A postscript is often used to highlight a particular point; it is not necessarily an item that has been omitted in the body of the letter. If a postscript is used, it is the last line entered. It is not necessary to precede the postscript with "P.S."; however, the postscript paragraph should be blocked or indented, depending on the style of letter used (Figure 9-8).

You were right, Daniel. The experience of working alongside my father in his practice has been invaluable. I only hope it has been as rewarding for him as it has been for me. Again, thank you for your continued interest in my success.

Very truly yours,

Ashley M Lake, DDS

je

Please make a note to join us for the Martinique Open on December 29th.

FIGURE 9-8 Letter with a postscript.

Second-Page Heading

When writing a patient referral letter, it is sometimes necessary to send a lengthy letter to provide adequate information about the patient. If a second page is necessary, the continuation is made on plain paper that is the same size, color, and quality as the letterhead. Leave a 1-inch bottom margin on the first page. Leave at least two lines of the paragraph at the bottom of the first page, and then continue with at least two lines of the same paragraph on the next page. A heading consisting of the addressee's name, the page number, and the date is set single-spaced 1 inch (line six) from the top of the sheet. The following are two acceptable arrangements for beginning the second page:

Block form (used when the letter is in block style):
Ms. Margaret Coady
Page 2
October 27, 2009
Horizontal form (used when the letter is in modified block style):
Ms. Margaret Coady 2 October 27, 2009 *(Three lines of space follow.)*

PUNCTUATION STYLES IN BUSINESS LETTERS

Two common styles of punctuation are used in business letters: open punctuation and mixed or standard punctuation. Open punctuation omits all punctuation (except for periods after abbreviations) in the salutation and complimentary close lines. Mixed or standard punctuation requires a colon after the salutation and a comma after the complimentary close. Either style of punctuation may be used with any of the basic letter styles.

The administrative assistant will frequently use titles and academic degrees in his or her writing. The traditional rules are to never omit the period after an element of an academic degree or religious order and to never include internal spaces (e.g., B.S., Ph.D., LL.B., D.M.D., C.D.A., R.D.A., R.D.H., Ed.D.). However, this rule may need to be altered in contemporary use when addressing envelopes or completing specialized federal, state, or insurance forms that limit space for computerization or scanning. In this case, all of the periods are deleted (e.g., BS, PhD). Addressing envelopes is discussed in greater detail later in this chapter.

Correct punctuation is based on certain accepted rules and principles rather than on the whim of the writer. Punctuation is also important so that the reader can correctly interpret the writer's thoughts. The summary of rules given in this chapter will be helpful to ensure the use of correct punctuation. The common use of periods, commas, colons, and other types of punctuation is reviewed in Table 9-1.

CAPITALIZATION

In addition to understanding the rules for punctuation, it is necessary to review the rules for capitalizing various initials and words. A summary of the rules for capitalization is convenient for reference purposes; this is provided as follows.

Common Usage

The following are examples of the most common use of capitalization:

- The first word of every sentence should be capitalized.
- The first word of a complete direct quotation should be capitalized.
- The first word of a salutation and all nouns used in the salutation should be capitalized.
- The first word in a complimentary close should be capitalized.

Outline Form

Capitalize the first word in each section of an outline form.

TABLE 9-1 Punctuation Styles in Business Letters

Uses	Example(s)
PERIOD	
The period indicates a full stop. It is used at the end of a complete declarative or imperative sentence.	*I need you to schedule this patient's appointment.*
It is also often used after an abbreviation and after a single or double initial that represents a word (this does not apply when addressing envelopes).	*acct. etc. Ph.D.* *U.S. viz. P.M.* *N.E. i.e. pp.*
Some abbreviations that are made up of several initial letters do not require periods.	*FDIC (Federal Deposit Insurance Corporation)* *ADA (American Dental Association)*
Insert a period between dollars and cents (a period and a cipher are not required when an amount in even dollars is expressed in numerals).	*$42.65* *$1.47* *$25*
Insert a period to indicate a decimal.	*3.5 bushels* *12.65%* *6.25 feet*
COMMA	
A comma separates coordinate clauses that are connected by conjunctions, such as *and, but, or, for, neither,* and *nor,* unless the clauses are short and closely connected. It sets off a subordinate clause that precedes the main clause, and it is also placed after an introductory phrase that contains a verb form. If an introductory phrase does not contain a verb, it usually is not followed by a comma.	*We have a supply on hand, but I think we should order an additional quantity.* *She had to work late, because the auditors were examining the books.* *Assuming that there will be no changes, I suggest that you proceed with your instructions.* *After much deliberation the plan was revoked.* *Because of the vacation period we have been extremely busy.*
A comma sets off a nonrestrictive clause or phrase. It separates from the rest of the sentence a word or a group of words that breaks the continuity of a sentence. It is also used to separate parenthetical expressions from the rest of the sentence. It can be used to set off names used in direct address or to set off explanatory phrases or clauses. It separates from the rest of the sentence expressions that might be interpreted incorrectly without punctuation. It is used with words or groups of words when they are used in a series of three or more. It can be used to set off short quotations from the rest of the sentence, and it separates the name of a city from the name of a state.	*Our group, which had never lost a debate, won the grand prize.* *The beacon, rising proudly toward the sky, guided the pilots safely home.* *The business manager, even though his work was completed, was always willing to help others.* *We have, as you know, two persons who can handle the reorganization.* *I think you, Mr. Bennett, will agree with the statement. Ms. Linda Tom, our vice president, will be in your city soon.* *Misleading: Ever since we have filed our reports monthly.* *Better: Ever since, we have filed our reports monthly.* *Most executives agree that dependability, trustworthiness, ambition, and judgment are required of their office workers.* *"The committees have agreed," he said, "to work together on the project."* *Our southern branch is located in Atlanta, Georgia.*
A comma can also be used to separate the abbreviations of titles from a person's name.	*William R. Warner, Jr.* *Ramona Sanchez, Ph.D.*
SEMICOLON	
Semicolons are used between independent groups or clauses that are long or that contain parts that are separated by commas. They may be used between the members of a compound sentence when the conjunction is omitted.	*He was outstanding in his knowledge of word processing, databases, spreadsheets, and related software applications; however, he was lacking in many desirable personal qualities.* *Many executives would rather dictate to a machine than to a secretary; the machine won't talk back.*
A semicolon precedes expressions used to introduce a clause, such as *namely, viz., e.g.,* and *i.e.* They are used with series of well-defined units when special emphasis is desired.	*We selected the machine for two reasons: it is as reasonable in price as any other, and it does better work than others.* *There are several reasons for changing the routine of handling mail: to reduce postage, to conserve time, and to place responsibility.Emphatic: The prudent secretary considers the future; he or she ensures that all requirements are obtained, and he or she uses his or her talents to attain the desired goal successfully.* *Less emphatic: The prudent secretary considers the future, ensures that all requirements are obtained, and uses his or her talents to attain the desired goal successfully.*

Continued

TABLE 9-1 Punctuation Styles in Business Letters—cont'd

Uses	Example(s)
COLON	
A colon is used after the salutation in a business letter, except when open punctuation is used. It is also used after introductory expressions (e.g., "the following," "thus," "as follows") and other expressions that precede enumerations.	*Ladies and Gentlemen:* *Dear Ms. Carroll:* *Officers were elected as follows: president, vice president, and secretary-treasurer.*
It separates hours and minutes when indicating time, and it introduces a long quotation.	*2:10 PM* *4:45 PM* *12:15 AM* *The agreement read: "We the undersigned hereby agree. . . ."*
Colons are used to separate two independent groups that have no connecting words between them and in which the second group explains or expands on the statement made in the first group.	*We selected the machine for one reason: in competitive tests, it surpassed all other machines.*
QUESTION MARK	
A question mark is used after each direct question. An exception to this rule is a sentence that is phrased in the form of a question merely as a matter of courtesy when it is actually a request. Question marks are also used after each question in a series of questions within one sentence.	*When do you expect to arrive in Philadelphia?* *Will you please send us an up-to-date statement of our account?* *What is your opinion of the IBM word processor? The Xerox? The CPT?*
EXCLAMATION POINT	
The exclamation point is ordinarily used after words or groups of words that express command, strong feeling, emotion, or an exclamation.	*Don't waste office supplies!* *It can't be done!* *Stop!*
DASH	
A dash indicates an omission of letters or figures. It is sometimes used in letters (especially sales letters) to cause a definite stop when reading the letter. Dashes separate parenthetical expressions when unusual emphasis on the parenthetical expression is desired.	*Dear Mr.—* *Date the letter July 16, 20—* *This book is not a revision of an old book—it is a brand new book.* *These sales arguments—and every one of them is important—should result in getting the order.*
APOSTROPHE	
An apostrophe indicates possession. It is used to form the possessive singular by adding *'s* to the noun.	*the patient's record* *the dentist's coat* *the assistants' responsibilities* *the dentists' records* *man's work* *bird's wing* *hostess's plans*
An exception to this rule is made when the word after the possessive begins with an "s" sound.	*for goodness' sake* *for conscience's sake*
An apostrophe forms the possessive of a plural noun that ends in an "s" or "z" sound by adding only the apostrophe to the end of the plural noun. If the plural noun does not end in an "s" or "z" sound, add *'s* to the plural noun. Proper names that end in an "s" sound form the possessive singular by adding *'s*.	*workers' rights* *hostesses' duties* *women's clothes* *children's toys*

TABLE 9-1 Punctuation Styles in Business Letters—cont'd

Uses	Example(s)
Proper names that end in "s" form the possessive plural by adding the apostrophe only. When reference is made to an entire family, the family name must first be made plural.	*Bob Williams's record* *Joan Fox's appointment* *Walterses or Joneses* *The Walterses' property faces the Joneses' swimming pool.*
An apostrophe indicates the omission of a letter or letters in a contraction. It also indicates the plurals of letters, figures, words, and abbreviations.	*it's (it is)* *you're (you are)* *we'll (we shall)* *Don't forget to dot your i's and cross your t's.* *I can add easily by 2's and 4's, but I have difficulty with 6's and 8's.* *More direct letters can be written by using shorter sentences and by omitting and's and but's.* *Two of the speakers were Ph.D.s.*
OMISSION MARKS OR ELLIPSES	
Ellipses marks (... or ***) are frequently used to denote the omission of letters or words in quoted material. If the material omitted ends in a period, four omission marks are used (....?). If the material omitted is elsewhere in the quoted material, three omission marks are used (...).	*He quoted the proverb, "A soft answer turneth away wrath: but...."* *She quoted Plato: "Nothing is more unworthy of a wise man ... than to have allowed more time for trifling and useless things than they deserved."*
PARENTHESES	
Parentheses are used when amounts expressed in words are followed by figures. They are placed around words that are used as parenthetical expressions and to indicate technical references. They are also used when enumerations are included in narrative form.	*He agreed to pay twenty-five dollars ($25) as soon as possible.* *Our letter costs (excluding paper and postage) are much too high for this type of business.* *Sodium chloride (NaCl) is the chemical name for common table salt.* *The reasons for his resignation were three: (1) advanced age, (2) failing health, and (3) a desire to travel.*

First Word After a Colon

Capitalize the first word after a colon only when the colon introduces a complete passage or a sentence that has an independent meaning.

In conclusion, I wish to say: "The survey shows that...."

If the material that follows a colon is dependent on the preceding clause, then the first word after the colon is not capitalized.

I present the following three reasons for changing: the volume of business does not justify the expense; we are short of people; and the product is decreasing in popularity.

Names

- Capitalize the names of associations, buildings, churches, hotels, streets, organizations, and clubs.

The American Dental Association, Merchandise Mart, Central District Dental Society, Peabody Hotel, Seventh Avenue, Administrative Management Society, Chicago Chamber of Commerce

- Capitalize all proper names.

Great Britain, John G. Hammitt, Mexico

- Capitalize names that are derived from proper names

American, Chinese

- Do not, however, capitalize words that are derived from proper nouns and that have developed a special meaning.

pasteurized milk, china dishes, moroccan leather

- Capitalize special names for regions and localities.

North Central states, the Far East, the East Side, the Hoosier State

- Do not, however, capitalize adjectives derived from such names or localities that are used as directional parts of states and countries.

far eastern lands, the southern United States, southern Illinois

- Capitalize names of government boards, agencies, bureaus, departments, and commissions.

Civil Service Commission, Social Security Board, Bureau of Navigation

- Capitalize names of deities, the Bible, holy days, and religious denominations.

God, Easter, Yom Kippur, Genesis, Church of Christ

- Capitalize the names of holidays.

    Memorial Day, Labor Day

- Capitalize words used before numbers and numerals, with the exception of common words such as *page, line,* and *verse.*

    The reservation is Lower 6, Car 27.
    He found the material in Part 3 of Chapter IV.

Titles Used in Business and Professions

The following are capitalization rules for businesses and professional titles.

- Any title that signifies rank, honor, and respect and that immediately precedes an individual's name should be capitalized.

    She asked President Harry G. Sanders to preside.
    He was attended by Dr. Howard Richards.

- Academic degrees should be capitalized when they precede or follow an individual name.

    Constance R. Collins, Ph.D., was invited to direct the program.
    Fred R. Bowling, Master of Arts

- Capitalize titles of high-ranking government officers when the title is used in place of the proper name when referring to a specific person.

    Our Senator invited us to visit him in Washington.
    The President will return to Washington soon.

- Capitalize military titles that signify rank.

    Captain Meyers, Lieutenant White, Lieutenant Commander Murphy

TELEPHONE NUMBERS

There are several ways of entering telephone numbers in a letter. The parentheses method—for example, (734) 956-9800—is frequently used, but it does not work well in text material when the telephone number as a whole has to be enclosed in parentheses. One reason it is suggested not to use parentheses is because of the growing use of the mandatory area code where there is a shortage of numbers. In these areas, the use of the parentheses with the telephone number may suggest that you would not need to use the area code. Three other methods of entering telephone numbers are 707-555-3998, 707 555 3998, and 707.555.3998. The latter system seems to be gaining popularity. It uses periods or dots to separate the elements, which resemble the dots used in e-mail addresses. In addition, phone numbers written this way are easier to type because the "Shift" key is not required, and the dot key is more accessible on the keyboard.

PREPARING AN EFFECTIVE LETTER

To prepare an effective letter, it is necessary to follow several basic steps:

- Collect the information.
- Make an outline.
- Develop the letter.
- Select a format style.
- Review and revise the letter.
- Produce the letter.
- Proofread the letter.
- Distribute the letter.
- Store the document.

Before beginning each step of the letter-writing process, it is necessary to determine who will receive the letter and what the person already knows about the subject. If a letter is to be written to another dentist about a patient, it will require the use of technical language. Alternatively, if a patient is to receive a letter about an unknown subject, the educational level of the person needs to be determined so that the letter can be written in understandable language.

Collecting Information

Before beginning to write a letter, gather the important facts that need to be included in the letter. In general, the following information will be needed: the name of the person to whom the letter is being sent, by whom the letter is being written, and the subject of the letter. If it is a letter of referral, the following information will be needed: the name of the patient, any necessary personal information for which consent to share has been given, the nature of the problem, any possible symptoms or diagnosis, any enclosures, the anticipated response, the deadline dates, and information regarding how the patient should contact the office. If it is a letter of inquiry, the nature of the inquiry, the product names (if available), the quantity or specifications of the product needed, and date of necessary reply should be included.

Making an Outline

One may ask, "Why is it necessary to make an outline if I know what I want to say?" After writing several letters, it may be natural to be organized. However, for a beginner or for someone who dislikes letter writing, making an outline will provide organization and a framework that forces a person to get his or her thoughts on paper. In the process, it may be discovered that all of the needed facts have not been gathered. An outline helps to clarify relationships among topics and to determine whether the letter is written in a logical sequence.

Developing the Letter

It is often said that, after the outline is completed, the letter is nearly finished. This is partially true, but special attention should be given to how each part of the letter is developed before determining the letter's format. A variety of format styles are illustrated in this chapter.

As the letter begins to develop, remember that the first paragraph is the most important one of any letter. It should get

PRACTICE NOTE

An outline helps you to see relationships among topics and to determine whether your letter is written in a logical sequence.

the reader's attention and set the tone for the letter. This paragraph places the emphasis on the reader and uses the "you" approach. Review each paragraph in the letter to determine if it gets the reader's attention and to be sure it clearly states the purpose of the letter. Make a natural transition from one paragraph to the next. Special consideration should be given to factors such as data and confidentiality that are included in various types of letters. Box 9-4 includes several suggestions for writing various types of letters.

Selecting the Format

The administrative assistant may select a template from the word processing software in the office, but the letter will still require decisions to be made regarding punctuation styles. Letter style is a personal choice that relates to a particular practice and that complements the office stationery most effectively.

BOX 9-4

Special Considerations for Letter Content

Order Letter

- Indicate the quantity.
- Provide a description of the material or product.
- List the price.
- Define the method of payment.
- Indicate the shipping preference.

Referral Letter

- Provide the complete and proper name of the patient.
- State the condition and expected type of consultation or examination.
- Always write out tooth names or provide an illustration; avoid using tooth numbers only.
- Refer to enclosures.
- Indicate timeliness, if necessary.
- Maintain confidentiality, and provide only information for which consent to share has been given.
- Extend a courteous expression of appreciation.

Inquiry Letter

- State the objective.
- Give all of the necessary facts.
- Close with good will.

Thank You Letter

- State the purpose.
- Explain your appreciation.
- Maintain confidentiality.
- Close with a sincere expression of good will.

Most word processing software provides several templates for a variety of letter styles. These can be modified to match the dentist's preferences and saved in the letter file as specialized templates. Several basic styles are shown in Figure 9-9, including the block style with mixed punctuation, the block style with open punctuation, the modified block style with mixed punctuation, the block style with attention line and enclosure, and the Administrative Management Society simplified style. The first styles are self-explanatory. The Administrative Management Society simplified style can be put to good use when informing all patients about a policy change or announcing that an associate will be joining the practice. The style has two basic rules:

1. The letter must have a subject line. The word *subject* is omitted, and the subject line is keyboarded in all capital letters, with three lines of space placed before and after the subject line.
2. The writer's name and title are keyboarded in all capital letters at least four lines below the last line of the letter.

Reviewing the Letter

After the letter has been written, determine whether it meets all of the criteria of an effective letter, as described in Box 9-1. If the letter does not meet most of these criteria, take time to modify it. If you are unsure about the quality of a letter, ask another person to review and evaluate it. Make the necessary changes until all of the effectiveness criteria are met.

Producing the Final Letter

Before the final printing of the letter, use the spell-checking and grammar-checking features of the word processing software, if available. Whether the letter is created from a template or is an original document, the letter needs to be produced on quality stationery that reinforces the professional image of the office.

Proofreading the Letter

Do not rely completely on an electronic system to proofread your letter. Although software packages provide spell-checking capabilities, many dental terms are not in the dictionary, unless they have been inserted. Likewise, English words are often misused or interchanged, such as *there* and *their.* Both of these words will come up as being spelled correctly, but they may have been misused. Not all word processing systems can be relied on for complete grammar accuracy. Therefore, make a final review of the letter to be sure that the grammar, spelling, and punctuation are correct. Proofreading a letter is much like performing the final check of the margins on a composite restoration. It is an individual creation, and it should be perfect.

PRACTICE NOTE

Do not rely completely on an electronic system to proofread your letters.

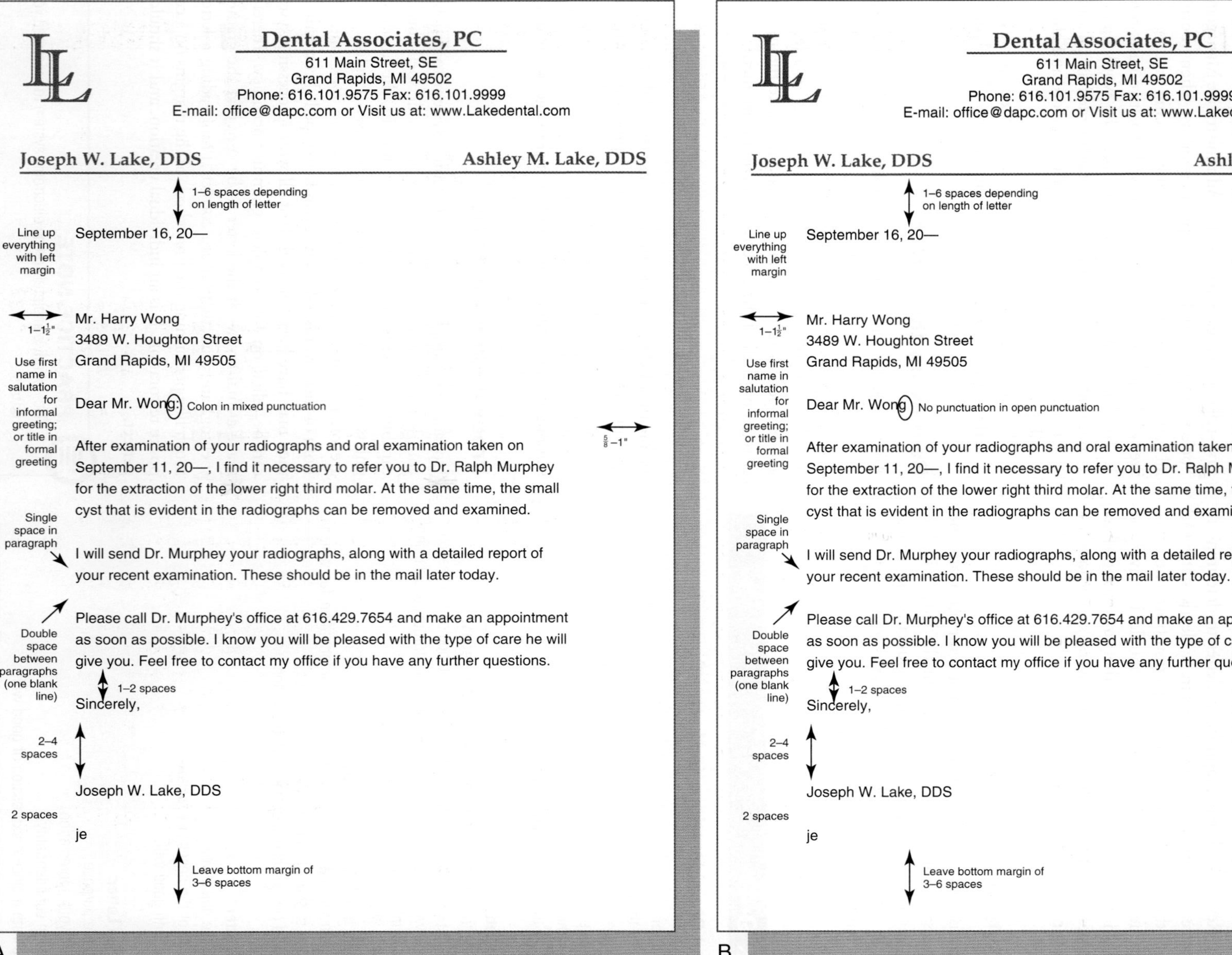

A

Dental Associates, PC
611 Main Street, SE
Grand Rapids, MI 49502
Phone: 616.101.9575 Fax: 616.101.9999
E-mail: office@dapc.com or Visit us at: www.Lakedental.com

Joseph W. Lake, DDS Ashley M. Lake, DDS

September 16, 20—

Mr. Harry Wong
3489 W. Houghton Street
Grand Rapids, MI 49505

Dear Mr. Wong:

After examination of your radiographs and oral examination taken on September 11, 20—, I find it necessary to refer you to Dr. Ralph Murphey for the extraction of the lower right third molar. At the same time, the small cyst that is evident in the radiographs can be removed and examined.

I will send Dr. Murphey your radiographs, along with a detailed report of your recent examination. These should be in the mail later today.

Please call Dr. Murphey's office at 616.429.7654 and make an appointment as soon as possible. I know you will be pleased with the type of care he will give you. Feel free to contact my office if you have any further questions.

Sincerely,

Joseph W. Lake, DDS

je

B

Dental Associates, PC
611 Main Street, SE
Grand Rapids, MI 49502
Phone: 616.101.9575 Fax: 616.101.9999
E-mail: office@dapc.com or Visit us at: www.Lakedental.com

Joseph W. Lake, DDS Ashley M. Lake, DDS

September 16, 20—

Mr. Harry Wong
3489 W. Houghton Street
Grand Rapids, MI 49505

Dear Mr. Wong

After examination of your radiographs and oral examination taken on September 11, 20—, I find it necessary to refer you to Dr. Ralph Murphey for the extraction of the lower right third molar. At the same time, the small cyst that is evident in the radiographs can be removed and examined.

I will send Dr. Murphey your radiographs, along with a detailed report of your recent examination. These should be in the mail later today.

Please call Dr. Murphey's office at 616.429.7654 and make an appointment as soon as possible. I know you will be pleased with the type of care he will give you. Feel free to contact my office if you have any further questions.

Sincerely,

Joseph W. Lake, DDS

je

FIGURE 9-9 **A,** Block style letter with mixed punctuation. **B,** Block style letter with open punctuation.

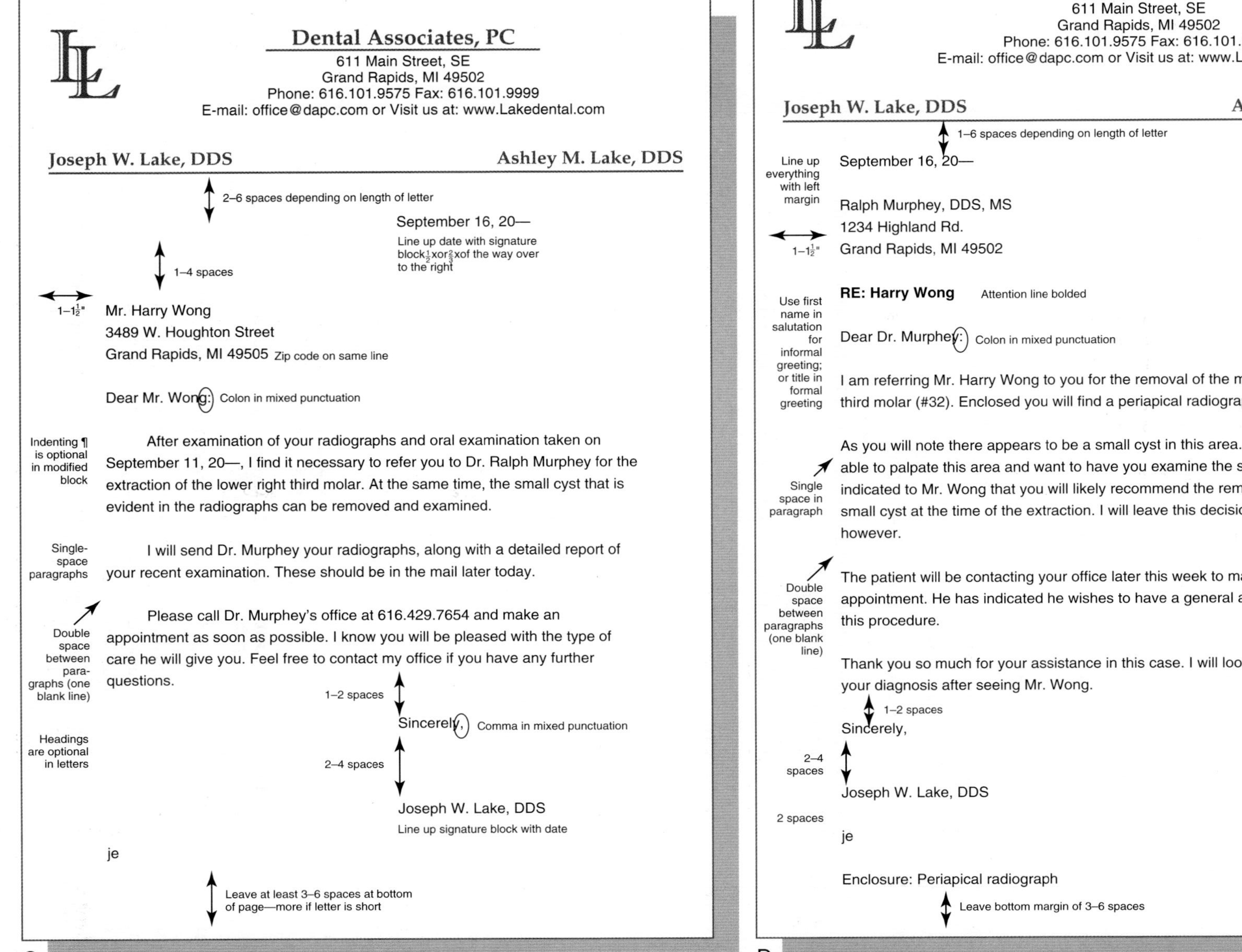

C

Dental Associates, PC
611 Main Street, SE
Grand Rapids, MI 49502
Phone: 616.101.9575 Fax: 616.101.9999
E-mail: office@dapc.com or Visit us at: www.Lakedental.com

Joseph W. Lake, DDS — Ashley M. Lake, DDS

September 16, 20—

Mr. Harry Wong
3489 W. Houghton Street
Grand Rapids, MI 49505

Dear Mr. Wong:

After examination of your radiographs and oral examination taken on September 11, 20—, I find it necessary to refer you to Dr. Ralph Murphey for the extraction of the lower right third molar. At the same time, the small cyst that is evident in the radiographs can be removed and examined.

I will send Dr. Murphey your radiographs, along with a detailed report of your recent examination. These should be in the mail later today.

Please call Dr. Murphey's office at 616.429.7654 and make an appointment as soon as possible. I know you will be pleased with the type of care he will give you. Feel free to contact my office if you have any further questions.

Sincerely,

Joseph W. Lake, DDS

je

D

Dental Associates, PC
611 Main Street, SE
Grand Rapids, MI 49502
Phone: 616.101.9575 Fax: 616.101.9999
E-mail: office@dapc.com or Visit us at: www.Lakedental.com

Joseph W. Lake, DDS — Ashley M. Lake, DDS

September 16, 20—

Ralph Murphey, DDS, MS
1234 Highland Rd.
Grand Rapids, MI 49502

RE: Harry Wong

Dear Dr. Murphey:

I am referring Mr. Harry Wong to you for the removal of the mandibular right third molar (#32). Enclosed you will find a periapical radiograph of this area.

As you will note there appears to be a small cyst in this area. I have been able to palpate this area and want to have you examine the site also. I have indicated to Mr. Wong that you will likely recommend the removal of this small cyst at the time of the extraction. I will leave this decision up to you, however.

The patient will be contacting your office later this week to make an appointment. He has indicated he wishes to have a general anesthesia for this procedure.

Thank you so much for your assistance in this case. I will look forward to your diagnosis after seeing Mr. Wong.

Sincerely,

Joseph W. Lake, DDS

je

Enclosure: Periapical radiograph

FIGURE 9-9, cont'd **C,** Modified block style letter with mixed punctuation. **D,** Block style letter with attention line and enclosure.

Continued

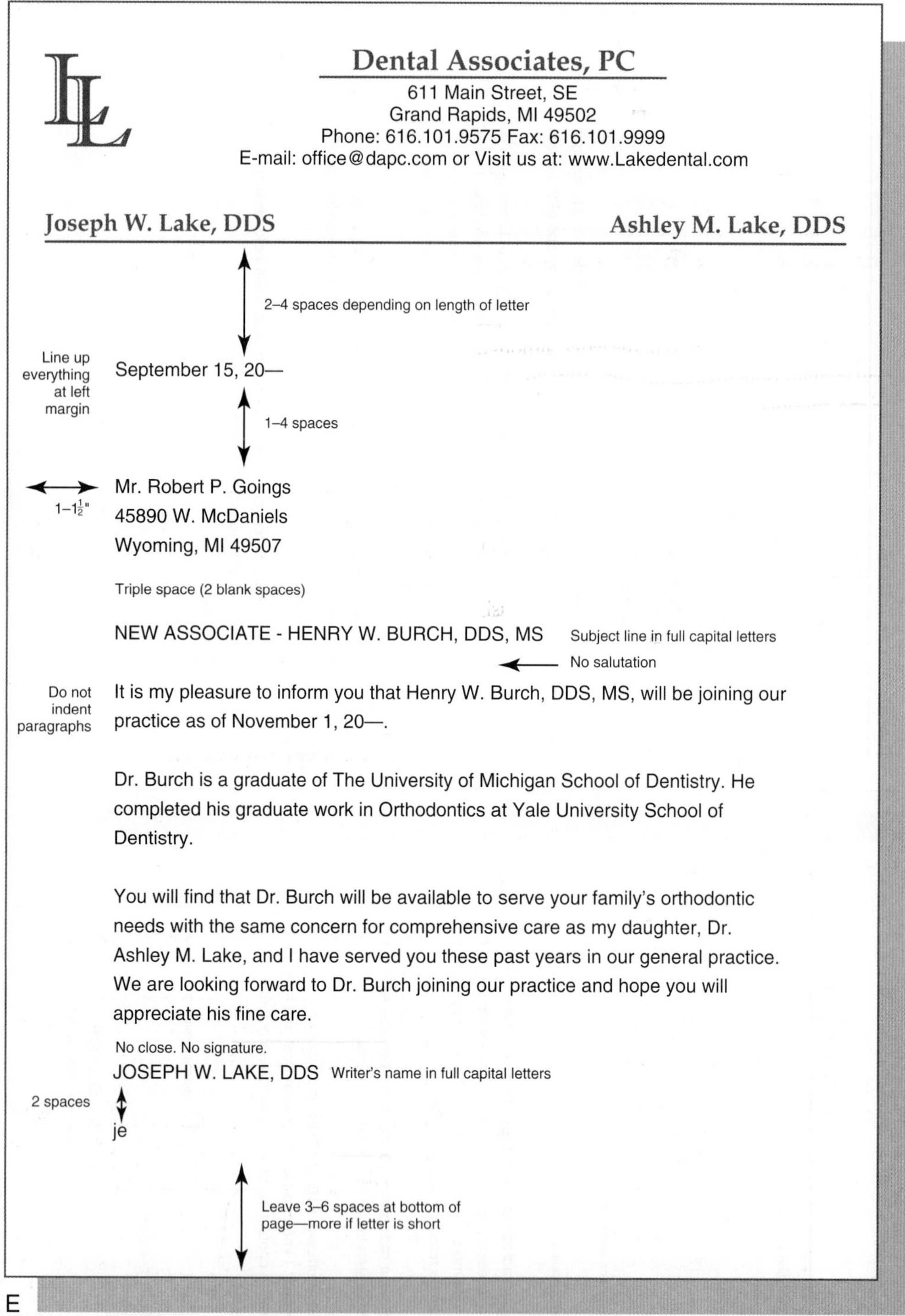

Dental Associates, PC
611 Main Street, SE
Grand Rapids, MI 49502
Phone: 616.101.9575 Fax: 616.101.9999
E-mail: office@dapc.com or Visit us at: www.Lakedental.com

Joseph W. Lake, DDS — Ashley M. Lake, DDS

September 15, 20—

Mr. Robert P. Goings
45890 W. McDaniels
Wyoming, MI 49507

NEW ASSOCIATE - HENRY W. BURCH, DDS, MS

It is my pleasure to inform you that Henry W. Burch, DDS, MS, will be joining our practice as of November 1, 20—.

Dr. Burch is a graduate of The University of Michigan School of Dentistry. He completed his graduate work in Orthodontics at Yale University School of Dentistry.

You will find that Dr. Burch will be available to serve your family's orthodontic needs with the same concern for comprehensive care as my daughter, Dr. Ashley M. Lake, and I have served you these past years in our general practice. We are looking forward to Dr. Burch joining our practice and hope you will appreciate his fine care.

JOSEPH W. LAKE, DDS

je

FIGURE 9-9, cont'd **E,** Administrative Management Society simplified style.

Distributing the Letter

There are several methods that can be used to distribute a letter: e-mail, traditional postal services, fax, or some form of specialized mail service. Each of these is explained in detail later in this chapter. Before creating the letter, be aware of the planned method of distribution to determine the type of envelope or mailing label necessary for production.

Storing the Document

If the letter is to be stored electronically, the procedure discussed in Chapter 8 should be followed. If not, a hard copy should be made and filed in the patient record or in another location that is appropriate for the document. Remember, if striving for a paperless office, maximize the use of the electronic filing system.

PREPARING THE ENVELOPE

It is possible to prepare the envelope as part of the word processing procedure. Larger mailing envelopes may require special labeling. In either case, it is necessary to prepare the envelope or package with a standardized delivery address. Most postal services use automatic sorting equipment, which begins with an automatic sorting process that involves an optical character reader. A standardized address that is readable by an optical character reader contains the correct city name, state, and zip+4 code. To obtain zip codes for any address, visit the U.S. Postal Service web site at www.usps.com, and then select the zip code navigation bar. The address on the envelope should agree with the inside address of the letter, although the inside address may contain punctuation not recommended by the postal service for the envelope.

The address should be single spaced, even if the address is only two lines. In this case, the name of the individual or firm is on the first line, and the city, state, and zip code are on the second line. The two-letter state abbreviations that have been approved and recommended by the U.S. Postal Service should be used; these appear in Box 9-5. For further information, request Publication 28, *Postal Addressing Standards,* from the local Postal Business Center or online at www.usps.gov. Figure 9-10 illustrates how an address should appear on various business envelopes.

Other important elements of the address are suffixes, directionals, apartment or suite numbers, post office box numbers, and complete rural/highway contract route addresses with box numbers. All of these elements must be spelled correctly and clearly written. If the address is not electronically readable, the letter or package will be delayed for manual handling. If the zip+4 code is not known, it can be obtained at www.usps.gov.

BOX 9-5

Two-Letter Abbreviations for States

State	Abbreviation	State	Abbreviation
Alabama	AL	Montana	MT
Alaska	AK	Nebraska	NE
Arizona	AZ	Nevada	NV
Arkansas	AR	New Hampshire	NH
California	CA	New Jersey	NJ
Colorado	CO	New Mexico	NM
Connecticut	CT	New York	NY
Delaware	DE	North Carolina	NC
District of Columbia	DC	North Dakota	ND
Florida	FL	Ohio	OH
Georgia	GA	Oklahoma	OK
Hawaii	HI	Oregon	OR
Idaho	ID	Pennsylvania	PA
Illinois	IL	Rhode Island	RI
Indiana	IN	South Carolina	SC
Iowa	IA	South Dakota	SD
Kansas	KS	Tennessee	TN
Kentucky	KY	Texas	TX
Louisiana	LA	Utah	UT
Maine	ME	Vermont	VT
Maryland	MD	Virginia	VA
Massachusetts	MA	Washington	WA
Michigan	MI	West Virginia	WV
Minnesota	MN	Wisconsin	WI
Mississippi	MS	Wyoming	WY
Missouri	MO		

Address Format

The use of the universal format for an address expedites the processing capability of automated equipment at the post office. The format requires the use of a uniform left margin. Type the address in uppercase letters as follows:

MS MARY BALL
3347 MAPLE RD
ROCKFORD MI 48167-2345

A secondary address unit, such as an apartment (APT) or suite (STE) number, should be printed as part of the address. Always use *APT* or *STE* rather than # (the pound sign) to note a specific number. Common designations are APT, BLDG FLOOR (FL), STE, UNIT, ROOM (RM), and DEPARTMENT (DEPT). When using this format, the address line may appear as follows:

1334 RIVERSIDE APT 201
or
3745 KINSEY DR STE 301
or
845 KELSAY BLVD BLDG 5
or
1234 KELLOGG PL RM 136

If the letter or package is sent to the attention of an individual, that information precedes the line giving the name of the firm

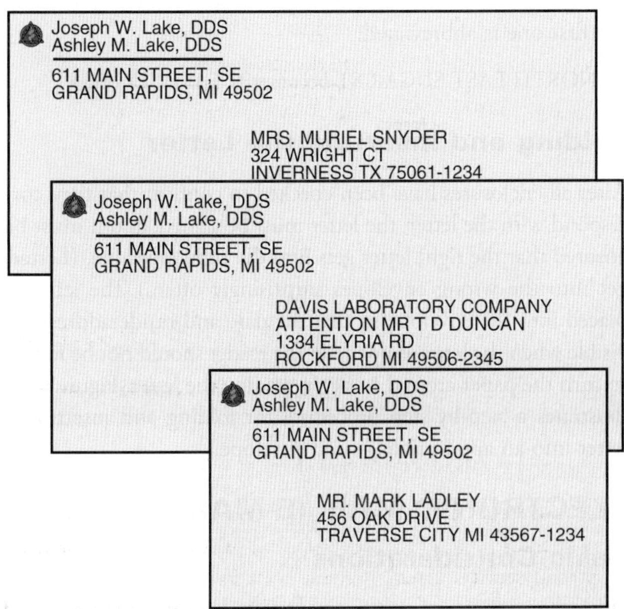

FIGURE 9-10 Address styles for different sizes of envelopes. Note the placement of the attention line.

or building. The attention line varies from the traditional format that many people have used. Consider the following example:

ATTN: MS MARY CUMMINS
ACME DENTAL COMPANY
134 FLETCHER
CUTLERVILLE MI 49504-2345

Avoid using dual addresses, although both a box number and street address may be available. Place the delivery address on the line immediately above the city, state, and zip+4 code.

Punctuation on Address Labels

The US Postal Service prefers that punctuation, special characters, or multiple blanks in the address not be used, with the exception of a hyphen in the zip+4 code or a hyphen that appears in the primary number of the delivery address, such as 51-234 HANCOCK ST. Spell out city names completely. If an abbreviation must be used because of labeling or space constraints, use existing abbreviations first for suffix or directional words:

EAST MARKET becomes E MARKET
JEFFERSON MOUNTAIN becomes JEFFERSON MT

The eight standard directionals can be abbreviated to one or two characters. For instance:

255 NW WASHINGTON ST
133 CHERRY DR S

If the first word in a street name is a directional word and no other directional is to the left of it, abbreviate it:

NORTH CHERRY ST becomes N CHERRY ST

or

LAKE DRIVE WEST becomes LAKE DRIVE W

When two directional words appear before the street name, the first one is abbreviated:

NORTH EAST SUGAR ST becomes N EAST SUGAR ST

Folding and Inserting the Letter

After all enclosures have been checked to confirm that they correspond with the letter, the letter must be signed, and it must be ensured that the right letter gets into the right envelope. (Letters get into the wrong envelopes surprisingly often.) The letter is placed into the envelope so that the date and inside address are visible when the letter is opened. The reader should not be forced to turn the paper around to begin reading the letter. Figure 9-11 illustrates a step-by-step procedure for folding and inserting a letter into an appropriately sized envelope.

ELECTRONIC MAIL (E-MAIL)

Basic Considerations

With the wide use of computers today, electronic mail (e-mail) has opened the doors to sending mail between computers within networked locations. E-mail within a large clinic or dental school has become the choice for sending memoranda to the staff. With more patients having e-mail, this becomes another source of communication between the office and the patient. As mentioned in Chapter 7, attention should be given to including a patient's e-mail address on the personal questionnaire during admission and asking the patient if this is a mode of communication that he or she would prefer to use. Some patients may even indicate that text messaging is also an option for them to receive messages. The patient's e-mail address can be integrated into various software programs, and it may even be used to confirm appointments or to send reminders for routine recall appointments. E-mail has many advantages as a communication tool, including the following:

- E-mail reaches its destination in a matter of seconds after it is sent, even if its destination is across the world.
- Multiple individuals may be sent the same message quickly, with all the recipients receiving the message instantly.
- Paper is saved. It is not necessary to make a hard copy of e-mail messages.
- E-mail may be filed electronically for later reference.
- E-mail may be forwarded to another party.
- E-mail may be destroyed immediately after it is read.
- E-mail takes less time to write than a paper letter. Only the receiver's name, the sender's name, and the body of the letter need to be entered. The date and time is entered automatically, and the letter and its envelope do not need to be printed.
- Other documents and graphic images may be transferred as attachments through e-mail.
- The recipient is notified of the arrival of an e-mail by a message that appears at the bottom of the computer screen or by an audio signal that is emitted through the computer.
- A hard copy of the e-mail may be printed if necessary for retention in a manual file.
- Notations such as "confidential" and "urgent" can be made on the e-mail message.

As with any new system, a person often overlooks the need to follow basic protocol. E-mail should not become a quick system for communication with no concern given to punctuation or formatting.

PRACTICE NOTE

E-mail should not become a quick system for communication with no concern given to punctuation or formatting.

Consider the following guidelines when using e-mail (Figure 9-12):

- Be sure to think about the purpose of the e-mail before beginning to write. In other words, know what it is that you want to achieve with the e-mail message.
- Be succinct. Before sending an e-mail, reread it. Delete unnecessary phrases, words, or sentences.
- Be polite. Think of an e-mail as a short letter, and follow etiquette rules. Use the words *please* and *thank you.*
- Be suitably formal when writing e-mail. The rule of thumb is to be almost as formal in e-mail as you would in a standard memorandum to employers, coworkers, or patients.

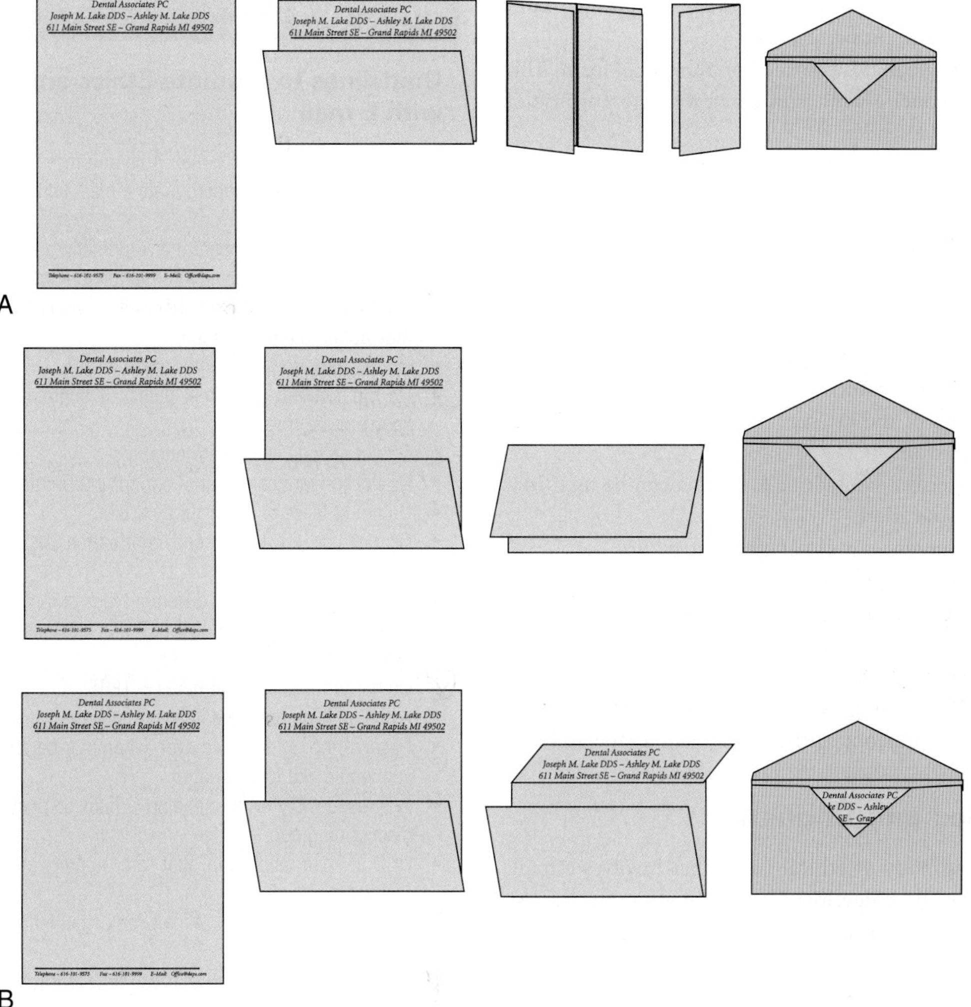

FIGURE 9-11 Folding and inserting a letter. **A,** Small envelope. **B,** Large envelope.

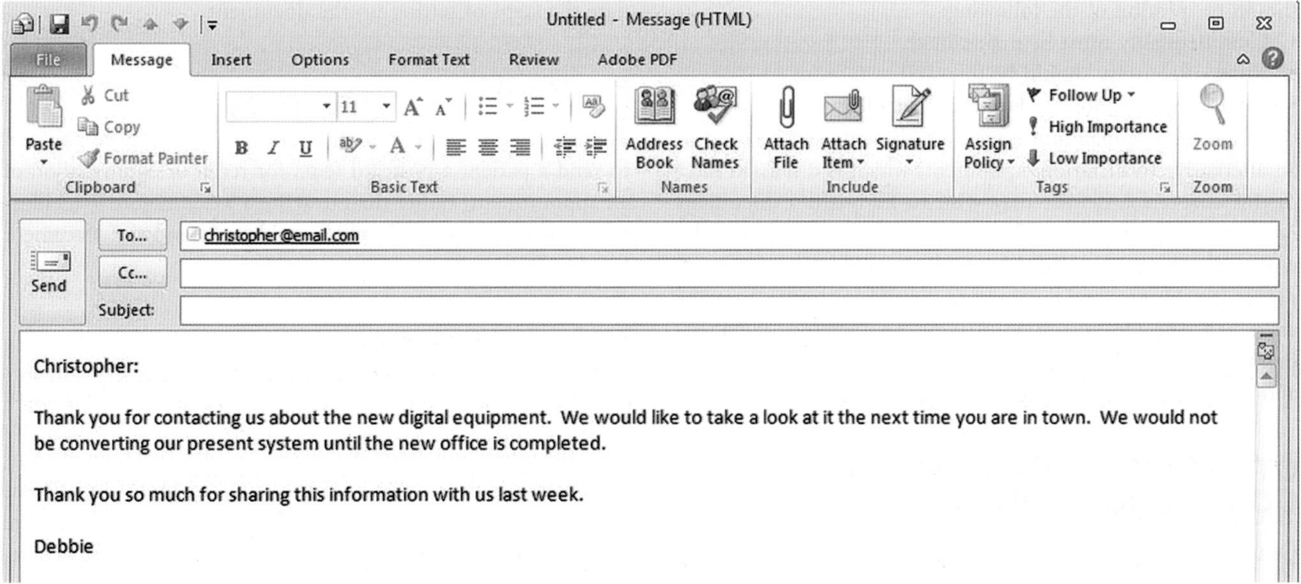

FIGURE 9-12 Screenshot of an e-mail message using suggested guidelines for e-mail.

- Always capitalize the appropriate words, be specific about your needs, and use proper closing.
- Use the subject line that is provided on the e-mail form. This line should be concise while still conveying the purpose of the message to the reader.
- If replying to a message but changing the subject of conversation, change the subject line as well.
- Edit and proofread carefully. Do not send an e-mail that contains inaccuracies or incorrect grammar.
- Use complete sentences.
- Capitalize and punctuate properly.
- Do not run sentences together; it is difficult to read e-mail constructed in this manner.
- Insert the nature of the message on the subject line.
- Include a salutation.
- Use a colon after the salutation. A comma can be used in a nonbusiness application.
- Use complete sentences and paragraph structure.
- Check the letter for spelling and grammatical errors.
- Insert a blank line after each paragraph.
- Always include the sender's name and title (if appropriate) when replying to an e-mail.
- Assume that any message sent is permanent. The message can be sitting in someone's private file or in a tape archive.

E-mail Ethics and Etiquette

There is a growing body of ethical issues that involves e-mail. Some organizations have developed a code of ethics for the use of e-mail. This form of communication should follow the same ethical guidelines used in any form of written communication in the dental office. Box 9-6 provides a checklist of items to help guide users in the ethical use of e-mail.

The content of an e-mail can be retained as a permanent record, so anything that you do not wish to be documented in writing should not be entered into an e-mail message. Users should be mindful of the following:

- Confidentiality must be maintained.
- Rules of courtesy should be followed.
- An appropriate closing should be included.

In addition, e-mail and e-mail attachments can be used as an alternative to dictation equipment, which is discussed later in this chapter. A dentist may wish to keyboard a document rather than to dictate it. This is often easier than physically writing the document. This keyboarding could be done in word processing software and then sent to the administrative assistant via e-mail. The administrative assistant can download the document, make any formatting corrections, print it if necessary, and then store it in the appropriate file.

BOX 9-6

Guidelines to Promote Ethics and Etiquette with E-mail

- Do not send personal e-mail from an office computer.
- When people send inappropriate e-mail, let them know politely that it cannot be received.
- Do not use e-mail to berate or reprimand an employee or patient.
- Do not use e-mail to send information that involves any type of legal action; third parties who should have no knowledge of the action may obtain the information.
- Do not forward junk mail or chain letters.
- Do not forward an e-mail unless it contains information that is known to be true.
- Do not include credit card numbers.
- Do not forward confidential patient information.
- Do not criticize or insult third parties.
- Do not use e-mail to send information that might involve legal action.
- Be cautious about using different types of fonts, colors, clip art, and other graphics in e-mail. It clutters the message, and it may be difficult for the reader to view.
- Do not write in ALL CAPITAL LETTERS.
- Avoid sending messages when angry.
- Observe the Golden Rule even when in cyberspace: treat others as you would like to be treated.
- Act responsibly when sending e-mail or posting messages to a discussion group.
- Use a style and tone that are appropriate for the intended recipients.
- Before replying to an e-mail, ask yourself if a reply is really necessary.
- Read through the e-mail that you have written before sending it.
- Use a meaningful subject line.
- Answer all e-mails promptly.

OTHER TYPES OF WRITTEN COMMUNICATION

Other types of written communication routinely prepared by the administrative assistant include postcards, interoffice memoranda, and manuscripts. For many of these documents, there are templates available that help with formatting and that eliminate the steps of setting up the document.

Postcards

There will be times in a dental office when it is more practical to send a patient a postcard (e.g., for recall or confirmation of an appointment) rather than to write a letter. Figure 9-13 illustrates how a postcard should be addressed and the placement for the message.

Interoffice Memoranda

Although most office correspondence is keyboarded on office letterhead, the interoffice memorandum is a timesaving form that is entered on plain paper (Figure 9-14). This type of communication is often used within a clinic or group practice or within a professional building in which several dental offices are located. The form provides space for the name of the department or individuals to whom the memorandum is being sent, the date, a subject or reference line, and the sender's name. The

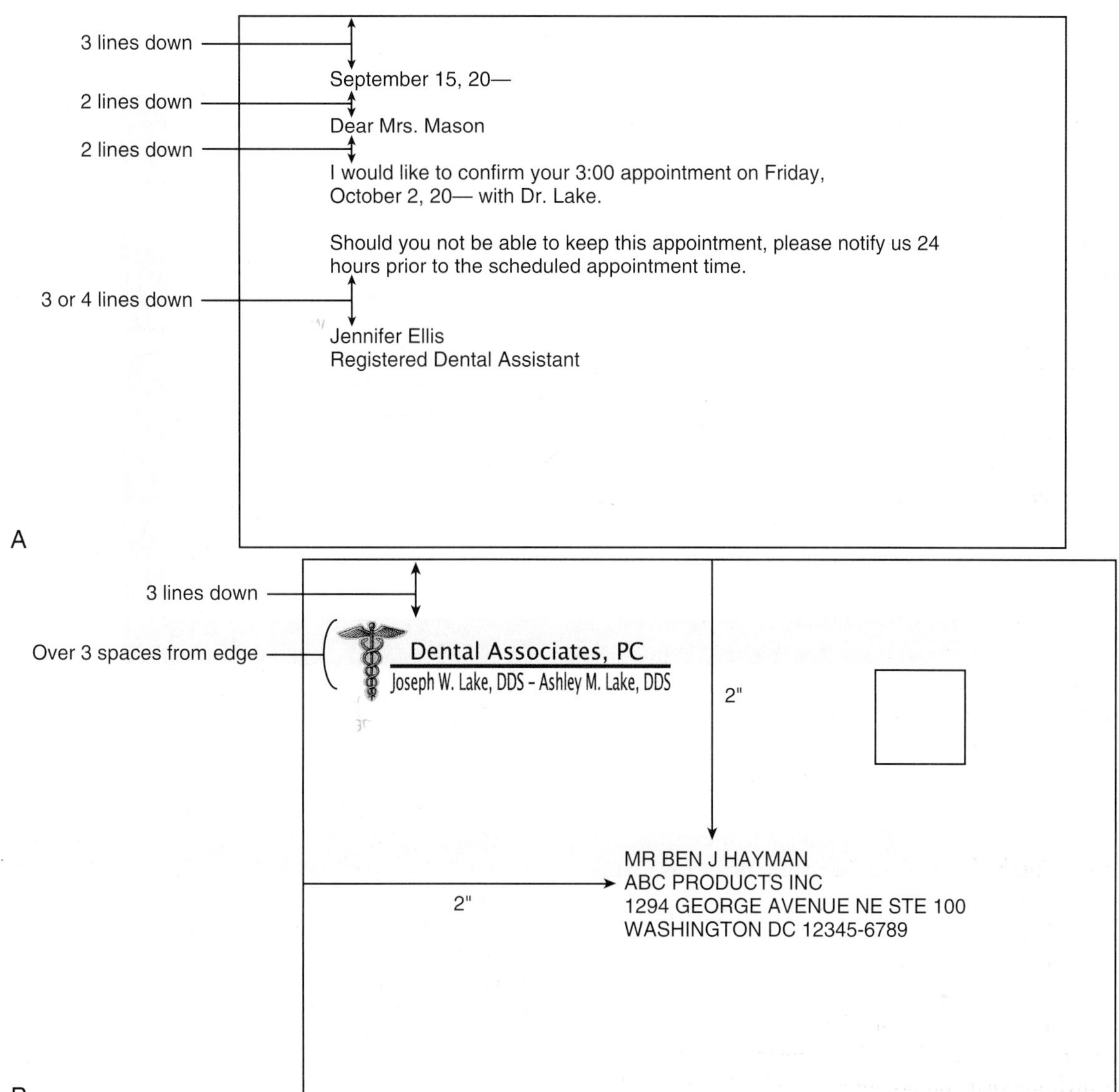

FIGURE 9-13 **A,** $5\frac{1}{2} \times 3\frac{1}{2}$-inch postcard message. **B,** Postcard address.

memorandum should be brief, clearly stated, well organized, and easy to read. A copy of the memorandum should be made for the office files. If several people are to receive the memorandum, their names are inserted in the space provided, or additional copies are made and the individual names entered on each memorandum.

Manuscripts

In the first part of this chapter, emphasis was placed on general correspondence. In both the academic and health environments, the administrative assistant may be asked to create a manuscript for the employer. Such reports could range from a business proposal to a research paper. Whether writing a business report or an academic report, follow standard style when preparing it.

Many styles exist for manuscript preparation, depending on the nature of the report. Each style requires the same basic information. For example, one style may use the term *Bibliography,* whereas another uses *References* and still another prefers *Works Cited.* Although a publisher may provide the author with a format for a manuscript, a popular documentation style used today for research papers is presented by the Modern Language Association (MLA), as shown in Figure 9-15. When preparing a paper, adhere to some form of documentation style. If none are given, it is wise to select the MLA style, which is summarized in Box 9-7.

Dictation and Transcription

Some dentists prefer to use dictation and transcription equipment as part of a written communication system. The use of dictation and transcription equipment (Figure 9-16) has

INTEROFFICE MEMORANDUM

TO: Jennifer Ellis, RDA

FROM: Dr. Ashley Lake

SUBJECT: Reassignment to business manager position

DATE: October 19, 20--

For some time I have been thinking that we should promote you to the position of office manager. After our discussion last Friday, I would like to confirm this reassignment. Both my father and I feel that you have considerable expertise in patient management and have excelled in the recent courses in small business management in which you have been enrolled. Both of us would like to discuss this transition with you.

Let's meet on Friday, October 25, at 2 P.M. to discuss this matter. If this date is inconvenient for you, please let me know.

FIGURE 9-14 Interoffice memorandum. (Note that this image is not to size; in reality, this would be placed on a letter-size piece of paper.)

BOX 9-7

Modern Language Association (MLA) Writing Style

- Use $8\frac{1}{2} \times 11$-inch paper.
- Double-space all pages of the letter, and use 1-inch top, bottom, left, and right margins.
- Indent the first word of each paragraph half an inch from the left margin.
- At the right margin of each page, place a page number half an inch from the top margin and 1 inch from the right margin. Add a line of space between the header and the body of the letter. Only use Arabic numbers. Do not use *pp, p,* or *#* (the pound sign).
- On each page, precede the page number with the author's last name.
- When a quote contains fewer than six lines, set it off with quotation marks, keep it within the normal text, and follow it with a reference citation. When a quote contains six or more lines, set it off by indenting it 1 inch from the right and left margins. Check MLA sources for other requirements regarding longer quotes, special circumstances, and quotes within quotes.
- *Each figure and table needs to be labeled and numbered.* Place the word *Figure* or *Table* and the corresponding number as well as one line of space before the actual figure or table. Other materials such as charts, photographs, and drawings also need to be labeled and numbered, and each one should include a caption.
- No title page is required. Instead, on the first page, place the author's name on the first line. Add a line of space, and then add the following with a line of space after each one: the instructor's name, the course name and number, and the date. This information should be in a block at the left margin that begins 1 inch from the top of the page.
- Center the title three lines below the date and other related information (e.g., the course number). The title's first, last, and principal words should be capitalized. Do not underline, italicize, or use all caps in the title. Do not end with a period. A question or exclamation mark may be used, if appropriate.
- Place author references in the body of the paper in parentheses within the text, and include the page numbers on which the referenced information is located. These parenthetical citations are used instead of footnoting each source at the bottom of the page. Footnotes are used only for explanatory notes. In the body of the paper, use superscripts (raised numbers) to signal that an explanatory note exists. Explanatory notes are optional. If such a note is used, it is placed either at the bottom of the page as a footnote or at the end of the paper as an endnote.
- MLA style uses the term *Works Cited* for bibliographic references. These are placed on a separate numbered page. Center the title 1 inch from the top margin. List the references in alphabetical order by each author's last name. Set all text in a double-spaced format. Works cited from books, journals, magazines, newspapers, letters, online sites, and compact discs each have their own MLA reference style that should be followed.

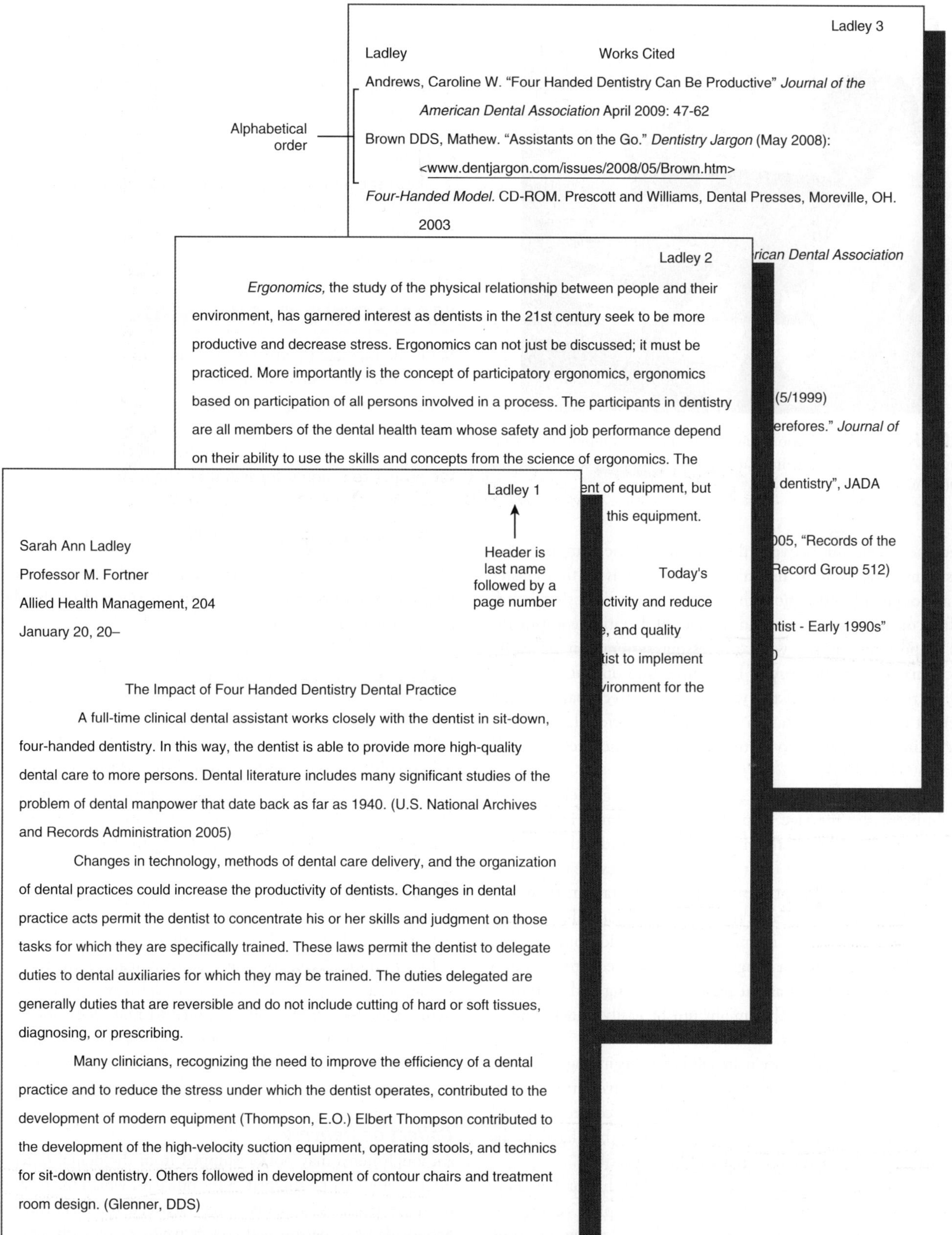
Ladley 3
Ladley Works Cited
Andrews, Caroline W. "Four Handed Dentistry Can Be Productive" Journal of the American Dental Association April 2009: 47-62
Alphabetical order
Brown DDS, Mathew. "Assistants on the Go." Dentistry Jargon (May 2008): <www.dentjargon.com/issues/2008/05/Brown.htm>
Four-Handed Model. CD-ROM. Prescott and Williams, Dental Presses, Moreville, OH. 2003
rican Dental Association
(5/1999)
erefores." Journal of
dentistry", JADA
005, "Records of the
Record Group 512)
ntist - Early 1990s"
Ladley 2
Ergonomics, the study of the physical relationship between people and their environment, has garnered interest as dentists in the 21st century seek to be more productive and decrease stress. Ergonomics can not just be discussed; it must be practiced. More importantly is the concept of participatory ergonomics, ergonomics based on participation of all persons involved in a process. The participants in dentistry are all members of the dental health team whose safety and job performance depend on their ability to use the skills and concepts from the science of ergonomics. The
ent of equipment, but
this equipment.
Today's
ctivity and reduce
, and quality
ist to implement
ironment for the
Ladley 1
Header is last name followed by a page number
Sarah Ann Ladley
Professor M. Fortner
Allied Health Management, 204
January 20, 20–
The Impact of Four Handed Dentistry Dental Practice
A full-time clinical dental assistant works closely with the dentist in sit-down, four-handed dentistry. In this way, the dentist is able to provide more high-quality dental care to more persons. Dental literature includes many significant studies of the problem of dental manpower that date back as far as 1940. (U.S. National Archives and Records Administration 2005)
Changes in technology, methods of dental care delivery, and the organization of dental practices could increase the productivity of dentists. Changes in dental practice acts permit the dentist to concentrate his or her skills and judgment on those tasks for which they are specifically trained. These laws permit the dentist to delegate duties to dental auxiliaries for which they may be trained. The duties delegated are generally duties that are reversible and do not include cutting of hard or soft tissues, diagnosing, or prescribing.
Many clinicians, recognizing the need to improve the efficiency of a dental practice and to reduce the stress under which the dentist operates, contributed to the development of modern equipment (Thompson, E.O.) Elbert Thompson contributed to the development of the high-velocity suction equipment, operating stools, and technics for sit-down dentistry. Others followed in development of contour chairs and treatment room design. (Glenner, DDS)

FIGURE 9-15 Modern Language Association manuscript format. Notice the setup for the first page, the footnotes, and the works cited page.

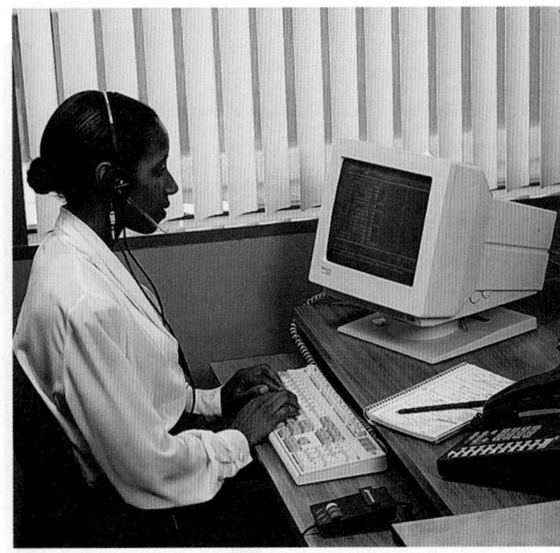

FIGURE 9-16 Dictation and transcription equipment. (From Young AP: Kinn's the administrative medical assistant, ed 6, St Louis, 2007, WB Saunders.)

become a vital link between the dentist and the administrative assistant. Studies show that machine dictation is six times faster than longhand and almost three times faster than shorthand. After considering the many advantages of dictation equipment, its importance in the word processing system can be easily recognized in the increase of both input and output.

At the conclusion of the workday or between patients, the dentist may use the dictation equipment for referral letters, for recording information to be transferred to clinical records, and so on.

Effective dictation requires following a few guidelines:

- Indicate the message disposition to the transcriber before beginning to dictate the message; this includes the number of copies to be made and to whom the copies are to be sent. If the material has priority over other dictation, then this too should be indicated at the beginning. State what is being dictated (e.g., letter, memo, report). In addition, indicate whether the item is a rough draft or finished product, and provide information about preferred spacing and margins.
- Spell out any words that might not be easily understood as well as names, streets, and cities.
- Organize correspondence materials before beginning to dictate.
- Dictate clearly, at an easy pace, and in a conversational tone. Most dictation equipment provides for the control of speed and volume, but the fewer adjustments that have to be made, the faster the material will be transcribed.

The administrative assistant can schedule his or her daily work to include transcription periods to complete correspondence and reports on a priority basis. The following are some guidelines for effective transcription:

- Assemble all materials and necessary equipment.
- Use reference sources such as a dictionary, a written communication reference book, a spelling and grammar checker, a thesaurus, and a name and address file.
- Listen to special instructions on the dictated material to determine priority. Some systems have audible indexing that gives a single tone signal to indicate the end of each document and two tones for special instructions. Determine whether other materials are needed for enclosures or if there are special mailing procedures to consider.
- If the dictation does not make sense or if there is a question about the information, ask the dentist rather than transcribing incorrect information.
- Proofread the entire transcription before printing the document.

MANAGING OFFICE MAIL

With the increase in written communications in today's dental office, more demands for efficient processing and the distribution of both incoming and outgoing mail must be met by the administrative assistant. Because of the constant flow of incoming and outgoing mail, the administrative assistant must know the proper techniques for handling the mail.

Processing Outgoing Mail

Outgoing correspondence may be prepared earlier in the day, but it is often organized for mailing at the end of the day as part of the daily routine.

Classification of Mail

Some of the outgoing mail will be sent as first-class mail, some will go out as fourth-class mail, some will be insured, and some will involve special handling using the address guidelines in Figure 9-17. The administrative assistant must be aware of these various classes of mail and services available to select the best classification for the type of item being mailed.

Certified Mail

Certified mail provides a receipt stamped with the date of mailing. A unique article number allows for the verification of delivery online. As an additional security feature, the recipient's signature is obtained at the time of delivery, and a record is maintained by the post office. Certified mail does not include insurance, and it is not available for international mail. For valuables and irreplaceable items, it is better to use services such as express mail, insured mail, or registered mail.

Collect on Delivery

Although items may not be shipped from the dental office very often, items may be shipped to the office for which the post office must be paid. With Collect on Delivery (COD), the Postal Service delivery person will collect payment by cash, check, or postage from the addressee for the items being delivered.

Delivery Confirmation

Delivery Confirmation is a special service that provides the date of delivery or attempted delivery for Priority Mail and Standard

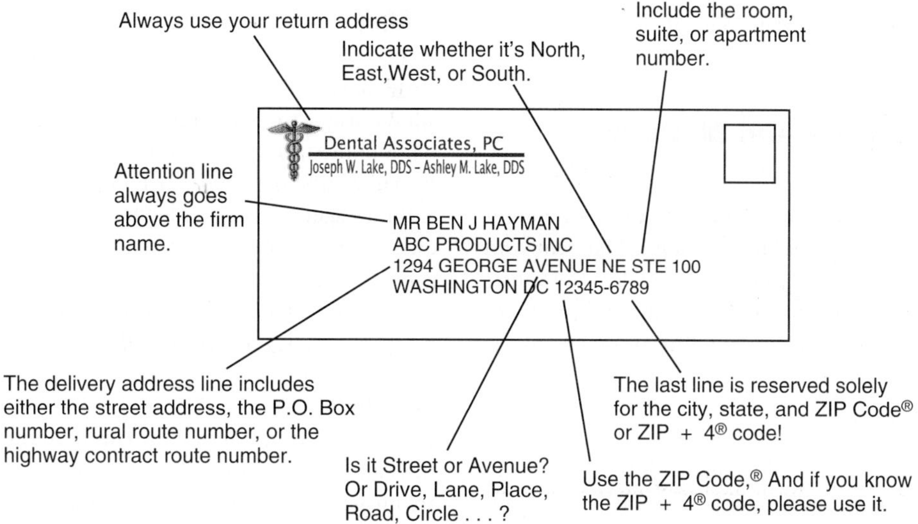
Follow these simple guidelines to help mail get where it's going faster.
Always use your return address
Indicate whether it's North, East,West, or South.
Include the room, suite, or apartment number.
Dental Associates, PC
Joseph W. Lake, DDS - Ashley M. Lake, DDS
Attention line always goes above the firm name.
MR BEN J HAYMAN
ABC PRODUCTS INC
1294 GEORGE AVENUE NE STE 100
WASHINGTON DC 12345-6789
The delivery address line includes either the street address, the P.O. Box number, rural route number, or the highway contract route number.
Is it Street or Avenue? Or Drive, Lane, Place, Road, Circle . . . ?
Use the ZIP Code,® And if you know the ZIP + 4® code, please use it.
The last line is reserved solely for the city, state, and ZIP Code® or ZIP + 4® code!

FIGURE 9-17 Guidelines recommended by the US Postal Service for addressing mail correctly.

Mail parcels, Bound Printed Matter, and Library Mail. Delivery Confirmation is available for a retail fee and an electronic fee. The retail fee can be purchased at the local post office and uses the fluorescent green Delivery Confirmation label, PS Form 152. Delivery information is available online and by phone (for retail fee customers only).

Express Mail

Express Mail is the Postal Service's premium delivery service, which provides guaranteed overnight delivery for documents and packages weighing up to 70 lb. Both domestic and international services are offered. This form of mail is automatically insured for US $100.

First-Class Mail

First-Class Mail includes letters, postcards, and all matter sealed or otherwise closed against inspection. This service is required for personal correspondence, handwritten or typewritten letters, and bills or statements of account.

Periodicals

Periodicals refers to a class of mail formerly called *Second-Class Mail,* which consists of magazines, newspapers, and other publications.

Insured Mail

This type of mail is insured against loss or damage to the articles being mailed. Security is key when sending valuable documents or materials from the office.

Priority Mail

Priority Mail is a 1- to 3-day nonguaranteed delivery service.

Registered Mail

Items sent with Registered Mail are placed under tight security from the point of mailing to the point of delivery and insured for up to US $25,000 against loss or damage. The date and time of delivery as well as information about delivery attempts can be verified online.

Return Receipt

A Return Receipt is available with Certified or Registered Mail when proof of delivery (information about the recipient's signature and actual delivery address) is wanted. A return receipt may be purchased before or after the mailing. A mailer who is purchasing Return Receipt service at the time of mailing may choose to receive the return receipt by mail or e-mail. (The e-mail option is available at most post offices. Contact your local post office for availability.)

Signature Confirmation

If mailing something important, the administrative assistant may want to be sure that it reaches not just the right address but the right hands as well. Signature Confirmation provides confirmation of delivery that includes the date, time, and location. The sender can ask to have a letter faxed or mailed to him or her with a copy of the recipient's signature.

Standard Mail

Standard Mail is a mailing service offered for any item, including advertisements and merchandise that weighs less than 16 ounces, that does not have to be sent via First-Class Mail. Standard Mail is typically used for multiple delivery addresses and bulk advertising.

Other questions that arise regarding outgoing mail can be answered by checking with the US Postal Service. Manuals are available from the Superintendent of Documents, Government Printing Office, Washington, DC 20402\MDomestic Mail Manual, 19 and International Mail Manual, 14 or by visiting the website at www.usps.gov.

Mailing Accessories and Methods

Postage Scale

A postage scale, which is used to determine the weight of outgoing mail, is an asset in the dental business office. Mail sent with insufficient postage might be returned to the sender. This causes a delay in the delivery of statements to patients and insurance forms to carriers, thereby delaying the return of money to the practice.

Postage Meter

A postage meter can be a time-saving device for the administrative assistant. Although various sizes of postage meters are available, a desk model is practical for a private practice. Group practices and clinics may need a larger meter that feeds envelopes through the machine automatically and both stamps and seals them. The meters are purchased outright, but the meter mechanism is leased. A meter license is obtained from the US Postal Service. With new electronic models, meter resetting is done by means of a telephone call. All that is needed is an active account with the Postage-by-Phone System and the appropriate meter. No special telephone hookups, computers, or software are required. The customer signs up for the system and then writes a check to put funds into an account to draw on as postage is ordered. Monthly reports listing the account activities are sent to the customer. In keeping with this new technology, postage scales are now available that weigh and automatically determine correct postage rates (Figure 9-18). The accuracy of electronic scales helps to eliminate the overpayment of postage. The meter can also be set for the amount of postage required for packages. The amount is printed on a tape, which is then affixed to the package.

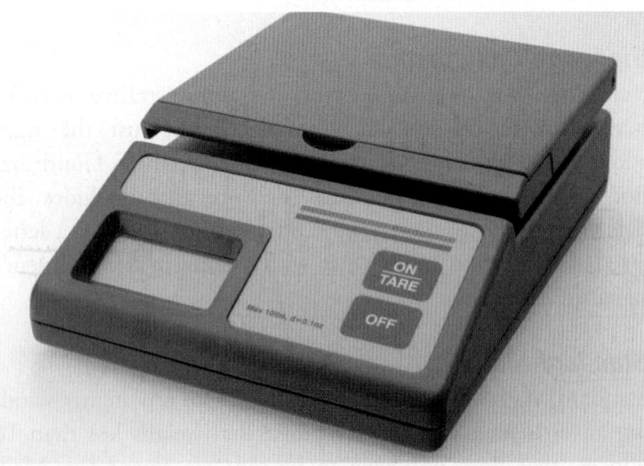

FIGURE 9-18 Postage scale. (Copyright © 2014 Didden, BigStock.com)

Outgoing mail that is addressed correctly, that has the proper amount of postage, and that is pre-postmarked goes through the post office faster and will arrive at its destination sooner.

E-Mail

Dental practices often make use of e-mail through a computer network system. This is a type of message service (software) that allows users to communicate directly with other users by sending messages electronically over communication channels. E-mail can be used to leave messages for other staff members, and messages are safeguarded because the users must have their own identification code to access the messages. E-mail has gained wide use for the processing of insurance claim forms. Turnaround time has been greatly reduced, and the result is an increase in cash flow for the office.

Facsimile

Another electronic means of communication is the facsimile (fax) machine. A fax machine is a scanning device that transmits an image of a document over standard telephone lines; it is described in detail in Chapter 10. The dentist may find this method of transmitting written communication to be very effective when it is necessary to have an immediate response or if the information involves an emergency procedure. The use of such a transmission requires a cover sheet, and it requires that the transmitted information be maintained confidentially. At the bottom of a fax cover sheet, some statement similar to the following should be included:

> **CONFIDENTIALITY NOTICE:** This fax cover sheet and the documents accompanying this fax transmission may contain confidential information belonging to the sender that is legally privileged. The information is intended only for the use of the individual or entity named above as recipient. If you are not the intended recipient, you are hereby notified that any disclosure, copying, or distribution or the taking of any action in reliance on or regarding the contents of this faxed information is strictly prohibited. If you have received this fax in error, please notify us immediately by telephone to arrange for the return of the original documents to us."

Mailing Services

Mailing services are service enterprises that specialize in mail communications. A mailing service is an independent postal service that is a complete business center that processes metered and bulk mail, first-class mail, UPS, FedEx, DHL, air freight, and so on. The use of such a service may be very useful for a dental practice with high-volume mailings. Some mailing services specialize in direct-mail advertising, promotional sales, and billings. Other types of services available from a mailing service might include data entry, file maintenance, labels and listings, and personalized letters.

Shipping Providers

Shipping providers such as United Parcel Service (UPS), FedEx, DHL, Greyhound Package Express, Purolator Courier, and many others are gaining popularity with businesses that need letters or packages delivered the next day or that need to send fourth-class material. When selecting a provider, it is important to consider the cost, the speed of delivery, and the convenience. Most providers will require the completion of a special form, and some are even moving toward the online generation of this paperwork.

The following list provides information about shipping providers:

- Rates are determined by the weight and size of the package, the distance to the destination, and the required time of delivery.
- Maximum weight varies with the carrier.
- Each package will be protected against loss or damage.
- Most general commodities may be shipped.
- Packages to be shipped can be picked up at the dental office or place of business. Deliveries are made to the exact address indicated on the parcel.
- Deliveries are not made to post office boxes.
- Delivery reattempts are typically made at no additional charge.
- The sender is not charged for the return of an undeliverable package.
- Shipping providers are available in most areas. Check local listings for providers near you.

Laboratory Services

For areas in which there is no local dental laboratory, certain material must be shipped to the laboratory via the US mail or commercial delivery services. The dental laboratory provides a dentist with a sturdy cardboard or plastic insulated mail carton. All impressions or devices that have been placed in the patient's mouth must be disinfected in compliance with Occupational Safety and Health Administration (OSHA) guidelines before packaging. The contents should be carefully wrapped. The case should be disassembled from articulators, and each item should be wrapped separately for reassembly when the package is received by the laboratory. The laboratory requisition is enclosed in the box, and a mailing label supplied by the laboratory is attached to the carton.

Processing Incoming Mail

The location of the dental practice may determine whether the mail is delivered to the office by a regular postal mail carrier or whether a post office box is rented and the mail is picked up at the post office or postal station. For a clinic within an institution, mail may be routed from a central mailroom within the building. Whatever the situation, the administrative assistant is responsible for the proper sorting and distribution of the mail.

When the mail is first sorted, the administrative assistant must distinguish among the various types:

- First-class mail, including priority mail, personal mail, special deliveries, registered or certified mail, payments, invoices, and general correspondence
- Printed matter, such as announcements of professional meetings, solicitations for contributions, collegiate newsletters, and other semiprofessional materials
- Magazines and newspapers for the reception room, professional journals, and periodicals
- Advertisements
- Samples of dental products and drugs
- Materials from laboratories
- Supplies ordered from a dental supply company

After the initial sorting, the personal mail should be distributed to the intended recipients and placed so that it will receive prompt attention.

When payments are received, attach the returned portion of the statement or note on the envelope the amount of money received. Enclosures should be clipped to the letter, invoice, or statement, and all incoming correspondence should be stamped with the date and time received. Many offices find that an automated time-stamp machine that stamps the date and time at which something was received is practical, especially if a question arises as to the time and date that a particular item arrived (Figure 9-19). If a time-stamp machine is not available, then the date and time that the correspondence was received have to be written on the correspondence. In addition, the administrative assistant may be responsible for opening and reading some first-class mail and highlighting the significant portions of the correspondence. When doing so, he or she should use a colored pen to make notations. This procedure saves the dentist valuable time when he or she reads through important mail. If the incoming mail item makes reference to previous correspondence, copies of the latter can be attached or clinical records pulled and attached. This will save the dentist time when replying, and it also serves as a reminder of previous conversations or correspondence. In a group practice or clinic, a routing slip may be used for a piece of correspondence when several people need to be informed of the contents (Figure 9-20). It should be noted that electronic mail can also be sent to a variety of people. When forwarding this type of mail, one can create an electronic routing slip with Microsoft Office documents by opening the file you want to route then going to File > Send to > Routing Recipient. Next, you click in the Address box and then choose the e-mail addresses of the people you want to appear on the routing slip. You can change the

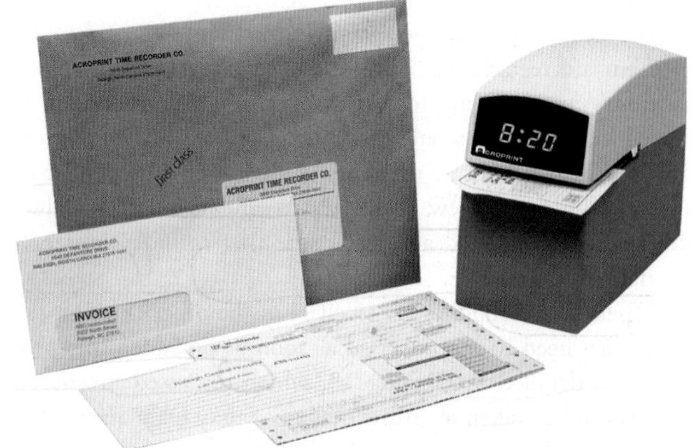

FIGURE 9-19 Automatic time-stamp machine. (Courtesy Acroprint Time Recorder Co., Raleigh, NC.)

Dental Associates, PC

Joseph W. Lake, DDS - Ashley M. Lake, DDS

INTEROFFICE

ROUTING SLIP

Please read the attached ______________________
and record the date passed on to the persons indicated.

Refer to:	Date Received	Date Passed on
Dr. Austin	________	________
Dr. Baker	________	________
Dr. Downing	________	________
Dr. Green	________	________
Dr. Mann	________	________
Dr. Powers	________	________
Routed by:	________________	

FIGURE 9-20 Mail routing slip.

recipient order by selecting the name and moving it with the arrow buttons located in the dialog box. Finally, select the options you want for that document, and then click "Route." The file will then be sent to the first name on the list.

When discarding the envelopes of incoming mail, be sure that the entire contents have been removed and that all important data (e.g., company name, individual's name, postmark date, time [if significant]) have been recorded. In some situations, the envelope may even be retained. If an envelope is to be discarded, it should be shredded so that personal information such as return addresses remain confidential.

Some printed material (e.g., meeting notices) will be opened by the dentist and should be placed on his or her desk along with the personal mail. The magazines for the office should be distributed to the reception room, and the older issues should be removed and recycled.

The administrative assistant may be asked to scan the professional magazines and make notes in the margins about special meetings and conferences that may be of interest to the dentist. This saves the dentist time when he or she is reading the magazine.

The dental office receives many advertisements, and many of them are regarded as "junk mail." It is the administrative assistant's responsibility to sort through the advertisements to determine which material should be examined by the dentist. The dentist will indicate the types of advertisements that he or she would like to review. If the advertisements are of no value, throw them away, and always be sure that confidential labels are destroyed properly.

When dental supplies are received in the office through the mail, they need to be processed as soon as possible. This procedure is detailed in Chapter 13, which discussed inventory. Care should be taken to ensure that any Safety Data Sheets that accompany the products remain with the products until the materials are checked in, stored, labeled appropriately, and entered into the practice's inventory system.

Open any samples received in the mail, and place them on the dentist's desk. Most of these samples accompany literature that should remain with the product.

Extreme care should be taken when opening materials from dental laboratories. Follow appropriate disinfection procedures, inform the dentist of the arrival of a lab case, and then confirm the patient's appointment.

Managing Mail in the Dentist's Absence

When the dentist is away from the office, the administrative assistant is responsible for handling all mail. Decisions will have to be made about the following:

- Contacting the dentist regarding any of the correspondence
- Forwarding mail to the dentist
- Answering mail and explaining that the dentist is away from the office
- Determining which correspondence can wait for an answer when the dentist returns

Before the dentist leaves the office for any length of time, a policy regarding the handling of mail should be established.

Please refer to the student workbook for additional learning activities.

LEARNING ACTIVITIES

1. List and explain the characteristics of an effective letter.
2. Outline the acceptable format for addressing envelopes.
3. Outline the procedures for sorting incoming mail.
4. List and define the four classifications of mail.
5. Discuss the special mail services that may be used by a dental office.
6. You need to mail a package, but you are not sure about the amount of the postage to attach. Explain how you would weigh the package and determine the cost of shipping.
7. List the advantages of using a commercial delivery service.
8. Explain a situation that could be handled through a fax process.

BIBLIOGRAPHY

FedEx Corporation: *FedEx service guide*, Dallas, 2014, FedEx Corporation.

Fulton-Calkins PJ, Rankin DS, Shumack KA: *The administrative professional*, ed 14, Mason, OH, 2011, Thomson South-Western.

Gibaldi J: *MLA handbook for writers of research papers*, ed 7, New York, 2009, Modern Language Association of America.

Locker KO, Kiensler D: *Business and administrative communication*, ed 10, New York, 2012, McGraw-Hill/Irwin.

U.S. Postal Service: *The domestic mail manual*, Washington, DC, 2013, U.S. Government Printing Office.

RECOMMENDED WEBSITES

www.albion.com/netiquette
www.fedex.com
www.mla.org/style
www.usps.gov

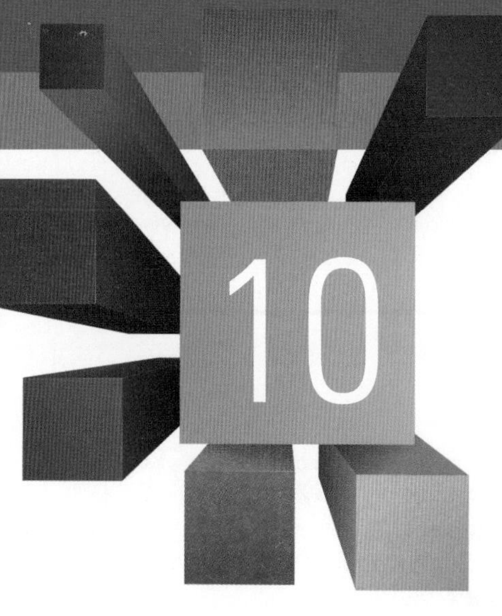

Electronic and Telecommunications

Kathy J. Zwieg

http://evolve.elsevier.com/Finkbeiner/practice

LEARNING OUTCOMES

1. Define the key terms in this chapter.
2. Discuss the application of electronic and telecommunications in a dental office, including:
   - Explain the special features of telephone equipment and services.
   - Describe various types of communication systems commonly used by the dental team.
3. Develop effective telephone etiquette to use in a dental office, including:
   - Discuss the components of a speaking voice and how to achieve a good telephone personality.
   - Describe the best way to manage incoming and outgoing calls encountered in the dental office.
   - Describe how to record phone messages correctly and discuss etiquette involving personal calls, cell phone, and social media.

KEY TERMS

Call forwarding A telephonic feature that automatically relays a call to another telephone number.

Call holding A feature of many telephone systems that allows a second call to be answered while the first caller "holds" on the line.

Caller ID A display that shows the number assigned to the telephone from which the person is calling.

Cellular technology A mobile telephone system that breaks down a large service area into smaller areas, called *cells.* Each cell is served by a low-powered receiver/transmitter. As the caller moves from one cell to another, a switching office automatically moves the call in a corresponding fashion.

Conference call A telephone call in which several people participate, often from a number of different locations. The call is arranged through a conference call operator, who is given the names and telephone numbers of the individuals to be included in the call and the time at which the call is to be made.

Facsimile (FAX) machine A scanning device that transmits an image of a document over standard telephone lines.

Facebook The world's largest social networking service that connects people with friends and others who work, study, and live around them.

Liquid crystal display (LCD) A device that allows the user to see the number dialed, that prompts the user with instructions, and that displays the number of minutes the individual remains on the telephone.

Mobile phone Another term for a cellular phone.

Pager A telecommunications device that allows a person to receive accurate messages instantly or that alerts the person to return a call.

Responsive web design A way of developing a single website that works effectively on both desktop browsers and mobile devices while providing the best-quality browsing experience, regardless of the operating system.

Smartphone A mobile telephone that also supports e-mail, text messaging, Internet use, photography, and a variety of other computer functions.

Social media The collective of websites and other online means of communication that are used by large groups of people to share information.

Speed dialing A feature that allows commonly called numbers to be stored in the telephone system's memory and subsequently dialed by keying in a one- or two-digit code.

Telecommunications The science and technology of communication via the electronic transmission of impulses as telegraphy, cable, telephone, radio, or television.

Time zones Geographic regions in which the same standard time is used. The United States is divided into four time zones: Eastern, Central, Mountain, and Pacific.

Twitter An online social networking and microblogging service that enables users to send and read short 140-character text messages called *tweets.*

YouTube A video-sharing website on which users can upload, share, comment on, and view videos.

Voicemail A telephone system that connects callers directly to an extension or a department and that can record messages for that person or department.

Website A virtual location on the World Wide Web that contains several subject- or company-related web pages and data files that are accessible through a browser.

Wi-Fi A technology that allows an electronic device to exchange data or connect to the Internet wirelessly.

A revolution is taking place in the field of communications. Trying to keep up with the latest devices and technology is like trying to keep up with all the new brands of composite restorative materials in clinical dentistry. New communications models are being introduced rapidly. Therefore, the materials presented here represent the current concepts, although a newer model may have been introduced only yesterday. It is often up to the administrative assistant in a busy dental office to complete the research regarding the most current models and to determine the application of the latest communications technology for the office.

If the patient is the most important person in the dental office, then certainly one can say that communications equipment is the most important system in the office. In the past, the telephone alone was the most common communication instrument for society. Modern electronic communications is now the most important communication system in the world, because it is the fastest and easiest way to transmit messages.

Considerable attention is paid to choosing modern equipment for the dental treatment rooms, hiring assistants highly skilled in business concepts or clinical procedures, and using the latest technological advances in diagnosis. Yet the most important system in the office—electronic communications—is often taken for granted and receives less consideration.

PRACTICE NOTE

Electronic communications is the most important system in the dental office.

The vast majority of today's patients will have done some form of electronic research before contacting the practice via telephone or electronically through the office website. Like it or not, this is where your office will have its one chance to make a positive first impression. Thus, communications management should not be entrusted to an inexperienced staff member. This responsibility should only be delegated to a person with a broad knowledge of dentistry and a high degree of self-confidence; he or she will be alert and able to make good decisions while possessing good verbal and written communication skills. Speaking with a smile in the voice, being enthusiastic, and having a cordial manner may not solve all problems automatically, but speaking with hostility or disinterest ensures that future communications with patients will be more difficult (Figure 10-1).

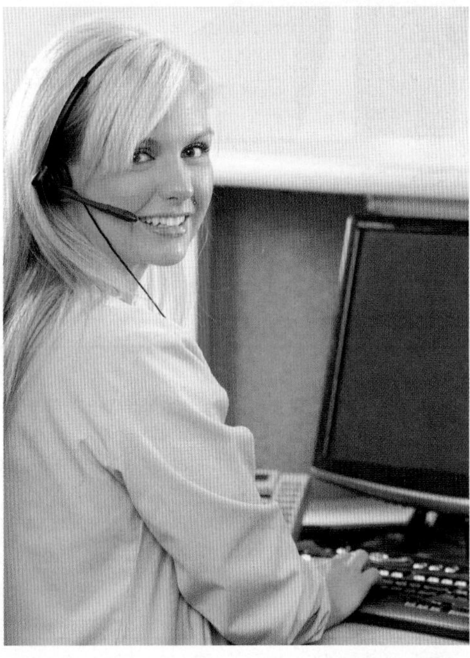

FIGURE 10-1 A voice that makes the caller feel as though a smile is coming through the receiver is a winning voice. (Copyright © 2014 Leaf, BigStock.com.)

PRACTICE NOTE

The majority of patients will have researched the dental office electronically before making contact.

FORMS OF COMMUNICATIONS IN DENTISTRY

Electronic telecommunications have grown and changed significantly in recent history. The term refers to the science and technology of communication that occurs via the electronic transmission of impulses by satellite, cable, telephone, radio, television, or computer. Wireless technology, or Wi-Fi, has enhanced the communications capabilities in the dental practice by providing the ability to eliminate bulky, sometimes hazardous cords or the need to be tethered to a desk. In a practical sense, electronic communications in a dental office refers to the different kinds of systems and communication that result from the use of them. It encompasses telephones, smartphones, mobile devices, websites, and a variety of ever-changing forms of social media. This chapter discusses the various types of communication hardware and how to manage communication using their capabilities for practice growth, profitability, and, of course, satisfied patients.

Telephones

With the array of specialized telephone equipment now available, the dental staff can take advantage of state-of-the-art equipment to become more efficient. For a modest price, dental business owners can buy sophisticated telephone systems that can improve the productivity and profitability of their enterprise. Telephone companies and agencies are usually very eager to help businesses determine their needs for telephone equipment and to make recommendations. Various types of equipment can also be explored at product websites (e.g., www.att.com, www.panasonic.com, www.apple.com). The equipment and services described in the following list can also be useful to the dental office:

- Integrated business communication systems offer features designed for a small business such as a dental practice. A system like the one shown in Figure 10-2 automatically redials the last outside number dialed at the touch of a button; easily establishes a conference call with the conference button; and, on most system phones, allows voice dialing and talking without picking up the handset. It includes basic transfer and hold functions as well as the programming of multiple numbers to allow for the speed dialing of frequently called numbers. Information can be displayed in multiple languages such as English, Spanish, and French. An alternative version of this system provides most of the same features but includes multiple handsets with only one base charger. A dentist may believe that only a basic, traditional telephone is required; however, a versatile telephone system with the features described allows for the more efficient handling of the many telephone calls the office receives daily.
- Communications can be improved between one area of the office or clinic and another through the paging and intercom features of this system. With single-button access, the person to be contacted can be reached quickly. Often the individual can answer intercom calls without touching the phone and creating infection control concerns or interrupting work.
- Computer-linked telecommunications systems allow businesses to manage incoming and outgoing calls, organize personal information, and store patient information (e.g., telephone numbers) in a database file that can be retrieved for autodialing. It also allows for the programming of phones from a computer database (Figure 10-3). With this type of computer/telephone integration, incoming calling information can be used to provide an automatic pop-up window on a personal computer that displays the caller's database file; this allows the administrative assistant to greet the caller by name and to have detailed information readily available to answer the caller's questions. This system brings the efficiency and productivity of advanced telecommunications technology to small and medium-sized businesses.
- Cordless telephone systems provide an extended mobility range in the office (Figure 10-4). This allows staff members to leave the base station and communicate with other areas

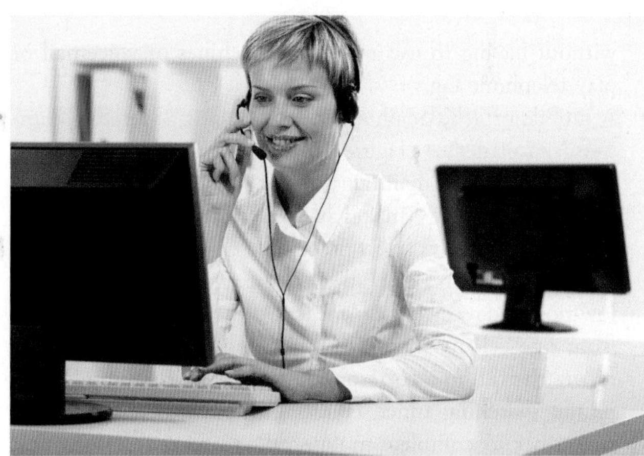

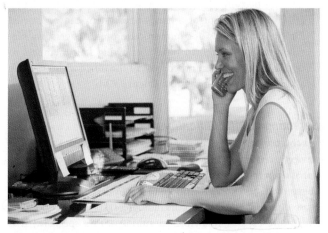

FIGURE 10-3 A telecommunications system linked to personal computers provides rapid access to patient data. (Copyright © 2014 Press Master, BigStock.com.)

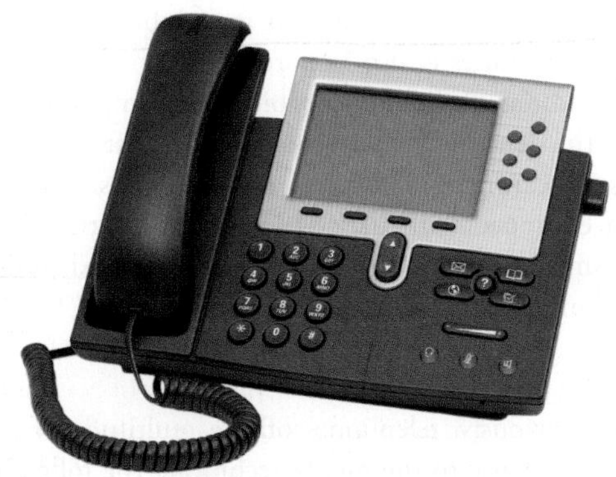

FIGURE 10-2 A basic, easy-to-use telephone system for a small business includes features such as a built-in speakerphone and a digital display for convenience as well as the ability to establish conference calls. (Copyright © 2014 Cflux, BigStock.com.)

FIGURE 10-4 A cordless telephone system allows for extended mobility in the dental office. (Copyright © 2014 Monkey Business Images, BigStock.com.)

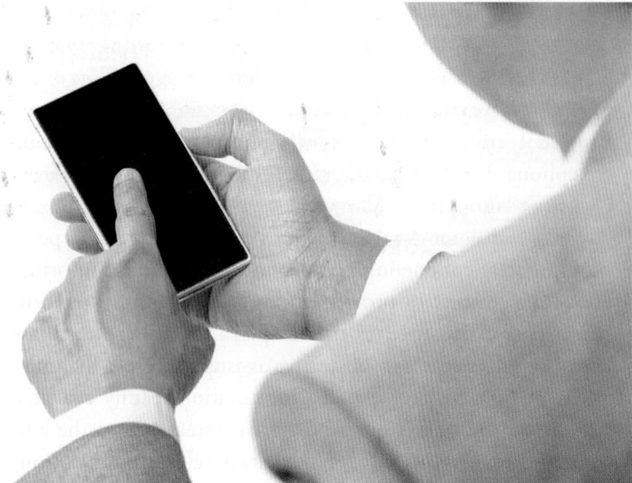

FIGURE 10-5 Smartphones allow dentists and staff members to communicate while outside of the dental office. (Copyright © 2014 Impak Pro, BigStock.com.)

without having to use answering machines or voicemail or play telephone tag.

- A mobile or cellular phone (cell phone) is a portable communication device (Figure 10-5). When a dentist or staff member needs to maintain contact with a central location, cellular technology makes it possible to use a fully functional telephone. This technology breaks down a large service area into smaller areas called *cells.* Each cell is served by a low-powered receiver/transmitter. As the mobile caller moves from one cell to another, a switching office automatically moves the call in a corresponding fashion. The mobile telephone switching office communicates with a land-based subscriber to complete mobile calls to fixed locations that are serviced by telephone lines.
- A hands-free telephone allows the administrative assistant to work on the computer, access records, or perform some other task while talking on the telephone. This time-saving device is becoming very popular in clinics and private dental offices. The concept of a hands-free system can be carried into other methods of communication (e.g., pagers, walkie-talkie types of systems), thereby allowing staff members to obtain messages from other areas of the office without using a keyboard or dialing system (Figure 10-6).

Selecting a Communications Carrier

When services are selected for an office or when an existing service is changed, consultation with a communications professional from the company responsible for service to the office may be required. Several factors should be considered before the purchase of a telephone system, including cost, flexibility, mobility, and future expansion. Before consulting with a specialist, it is wise to do a task analysis to determine present and future needs.

Generally cost is the primary factor when selecting a system. Today, hardware such as telephones and other equipment can be purchased at a variety of stores. However, be sure that the operating system purchased is from a reliable source that will provide support when needed. The equipment market is cost-competitive, but costs can vary considerably. Before selecting a system, examine the specifications carefully to determine the cost of the standard features and the cost of each of the optional features. In addition, be sure to consider the cost of operating and maintaining the system. A reliable system often saves money in future maintenance. In some areas, suppliers provide maintenance contracts as insurance for multiple service calls.

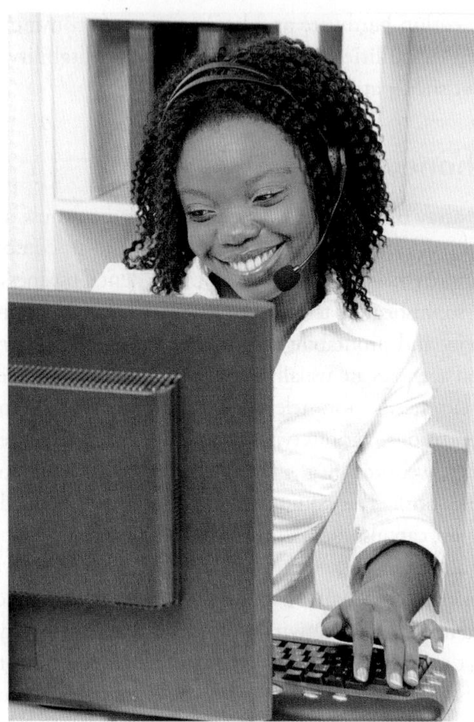

FIGURE 10-6 A hands-free telephone system allows the administrative assistant to perform other tasks while speaking on the telephone. (Copyright © 2014 Pic Hunter, BigStock.com.)

Flexibility should also be a major consideration. Expansion or updating of the communications system must be possible as the practice grows. The ability to move equipment between systems and facilities is also important.

Voice and data switching capabilities are important considerations. The dental office staff must be sure that a communications system can meet existing and future needs. For example, a system equipped with data-handling capabilities allows for data transmission and reception between users and equipment, such as computers linked to the system.

Telephone Features

As noted previously, telephones offer a multitude of features, from the very basic to the highly technical. The following sections describe some of the basic features.

Speakerphone. The dentist may find the hands-free speakerphone feature very convenient. With most systems, with just a push of a button, the speaker's voice is picked up by a microphone and then can be heard anywhere in the office. The handset need not be picked up, and the volume of the loudspeaker is adjustable. The speakerphone function can be canceled, even in the middle of a conversation, by picking up the handset. Speakerphones are particularly valuable for group meetings.

Voicemail Messaging. Voicemail messaging, or phone mail, uses advanced recording and routing functions to combine the features of a telephone, a computer, and a recording device. This feature can be learned quickly, and it is simple to use. The only equipment needed is a touch-tone telephone.

Users of voicemail can dial their voice mailboxes at any time, regardless of the location. A caller may hear previously recorded messages or may leave a message with such options such as replaying the message, erasing it, adding to it, sending it by normal or urgent delivery, switching the call to another line, or having it directly recorded to a voice mailbox. Dental office applications include voice-recorded daily updates of office activities and directions to callers regarding ways to obtain emergency care.

The dentist usually decides which type of message service meets the particular needs of the practice. Alternatives to voicemail include an answering machine or service. At this point in time, most answering machines are built into telephones and function much like a voicemail system; messages are retrievable from outside of the dental office.

An answering service with operator-answered calls can be used when patients call after office hours, on weekends, or on scheduled days off. The answering service operator informs the caller where the dentist can be reached for emergencies or takes the information from the caller and then notifies the dentist. This type of service is frequently used in an oral surgery practice, in which the likelihood of emergencies is greater than in a general practice.

Regardless of whether a voicemail system or a separate automatic answering device is used, some basic courtesies must be observed:

- If an answering machine is used, turn it on before leaving the office.
- In the outgoing message, indicate that the caller has reached an answering system. Give the name of the office rather than the telephone number so that the caller knows she or he has reached the correct office.
- Give clear information about office hours or ways to contact the dentist.
- Ensure that the answering message includes specific information about emergency contacts.
- Make sure that the caller has adequate time to record a message.
- Arrange to have messages checked periodically by the dentist or a staff member if the administrative assistant is out of the office for a period of time.
- Upon returning to the office, check the calls on the voicemail.
- Take care of any necessary follow-up related to the recorded calls. Most systems allow the user to access the answering machine or voice mailbox to receive messages, even when he or she is off site.
- Update the outgoing message regularly.
- Do not leave nonprofessional messages that may distract the caller.

Conference Calls. If the dentist or the administrative assistant needs to talk to several people in various locations simultaneously (i.e., insurance carriers), a conference call may be placed. Most telephone systems are equipped with this technology, and staff can establish conference calls very easily and quickly.

Caller ID. The caller ID feature can help to identify a caller before the telephone is answered by displaying the number of the telephone from which the person is calling. A number may be blocked from appearing by pressing a special key.

Call Forwarding. A telephone call can be automatically forwarded to another telephone number with call forwarding.

Call Holding. Call holding is frequently used in dental offices, which often receive calls in rapid succession. This feature allows for the answering of a second call while the first caller holds on the line. Care should be taken to extend maximum courtesy to the caller who has been asked to hold (Box 10-1).

Music on Hold. The music on hold system provides the caller with music or a short narrative about treatment in the dental office while the person is on hold. The system can be personalized to address specific types of treatment in the office and then revert to music periodically. This feature tends to ease the caller's impatience and can offer short educational clips that may market certain aspects of the practice.

Automatic Call Back. A caller can give instructions to a busy station to call back as soon as the busy station is free.

Automatic Call Stacking. Calls that arrive at a busy station are automatically answered by a recorded wait message.

Speed Dialing. Commonly called numbers can be stored in the telephone's memory, and the call can be made by keying in a one- or two-digit code. Speed dialing cuts down on the time that the administrative assistant spends dialing other offices or laboratories that are contacted frequently.

Call Timing. This feature is used in professional offices that charge clients by the time spent handling their business on the telephone. It is common in law and accounting firms and in other professional offices that bill for consultation on the telephone.

BOX 10-1

Using Call Holding

- Excuse oneself from the first caller before answering a second call.
- Greet the second caller with the standard office greeting.
- If the second caller requires only a short response, complete the call, and then return to the first caller.
- If the second caller appears to need more extensive assistance, explain that there is another call, ask the caller if he or she can wait, and then place the call on hold. If the caller does not want to wait, ask where the person can be reached, and say that the call will be returned. Always return the call promptly.
- When returning to the first caller, always thank the person for waiting before proceeding with the conversation.

Call Restriction. Unauthorized long-distance telephone calls can be eliminated with this feature. If an individual is authorized to make a long-distance call, the call is given an authorization code that must be keyed into the telephone before the call can be processed. The telephone may also be programmed not to accept or make long-distance calls, such as a telephone placed in the reception area for patient use.

Identified Ringing. This feature provides distinctive ring tones for different categories of calls. For example, internal calls may have one long ring, whereas outside calls may have two short rings.

Liquid Crystal Display. A liquid crystal display (LCD) allows the user to see the number dialed, prompts the user with instructions, and displays the number of minutes the individual remains on the telephone. When used for incoming calls, an LCD also displays the number of the caller.

Multiple Lines or Key Telephones. Multiple lines are a standard feature on most telephones in a dental office. Special care must be taken when using them to ensure privacy and to avoid interfering with other calls that are in progress.

If multiple lines are available for receiving or placing calls, one of the lines is often for a number that is not listed in the telephone directory or printed on the business stationery; this line should be used for outgoing calls, thus leaving the other lines available for incoming calls.

A telephone system with multiple lines can be used for both inside and outside calls. This can be a very efficient system, but the administrative assistant must remember several key points, which are presented in Box 10-2.

BOX 10-2

Using a Multiple-Line Telephone System

1. Determine which line is to be answered; this is usually indicated by a ring or a buzz, and the button flashes until the line is answered. Depress the key to be answered before lifting the receiver.
2. If placing an outside call, determine which line is available; this is indicated by an unlighted button. Depress the key for that line, and then dial the number. If accidentally selecting a line that has been placed on hold, depress the hold key again to put the call back on hold.
3. If placing an incoming call on hold, indicate to the caller that this is being done. Depress the hold key, which keeps the caller on the line. (The hold key then returns to its normal position.) The line key remains lighted, which indicates that the line is in use. Other calls then can be placed or received on another line.
4. Before transferring a call, be sure to inform the caller that this is being done, because the person may not want the call transferred. Give the caller the extension number to which he or she is being transferred in case the call is disconnected. This allows the caller to call the person back directly.
5. To transfer an outside call with the button system, first place the call on hold. Then push the button for local, which lights when in use (the local button is for in-office transfers only). Dial or buzz a number in the office telephone system; the telephone is answered on local in another office. Inform the dentist of a call on a particular line, and then the dentist will complete the call from that telephone. If returning to the incoming line, remember which line the caller used. "Hold reminder" is a feature on advanced telephone systems that gives a reminder tone at various intervals to indicate that a caller is still waiting. Depress that button, which opens the line once more and allows for the completion of the call.

Pagers

A pager is a telecommunications device that allows a person to receive accurate messages instantly. The pager can receive numeric messages, including phone numbers and special codes that have been devised, or it may receive alphanumeric messages. It may be used by a dentist when he or she is on call or after business hours to handle any emergency patient needs. Most pagers, such as the one shown in Figure 10-7, are easy to read, have various alert tones, display the date and time, offer various-size message slots, and retain messages in memory.

Smartphones

A smartphone is a mobile phone with more advanced computing capability and connectivity than basic feature phones (Figure 10-8). Smartphones typically combined the features of a mobile phone with those of other popular consumer devices, such as a personal digital assistant (PDA), a media player, a digital camera, a Global Positioning System (GPS) navigation unit, and a touchscreen computer. Smart phones have built-in keyboards that enable the user to type and then send messages. Two very popular brands include the iPhone from Apple and phones that use the Android operating system from Google.

Smartphones have gained a reputation for their ability to send and receive e-mail wherever they can access the wireless networks of certain cellular phone carriers. In addition, they have almost eliminated long-distance calling charges within the United States.

Instant Messaging System

The intercom system is discussed in Chapter 6 as a method of nonverbal interoffice communication by means of a light system. A more comprehensive messaging system can be established through part of the DataMate family or other compatible software. IMiN Lite is one example of an instant messaging program designed specifically for the small office. It provides secure instant communication within the dental office. The result is a cost-effective, local area network (LAN) messaging program that delivers the benefits of larger, more expensive messaging systems. This system is easy to use and easy to administer; it can support one person or networks of multiple users.

How Does It Work?

While the dentist is at chairside, an important telephone call comes in. To let the dentist know who is calling, the administrative assistant uses IMiN (Figure 10-9) to type a message, such as "The patient is ready," and sends it to the dentist in

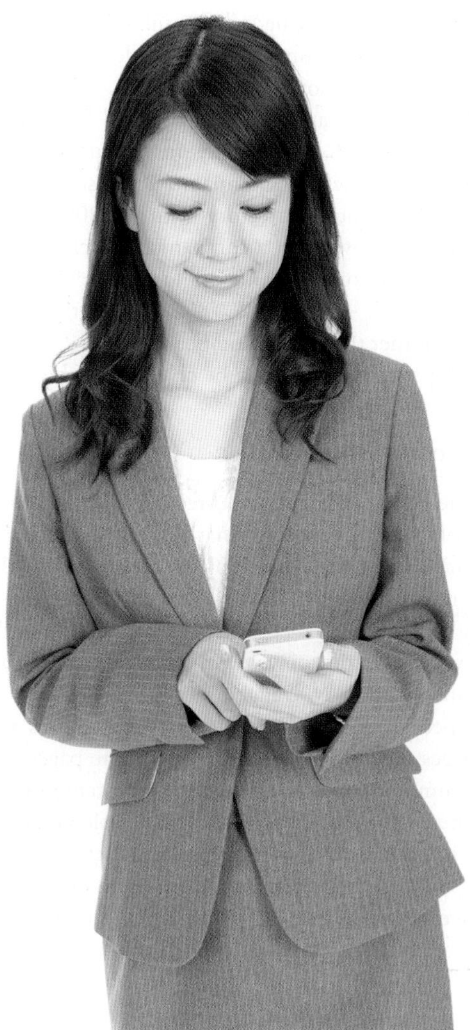

FIGURE 10-7 A dentist calls the office from a smartphone after receiving a message. (Copyright © 2014 Yo-Ichi, BigStock.com.)

the treatment room. The message instantly pops up on the computer screen in the treatment room. To reply, the dentist simply selects the desired response from the customizable message palette with a click of the mouse or by hitting the corresponding function key. The reply, such as "I'll be right there" or "I'll be just another 5 minutes," now appears on the administrative assistant's screen. This system prevents frantic waving, running back and forth, obvious patient interruption, and cryptic hand signals about what to do with the call. The system is clear, crisp, and professional, and the keyboard, mouse, and other hardware components can be protected with a barrier to prevent cross-contamination.

Facsimile (FAX) Communication System

Another electronic means of communication is the **facsimile (FAX) machine** (Figure 10-10). A facsimile transmission machine is a scanning device that transmits an encrypted image of a document over standard telephone lines. The machine

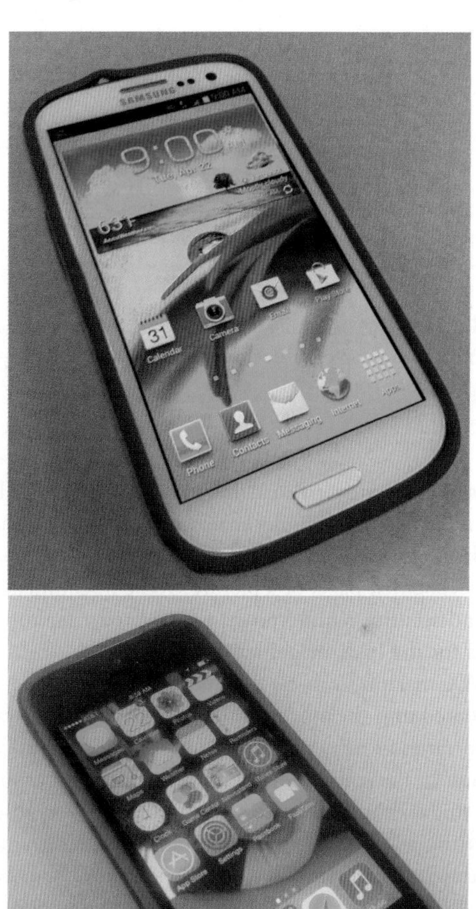

FIGURE 10-8 iPhones and various Android phones both feature a touch screen and provide the user with multiple technologies in a single device.

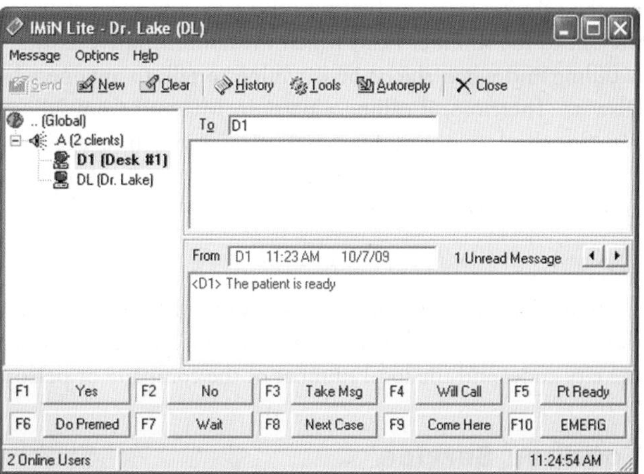

FIGURE 10-9 The IMiN screen indicates a message has been sent from the business office to the treatment room. (IMiN screenshot courtesy JustWrks, Inc, www.justwrks.com.)

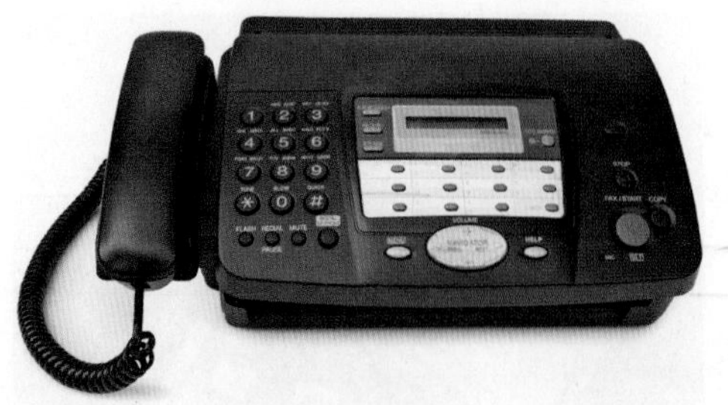

FIGURE 10-10 A facsimile (FAX) machine uses a dedicated telephone line to send copies of documents. (Copyright © 2014 Ruslan Ivantsov, BigStock.com.)

operates like a photocopy machine that sends an image by wire. At the receiving end, a similar machine receives the transmitted copy. The message may be a document handwritten in ballpoint pen, a keyboarded page, or a picture. To be in compliance with safety and security requirements, a dedicated telephone line is required for the FAX machine.

A FAX machine can be a stand-alone unit, or it may be incorporated into the office computer. The cost of the facsimile machine varies greatly, depending on its added features.

In case of an emergency or for consultation purposes, the dentist might find FAX telecommunications very useful for transmitting a patient's clinical dental record either locally or out of town. Documents that require signatures can be transmitted via the FAX system, but most legal transactions require the signing parties to eventually sign the original document.

It should also be noted that, in some cases, the FAX machine is not used. Instead, a document may be scanned on the computer and sent to the receiver via e-mail.

Direct Distance Dialing

With direct distance dialing (DDD) from the office telephone, long-distance numbers in other parts of the United States or other countries can be dialed on a station-to-station basis. To use the DDD system, dial a 1 plus the area code when charging the call to the number from which the administrative assistant is calling and when she or he is willing to talk to anyone who answers. Therefore, if calling a party in Missouri from Michigan, first check an online directory such as www.whitepages.com or the front pages of the telephone directory to determine the area code, and then do the following:

Key: 1 + 314 (or 636) + local number

To access a number in a foreign country, key the international access code (also available online) plus the country code, the city code, and the local number of the company or person.

Toll-Free Service

A toll-free number that begins with 800, 888, 877, or 866 allows callers to reach businesses and individuals without being charged for the call. The charge for using a toll-free number is paid by the called party (the toll-free subscriber) instead of the calling party. Toll-free numbers can be dialed directly to a business or personal telephone line.

Toll-free numbers are very common and have proved successful for businesses, particularly in the areas of customer service and telemarketing. Companies that use this service are listed in the telephone directory with an 800/888/877/866 number. If it is known that a company has such a number but it is not available online or in the local directory, it may be obtained through 800/888/877/866 information by keying 1-800 (or another three digit number)-555-1212. As with most information services, a fee may be charged for this service.

Telephone Directories

The online or paper telephone directory is a vital tool in the business office. It is important that the administrative assistant become familiar with the type of directory used in the office and the information available so that he or she can use the directory as efficiently as possible. If using an online directory such as www.411.com or www.whitepages.com, virtually any contact information is available at your fingertips. In some cities, paper telephone directories are available as well. The yellow pages may be separate from the white pages, and areas of the community may be divided into separate directories.

In general, the front pages of a paper telephone directory provide important information, such as emergency phone numbers for the police department, the fire department, and ambulance services. Suicide prevention and poison control numbers are often included as well.

DEVELOPING EFFECTIVE TELEPHONE ETIQUETTE

Most people take great care to exude a professional business appearance, but few people take as much pride in developing their telephone image. This is unfortunate for an administrative assistant who takes responsibility for telephone calls, because people spend more time listening to him or her than looking at him or her.

When using the telephone, people often forget that the person on the other end of the line is a human being. It is important to take time to develop a professional telephone personality. To be effective on the telephone, keep a smile in the voice, answer calls promptly, be attentive and discreet, be cordial and responsive, ask questions tactfully, take messages courteously, speak distinctly, transfer calls carefully, place calls properly, avoid sexism, and be considerate to the caller. The techniques for successful telephone contact, which involves a voice-to-voice relationship, are somewhat different from those of successful personal contact, which involves a face-to-face relationship (Figure 10-11).

PRACTICE NOTE

To be effective on the telephone, keep a smile in your voice.

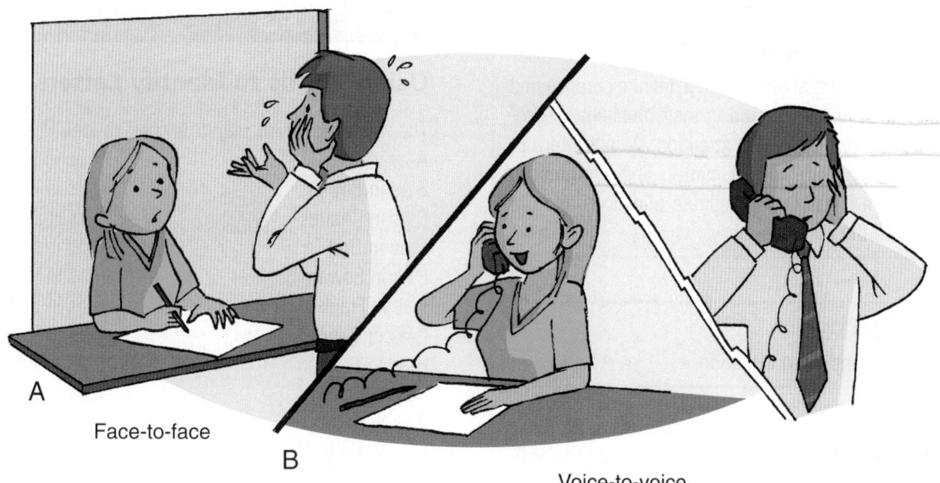

FIGURE 10-11 **A,** Face-to-face conversation. Nonverbal cues are apparent; the person smiles or makes gestures to be understood. Poise, interest, and sincerity provide observable feedback. Facial expressions help to indicate the degree of understanding. Discussion is extemporaneous, and notes generally are not used. **B,** Voice-to-voice conversation. The impression of the person is acquired only through hearing, and interpretation comes only from the tone of voice. The degree of understanding is determined by questioning and by rephrasing statements. Notes are advantageous in this situation.

Speaking Voice

The speaking voice has four separate but interrelated components: loudness, pitch, rate, and quality.

Loudness refers to the volume of the voice. If the speaker talks too loudly, the listener may be uncomfortable. (Have you ever talked on the telephone with someone who spoke so loudly you had to hold the receiver away from your ear? If you have, then you know how unpleasant excessive volume is to the listener.) The opposite situation can be equally unpleasant. If the speaker lacks confidence, the voice may be so quiet that people will ask for a repetition of what has been said. If this happens, the speaker should try to increase both confidence and volume.

The *rate* of speaking can determine how well someone is understood. When discussing familiar procedures with a patient, dental assistants may tend to speak rapidly, forgetting that this is new material to the patient. There is no ideal rate, but a general rule is to speak at a rate that does not detract from the clarity of the message and that is easy and comfortable to listen to for an extended period.

Pitch is the tone of the voice. This is more difficult to change, because once it has been developed, persistent discipline is required to alter it. A low, gravelly voice or a high, squeaky voice may be unpleasant to listen to and be hard on the throat. Many exercises for improving voice pitch are available online and from reference libraries.

The *quality* of a voice is a combination of physical and psychological factors. Changes in each of these alter the effectiveness of the speaking voice. Daily experiences affect quality, and care should be taken to withhold depression, excitement, and anger from the voice when speaking on the dental office telephone.

To achieve a good telephone personality, develop the qualities of alertness, expressiveness, interest, naturalness, and distinctness.

A patient who calls the dental office expects to have the call answered promptly. Answer the phone within the first two rings. Everyone enjoys being recognized, so be attentive to the patient's identity, and express this in the voice. When a patient calling the office identifies himself, the alert assistant replies, "Yes, Mr. Jones, how may I help you?"

Furthermore, when the patient presents a problem, do not stammer and stutter and say, "Yeah, well, uh, I don't know." Such a response indicates inexperience to the patient. "I will be glad to check your record" or "Let me check with the dentist and call you back within the next hour" is the type of response that indicates a sincere effort to help and a willingness to seek a solution to the problem. Remember, if a patient is promised a call back, do it at the time promised. Offer to find an answer if information is not known. Do not force the patient to seek the information himself or herself.

Nothing is more boring than listening to a person who speaks in a monotone. Put expression into what is being said. Add enthusiasm to the voice by using natural voice inflections. To create a smile in the voice, place a mirror in front of the telephone. This ensures that there is a smile on the face before answering the telephone. Try it—it works! If one acts enthusiastic, one becomes enthusiastic.

To be natural, be yourself; do not be a phony. An unnatural voice is easily detected. Keep the breathy "daaarhling," "sweetie," "honey," and "dear" words out of your vocabulary. Remember, "sugar and syrup" have no place in dentistry, so keep them out of your voice.

To speak distinctly, pronounce each syllable of the word completely. When using a telephone, speak directly into the

PRACTICE NOTE

If one acts enthusiastic, one becomes enthusiastic.

Patients who call the dental office have a definite purpose and expect the assistant to be interested in their problems. Therefore, give the patient your undivided attention. Do not interrupt or become preoccupied with another matter. Show interest in the patient's problem by asking appropriate questions and not rushing to terminate the conversation.

PRACTICE NOTE

Give the patient your undivided attention.

PRACTICE NOTE

To be natural, be yourself.

transmitter, which should be 0.5 to 1 inch from the lips. Do not chew gum, eat, bite on a pencil, or cover the mouth with a hand; these all create mumbled conversation and do not present a good image for the dental office. Avoid slang; it is neither businesslike nor in good taste. Some examples of what to say and what not to say include the following:

Avoid	Say
Bye-bye	Goodbye
Huh?	I do not understand. Would you please repeat that?
Uh-huh	Yes Of course
Yeah	Yes Certainly I agree
OK	Yes

Creating a Good Image

In addition to achieving good voice qualities, choose the word or phrase that best communicates the message and makes the best impression. In general, to promote better understanding, use short, simple, descriptive words that are appropriate to the situation. When using technical dental terms, names, numbers, formulas, foreign words, or dictated material, the information should be given slowly and distinctly. Suggestions for identifying letters are presented in Box 10-3; those for identifying numbers are shown in Table 10-1.

A variety of words and phrases in the dental office can convey an unfavorable image to the patient (Figure 10-12). Table 10-2 lists suggestions for appropriate telephone responses that will create a more positive image. Each time the assistant speaks on the telephone, he or she needs to think about what is being said and consider whether that is what is really meant. See things from the patient's point of view and his or her culture to decide whether connotations that should be avoided are being communicated.

BOX 10-3

Using Words to Identify Letters

The following words might be used to identify letters for a caller:

A as in Alice	N as in Nancy
B as in Boy	O as in Old
C as in Charles	P as in Peter
D as in Dog	Q as in Queen
E as in Edward	R as in Robert
F as in Frank	S as in Susan
G as in George	T as in Thomas
H as in Hat	U as in Union
I as in Ida	V as in Victory
J as in Jack	W as in William
K as in King	X as in X-ray
L as in Lion	Y as in Young
M as in Mary	Z as in Zero

TABLE 10-1 Pronouncing Numbers Clearly

Number	Sounds Like	Formation of the Sound
0	Zir-o	Well-sounded Z, short I, rolled R, long O
1	Wun	Strong W and N
2	Too	Strong T and OO
3	Th-r-ee	Single roll of the R, long EE
4	Fo-er	Long O, strong R
5	Fi-iv	I changes from long to short; strong V
6	Siks	Strong S and KS
7	Sev-en	Strong S and V, well-sounded EN
8	Ate	Long A, strong T
9	Ni-en	Strong N, well-sounded EN

Managing Incoming Calls

Although each call to and from the dental office presents a unique situation, most calls can be placed in specific categories, and certain conditions remain constant in each situation. As a result, the administrative assistant is able to formulate certain questions and answers for each situation. Care should be exercised not to use these statements in a rote manner but rather to incorporate the ideas into one's own words and develop a technique that fulfills the philosophy of the dental office. This is especially important when training new personnel who are unfamiliar with the common situations that may arise on the dental office telephone.

The following are examples of typical conversations that illustrate the efficient management of the telephone in a dental office. Some suggestions for managing incoming calls are presented in Box 10-4.

PRACTICE NOTE

Each time the administrative assistant speaks on the telephone, he or she should think about what is being said and ask himself or herself whether that is what is really meant.

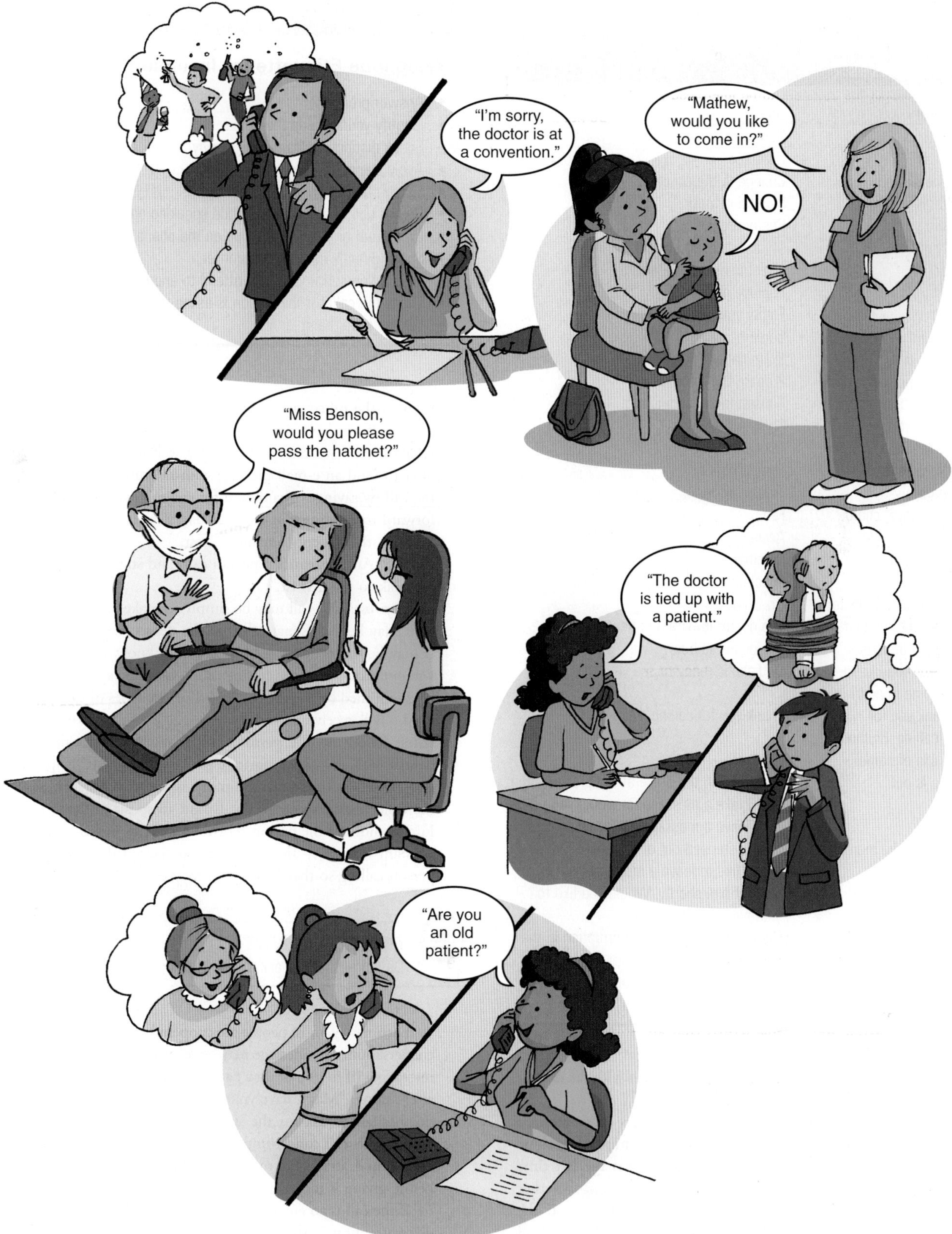
"I'm sorry, the doctor is at a convention."
"Mathew, would you like to come in?"
NO!
"Miss Benson, would you please pass the hatchet?"
"The doctor is tied up with a patient."
"Are you an old patient?"

FIGURE 10-12 Words and phrases that the administrative assistant should avoid using.

TABLE 10-2 Appropriate Words and Phrases to Use in Personal and Telephone Responses

Avoid	Say
Work	Dentistry
Plates	Dentures
Cancellation	Change in the schedule
Waiting room	Reception room
Filling	Restoration
My girl	My assistant or hygienist
Cost	Investment
Pull	Remove or extract
Spit	Empty your mouth
Remind	Confirm
Check-up	Examination
Grind the tooth; drill	Prepare the tooth
Case presentation	Consultation appointment
Rehabilitation	Complete dentistry
Hurt; pain	Uncomfortable
Old patient	Former patient
Operatory	Treatment room
Cost; price; charge	Fee
Bill	Account
Convention	Seminar
Shot	Injection
Joe; Doc; the doctor	Dr. Lake
The doctor is tied up, I'm sorry.	The doctor is with a patient. The doctor is busy.
Would you like to come in now?	Dr. Lake is ready to see you, Mrs. Ward.
Thank you for calling. (without use of name)	Thank you for calling, Mrs. Main.
She is out.	She is not in the office at the present time. May I take a message, or would you prefer to leave a message on her voicemail?
He is in the men's room.	He has stepped out of the office. Would you like to leave a message?
He hasn't come in yet.	I expect him shortly. Would you like to leave a message?
The doctor is running late.	The doctor has had an interruption in the schedule.
When would you like to come in?	Do you prefer mornings or afternoons?

The call: "I would like to make an appointment with the dentist to have my teeth cleaned."
The response: The caller has indicated the nature of the desired treatment, but the administrative assistant must determine whether this is a new patient. Ask, "When was the last time you were seen by Dr. Lake?" This indirectly determines whether this is a former patient (not an "old patient," please). If the patient has never seen Dr. Lake, then further information should be obtained. First, obtain the person's name by asking, "How do I spell your name?" Next, ask the patient who referred him or her; obtain the patient's home and business telephone numbers, his or her home address, and the approximate date of his or her last dental treatment. Because the person has never been to the office, ask if he or she knows where the office is located; if not, give simple and explicit directions. If available, refer the new patient to the office's website for directions, or offer to send an e-mail message with the directions. Conclude the call by saying, "Thank you for calling, Mr. Jones. We look forward to meeting you on Thursday, February 8, at 1:30 PM." Wait for the patient to hang up first.
The call: An unidentified person calls and states, "I would like to speak to the dentist."
The response: This call may be simply to make an appointment, or it may be a personal call that the dentist wishes to receive. It may be someone the dentist does not know, and the person will not state the reason for the call. It is important that a policy be established by the dentist regarding the types of calls that he or she will receive personally. Regardless of the form the call takes, follow up the person's initial request to speak to the dentist with, "Dr. Lake is with a patient. How may I help you?" The "how" is important; if simply asking, "May I help you?" the caller may respond, "No, I want to speak to the dentist." Furthermore, if the person refuses to give his or her name, the assistant may say, "The dentist has requested the name of the person calling so that he (or she) may return your call."

BOX 10-4

Telephone Etiquette for Incoming Calls

- Answer promptly.
- Identify yourself and the office.
- Speak distinctly, clearly, and slowly.
- Avoid slang.
- Listen attentively. Do not interrupt.
- Do not talk to anyone else while speaking on the phone.
- Do not eat or chew gum while on the phone.
- Speak directly into the transmitter.
- Excuse yourself if you must attend to another call.
- Thank the caller if the person is asked to hold.
- Let the caller hang up first.

PRACTICE NOTE
Do not hesitate to ask for the spelling of the caller's name.

Fortunately, most people are cooperative at the outset of the conversation. Any message may be recorded via office electronic messaging (if in use) or on a paper message form (Figure 10-13) after asking, "May I have your name and phone number?" Do not hesitate to ask for the spelling of the caller's name. Then ask, "Is this call concerning dental treatment?" If so, the assistant should attach the message to the patient's clinical record before giving it to the dentist.

If the call is an emergency that warrants the dentist's immediate attention, a short message may be written and given to him or her in the treatment room. Remember, do not discuss other patients or business in front of the person undergoing treatment.
The call: "Hello, this is Mrs. Harris, and I need to see the dentist today to have him look at a tooth that is bothering me."

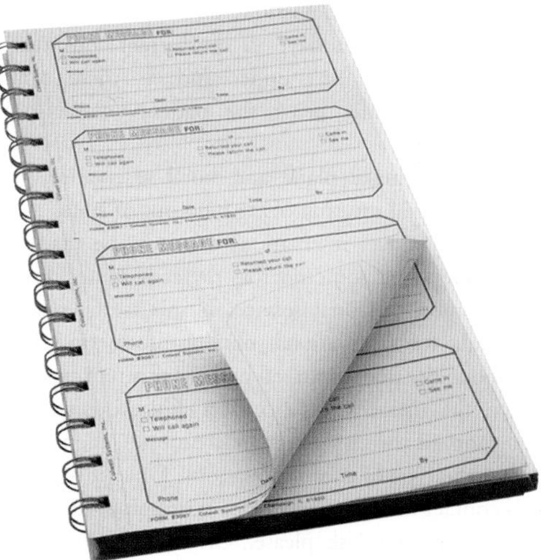

FIGURE 10-13 Message forms allow the administrative assistant to keep accurate records for other dental team members. (Courtesy Patterson Office Supplies, Champaign, Illinois.)

The response: This type of call may or may not be an emergency. Therefore, it is necessary to ask the patient, "How long has the tooth been bothering you?" "How severe is the discomfort?" "Is the tooth sensitive to extreme hot or cold?"

These questions help to determine whether an emergency exists. If the situation is an emergency, the patient should be seen immediately, during reserved buffer time. The patient should be informed that this appointment will be given to relieve the immediate discomfort and that, if further treatment is necessary, an additional appointment will be scheduled. (If this is not done, the patient may anticipate having all of the treatment completed at the emergency appointment.)

If the existing condition is not an emergency, an appointment may be scheduled on another day in the near future.

The call: "This is Mrs. Alvarez. My daughter, Juanita, just fell off her skateboard and broke her front tooth. It's bleeding. What should I do?" (Caller is frantic.)

The response: Patients with emergencies such as this should be seen immediately. The anxious mother should be told to bring the child into the office as soon as possible. Remain calm and reassure the frantic mother by saying, "Place some cold compresses on the area." Evaluate the situation further, and, if the schedule is filled, call some of the later patients and detain them. Do not tell them that the office is "running late"; instead, inform them that there has been an unexpected emergency, and ask them to come in a half-hour later. Patients appreciate consideration of their time and understand that the same care and treatment would be provided to them and their families if they were to have a similar situation.

The call: An unidentified person calls and asks, "How much does Dr. Lake charge for fillings?"

The response: Generally, fees should not be quoted on the telephone. However, fees for basic treatment are often quoted, and some states have a requirement that certain general fees be made available. For major treatment, the patient should come to the office for an examination to determine the extent of treatment needed, because diagnosis cannot be done on the telephone, and the dentist cannot see the conditions in the patient's mouth. It should be remembered that the patient as a consumer has the right to know the basic fees before treatment. In complex situations, the patient should be given an estimate of fees. These factors must be considered when the dentist establishes a policy for quoting fees.

The call: "This is Mr. Huang, and I just received my statement. I think it is awfully high. You must have made a mistake."

The response: Two possibilities exist here: (1) the patient is right, and there is an error on his statement; and (2) there has been a lack of communication with the patient regarding the fee. Regardless of the reason, do not become defensive on the telephone. This always seems to be the first reaction when challenged. Instead, reply, "I'm sorry, Mr. Huang, perhaps I can clarify the statement for you. What is your specific question?" This focuses on the particular problem. Do not make comments until the patient's concern is thoroughly understood. The patient may state, "I sent a check in the mail on the 28th, and you didn't deduct it from the statement." To this, you can respond, "Perhaps we didn't receive it before the billing date, Mr. Huang. If you will wait just a moment, I will be glad to get your record and check it for you." Depress the hold button, and check the patient's record. When you return to the telephone, thank the patient for waiting, and inform him whether the check was received. If an error has been made, tell the patient that it will be corrected and that he will be sent a corrected statement in the mail immediately.

However, if the statement is correct and the patient feels that the fee is too high, return the patient's call rather than keeping him on hold. Such calls are often the result of the dentist's failure to inform the patient of the fee before rendering the service. "Inform before you perform" is a rule that saves many hours on the telephone attempting to explain a patient's statement. In addition, the patient may have been informed of the original treatment plan, but, because of a change in the plan, the fee was higher than originally quoted. It is also possible that the patient still does not understand the treatment plan. In any case, this type of problem is difficult to resolve on the telephone. It is best managed by asking the patient to come into the office, where the treatment plan can be reviewed once again in person.

PRACTICE NOTE

Do not become defensive when dealing with callers.

Managing Outgoing Calls

An administrative assistant places many outgoing calls. The following tips are helpful for the making of such calls:

1. Plan ahead. Be sure to have the telephone numbers programmed or written correctly. If calling a patient, list the name with the telephone number; if calling another dentist's office or business, have that number written down or easily accessible. Be sure to consult the telephone directory if in doubt about a correct telephone number. Names appear in the telephone directory in alphabetical order; however, some public services or governmental agencies may be listed differently. For example, state offices are listed under the state name first and then alphabetically according to office. County and city offices are also listed by county or city name first and then alphabetically according to the office. Federal

offices are listed under "Government" first and then alphabetically according to the office. Parochial and other private schools are listed alphabetically by the name of the school.

Another source for obtaining the correct telephone number for most businesses is the business white pages or yellow pages directory or a directory search if looking online. If the name of the business is known, check in the business white pages in alphabetical order. If the name of a particular dental laboratory is not known but the location is, find the number by consulting the yellow pages under "Dental Laboratories."

2. If the telephone being used is a lighted push-button system, make sure that the line is free before placing the call (the light signals when the line is in use). As the telephone receiver is lifted, make sure that the dial tone is heard before starting to dial. When the call is answered, the administrative assistant must identify himself or herself and then state the name of the dentist for whom he or she is calling.
3. State the reason for calling. If changing a patient's appointment, have another appointment time available. Indicate why the change is being made, because it may cause a disruption in plans, and the patient may also have to adjust another appointment or his or her work schedule.
4. The person who placed the call should also terminate it. It is discourteous to hang up without an indication that the conversation is finished. End the conversation with a courteous "goodbye," and then replace the receiver gently.
5. If a wrong number is reached, apologize for the inconvenience, verify that the number was dialed correctly, and recheck the number before redialing.

PRACTICE NOTE

The person who placed the call should also terminate it.

Examples of common outgoing calls are provided in the following scenarios:

The purpose: To confirm a patient's appointment for the following day.

The call: When the patient answers the telephone, identify yourself, and state the reason for the call: "Hello, Mrs. Thompson, this is Ms. Benson from Dr. Lake's office." (Do not say, "This is Dr. Lake's office calling." Offices do not make calls—people do!) You may then continue with your message, stating it briefly and completely: "I would like to confirm (not "remind you of") your appointment for tomorrow at 1:30 PM with Dr. Lake." When the patient acknowledges it affirmatively, you may simply say, "We look forward to seeing you tomorrow at 1:30," and then conclude the call by saying, "Goodbye." Wait for the patient to hang up.

Sometimes patients send up a "trial balloon" and simply state, "I won't be able to keep the appointment tomorrow, and I'll call you later for another one." Although this may be a legitimate statement and the patient does plan to call you at a later date, you should pursue the conversation, because it may be a signal that there has been a lack of communication with the patient. Instead of abruptly concluding the conversation, ask the patient, "Would it be possible to reschedule your appointment for a week from today?" If the patient continues to be negative, saying, "I don't understand. Is there something wrong?" will generally bring the patient to the point of explanation.

The purpose: To make plane and hotel reservations for the dentist for a dental meeting being held out of state.

The call: Many travel reservations can now be made on the computer. However, some doctors prefer working through an agency for more personal service. If this is the case, before making calls for reservations, obtain information from the dentist about the desired arrival and departure times, the type of service, the airline preference (if a choice exists), the name of the airport (if the city has more than one), the name of the hotel, and the type of accommodations. Once this preparation is done, contact the travel agency or the appropriate airline and ask for "Reservations desk, please." Give the person who answers the necessary information: "I would like to make a reservation for Thursday, January 27, for a flight to Los Angeles, California, from Grand Rapids, Michigan, in the morning, returning on Tuesday, February 1, in the afternoon." After the clerk has provided the available times, decide which flights will be agreeable to the dentist, and then tell the clerk which ones are preferred. For example, "I would like to make a reservation in the business-class section for the flight leaving Grand Rapids at 8:20 AM and arriving at Los Angeles International Airport at 10:57 AM (California time), and returning on the nonstop flight leaving on Tuesday, February 1, at 3:30 PM and arriving at Grand Rapids at 12:35 AM." The reservation is made in the dentist's name. Obtain all flight numbers and details regarding how the confirmation and boarding passes will be transmitted to the office, and send an interoffice memorandum to the dentist via e-mail that contains the information shown in Box 10-5, which includes the itinerary.

Many hotel reservations can be made through a local office, an 800 number, or online. For example, because Dr. Lake preferred to stay at an Ocean Inn, his assistant contacted a local Ocean Inn and made the reservation through this office. Specific information should be given to the clerk regarding the dentist's choice of accommodations, such as preference for a smoking or nonsmoking room or single or double occupancy. After the reservation has been made and a confirmation number given, obtain information about the location of the facility. This

BOX 10-5

Travel Arrangements Memorandum

Departure

Leave: Grand Rapids, Thursday, January 27, Spirit Airlines—Flight #846—8:20 AM (nonstop)

Arrive: Los Angeles National Airport—10:57 AM

Hotel: Ocean Front Inn, 2100 Wilshire Boulevard

Return

Leave: Los Angeles National Airport, Tuesday, February 1, Spirit Airlines—Flight #546—3:30 PM (nonstop)

Arrive: Grand Rapids—12:35 AM

information is included on the itinerary. E-mail verification is typically sent to the dentist and practice, if requested.

The procedure for DDD calls was described previously. However, several factors should be considered when making this type of call. First, when placing a long-distance call to another time zone, the time difference must be kept in mind. The United States is divided into four time zones: Eastern, Central, Mountain, and Pacific (Figure 10-14). For example, if it is 2 PM in Grand Rapids, Michigan (Eastern time zone), it is 1 PM in St. Louis, Missouri (Central time zone), 12 PM in Denver (Mountain time zone), and 11 AM in Los Angeles (Pacific time zone). If in doubt about a time zone, check the time at www.time.gov for any area of the country.

Recording Telephone Messages Carefully

Although many offices have voicemail systems to handle messages, you may need to record messages for the dentist and other staff members. Be prepared for incoming calls by keeping a pencil and message pad handy. Obtaining the correct information when taking a message is of utmost importance. Repeat the message, the spelling of names, and the telephone number if the dentist is to return the call. Take sufficient time to obtain the correct information for the message. Be sure to date the message, indicate the time it was written, and sign it with your name or initials. The message should always be signed by the person taking it in case questions arise later about the information. If the dentist must first find out who took the message, it takes extra time. Forms similar to the one shown in Figure 10-13 may be ordered from most stationery suppliers.

PRACTICE NOTE

Be prepared for incoming calls by keeping a pencil and message pad handy.

Personal Telephone Calls

The telephone in the dental office is installed as a service for the dental patients and should be maintained as a business telephone. Consequently, staff members should refrain from using the telephone for personal calls, and only emergency calls should be made.

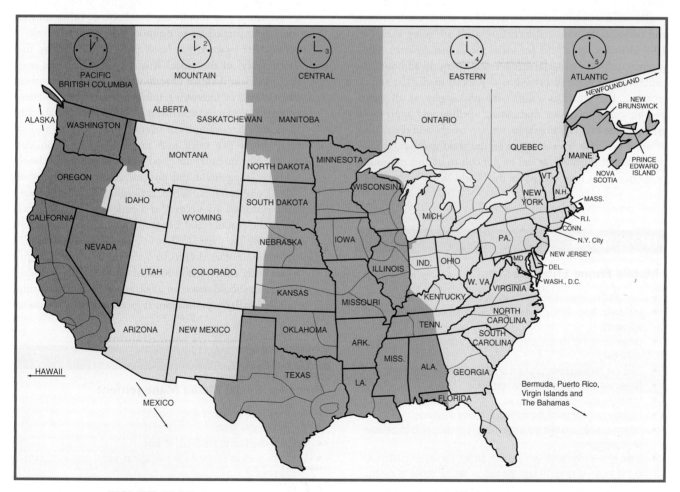

FIGURE 10-14 Time zones in the United States. (From Proctor DB, Adams AP: Kinn's the administrative medical assistant: an applied learning approach, ed 12, St. Louis, 2014, Saunders.)

Cellular Telephone Etiquette

Although most of the calls for the dental office will be made on the traditional telephone, a mobile phone may be used when out of the office. All of the rules regarding voice and telephone use mentioned in the preceding apply to the cellular phone. However, because the cellular phone is used in public spaces, you need to be aware of special etiquette for its use. It is also important to be aware of how to appropriately manage a personal cell phone when at work and in accordance with office policy. Box 10-6 presents a list of suggestions to follow when using a cellular phone.

Social Media

The face of communication in the dental office has been forever changed by the addition of the collective of websites and other online means of communication on the Internet called *social media*. Conversations about dentistry and your practice are likely taking place on the Internet in some fashion, whether or not you are contributing to them. The administrative assistant may be responsible for the oversight of the office's social media plan and schedule, so he or she needs to be very familiar with every aspect in which the practice chooses to participate.

The office's social media plan should be well defined, written, and periodically evaluated to ensure goals are being met. Box 10-7 identifies some rules for social media management. Consistency is the key to social media engagement. In addition, the content of all material posted to any social media site should represent the practice's values and philosophy at all times. Double check to ensure that correct spelling and appropriate grammar are used. Photographs, written words, and the sharing of other materials have an effect on the good name and online reputation of the office. It can be difficult to undo a misguided post after it has been placed on the World Wide Web.

BOX 10-6

Mobile Phone Etiquette

- Turn off the ringer or set to vibrate while in the office.
- Let calls from family members and unimportant calls go to voicemail.
- When using the mobile phone, find a private and quiet place to make calls.
- Turn the mobile phone to silent or vibrate while in meetings.
- Never use the mobile phone in restrooms.
- Eliminate embarrassing ringtones.
- Maintain a quiet voice during mobile phone conversations.
- When possible, use text messages instead of voice calls to maintain professionalism.
- If the phone rings while you are with others, excuse yourself, move out of listening range to take the call, or set the phone to vibrate.
- Do not use the mobile phone while driving.
- Maintain a courteous but succinct introductory message.

Practice website: As the base hub for all social media for the practice, the website should be current and draw potential patients in to want to see more. Several studies indicate that it takes a visitor to your office website less than 1 second to form an impression. The main home page should contain the office logo, a main photo or image, the main navigation menu, a search box, links to other sites in which you participate (e.g., Facebook, Twitter), and minimal written content, because patients do not tend to spend much more than 5 seconds reading this page. Ideally, the website should include a responsive design so that it functions effectively on both desktop browsers as well as mobile devices (e.g., iPad, Android phone).

Practice blog: Your practice blog should be connected to your practice website and identified on the main navigation menu. Blog posts are typically more than 100 words long, and they should be entered at least once a week. They appear in reverse chronological order and contain original or shared information that is relevant to the office or to dentistry; they may also relate to the betterment of the community or support charities and events that are in line with the practice's values. Blogs should be enjoyable, stimulating, enlightening, and engaging. When you post a new entry, you should use Facebook or other sites in which you participate to promote it by posting a link.

Facebook: The practice Facebook page should display the "personality" of the office. This is a site where you may post photos and videos of staff and community events or share a link to interesting information. Office updates, emergencies (e.g., a snowstorm closing), and special occasions are other examples of relevant posts. Posting two to three times per week and remembering to consider quality over quantity are good rules of thumb. Facebook is about engagement and not just about the number of "likes" one receives. When reviewing the office's Facebook postings, ask yourself if a patient will know more about the practice and hopefully be engaged as a result of viewing the page.

Twitter: If your office decides to maintain a Twitter account, it is a daily conversation focused on nurturing relationships; you should shoot for a balance of 90% relationship building to 10% promotion. It gives patients a reason to

BOX 10-7

Rules for Social Media Management

- Set a schedule and stick to it.
- Set measurable goals.
- Set up a checklist of posts and shares.
- Use tools such as Hootsuite to manage all social media accounts in one place.
- Consider that there may come a time when the office will need to outsource the management of its social media.

follow the practice when you "tweet" and "retweet" interesting things. One tip is to follow key leaders in the industry and then retweet posts that are consistent with your office goals and objectives. Twitter requires daily monitoring and posting.

Other sites: YouTube, Google+, and Instagram are other examples of social media sites that could prominently figure into your social media communications. As other sites are developed, the administrative assistant should review and make recommendations regarding whether the office should consider adding them to its social media portfolio.

LEARNING ACTIVITIES

1. List and briefly explain five qualities of a good telephone service.
2. Explain the management of the following calls:
   a. Mr. Sanchez calls the office and says that he has broken a tooth and needs to see the dentist right away.
   b. Mrs. Alvarez calls the office and states that she is new in town. She wants to make an appointment for her son, Jim, who needs to have his teeth cleaned.
   c. Mr. Hubbard calls and states that his daughter was just hit in the mouth with a softball bat and has some broken teeth. He asks, "What do I need to do?"
3. Replace the following statements with statements that would create a better image.
   a. "I'm sorry, the dentist is tied up with a patient."
   b. "Johnny, would you like to come in now?"
   c. "Jennifer, this shot won't hurt much."
   d. "He just went to the men's room."
   e. "I'm sorry, the dentist is running late."
4. Complete a message form for the following telephone conversation: Mr. Schultz from Pine Mutual Insurance Company calls the office and wants the administrative assistant to tell the dentist he will meet her at the Yacht Club at 4:30 PM today. If this is not agreeable, Mr. Schultz can be reached at 495-8272.
5. List and briefly define different telephone systems or services available for use in a dental office.
6. List and briefly describe the various social media sites that may be used by a dental office.

Please refer to the student workbook for additional learning activities.

BIBLIOGRAPHY

Fulton-Calkins PJ, Rankin DS, Shumack KA: The administrative professional, ed 14, Mason, Ohio, 2011, Thomson South-Western.

RECOMMENDED WEBSITES

www.time.gov
www.kellyservices.com
www.ada.org
www.healthgrades.com
www.pewinternet.org
www.ritazamora.com
www.sesamecommunications.com

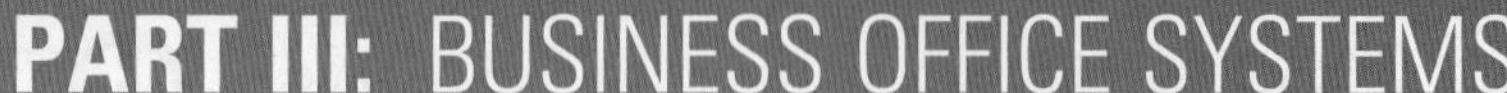

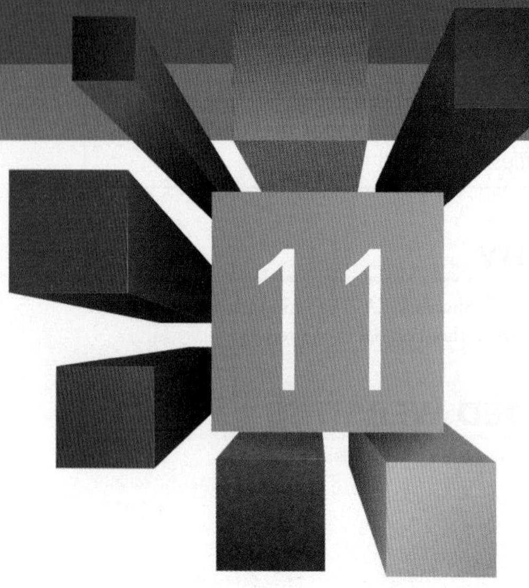

11 Appointment Management Systems

http://evolve.elsevier.com/Finkbeiner/practice

LEARNING OUTCOMES

1. Define the key terms in this chapter.
2. Demonstrate knowledge of appointment management, the advantages of an electronic appointment book, and basic scheduling concepts.
3. Describe the components of an appointment matrix.
4. Demonstrate an understanding of time allocation and other important factors in scheduling appointments.
5. Explain the importance of understanding the dentist's biological clock when scheduling appointments and discuss several scheduling considerations to keep in mind.
6. Apply the basic steps of entering appointments into an appointment system and additional activities included with appointment entries.
7. Demonstrate knowledge of the daily appointment schedule and scheduling patients in an advanced-function practice.

KEY TERMS

Appointment book A hard copy book or scheduling software into which patients and data are entered for appointment times.

Appointment matrix An outline of various activities that routinely occur in the dental practice.

Appointment card The form on which the patient's next appointment is scheduled; the information entered includes the day, date, and time of the appointment.

Buffer period A small amount of time set aside to absorb the hectic workload of the day or to allow for emergencies.

Daily appointment schedule A chronological listing of the day's activities.

Dovetailing Working a second patient into the schedule during another scheduled patient's treatment.

Prime time The busiest time of day in the dental practice.

Treatment plan A sequential listing of the treatment to be completed for a patient.

Unit (u) A given amount of time (generally 10- or 15-minute increments) into which each day of the appointment book is separated.

As mentioned in previous chapters, dentistry is both a business and a healthcare profession. This concept becomes critical when it comes to appointment management. The administrative assistant must be certain that there is a patient being treated in every chair in the office all day long and that the needs of the patient are met to ensure quality care. If there is an empty chair, then there is no production and no revenue, but the overhead continues. However, if the needs of the patient are not met, it is likely that the patient may seek care elsewhere. This chapter describes how to manage an appointment system and how to be aware of common situations that arise in most dental offices.

Appointment management in the modern dental practice most often takes the form of a software system. The traditional appointment book, although still available, is used less frequently (Table 11-1). Appointment management on the computer was one of the last holdouts for many dentists, but today most dentists have realized that electronic appointment scheduling is more efficient and provides a variety of additional benefits that the traditional appointment book does not. Box 11-1 lists the advantages of an electronic appointment book.

PRACTICE NOTE

The dental practice should be controlled through the appointment system but not by it.

Today, the prediction that Bill Gates once made that someday there would be a computer in every household is quite realistic. And in today's dental practice, you will find that there is likely

TABLE 11-1 Symbols for Traditional Appointment Book Entries

Symbol	Meaning
N	New patient
*	Patient prefers an earlier appointment
B	Business phone number
H	Home phone number
L	Case at the laboratory
Ⓛ	Case returned from the laboratory
PM	Premedication required (i.e., medicate patient before treatment)
÷	In red, denotes a confirmed appointment
↓	Length of appointment

BOX 11-1

Advantages of an Electronic Appointment System

- Production goals can help with appointment scheduling.
- Production data are visible daily.
- Data entries are easier to read.
- Autoscheduling eliminates paging through the book.
- Various screen-viewing modes are available.
- Cross-referencing saves time and motion.
- Patient data are more likely to be accurate.
- Searching for appropriate appointment openings is easier.
- Procedures can be posted to several different records from one entry.
- Patient follow-up is easier.
- No manual record filing is necessary.

to be a computer terminal in every treatment room as well as in the business office. For the dental hygienist, this direct access to the appointment scheduler allows for more freedom in scheduling appointments and managing the hygiene schedule.

The appointment system, which contains lists of all the scheduled patients and events for the dentist and the staff, is the control center of the office and an important factor in the success or failure of a dental practice. The practice should be controlled through the appointment system but not by it. Each dental practice should have a scheduling coordinator who maintains the schedule and keeps patients in the dental chairs. In a dental practice in which there is more than one business assistant with no real defined duties, these individuals are likely to perform the same basic functions in the business office, such as answering the phone, collecting money, opening mail, filing, verifying insurance, and making appointments. When no one person is held accountable for any particular assignment, as long as the schedule is full, collections are good, and the practice overhead falls within defined goals, then inefficiencies in the business office are not noticeable. That does not mean that there are no inefficiencies; however, these inefficiencies are not glaringly obvious.

BOX 11-2

Tips for Efficient Appointment Management

1. Put one person in charge of the appointment system.
2. In a traditional appointment book, make accurate and neat entries.
3. Accommodate the patient as much as possible, but maintain control of the appointment schedule.
4. Always have a patient being treated in each dental chair.
5. Avoid scheduling repetitive procedures over long periods.
6. Be aware of production goal criteria.
7. Be aware of scheduling in "power blocks."
8. Schedule the workload according to the staff members' body clocks.
9. Assign clinical tasks only to legally qualified personnel.
10. Avoid leaving large blocks of time between appointments.
11. Establish guidelines for problem situations.
12. Make sure that the practice is controlled through the appointment system rather than by it.

An efficient arrangement for the business staff would be to have one person designated as the scheduling coordinator and one person assigned as the financial coordinator, unless this latter role is fulfilled by a management company. With this arrangement, each staff person can be held accountable for specific assignments, such as scheduling and collections. Job performance, whether good or bad, can then be measured by the amount of downtime (5% or less) and the percentage of collection (a goal of 96% or more).

Poor management of the appointment system can result in mounting tension among staff members, and it can turn the reception room into a waiting room of discontented patients. Basic scheduling concepts are listed in Box 11-2. The entire staff of a dental office should analyze the practice and determine an organized system of appointment control that maximizes productivity, reduces staff tension, and maintains concern for patients' needs.

THE ELECTRONIC APPOINTMENT BOOK

There are a variety of companies that provide electronic appointment scheduling systems, including Curve Dental, Dentrix, Easy Dental, and Eaglesoft. It is not feasible to provide instructions for all of these programs, but the concepts of appointment scheduling are similar for all of them. If a user learns one system, then he or she should be able to adapt easily to scheduling with the use of almost any other software product. The websites for these companies are listed at the end of this chapter.

With an electronic appointment system, appointments can be entered, canceled, rescheduled, and moved easily with one keystroke. Electronic scheduling can be goal oriented, with the use of state-of-the-art technology to set production goals for the practice. With income a consideration (rather than just filling the book), the dentist can begin to maximize profits while controlling where and when certain procedures are performed.

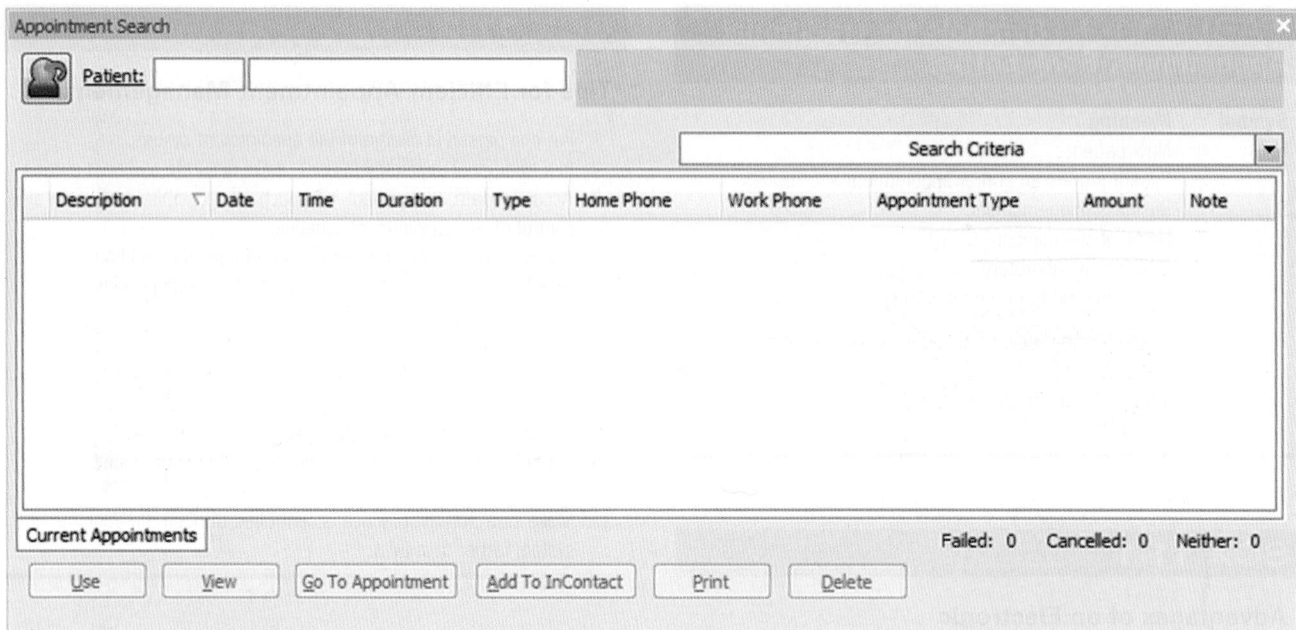

FIGURE 11-1 Search screen for locating an available appointment opening. (Courtesy Patterson Office Supplies, Champaign, Ilinois.)

Common electronic software scheduling packages generally have a number of components, including the following:

- *Finding the next available appointment:* This feature allows the staff member to find an open appointment time in a matter of seconds. It lets the person scheduling the appointment search on specific days, during specific hours, and for selected providers; it then provides a list of available appointments so that the patient may select what works best for him or her. Figure 11-1 shows a screen that will enable the appointment coordinator to search for an available appointment.
- *Daily appointment screen:* Most software programs allow for a wide variety of setup and viewing options for the office schedule. This allows the office staff members to select the options that work best for them. Generally these views show the treatment rooms in a column format with each patient's name, his or her treatment information, and a list of resources needed for each time unit (Figure 11-2). An expanded view will offer more details about the appointment. There is often an easy way to advance from date to date or to show the schedule in a weekly format (Figure 11-3).
- *Patient information window:* In most systems, the patient information screen (Figure 11-4) shows many types of information, including demographic, financial, insurance, recall, and appointment details. Patient information that can be entered on this record includes the patient's complete name, marital status, gender, age, date of birth, and work, cell, and home phone numbers. There is often an easy way to view the patient's current balance, pharmacy and medication histories, examination history, treatment plan, financial information, referrals, medical alerts, treatment completed, and appointment time preferences, each of which are updated on the patient screen after being entered in different areas of the program.
- *Locate appointment feature:* Most scheduling software allows the user to search to see whether a patient has an existing appointment. This is very valuable when a patient calls and thinks he or she has an appointment but cannot remember the date (Figure 11-5).
- *Goal tracking:* The dental staff can set monthly goals by provider and enter these goals into the system. The software can then report a summary of the scheduled production, the monthly goal, the percentage of the goal that was attained, any new patients, the total number of appointments, and the production totals so that the staff can track how they are performing toward the meeting of the goal (Figure 11-6).
- *Short call list:* Electronic appointment books allow for the excellent tracking of any appointments that were canceled and not rescheduled, for patients who want to come in earlier if an appointment opens up, or for patients who want to be called if there is a cancellation. Figure 11-7 illustrates a short call list of people who can be contacted quickly to fill an opening in the appointment book.
- *New calendar year:* Electronic appointment books usually will automatically load each year's calendar based on the preference set. The calendar is perpetual but, at the beginning of each year, the calendar should be reviewed for possible changes.

DESIGNING THE APPOINTMENT BOOK MATRIX

An appointment book matrix, which is an outline of the appointment book, functions like the matrix of a restoration:

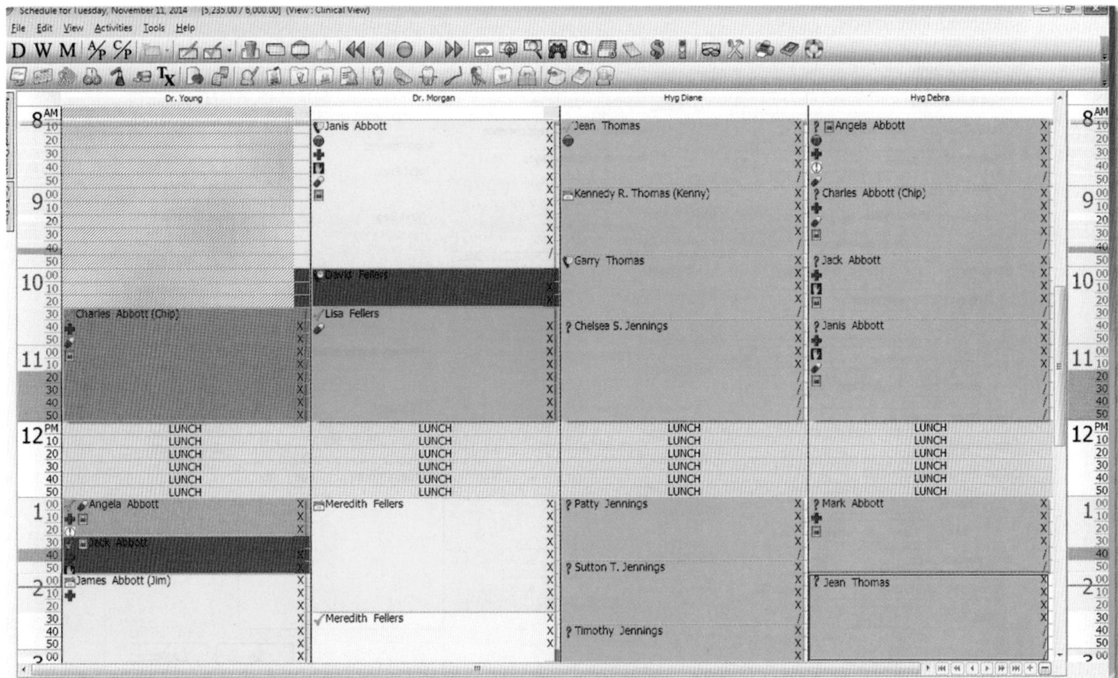

FIGURE 11-2 Daily appointment screen (expanded view). (Courtesy Patterson Dental, St. Paul, Minnesota.)

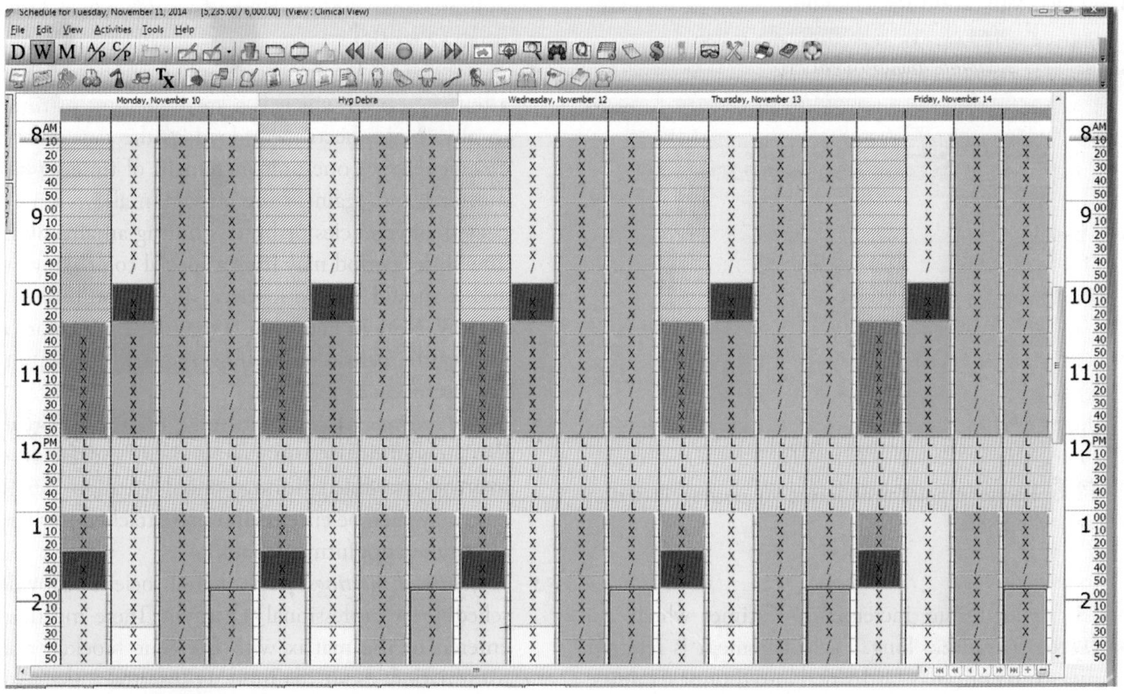

FIGURE 11-3 Quick-glance screen showing a week at a glance. (Courtesy Patterson Dental, St. Paul, Minnesota.)

it provides support (see Figure 11-8 for the components of an electronic appointment book). This is the framework around which appointments are made. A new matrix should be completed before each new year begins. The use of color-coding in the electronic system allows the scheduling coordinator to use a variety of colors for various activities. The matrix should include the following elements:

- *Columns:* Columns are provided for each of the treatment rooms. They may be numbered or assigned by the name of the operator, the dentist, or the hygienist. Each of the

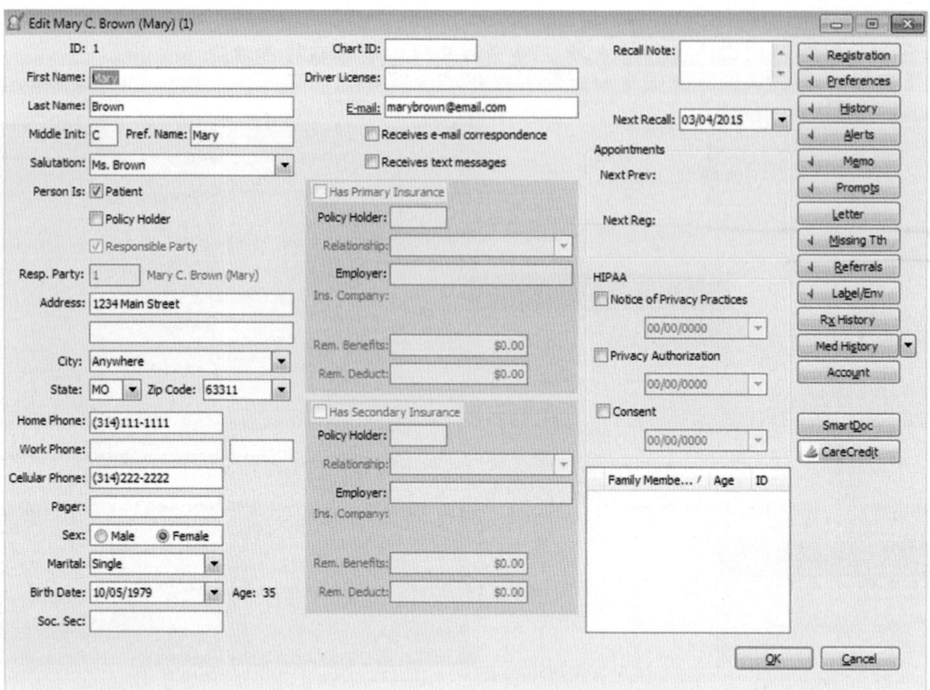

FIGURE 11-4 Patient information screen. (Courtesy Patterson Dental, St. Paul, Minnesota.)

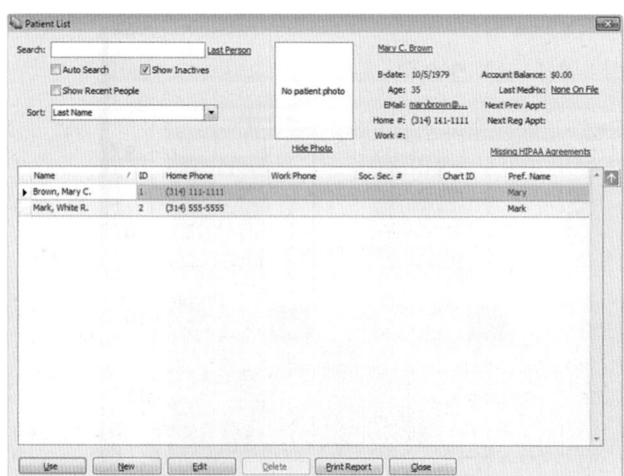

FIGURE 11-5 Locate appointment screen. (Courtesy Patterson Dental, St. Paul, Minnesota.)

columns is divided into increments of time, which are usually 10 to 15 minutes long. Each increment is referred to as a **unit**, so an hour may be divided into four or six units, depending on the time increment of the column. The 10-minute unit has become generally accepted for expanded function practices. The illustration in Figure 11-8 shows columns in which each unit is 10 minutes in length.

- *Holidays:* Holidays can be noted in the electronic appointment book, and they may be part of the template set up by the office staff.
- *Lunch hours:* Computerized scheduling will follow the template and will automatically insert lunch hours. Figure 11-8 indicates that the lunch hour for this particular practice is from 12 to 1.
- *Buffer periods:* Again, the template can automatically insert a **buffer period**, which is a small amount of time set aside to absorb the hectic workload of the day or to allow for emergencies. A one-unit increment of time set aside in the morning and again in the afternoon allows time for unexpected emergencies or buffers during an already hectic day. The buffer period may have a special color designated for it, and it should not be inserted during the busiest period of the day. Note in Figure 11-9 that there is a color-coded unit for a buffer period in the morning at 11:45 AM and again in the afternoon at 2:30 PM.
- *School calendar:* A school calendar may be obtained from the local school districts so that students and faculty members may be scheduled during school vacation periods. These data may then be entered in notes attached to the day in the electronic appointment book.
- *Professional meetings:* Most dental societies provide a yearly schedule of professional meetings. These meetings may be entered in the matrix with the time blocked out and the information about the meeting inserted.
- *Staff meetings:* Morning huddle time need not be part of the matrix, because it is routinely done each morning. However, time should be set aside regularly (e.g., weekly, once or twice a month) for all members of the staff to meet and discuss office activities and goals. This time should not be scheduled during the lunch period or after office hours but should instead be integrated into regular office hours and indicated on the schedule (see Chapter 2 for suggestions about scheduling staff meetings).

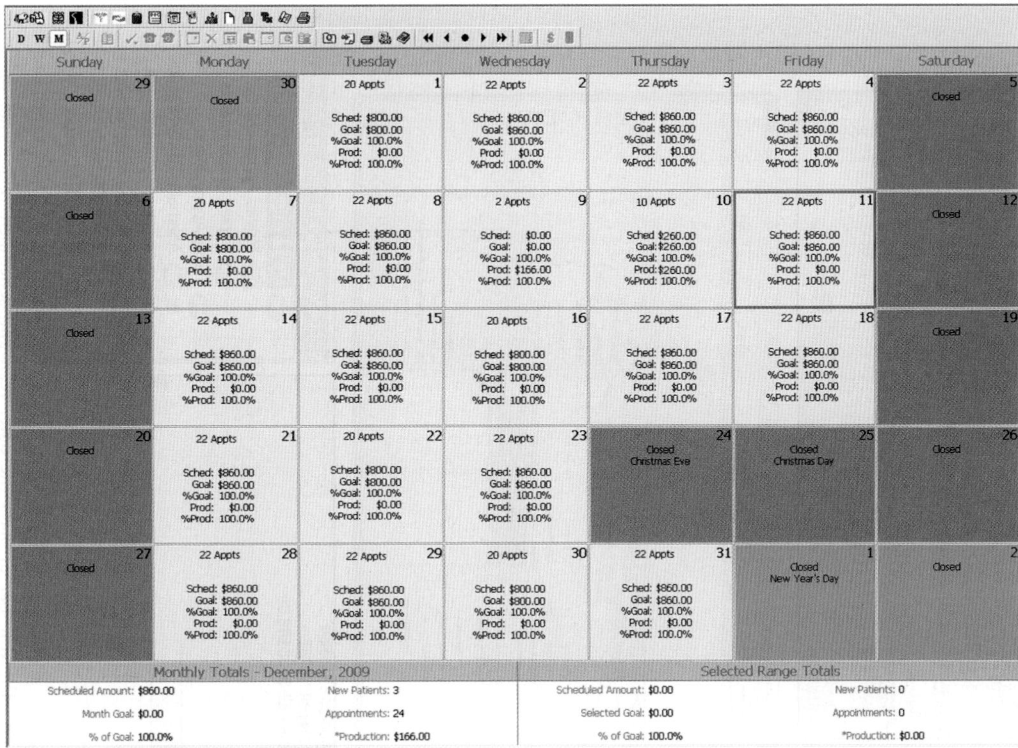

FIGURE 11-6 Goal-tracking screen. (Courtesy Patterson Dental, St. Paul, Minnesota.)

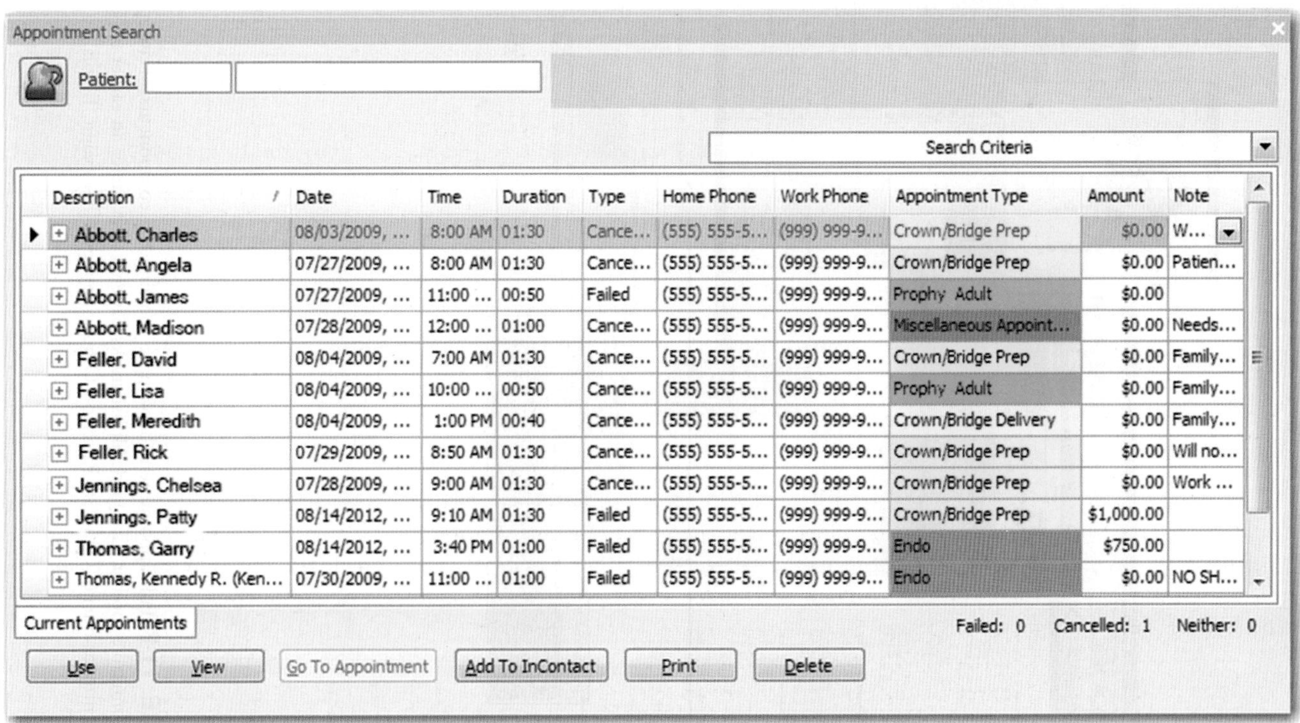

FIGURE 11-7 Short call list feature. (Courtesy Patterson Dental, St. Paul, Minnesota.)

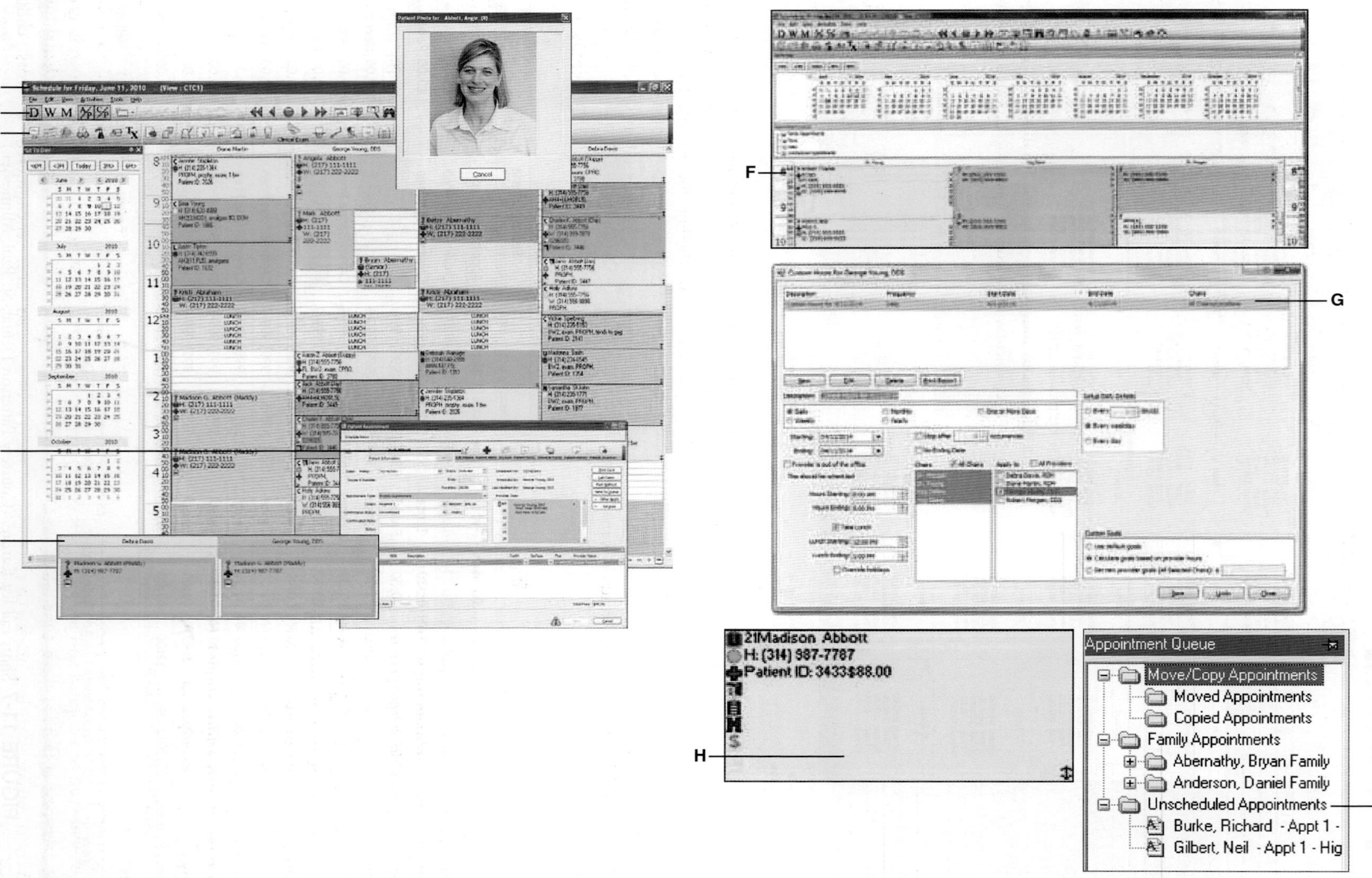

FIGURE 11-8 Full appointment book page showing the components of an appointment book. **A,** The title bar displays the date, year, and scheduled versus goal summary. **B,** Customizable toolbar. **C,** Quick fill list tracks patients who prefer an earlier appointment. **D,** Patient bar. **E,** Provider view. **F,** Dockable panels. **G,** Custom hours. **H,** Indicators. **I,** Appointment queue (Courtesy Patterson Office Supplies, Champaign, Ilinois.)

Tuesday, April 24	
8	
15	
30	
45	
9	
15	
30	
45	
10	
15	
30	
45	
11	
15	
30	
45 JOHN FLETCHER FR #8	
12	
15	
30	
45	
1	
15	
30	
45	
2	
15	
30	
45	
3	
15	
30	

FIGURE 11-9 A one-unit buffer is highlighted. Note the color-coding used in the appointment book.

- *Vacation days:* There may be times when the entire staff will be on vacation, and this time should be blocked out. This type of scheduling should be done with as much advance notice as possible.

APPOINTMENT TIME SCHEDULE

Time allocation for each type of treatment should be determined by the staff and a template provided so that all those responsible for appointment management understand the number of units that need to be scheduled for each type of treatment. Basically, the same type of treatment should take the same amount of time (e.g., a full gold crown preparation on a molar may take a dentist two or three units, 30 to 45 minutes, depending on the type of unit). However, not every patient is the same. What may take three units with one patient may require four units for another. An average amount of time for each type of procedure should be determined; when a complex procedure is anticipated, the dentist needs to identify this with the appointment scheduler so that a time adjustment can be made.

After the average time is determined for a variety of services provided, then a schedule can be designed and provided to the entire staff so that everyone is familiar with time allocations. Care should be given to consider the time needed to clean and prepare a treatment room when making this schedule. Once the appointment lengths are determined, appointment types can be added to the computer, which are then templated for these times, to make scheduling consistent and easy.

IMPORTANT FACTORS TO CONSIDER WHEN SCHEDULING APPOINTMENTS

The administrative assistant must deal with a variety of situations when scheduling appointments. The management of the appointment book requires a well-defined treatment plan, an established appointment sequence, and an ability to maintain strict control over the appointment book while still meeting the needs of patients.

Several of these situations are common to all dental offices. For an assistant with several years of experience, managing such problems is fairly easy, but it may be more difficult for an inexperienced individual. The office staff should identify situations that commonly occur and develop a policy for managing appointments for these situations.

Emergency Patients

Patients who call the office for emergencies should be seen by the dentist during designated buffer periods. When a patient calls and requests an immediate appointment for a toothache, ask the patient the following questions: "How long has the tooth been bothering you?," "Which tooth is it?," "What type of discomfort are you experiencing: a sharp pain or a dull ache?," and "Is the tooth sensitive to hot, cold, or pressure?" At this point, determine whether the patient has a true emergency. It is then prudent to say, "The dentist's schedule is filled for the day, but Dr. Lake could see you to relieve the discomfort at 10:30 this morning. Then, if further treatment is necessary, we can schedule an additional appointment." This eliminates any preconceived idea that the dentist's schedule permits time for extensive treatment that has not been scheduled. If the patient finds it difficult to come in at the suggested time, it may be necessary to schedule the appointment for a later date.

A dentist should always be prepared to see patients of record for emergencies or to make provisions for such coverage in his or her absence. Emergency treatment for new patients can become a lifeline for a dental practice. These patients often become excellent patients in the future. They appreciate being seen by the dentist on an emergency basis and often accept treatment plans willingly to avoid future emergencies.

Young Children

Young children should be scheduled at times that will not interfere with their nap periods or their regularly scheduled activity times. For these reasons, early morning is generally considered a good time for a young child's dental appointment. Have you ever encountered a cross child just before nap time, or have you ever had to call a child in from play to go to the dentist? Ask the mother about the child's daily routine, and be considerate when scheduling these appointments.

Older Adults

Older patients often require special attention. Although they may arise early, these patients may find rush-hour traffic very disconcerting, whereas others may find it difficult to get out the door quickly in the morning. Although many older patients require special considerations, remember not to embarrass them by calling attention to their age.

THE DENTIST'S BODY CLOCK

Complex cases, such as crown and bridge work, are best scheduled at a time when the dentist is experiencing a peak energy period. Not all people are at their best at all times of the day. Early morning has generally been considered the best time for extensive treatment. However, some dentists do not reach their peak period until 1 or 2 PM, when the early birds who were dynamic at 8 AM have begun to lose energy. This becomes an important factor to consider to determine when certain types of treatment should be scheduled. As a rule, appointments for extensive operative and surgical treatment and those that involve the management of difficult children should be made at the dentist's peak time.

Scheduling for Productivity

One of the most effective ways for a business such as a dental office to be profitable is to increase productivity. The dentist should focus on procedures that are most profitable while performing the routine tasks or delegating them when this is legally possible. Theodore Schumann, a noted Certified Public Accountant (www.dentalbusinesssuccess.com), explains that the typical practitioner produces about $300 to $500 per hour. It is not uncommon to produce even less than this if the scheduling system is not managed effectively. Over the course of the year, if the dentist increases production by just $50 per hour, annual production could increase by $76,000, of which about $60,000 would be additional profit. These amounts may fluctuate depending on the region of the country where the office is located, but the concept remains the same.

This is where the administrative assistant needs to think outside the box and modify the old ways of scheduling. To achieve this increased productivity, hourly production must increase. When this concept is considered in conjunction with the dentist's body clock, the way scheduling is done can begin to be modified. If "power blocks" of time are set aside for high-productivity and high-profit procedures, production will increase. Therefore, if the dentist's body clock means that he or she is most productive from 10 AM to 2 PM, then all high-productivity procedures (and *no* other types of treatment) must be scheduled during that period. This time must be reserved for productive and profitable procedures, and all attempts to break into these power blocks must be forestalled. It takes time to make this system work, and it requires a different mindset at first. However, after about 6 months, this concept will be found to be very effective, and the practice will begin to reap the profits.

Extended Office Hours

Many offices develop a schedule that includes extended office hours, which are hours beyond the traditional work day. These may include early morning, evening time, or weekend days. There is no significant difference in scheduling appointments for this type of practice, but it requires special attention in the selection of an appointment book and designing the matrix. Care should be taken that the days identified for extended hours include times to cover all the hours the office will be open. This situation may require an unmarked appointment book that allows insertion of days and times in accordance with the office schedule. Computer scheduling should easily accomplish extended office hours.

Management of Prime Time

Prime time is the time period that is most often requested by patients; in most offices, it is generally after 3 PM. Obviously, not all patients who request appointments during this time will receive them; therefore, patients must be informed of the need to schedule this time on a rotating basis. Forms are available for students who will need to be excused from class time to attend their dental appointments.

Habitually Late Patients

A small number of patients are continually late for their appointments. Stress the importance of being on time for the appointment by explaining, "Mr. Campbell, the nature of your treatment requires all of the time allotted; therefore, we must ask your cooperation in being on time for your appointments." This should be done in a firm but pleasant manner. Another way of handling this situation is to enter an earlier time on the **appointment card** than is entered in the appointment book. However, be careful, because this could backfire! Care should be taken to enter a code in the appointment block that indicates the patient was told an earlier time. "TP" is a code that could be used to indicate that the patient was told to come one unit earlier than the time shown in the appointment entry. In this way, all staff members would know what the patient had been told.

Series Appointments

Care should be taken to not schedule too many appointments for a patient at one time. The patient who has a long series of appointments is likely to cancel more readily; he or she may believe that the treatment scheduled for the current appointment can be done during his or her next scheduled appointment when in fact the appointments may not be of the same length. This disrupts the treatment schedule. It is acceptable to make tentative appointments beyond 2 to 3 weeks, but do not list them on the appointment card until the patient has completed the first series.

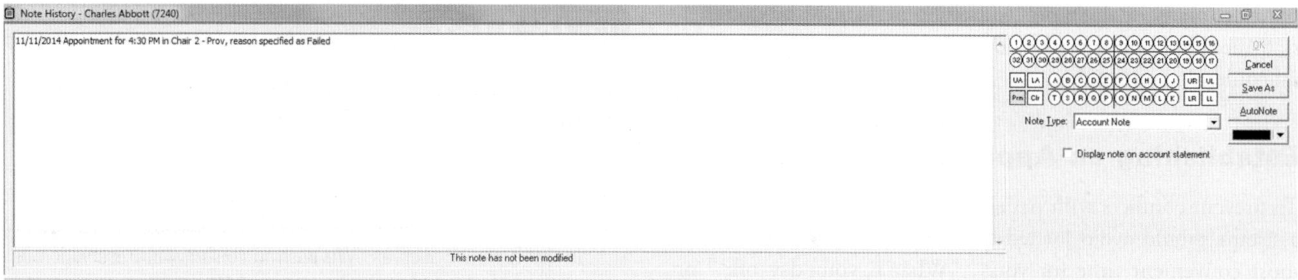

FIGURE 11-10 Clinical chart showing a broken appointment. (Courtesy Patterson Dental, St. Paul, Minnesota.)

Patient Who Arrives on the Wrong Day

No office would be complete without a patient who arrives on the wrong day or at the wrong time. The error may be the patient's, or the assistant may have written the wrong date on the appointment card. Ask to see the appointment card and, if the patient has made the mistake, indicate the actual date and time of the appointment. Of course, if the administrative assistant or another staff member made the error, an apology is necessary, and the patient should be seen by the dentist. The scheduled patients may be contacted to explain that an "unexpected change has occurred in the schedule" and thus asked to delay their arrival. Regardless of who is responsible for the error, the assistant should remain tactful and helpful when correcting the mistake.

Drop-Ins

Nothing is more frustrating than to have a patient drop by the office and say, "I was just in the area, and I thought I'd drop in and see if Doc could do something to this tooth that's been bothering me." Seeing a patient on this basis can open a Pandora's box and create the notion that the patient can just drop in at any time. Tactfully inform the patient that the dentist sees patients by appointment, and then tell him or her when the next appointment is available. However, if the drop-in patient is a patient of record and has a legitimate emergency, try to accommodate him or her.

This practice does not apply to the many walk-in (convenience) dental clinics that have been established during the past few years. One of the prime objectives of these clinics is to accommodate patients who do not have appointments.

Broken Appointments

At times a patient absolutely must cancel an appointment or is prevented from keeping the appointment by some unforeseen circumstance. Most patients respect the dentist's time, and the dentist should understand when a cancellation occurs. Other patients, unfortunately, always seem to find an excuse for breaking an appointment. Although most dentists' initial reaction is to charge for broken appointments, this becomes difficult to

Friday, April 22		
8	MS. HAZEL GATES	(JOHN)
15	PREP. #7 PVC	
30	↓ H-459-7252	B-454-2100 EXT. 29
45	MR. JOHN MON	ROE
9	PREP. #31 F.C.	
15	↓ H-243-6410	B-454-6300
30		
45		

FIGURE 11-11 Dovetailing on an appointment page in a traditional appointment book.

accomplish and results in poor public relations. The patient should be informed of the importance of keeping the appointment: "Mr. Ward, since you failed to keep your 2-hour appointment, the treatment schedule has been delayed. I can only reschedule such a lengthy appointment if we can be assured that you will be here." Such cancellations should be noted on the patient's clinical chart (Figure 11-10).

If the patient continues to cancel appointments, the following statement could be made: "Mr. Ward, we are unable to continue to make appointments for you because you have failed to cooperate with us." However, such a policy should be exercised only after it has been approved by the dentist, and be certain to follow the recommended guidelines of state law regarding dismissing a patient from the practice.

Dovetailing

Minor types of treatment can easily be accomplished in less than one unit of scheduled time. **Dovetailing** means working a second patient into the schedule during another scheduled patient's treatment (e.g., while the first patient waits for an anesthetic to take effect or an impression to set). The appointment page shown in Figure 11-11 has four places for dovetailing: at 8 AM, while waiting for anesthesia for Hazel Gates; at approximately 8:30 AM, while waiting for the final impression to set; at 8:45 AM, while waiting for anesthesia for John Monroe; and at 9 AM, while waiting for John Monroe's final impression to set.

Many types of appointments can be dovetailed, such as denture adjustments, suture removal, healing checks, restoration polishing, and dressing changes. In an expanded-duties practice, many of these procedures are performed by qualified staff members and must be dovetailed appropriately into their schedules.

Establishing an Appointment Time

To prevent conflicts with patients over appointment times, the assistant should avoid loaded questions, such as "What is the most convenient time for you?," "What is your day off?," or "When does Frank get out of school?" It is wiser to ask, "Is morning or afternoon better for you?"; the patient can then be presented with two appointment options. By encouraging the patient to make a choice that is realistic for the office's schedule, the assistant will not be forced to say "I'm sorry" to each of the patient's suggestions.

Confirming Appointments

The practice of confirming an appointment versus not confirming it is often a reason for debate. Regardless of the approach that the dentist chooses for the practice, it is vital to use the term *confirm* rather than *remind;* the word *remind* does not quite sound professional, especially to an adult. However, most patients appreciate the confirmation of an appointment.

The issue with confirming an appointment is that few other professionals make such calls. Over the years, dentistry has adopted the policy of confirming appointments, and this practice has been perpetuated. Many practice management consultants believe that, when a patient is well educated about the need for complete and thorough dental care, he or she will respect the appointment time and follow through with all appointment times. With the use of e-mail, text messages, and answering machines, it is easy to confirm appointments if a few basic rules are followed. Before dismissing the patient when a future appointment is needed, ask the patient whether he or she needs a courtesy confirmation call or notice. This will retrain the patient to accept responsibility for the appointment. Box 11-3 lists some suggestions for placing confirmation calls or sending notices by e-mail.

BOX 11-3

Suggestions for Placing Confirmation Calls or Sending Notices via E-mail

- Ask patients if they would like a courtesy confirmation call or e-mail.
- If the confirmation is for a preventive recall appointment, do not trivialize that appointment by calling it a "cleaning." You may wish to use a phrase such as "We wish to confirm your reservation in our hygiene department on Tuesday at 3:00 p.m."
- Avoid leaving confirmation messages on an answering machine for any patient who has a history of broken appointments.
- Do not allow patients to leave messages of cancellation on the office answering machine over the weekend.
- Avoid leaving a message on a patient's answering machine that requires the patient to call back to confirm receipt of the message. This is disruptive to the office's schedule, and it can be annoying to the dependable patient.
- Use a short and succinct message of confirmation: "Hello, Mrs. Gomez. This is Mary at Dr. Lake's office. I'm calling to confirm your reservation with our dental hygiene department on Wednesday, May 5, at 10 AM. Please call our office within 24 hours of the appointment if there is a change in your schedule. Thank you for your consideration." When sending an e-mail confirmation, the message should be as succinct as it is for the telephone.

ENTERING APPOINTMENTS

Overview

As mentioned previously, one person should be in charge of the appointment system at all times. This does not mean that no one else can make appointments, but this person must routinely check the appointment book and manage it according to the guidelines that the staff has determined. The dentist should never encourage friends or relatives to "drop by the office"; rather, he or she should direct everyone to contact the administrative assistant or appointment manager for an appointment. Great effort should be made to schedule the next appointment for a patient when the patient is in the office. Never let the patient say "I will call you," because the person will forget and get distracted by many other activities at home and in his or her personal life.

When new patient appointments are made, the sequence normally followed in a dental office is the initial examination and prophylaxis, radiographs, and diagnostic models. After the dentist has concluded the diagnosis and treatment plan, the patient returns for a consultation appointment. At this time, the patient accepts the original or modified treatment plan, and the assistant makes the necessary appointments in the recommended time and sequence.

After treatment is complete, the patient is recalled periodically via the preventive recall or recare system outlined in Chapter 12. An appointment sequence must be established in coordination with the treatment plan. To do this, the dentist needs to establish the sequence and the amount of time needed for each appointment for all types of treatment. In an electronic system, the information is entered when the system is set up, and the appointment time is entered automatically (Box 11-4).

After establishing the appointment sequence, refer to the patient's **treatment plan** to determine what must be done. The treatment plan is completed at the time of the diagnosis by the dentist and recorded on a treatment plan shown similar to the one shown in Figure 11-12. The template for sequencing will enable the assistant to make appropriate and properly sequenced and timed appointments.

At this point, the times for the appointments should be determined by using the suggestions made previously. Care should be taken to eliminate useless voids in the schedule by always beginning to schedule appointments at the bottom or top of a large block of time (never in the middle) and not leaving units of time (except for buffers) vacant between appointments.

The following steps provide an outline of how to make an appointment entry using the Eaglesoft *OnSchedule* system. Please note that this procedure is common to many other electronic systems.

BOX 11-4

Information to Include in an Appointment Book Entry

- The patient's full name, with cross-references in case of the duplication of names
- The patient's home and business phone numbers to confirm the appointment or to reach the patient in case of an emergency
- The treatment to be done
- The age of the patient (if he or she is a child)
- The length of the appointment (indicated with an arrow)
- Any special notations (e.g., new patient, premedication required, case at the laboratory)

New Appointment

Select the date and time you would like to make the appointment by clicking on the cell in the appointment book. Select the patient from the *Patient* hyperlink, or use the *Last Patient* button (Figure 11-13).

Patient Information

Use the *Patient bar* to open other features such as *Alerts and Treatment Plan* that you may want to review before making the appointment such as *Patient Details* and *Insurance Information* (Figure 11-14). Select the *Insurance Information* tab; review the *Primary* and *Secondary* information (Figure 11-15, *A* and *B*).

Appointment Entry

Use the dropdown arrows to select the *Appointment Type* and *Provider* for the appointment. This should fill most of the appointment fields with your predetermined appointment guidelines. Use the dropdown arrow to select the *Confirmation Status,* and enter a *Confirmation Note* if desired (Figure 11-16).

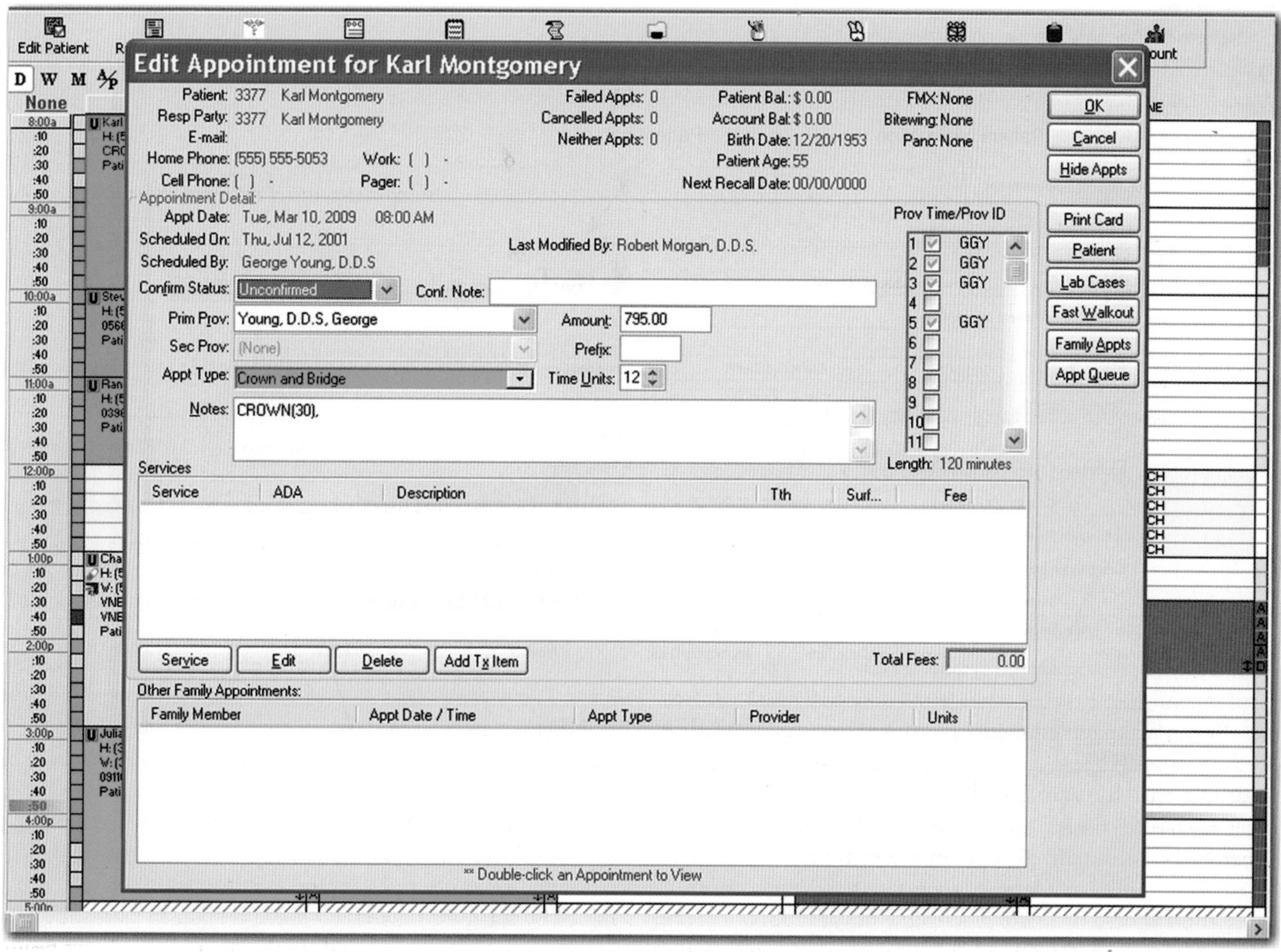

FIGURE 11-12 Electronic treatment plan screen. (Courtesy Patterson Dental, St. Paul, Minnesota.)

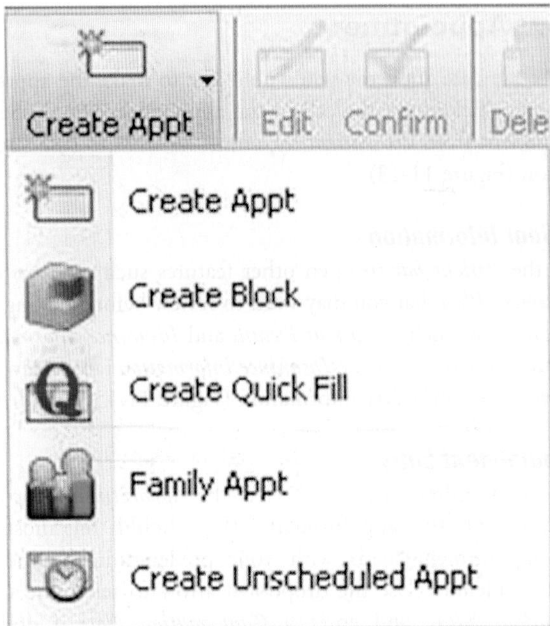

FIGURE 11-13 Create a new appointment in *OnSchedule.* (Courtesy Patterson Dental, St. Paul, Minnesota.)

Provider Time on Appointment

Click and drag in the *Provider Time* area to change the time allotted per provider (Figure 11-17).

Double-click or right-click on an empty space to add another provider to the same appointment.

Services

Select the *Services* button to pin the *Services* window to the bottom of the appointment. The *Services* window defaults to the provider attached to the appointment and to the time units selected previously. Use the *Add Services* button to add more service codes to the current appointment. Select *Add Tx Item* to select an item from an existing *Treatment Plan.* To delete a service, select the checkbox and then select *Delete.* Edit the provider for individual services by selecting the *Provider* field.

Tabs

In order to make the best use of the available space on a computer screen but still offer options and features, computerized schedules often have tabs on the scheduler window.

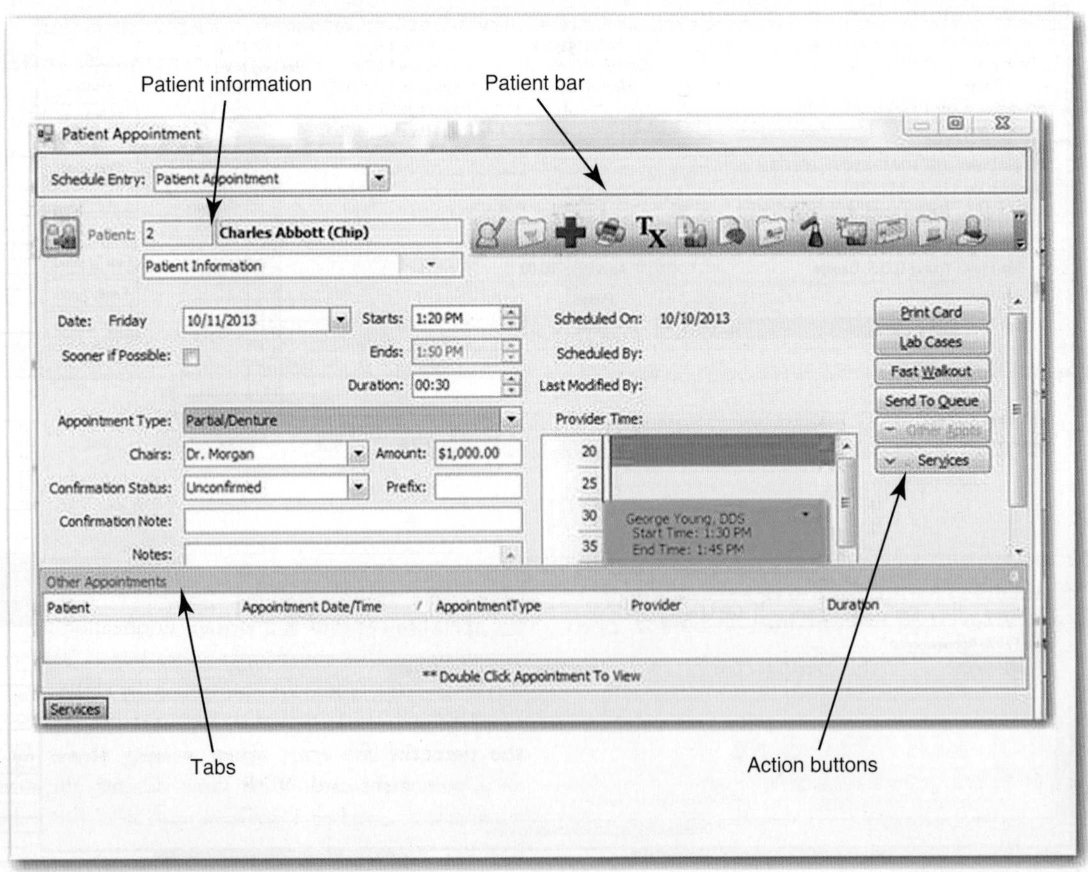

FIGURE 11-14 The patient information screen provides patient details. (Courtesy Patterson Dental, St. Paul, Minnesota.)

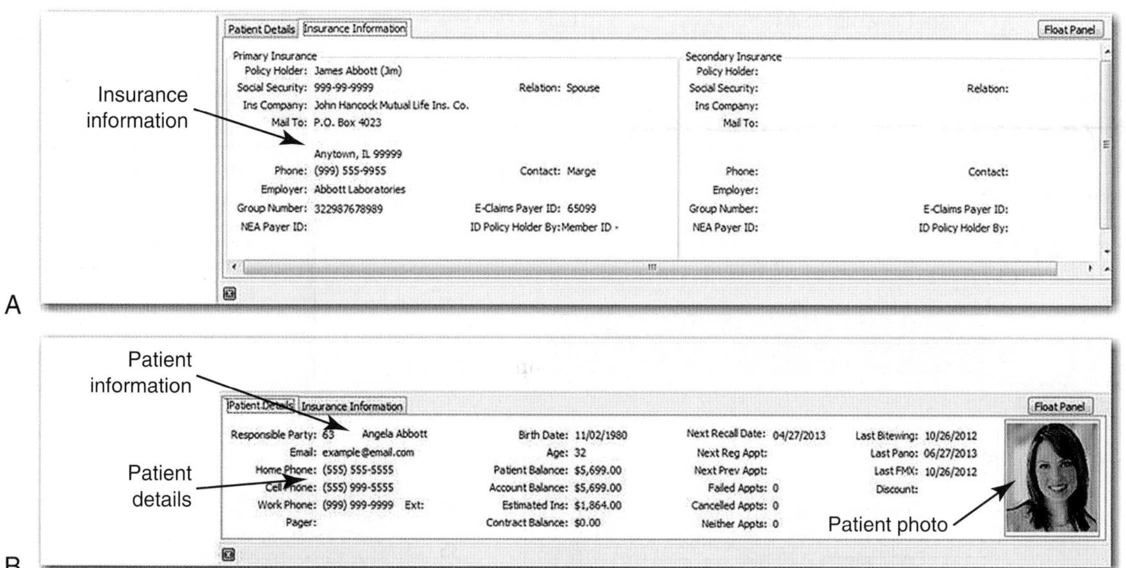

FIGURE 11-15 Floating the information panel. **A,** Insurance information. **B,** Floating the panel. (Courtesy Patterson Dental, St. Paul, Minnesota.)

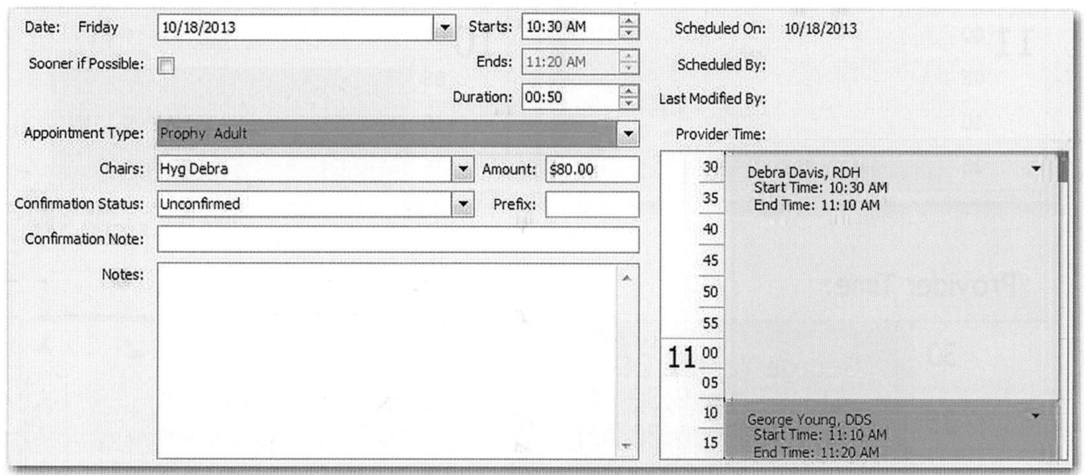

FIGURE 11-16 Templates with appointment details are available to make appointment scheduling quick and easy. (Courtesy Patterson Dental, St. Paul, Minnesota.)

When the functionality of the tab is desired, the operator can hover over the tab and it will expand to view the information/functionality on the tab. These tabs can often be "pinned" open if the staff would prefer (Figure 11-18).

ADDITIONAL ACTIVITIES IN APPOINTMENT ENTRIES

Appointment Search

Select the *Appointment Search* button to locate any existing appointments for an individual patient, or enter search criteria to find available appointment times (Figures 11-19 and 11-20).

Appointment Card

An appointment card is a written notification of the patient's appointment that the patient takes home. This card can be made directly from the computer by following the steps listed below. The use of the electronic system does eliminate the potential for error when writing things by hand on an appointment card. With some systems, the next appointment can be listed on a walkout statement, but many patients like the security of a separate appointment card; thus, this can easily be printed from the computer. It is always wise to recheck the appointment card just in case the wrong key has been depressed.

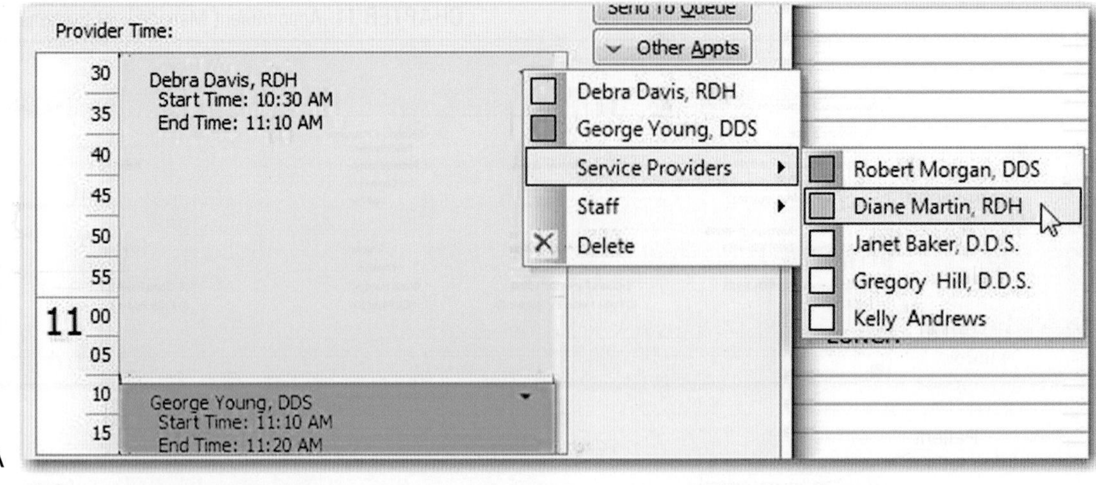

A

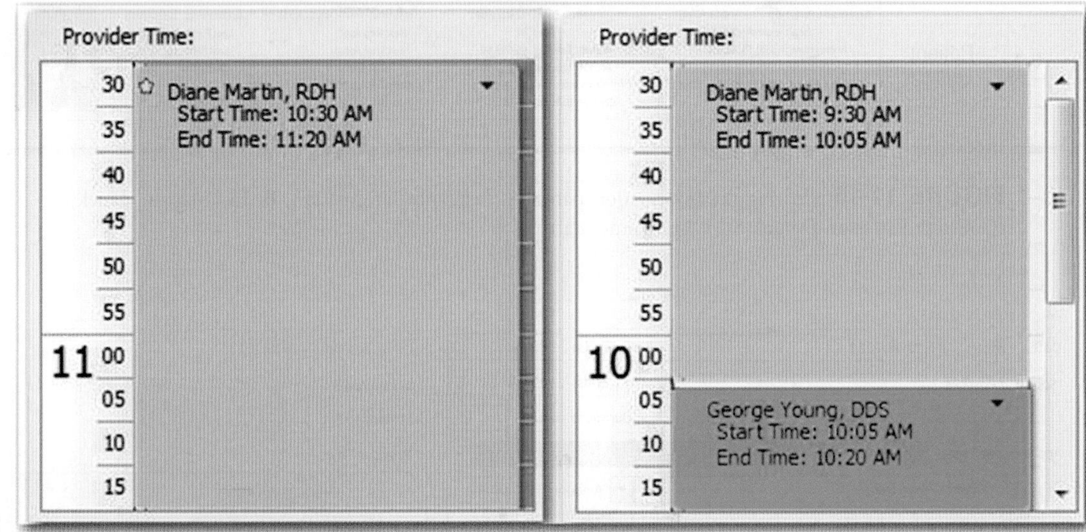

B

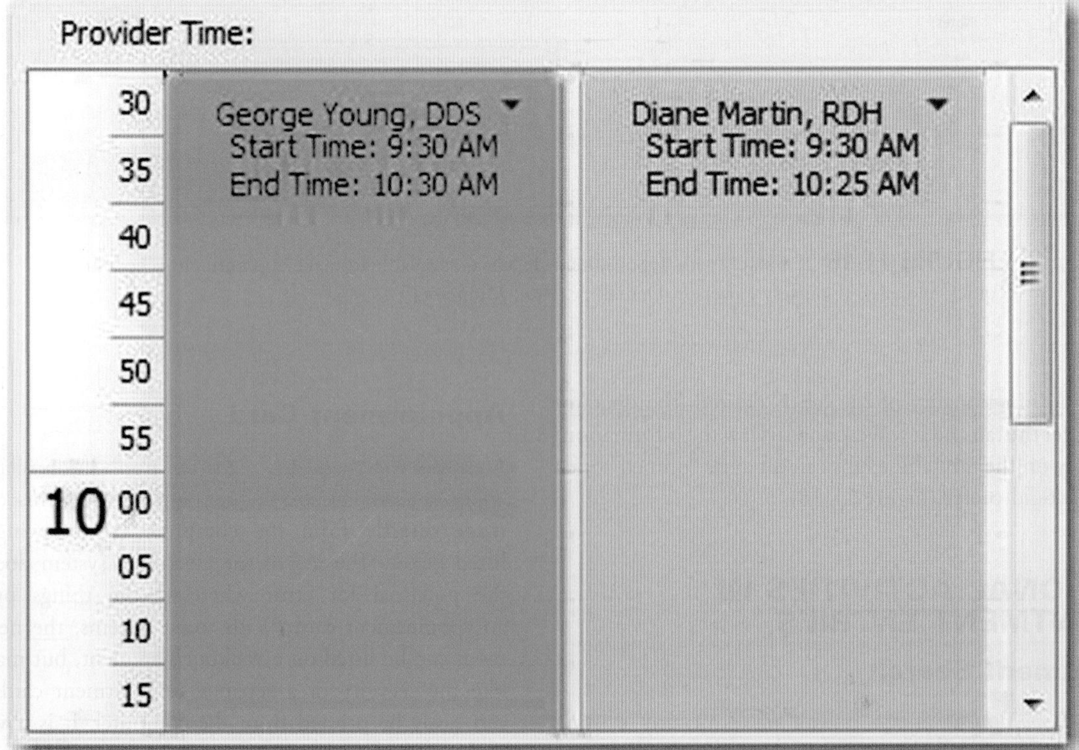

C

FIGURE 11-17 **A,** Making the entry using arrows to select the date and time of the appointment. **B,** Selecting the provider screen. **C,** Sending the appointment into the queue by dragging and dropping. (Courtesy Patterson Dental, St. Paul, Minnesota.)

Other Appointments
Patient
Appointment Date/Time
AppointmentType
Provider
Duration
Fellers, Lisa
Fri, Nov 22, 2013 @ 1:40 PM
Prophy Adult
Diane Martin, RDH, George Youn...
0:50
** Double Click Appointment To View
Other Appointments
Services
Save
Cancel

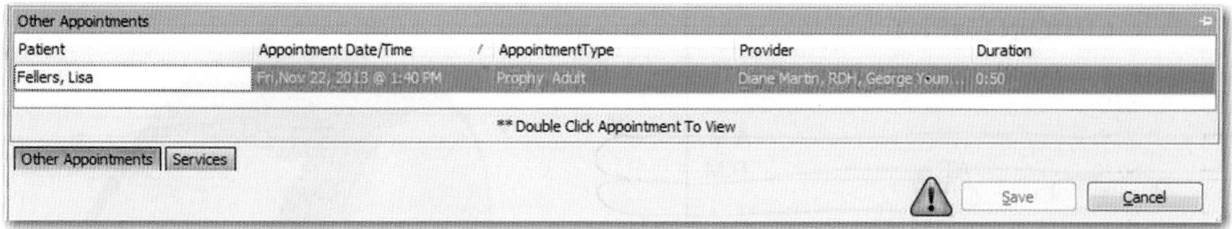

FIGURE 11-18 Using tabs to access other appointments and services within the appointment window.

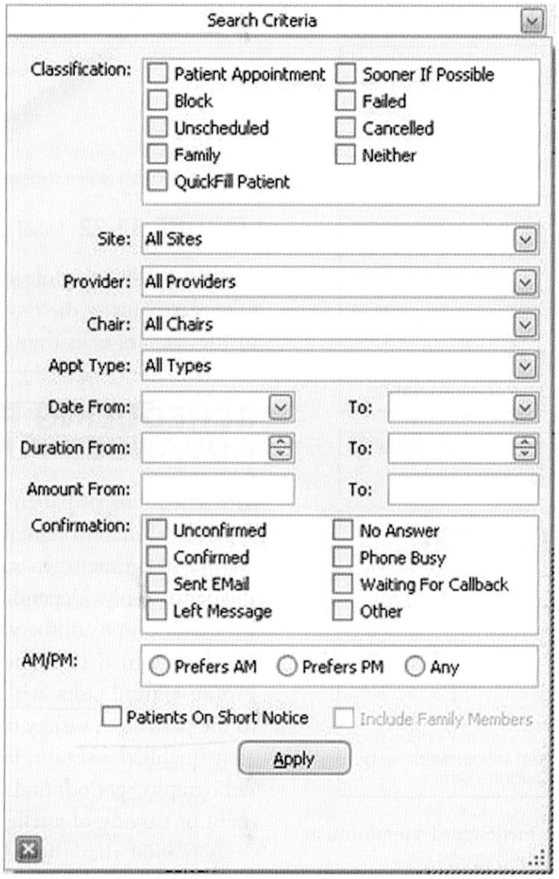

Search Criteria
Classification:
Patient Appointment
Sooner If Possible
Block
Failed
Unscheduled
Cancelled
Family
Neither
QuickFill Patient
Site: All Sites
Provider: All Providers
Chair: All Chairs
Appt Type: All Types
Date From:
To:
Duration From:
To:
Amount From:
To:
Confirmation:
Unconfirmed
No Answer
Confirmed
Phone Busy
Sent EMail
Waiting For Callback
Left Message
Other
AM/PM:
Prefers AM
Prefers PM
Any
Patients On Short Notice
Include Family Members
Apply

FIGURE 11-19 Screenshot with search to find a patient's existing appointment.

Before	After
Limited options for searching No filtering options	Search criteria allow for greater control. Add to *Incontact* option. Current and past appointments are separate.

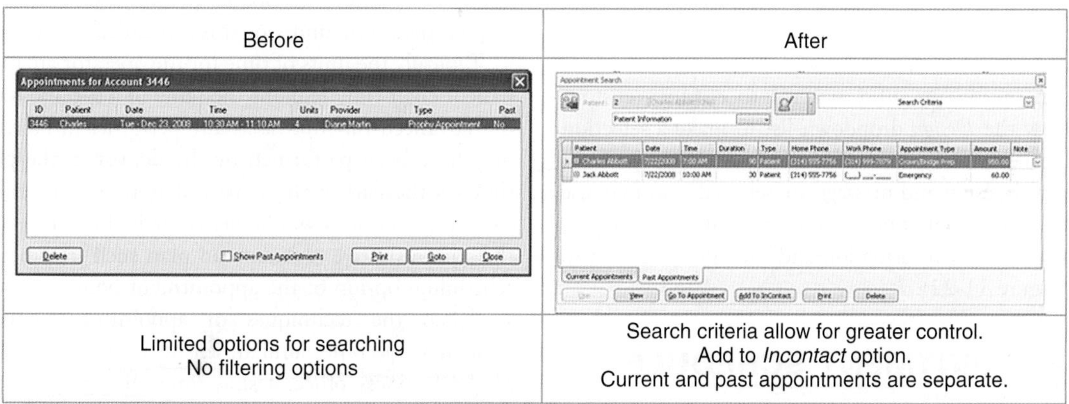

FIGURE 11-20 Screenshot of *OnSchedule* to search for available appointment times.

APPOINTMENT

FOR ____________________

____________ AT ____________ A.M. P.M.

Dental Associates, PC
611 Main Street, SE
Grand Rapids, MI 49502
TELEPHONE (616) 101-9575

IF UNABLE TO KEEP APPOINTMENT KINDLY GIVE 24 HOURS NOTICE

Dental Associates, PC
611 Main Street, SE
Grand Rapids, MI 49502
TELEPHONE (616) 101-9575

____
HAS AN APPOINTMENT ON

____
DAY MONTH DATE

AT ________ A.M. ____ P.M. ____

IF UNABLE TO KEEP APPOINTMENT KINDLY GIVE 24 HOURS NOTICE

Dental Associates, PC
611 Main Street, SE
Grand Rapids, MI 49502
(616) 101-9575

APPOINTMENT

Name: ____________
Date: ____________
Time: ____________
With: ____________

IF UNABLE TO KEEP APPOINTMENT KINDLY GIVE 24 HOURS NOTICE

FIGURE 11-21 Choosing from three predesigned appointment card layouts when using this feature.

Appointment Card Form and Preview Button

Choose from three predesigned appointment card layouts when using this feature; use the *Preview* button to view the templates (Figure 11-21).

There is an option on most systems to create a custom message. Follow the *Design* dropdown list to make a selection for the appropriate situation.

Once the card design and message are selected, you may use a label printer to print an appointment card with the patient's name and appointment information and then give the card to the patient (Figure 11-22).

DAILY APPOINTMENT SCHEDULE

To observe the day's appointment schedule, it is only necessary to view the day's appointments. It is possible to print this schedule and post it in areas where a computer monitor is not available. This schedule should be updated regularly as changes take place during the day and the clinical staff must be notified of these changes as they occur (Figure 11-23).

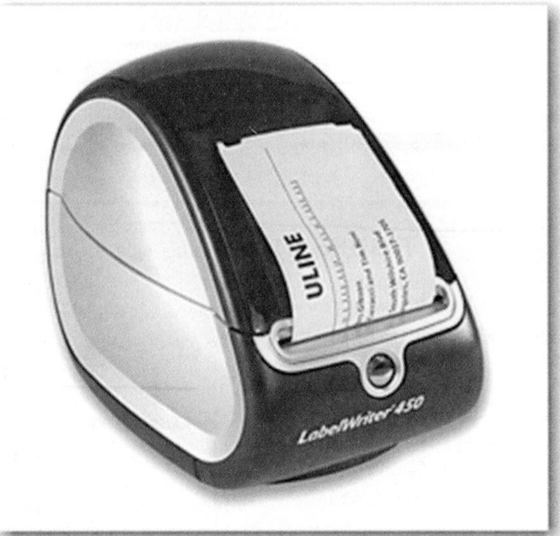

FIGURE 11-22 Label printer to produce an appointment card.

SCHEDULING PATIENTS IN AN ADVANCED-FUNCTION PRACTICE

The scheduling of patients in an office that has an advanced- or expanded-function dental auxiliary requires a different concept of time assignment. In such practices, the patient does not see the dentist only. Depending on the state dental practice act and the qualifications of the various clinical staff members, time may also be assigned to the advanced-function assistant to perform various clinical tasks, without the dentist needing to be assigned to the patient. A variety of tasks can be assigned to the appropriately qualified assistant, including diagnostic impressions, dental radiographs, periodontal dressing placement or removal, placement or carving of amalgam, and various other specialty tasks.

It is vital that the administrative assistant understand the legal ramifications of assigning an unqualified or noncredentialed person to perform various clinical tasks. The administrative assistant must have a thorough understanding of the state law, and the clinical assistant's qualifications for a task must be verified before the individual is scheduled to treat patients.

Typically the units of time for the operator are modified, but patient chair time remains the same in a specific room because the advanced-function assistant performs intraoral tasks that may have been performed by the dentist in the past. It takes time on the part of the staff to determine how and by whom the intraoral duties will be performed; after this is determined, the administrative assistant can plan such treatment using the scheduling option of the appointment book.

When the techniques of appointment book management have become familiar, this can be a very enjoyable part of the business office. Using time efficiently can make each day in the office more productive and reduce tension while still meeting the patients' needs. If the rules in Box 11-2 are followed, the dental office can maintain efficiency.

8/4/2014 Schedule for Wednesday, December 04, 2013 [7,955.80 / 5,000] 3:14 PM

Time	Dr. Young	Dr. Morgan	Hyg Diane
8 AM	? Charles Abbott (Chip)	? Tyler K Davies	
10	+ CERCR(19),	+ FPC(8),	
8:50			? Olivia D. White (Livie)
9 00			BWX 4, PRO A, PEXAM,
20	? Sabrina R. Alexander		
30	ONLAY(5,MODB),		
50		? Kennedy R. Thomas (Kenny)	
10 00		FPC(8)	
30	? Rebecca B. Carson		? Chelsea S. Jennings
40	ENDO (15)		FL2, EXAM,PRO,4BWX
11 30	? Richard Ballard	? Jack Abbott	
40	+ PAX, LEXAM,	+ LEXAM, broken tooth #14	
12 PM	LUNCH	LUNCH	LUNCH
10	LUNCH	LUNCH	LUNCH
20	LUNCH	LUNCH	LUNCH
30	LUNCH	LUNCH	LUNCH
40	LUNCH	LUNCH	LUNCH
50	LUNCH	LUNCH	LUNCH
1 00	? Jack Eaton	? Denise Schultz	
10	CNSLT,	Bridge del #2-4	
30	? Garry Thomas		? Sammy Murphy
40	PAX, PRExm, pain upper right gums	? <NP> Miranda Myers (Mandy)	BWX 4, PRO A, PEXAM,
50		PAX, LEXAM, pain upper right	
2 00	? Jim Carson		
10	RCT(31,DM)	? Roslyn Ballard	
20		FPC(10),	? Jean Thomas
30			FL2, EXAM,PRO,4BWX
3 10	? Keith Davies		? Cole Walden
20	COM P(30,MO),		FL2, EXAM,PRO,4BWX
40		? Harrison R. Wilson (Harry)	
50		S EXT(15),	
4 10	? Lynn J. Roberts (Lynnie)		
20	COM P(5,DO), COM P(4,MO),		

FIGURE 11-23 Electronic day schedule. (Courtesy Patterson Dental, St. Paul, Minnesota.)

LEARNING ACTIVITIES

1. Discuss the types of appointment systems available for use in the dental office.
2. Explain the advantages of an electronic appointment system.
3. Explain the components of an **appointment matrix**.
4. Explain the management of the following appointment scheduling situations:
   a. A mother calls the office in hysterics because her 8-year-old has just fallen off his bicycle. She states that there is a great deal of bleeding and that his teeth are broken.
   b. A patient who has not been treated by the dentist for more than a year comes into the office around 2:30 PM. He states that he is having some discomfort around a bridge abutment and that he has severe bleeding when he brushes. The schedule for the remaining part of the day is full.
   c. A patient comes into the office on Monday, January 23, at 10 AM. The assistant greets her, and she says she has a 10 o'clock appointment. The assistant checks the appointment book, but the patient's name is not listed for that day.
   d. A patient's appointment was confirmed for 1 PM today. The patient does not show up for the appointment.
5. What information is included on the following forms?
   a. Appointment card
   b. Appointment daily schedule
   c. Call list
   d. Treatment plan

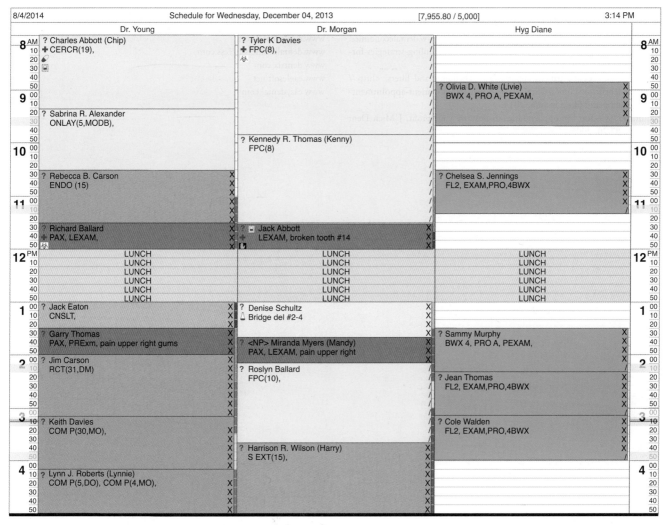

Please refer to the student workbook for additional learning activities.

BIBLIOGRAPHY

Banta L: Scheduling strategies for success. <http://www.dentaleconomics.com/articles/print/volume-103/issue-6/practice/scheduling-strategies-for-success.html/>, 2013.

Brady LA: New dental patient appointment scheduling and filters. <http://www.dentistryiq.com/articles/2013/03/new-dental-patient-appointment-scheduling-and-filters.html/>, 2013.

Schumann TC: Top five opportunities to improve your profit, J Mich Dent Assoc 87:20, 2005.

RECOMMENDED WEBSITES

www.curvedental.com
www.dentalbusinesssuccess.com
www.dentrix.com
www.eaglesoft.net
www.easydental.com

12 Recall Systems

Carol Chapman

http://evolve.elsevier.com/Finkbeiner/practice

LEARNING OUTCOMES

1. Define the key terms in this chapter.
2. Describe the purpose of a recall or re-care system and why patients need to understand the importance of the system.
3. Identify different types of recall or re-care systems.
4. Explain how to establish a recall or re-care system.

KEY TERMS

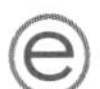

Advanced appointment system A recall or re-care system in which appointments are scheduled at the time that the patient leaves the office.

E-mail or text-messaging system A recall or re-care system that electronically notifies the patient that it is time to make an appointment for recall or re-care.

Mail system A recall or re-care system in which the patient receives a card that either asks the person to contact the office to make an appointment for a preventive recall visit or gives the patient an appointment time and asks the individual to contact the office to confirm it.

Recall or re-care system A system by which patients are notified of the need to make an appointment for routine prophylactic dental care.

Telephone system A recall or re-care system in which the patient is contacted by telephone for a recall appointment.

A **recall or re-care system** notifies patients of the timing of routine dental hygiene care. Some practitioners have adopted the term *re-care* rather than *recall* because they believe it infers a more caring approach. Other terms for routine dental hygiene care include *maintenance therapy* and *supportive therapy.* No matter which term is used in the office, this system is an integral part of every modern dental practice, and it is essential to both the patient and the dentist. A recall or re-care system is the lifeline of the dental practice. It helps to achieve one of the primary objectives of dentistry: helping patients to maintain good oral health for a lifetime. Each dental professional in the practice must assume a role in maintaining and promoting a successful recall system.

PRACTICE NOTE

A recall system is the lifeline of the practice. It helps to achieve one of the primary objectives of dentistry: helping patients to maintain good oral health for a lifetime.

Patients often associate routine dental hygiene care with prophylaxis, but the recall or re-care appointment should not be viewed from this limited perspective. Many other procedures are performed by the dental hygienist during this appointment time, including the following:

- Taking vital signs
- Exposing radiographs
- Performing extraoral and intraoral cancer screening
- Detecting carious lesions
- Evaluation of the supporting structures of the teeth
- Examination of the eruption patterns for possible orthodontic referral
- Examination of the fixed and removable prosthetic devices (e.g., full or partial dentures, implants, crowns, bridges)
- Taking intraoral photographs
- Reviewing patient oral hygiene

The dentist may need to verify certain procedures performed by the dental hygienist and determine whether any follow-up care is indicated. The importance of the tasks performed during the recall or re-care appointment should be emphasized to the patient by the administrative assistant, as well as by other staff members, because this promotes routine dental hygiene care.

The success of a recall or re-care system depends on three factors: (1) educating the patient about his or her dental health; (2) motivating the patient; and (3) providing consistent follow-up. The entire staff must help patients develop a sense of responsibility toward their own dental health. In addition, the patient must be aware of how the practice's recall or re-care system operates.

PRACTICE NOTE

The success of a recall system depends on three factors: (1) educating the patient about his or her dental health; (2) motivating the patient; and (3) providing consistent follow-up.

Education begins when the patient first visits the office. In addition to asking for the patient's basic health information, the health questionnaire should address the patient's views toward maintaining or improving his or her oral health. Questions such as "Are you happy with your smile?" or "How do you think your smile could be improved?" can lead to discussions about oral health and help the dentist or hygienist determine the patient's oral health goals

Asking a patient if he or she would like to discuss developing a lifetime approach toward his or her dental health and appearance is vital to determining long-range plans for the patient's dental care. By talking about a lifetime strategy toward good dental health and appearance, patients think about lifetime plans rather than simply fixing a problem found during routine prophylaxis. Thus, the dentist and the hygienist are able to include the routine recall or re-care appointment as part of total lifetime care. In fact, some dentists have adopted the approach of including the first recall or re-care appointment after extensive dental care as part of the total fee. This lets the patient know how important it is to return to the office for complete prophylaxis and routine care.

The timing of a recall/re-care appointment is determined on an individual basis. Consultation between the dentist and the dental hygienist will determine whether the patient needs to return on a 3-, 4-, or 6-month recall/re-care. This can help the patient to stop thinking solely of dental visits as something that occurs every 6 months; this elevates the appointment to higher therapeutic ground.

Remember that a successful recall or re-care system requires that the administrative assistant use effective communication skills. For example, when a patient returns to the business area after a routine oral prophylaxis, the administrative assistant might say, "We're looking forward to seeing you at your next re-care appointment. You know you want to keep that beautiful smile."

The motivation of patients, which is critical to the effectiveness of the recall or re-care system, is the responsibility of the entire dental staff. After a patient has been educated and motivated to accept a recall or re-care system, the administrative assistant is responsible for maintaining the system efficiently. The importance of this step cannot be overemphasized. If an assistant ignores the system even for 1 month, the effect on the patient flow becomes noticeable within a short time, and patients begin to feel ignored.

KEEPING PATIENTS INFORMED

Patients in the dental practice must understand the importance of recall or re-care. Patient education should promote the recall or re-care system and at the same time inform the patient about the dental procedures that the office offers. Some practical and easy ways to keep patients informed about the office include the following:

- Updated practice brochures
- Newsletters
- Audiovisual materials in the reception room
- Intraoral cameras
- Before-and-after photographs
- Bulletin boards
- Follow-up e-mails
- Social media web pages

TYPES OF RECALL OR RE-CARE SYSTEMS

Any of several types of recall or re-care systems can be used. Most dentists find that no one system is perfect; therefore, they often use more than one. The most common systems are the advanced appointment system, the telephone system, the mail system, and, more recently, the telecommunications system, which involves e-mailing and text messaging patients.

Advanced Appointment System

With the **advanced appointment system**, recall or re-care appointments are scheduled before the patient leaves the office. Most dental management companies promote advanced scheduling as the most efficient method to schedule recall/re-care appointments. The downside to this type of scheduling is that certain groups of patients, such as professionals with their own schedules (e.g., physicians, attorneys), may not know their schedule 3, 4, or 6 months in advance. Advocates of this system contend that most patients know their routines as well as the appointment times that are generally best for them.

One of the most important points when using the advanced recall/re-care system is to leave room in the dental hygienist's schedule for new patients and for patients who are not able to schedule in advance. Selectively blocking appointment times in advance will allow for appointment times for these patients. Several morning and afternoon appointments on alternate days should be made available. If these blocks are not scheduled, the administrative assistant can use these times to schedule patients on a short call list. This is a list where patients have indicated they are available on short notice to fill the appointment time.

The office staff should weigh the advantages and disadvantages listed in Box 12-1.

Even if a patient states, "I don't know what I will be doing in 6 months," whoever is scheduling the appointment can say, "I can schedule you now, and then you *will* know what you'll be doing in 6 months." The scheduler should never make statements such as, "If the appointment presents a problem, just

BOX 12-1

Advantages and Disadvantages of an Advanced Appointment System

Advantages

- No cost involved
- 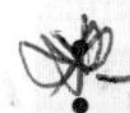 Little time required of the administrative assistant
- Simple

Disadvantages

- Patients do not know what their future commitments might be

give us a call, and we'll reschedule." That creates havoc in the business office. Not only does the scheduler have to find a new appointment for the patient who is rescheduling but it also creates an opening in the hygiene schedule. A more appropriate response would be, "I've set aside this time in the schedule for you so that we can maintain your oral health."

Scheduling a re-care or recall appointment can be done at the chairside by the dental hygienist. It is the most efficient and effective method to ensure that the patient returns for routine care. The hygienist is the staff member who is most aware of any problems that the patient may present with at the next recall or re-care appointment. For example, if a patient presents with a great deal of stain or calculus at each visit, then the hygienist knows that particular patient requires a longer appointment time. The dental hygienist is also aware of any specific need that has been addressed during the current prophylaxis appointment and thus that should be addressed at the next recall or re-care visit. For example, to emphasize the importance of the re-care appointment, the hygienist might say, "Mrs. Ortiz, at your next visit with me, I want to review how you are doing with the power toothbrush I recommended."

Telephone Recall or Re-care System

The **telephone recall or re-care system** allows for the most immediate response, because the administrative assistant contacts each patient by telephone to schedule a recall or re-care appointment. This can be a good practice builder for a new practitioner, but it can be an exhausting and time-consuming task in a large, well-established practice.

When contacting a patient by telephone, use phrases that do not devalue the service. Eliminate such phrases as *for your checkup* or *for your cleaning*. Some assistants find it cumbersome to use the words *prophylaxis* and *examination,* because they feel that these terms are too technical. In addition, these words do not accurately convey the importance of the recall or re-care visit, which includes a complete dental examination, an examination of all oral tissues (to detect oral diseases early), and the complete scaling and polishing of teeth. Take the time to inform patients that this is an important preventive service, or try using the phrase *preventive recall* or *re-care appointment.*

Because many people have answering machines or voicemail, which allow for the leaving of messages, the telephone system can be an effective technique that provides personal contact with the patient. Care should be taken to avoid leaving personal messages on the telephone unless the patient has indicated in a signed permission form that personal messages may be left on the answering machine or via voicemail. Box 12-2 lists a few suggestions for successfully using the telephone in a recall or re-care system. The advantages and disadvantages of the telephone system are listed in Box 12-3.

BOX 12-2

Suggestions for Using a Telephone Recall or Re-care System

- Do not call patients too early in the morning.
- Make sure that your voice conveys a positive attitude; do not make calls if you are tired or grumpy.
- Make the calls in private and out of the hearing of other patients.
- Do not pester patients. If they say they will call back, record it on the recall file cards, and wait 2 to 3 weeks before contacting them again. If they do not respond after three calls, ask them if they wish to remain on the active recall program.
- Have the patient's recall record in front of you so that you will be well informed.
- Try calling on inclement days; patients are likely to be indoors on such days.
- If an answering machine is reached, speak clearly, and leave a complete message that includes the reason for the call, the times that the office will be open, the office's telephone number, and a cordial "Thank you." Be sure that you have permission to leave messages on the patient's answering machine.

BOX 12-3

Advantages and Disadvantages of a Telephone Recall or Re-care System

Advantages

- Immediate response from the patient
- Practice builder

Disadvantages

- May get no answer
- May be unable to reach the patient
- May disturb the person called
- Time-consuming for a large practice
- Places responsibility on the hygienist or administrative assistant for follow-up

Mail Recall or Re-care System

With the **mail recall or re-care system**, the patient is responsible for making the appointment. Patients receive a card that (1) asks them to contact the office to schedule a preventive appointment or (2) gives them an appointment time and asks them to confirm it (Figure 12-1). The card should emphasize the importance of the prophylaxis and should not use words such as *cleaning* or *checkup.* The office manager addresses the card or the patient addresses the card at the previous visit. The latter arrangement can be especially effective, because patients recognize their own handwriting when they receive the card, and this may confirm their interest in the recall/re-care system. If the office has a computerized system, address labels can be printed to adhere to postcards. Despite some drawbacks (Box 12-4), the mail system can be advantageous in a large practice.

BOX 12-4

Advantages and Disadvantages of a Mail Recall or Re-care System

Advantages

- Places responsibility on the patient
- Visible reminder

Disadvantages

- Possible to ignore notice
- Cost of postage
- Lack of immediate response

Date:________________

As you requested, we are reminding you that it is now time for your next visit. The appointment schedule at the right shows your next appointment.

If the date or time is not convenient for you, please call this office immediately for a more suitable time.

Sincerely,

____

____
HAS AN APPOINTMENT WITH

LEONARD S. TAYLOR, D.D.S.
201 KENYON ROAD
CHAMPAIGN, ILLINOIS 61821
TELEPHONE (217) 555-0000

FOR
MON.______AT______
TUES.______AT______
WED.______AT______
THURS.______AT______
FRI.______AT______
SAT.______AT______
IF UNABLE TO KEEP THIS APPOINTMENT, KINDLY GIVE 24 HOURS NOTICE

FIGURE 12-1 Recall card sent to a patient to confirm a previously made appointment. (Courtesy Patterson Office Supplies, Champaign, Ilinois.)

Telecommunications (E-mail or Text Messaging) Recall or Re-care System

The e-mail or text-messaging system is becoming more widely used in dental offices today. As patients become accustomed to using e-mail and text messaging for appointment management, they will welcome the use of this format from the dental office. Busy patients who often rely on their e-mail and text-messaging systems to obtain their daily schedules and messages are often closely linked to these systems and would rather rely on this method of communication than on the telephone or the postal service. The advantages and disadvantages of an e-mail or text messaging system are shown in Box 12-5.

Several types of recall or re-care messages can be used (Figure 12-2). Take care to not underestimate a child's maturity when deciding which type of message to send to pediatric patients.

BOX 12-5

Advantages and Disadvantages of an E-mail and Text Messaging Recall or Re-care System

Advantages

- Message reaches its destination in a matter of seconds after it is sent, even if its destination is across the world
- Places responsibility on the patient to contact the office for an appointment
- Visible reminder
- Good communication tool for those who routinely use this
- Paper is saved; it is not necessary to make a hard copy of e-mail
- E-mail may be filed electronically for later reference

Disadvantages

- Time consuming for the hygienist or administrative assistant
- Not all patients prefer this technology
- Patient may quickly delete the message

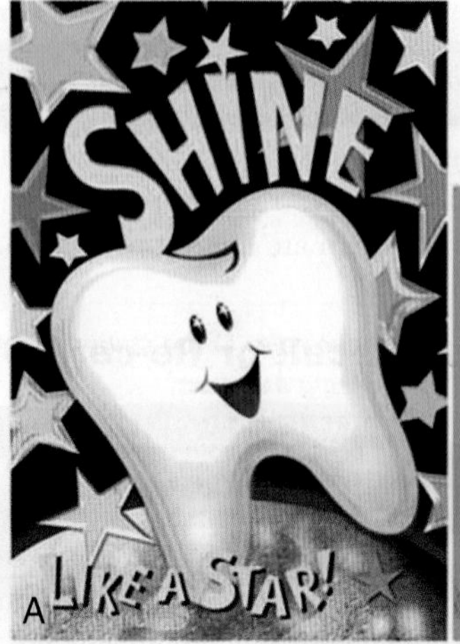

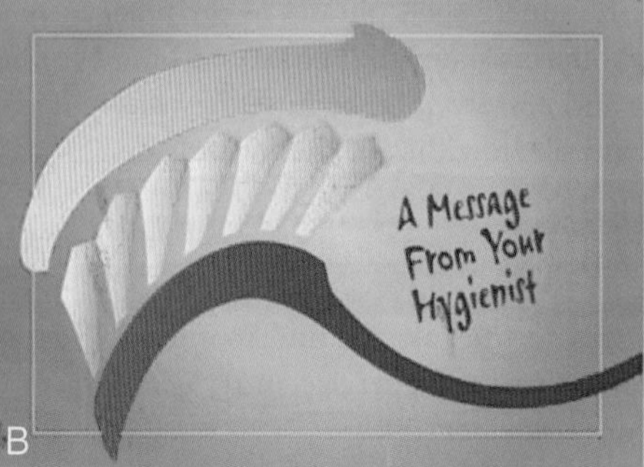

FIGURE 12-2 **A** and **B,** Two styles of recall or re-care cards. **C,** The back of a recall card has a message for the patient. (**A** and **B,** Courtesy Patterson Office Supplies, Champaign, Ilinois.)

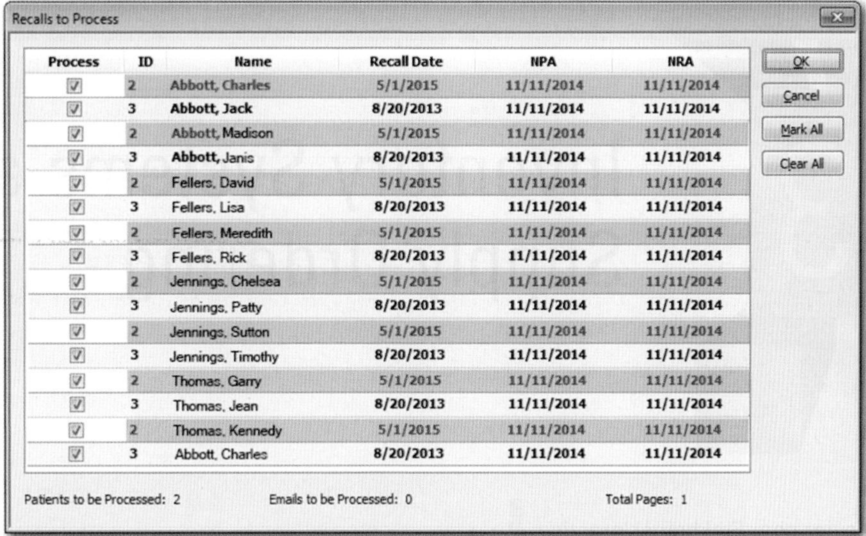

Recalls to Process

Process	ID	Name	Recall Date	NPA	NRA
☑	2	Abbott, Charles	5/1/2015	11/11/2014	11/11/2014
☑	3	Abbott, Jack	8/20/2013	11/11/2014	11/11/2014
☑	2	Abbott, Madison	5/1/2015	11/11/2014	11/11/2014
☑	3	Abbott, Janis	8/20/2013	11/11/2014	11/11/2014
☑	2	Fellers, David	5/1/2015	11/11/2014	11/11/2014
☑	3	Fellers, Lisa	8/20/2013	11/11/2014	11/11/2014
☑	2	Fellers, Meredith	5/1/2015	11/11/2014	11/11/2014
☑	3	Fellers, Rick	8/20/2013	11/11/2014	11/11/2014
☑	2	Jennings, Chelsea	5/1/2015	11/11/2014	11/11/2014
☑	3	Jennings, Patty	8/20/2013	11/11/2014	11/11/2014
☑	2	Jennings, Sutton	5/1/2015	11/11/2014	11/11/2014
☑	3	Jennings, Timothy	8/20/2013	11/11/2014	11/11/2014
☑	2	Thomas, Garry	5/1/2015	11/11/2014	11/11/2014
☑	3	Thomas, Jean	8/20/2013	11/11/2014	11/11/2014
☑	2	Thomas, Kennedy	5/1/2015	11/11/2014	11/11/2014
☑	3	Abbott, Charles	8/20/2013	11/11/2014	11/11/2014

OK
Cancel
Mark All
Clear All

Patients to be Processed: 2 Emails to be Processed: 0 Total Pages: 1

FIGURE 12-3 An electronic file generates a list of all patients due for recall during a specific month. (Courtesy Patterson Dental, St. Paul, Minnesota.)

ESTABLISHING A RECALL OR RE-CARE SYSTEM

After the type of system has been determined, the administrative assistant should set up a recall file that is simple, efficient, and accurate. The most efficient recall system is managed electronically. In today's dental practice, this management tool is simply too important to rely on a manual system.

Electronic Recall or Re-care Files

The computer is a valuable component of recall or re-care management. With an electronic file, the software system generates a list of patients who need to be contacted (Figure 12-3). The computer also can produce an actual letter or card or create mailing labels for preprepared cards. If the office uses a telephone system, the computer can generate a master list of patients and their telephone numbers.

Follow-Up Care

As mentioned previously, it is critical that patients be recalled routinely. Patients need to be informed of how the recall or re-care system works and how they will be notified before they leave the office. For example, "Mr. Hamilton, you will receive a postcard several weeks before your next re-care visit to confirm the date and time of your appointment." The word "confirm" is a more appropriate choice than "remind," which suggests the patient is forgetful. No matter which re-care system is selected, it is imperative that the administrative assistant maintain flawless records and manage the system to ensure that the patient returns to the office in a timely manner.

Purging the System

As with any records management system, the recall records must periodically be purged. This can be done electronically for patients who have not been in the practice recall system for a period of years. To avoid the possibility of litigation for negligence, the dental office should inform the patient that the record is being removed from the system. A letter should be sent to the patient (and included in the patient's record) to inform the person that he or she is being removed from the recall system. This protects the practice and reminds the patient one last time of the importance of a preventive recall or follow-up appointment.

LEARNING ACTIVITIES

1. Explain the value of a recall or re-care system to both the patient and the dentist.
2. Describe the concept of re-care versus recall.
3. What are the components of a successful recall or re-care system?
4. Explain the advantages and disadvantages of each of the three basic recall or re-care systems.
5. What effect would a computer have on a recall or re-care system in a dental office?

Please refer to the student workbook for additional learning activities.

BIBLIOGRAPHY

Bird DL, Robinson DS: *Modern dental assisting*, ed 11, St. Louis, 2015, Elsevier.

Gaylor LJ: *The administrative dental assistant*, ed 3, St. Louis, 2012, Elsevier.

Goldstein J: The search for a more productive recall system, <http://www.rdhmag.com/articles/print/volume-23/issue-5/feature/the-search-for-a-more-productive-recall-system.html/>, 2003.

13 Inventory Systems and Supply Ordering

 http://evolve.elsevier.com/Finkbeiner/practice

LEARNING OUTCOMES

1. Define the key terms in this chapter.
2. Identify three types of dental supplies.
3. Describe various types of inventory systems.
4. Discuss establishing an inventory system.
5. Discuss the factors involved in maintaining an inventory supply, including a technique for receiving supplies and the storage of hazardous materials.

KEY TERMS

Back-order memo A form that accompanies an order to notify the purchaser that an item ordered is not currently in stock at the supply house and will be sent at a later date.

Capital supplies Large, costly items that are seldom replaced; these include equipment such as computers, sterilizers, and dental units.

Credit memo A form that indicates that the dentist's account has been credited for the cost of a returned item; the amount appears as a credit on the statement at the end of the month.

Expendable supplies Single-use items, such as dental cements, stationery, local anesthetics, and gypsum products.

Invoice A list of the contents of a package, the price of each item enclosed, and the total charge.

Safety Data Sheets (SDSs) Forms supplied by the manufacturer that provide information about a hazardous material; these forms are required by the U.S. government.

Nonexpendable supplies Reusable items that do not constitute a major expense; this category generally includes most dental instruments.

Packing slip An enumeration of the items included in an order; this does not include the cost per item.

Purchase order A standardized form for ordering supplies.

Statement A request for payment submitted by the dental supplier.

The day-to-day activity of the busy dental office is stressful enough without worrying about supplies. Stress increases when a necessary item is out of stock. Whether it is the dental hygienist reaching for the fluoride rinse and finding none available or the clinical assistant suddenly realizing that there is no more of a specific dental cement, it is a factor that diminishes productivity and profitability. An effective inventory control system is invaluable, and it does not have to be complicated. An important issue in inventory control is organization. There must be a plan; each member of the team must understand how it works, and each person must assume responsibility to carry through with his or her part of the system. In this chapter, the reader will learn about a variety of factors that can expedite inventory control and have the opportunity to review several systems.

Although one person may be assigned to ordering and maintaining supplies, the actual inventory control is the responsibility of the entire staff. In some dental offices, the dental hygienist is responsible for ordering supplies related to the preventive area of practice. Those individuals responsible for the clinical areas of the office must note how much product is left when restocking the treatment rooms each day. When the product is low, there must be a communication system in place to indicate that it is time to reorder the product. Most systems enable the administrative assistant to keep a record of order dates and product costs. This helps track when a supply is received and how much of a product is being used. In most situations, the person using the last item is required to add the product to the purchasing list or to be certain that an automated system has logged it into an order.

One person should be in charge of ordering, receiving, and storing supplies; managing hazardous waste; and maintaining Safety Data Sheets (SDSs). Because the practice has both a business side and a clinical side, a business staff member may order all the business supplies, and a clinical staff member may be responsible for managing clinical supplies and hazardous materials. However, as mentioned previously, all staff members are responsible for noting whether supplies are low or exhausted as they perform their daily tasks.

PRACTICE NOTE

Whether at chairside, in the laboratory, or in the business office, dental professionals find it frustrating to reach for an item and find only an empty box.

TYPES OF SUPPLIES

Basic Categories

Supplies can be divided into three basic categories: expendable supplies, nonexpendable supplies, and capital supplies. Expendable supplies are single-use items such as dental cements, stationery, local anesthetics, and gypsum products. Nonexpendable supplies are reusable items that do not constitute a major expense; this category includes most dental instruments. Capital supplies are large, costly items that are seldom replaced, such as computers, sterilizers, and dental units.

Selecting Supplies

Not all materials can be purchased from one supplier, and buying from several suppliers may be more economical. Shopping locally promotes good relations and stimulates the local economy, but for economic reasons a dentist may order supplies from a larger catalog or a discount house.

PRACTICE NOTE

Much of the efficiency of a dental office depends on a systematic and economical approach to the ordering of supplies.

A dental supply house can provide all of the basic dental supplies, both brand name and generic. Purchasing from the dealers in a local area is convenient, but many large wholesale supply houses provide quick service and special rates. Making use of toll-free telephone numbers or ordering online can also speed up service. Make sure that the vendor is reliable; the materials must be quality products, and, where applicable, they must meet American Dental Association specifications.

Many dealers routinely send representatives to dental offices to obtain orders. The administrative assistant should have the order prepared or information available about what is needed in one of the inventory management systems. A manufacturer's representative who wants to see the dentist about a new product may accompany the supply person. If the dentist's schedule does not allow time to meet with the representative, information about the new products can be obtained and relayed to the dentist later.

Medicaments, which are not specifically dental items, can be purchased from a local pharmacy. Surgical supply companies sell materials such as thermometers, surgical scissors, and hemostats.

Business materials are available from local business office supply stores or online. Some supplies, such as cleaning materials, must be purchased at local businesses or specialty companies.

For convenience, a file of the business addresses and telephone numbers of all of the companies patronized routinely can be kept on the computer (see Chapter 8).

DESIGNING AN INVENTORY SYSTEM

The first step in inventory control organization is to streamline inventory management. An *inventory system* is a list of the stock and assets in the dental office. This list is divided into two parts: capital equipment and expendable and nonexpendable supplies. Become familiar with the types and quantities of products and materials used in the office. In addition, become quickly familiar with the monetary value of the current inventory and what the minimum and maximum quantities of the products are for the office. With a manual system, this can be done using a spreadsheet, as will be discussed later in this chapter. With a computer system, a formulary can be set up to identify all of the products commonly used in the office. This is done primarily for the expendable and nonexpendable products. However, some systems provide a component in the software for capital equipment to be listed as well.

Capital Equipment Inventory Control

A spreadsheet can be used to maintain an inventory of capital equipment. For a spreadsheet, software such as Excel or Access can be used. The administrative assistant can track all of the major categories of capital supplies and have vital purchase and warranty information at his or her fingertips. Figure 13-1, *A*, illustrates the headings on a spreadsheet for each capital item and details important information about the item, including date of purchase, serial numbers, and any comments about the product, including warranty dates. The system shown in Access in Figure 13-1, *B*, allows for the development of a cardlike system within the software for each room or category desired. In both Excel and Access software, templates are available that can be adapted for the individual needs of a specific office. A spreadsheet system can save much time and guesswork regarding the servicing of equipment, and it can be helpful to the accountant for determining depreciation. This information should be reviewed frequently for necessary preventive maintenance service. Such service is best scheduled when the dentist is out of the office.

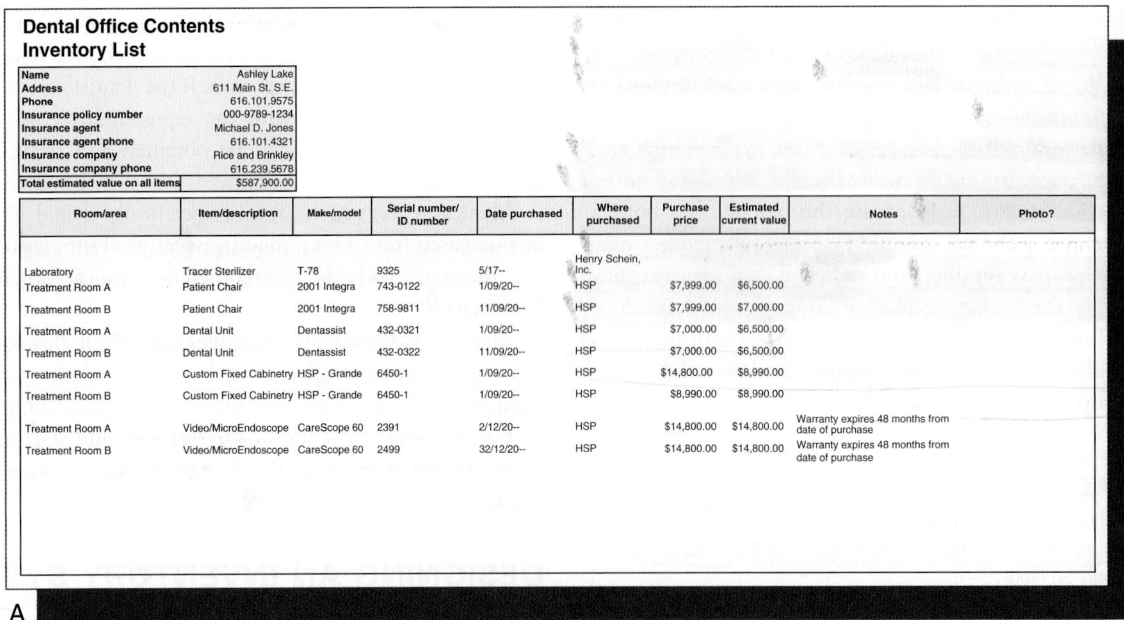

Dental Office Contents
Inventory List

Name	Ashley Lake
Address	611 Main St. S.E.
Phone	616.101.9575
Insurance policy number	000-9789-1234
Insurance agent	Michael D. Jones
Insurance agent phone	616.101.4321
Insurance company	Rice and Brinkley
Insurance company phone	616.239.5678
Total estimated value on all items	$587,900.00

Room/area	Item/description	Make/model	Serial number/ ID number	Date purchased	Where purchased	Purchase price	Estimated current value	Notes	Photo?
Laboratory	Tracer Sterilizer	T-78	9325	5/17--	Henry Schein, Inc.				
Treatment Room A	Patient Chair	2001 Integra	743-0122	1/09/20--	HSP	$7,999.00	$6,500.00		
Treatment Room B	Patient Chair	2001 Integra	758-9811	11/09/20--	HSP	$7,999.00	$7,000.00		
Treatment Room A	Dental Unit	Dentassist	432-0321	1/09/20--	HSP	$7,000.00	$6,500.00		
Treatment Room B	Dental Unit	Dentassist	432-0322	11/09/20--	HSP	$7,000.00	$6,500.00		
Treatment Room A	Custom Fixed Cabinetry	HSP - Grande	6450-1	1/09/20--	HSP	$14,800.00	$8,990.00		
Treatment Room B	Custom Fixed Cabinetry	HSP - Grande	6450-1	1/09/20--	HSP	$8,990.00	$8,990.00		
Treatment Room A	Video/MicroEndoscope	CareScope 60	2391	2/12/20--	HSP	$14,800.00	$14,800.00	Warranty expires 48 months from date of purchase	
Treatment Room B	Video/MicroEndoscope	CareScope 60	2499	32/12/20--	HSP	$14,800.00	$14,800.00	Warranty expires 48 months from date of purchase	

A

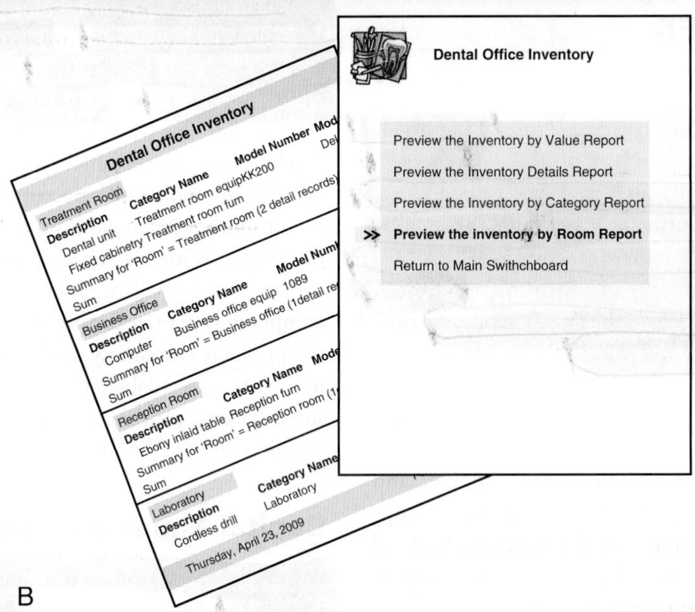

FIGURE 13-1 A, Capital equipment inventory spreadsheet produced in Microsoft Excel. **B,** Two components of a category-type system generated by computer software.

EXPENDABLE AND NONEXPENDABLE SUPPLIES INVENTORY CONTROL

Dental offices generally do not keep a large stock of nonexpendable supplies on hand; however, a list may be included in an inventory system if the dentist wishes. Because the expendable supplies require more attention, an inventory of these items is important. The inventory can be automated on a computer through the formulary or maintained manually.

AUTOMATED INVENTORY SYSTEMS

Most dental supply dealers provide inventory management systems for their customers. The type of system may vary, but one manual system involves products being placed in bins or containers with tags that identify the product, the quantity to order, and the reorder point for the product. When a product needs to be reordered, the tag is removed from the container and placed in a location, where the order can then be created from the various tags. Other dealers provide systems that reference bar codes on products so that, when a product is used, the bar code (Figure 13-2) is scanned and the data goes directly to the supply house through the database that is linked to the office.

Many systems like this are Internet based, and the company will provide bar coding or other techniques that staff members can use when taking items out of inventory. When the reorder point is reached, the product information is scanned with the reader (see Figure 13-2) and stored until it can be uploaded from the office computer, via the Internet, to the appropriate dealer site. Many programs will give a cost comparison for purchasing products from the company and can complete an order with just a few extra steps.

When all products have been entered into the system, a total value of the inventory can be provided; this is helpful for tax returns, financial management, and budgeting. The system can also track money spent for supplies by category on an ongoing basis. Some systems provide reports in a list or in a graph or chart format, which is helpful for making monthly or yearly comparisons. When analyzed, these comparisons can provide valuable data for the practice in terms of the amount of money invested in certain types of products and supplies; they can also help to identify where changes might be necessary to increase profitability.

An office that uses an automated system will find that it is relatively easy to place orders and that the staff can be assured that products will always be available. Consider the following example:

The dentist makes an agreement with the supply house and is logged into the supply house's system. An account is established, and a formulary (i.e., a list of approved and preferred items) is created. The administrative assistant or another staff member can then log into *My Account* with a username and password (Figure 13-3). From the screen, the user selects *My Account,* which then enables the person to choose from a list of categories. These may include the following:

My Account allows the user to review subaccounts, to search orders and invoices, and to filter through records by item, description, or manufacturer.

Shopping list is a tab that enables the user to create a new shopping list or to add or remove items from an existing shopping list (Figure 13-4).

Shopping cart and *Checkout* allow the user to check items in the cart, to edit the item quantity, and to add or delete items from the shopping list (Figure 13-5).

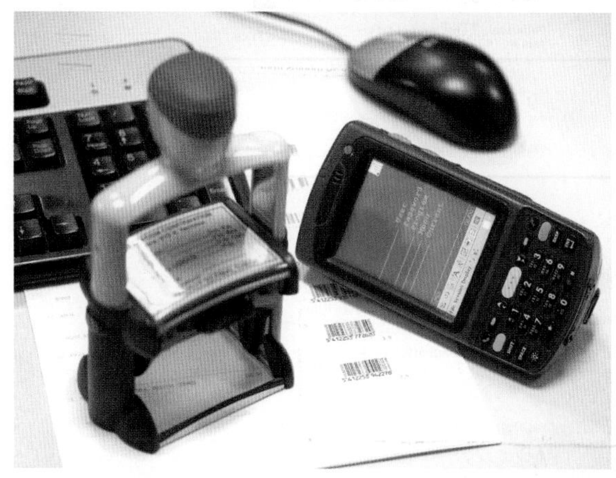

FIGURE 13-2 Bar code used with a scanner for computerized inventory. (Copyright © 2014 J. Markow, BigStock.com.)

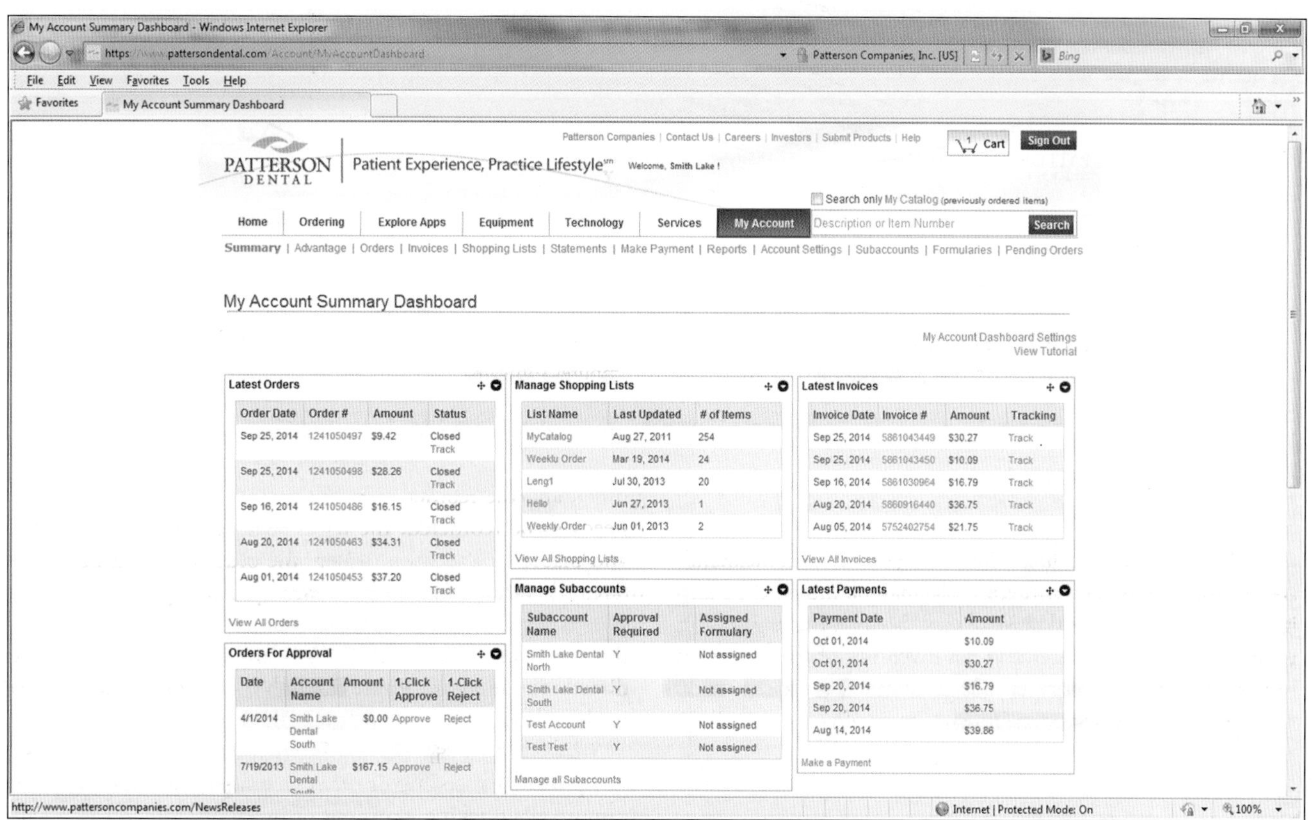

FIGURE 13-3 Inventory screen from which the user selects *My Account.* (Courtesy Patterson Dental, St. Paul, Minnesota.)

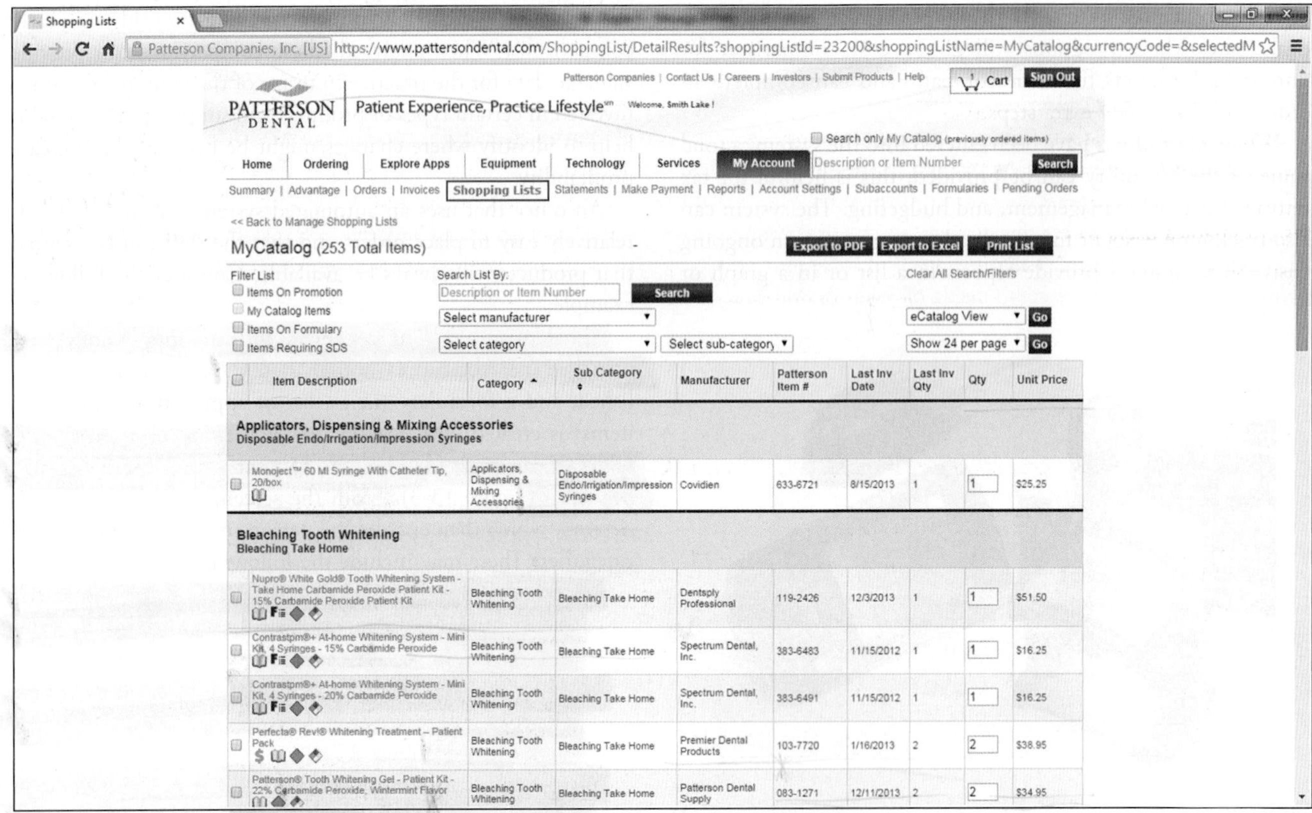

FIGURE 13-4 Screen showing an inventory shopping list. (Courtesy Patterson Dental, St. Paul, Minnesota.)

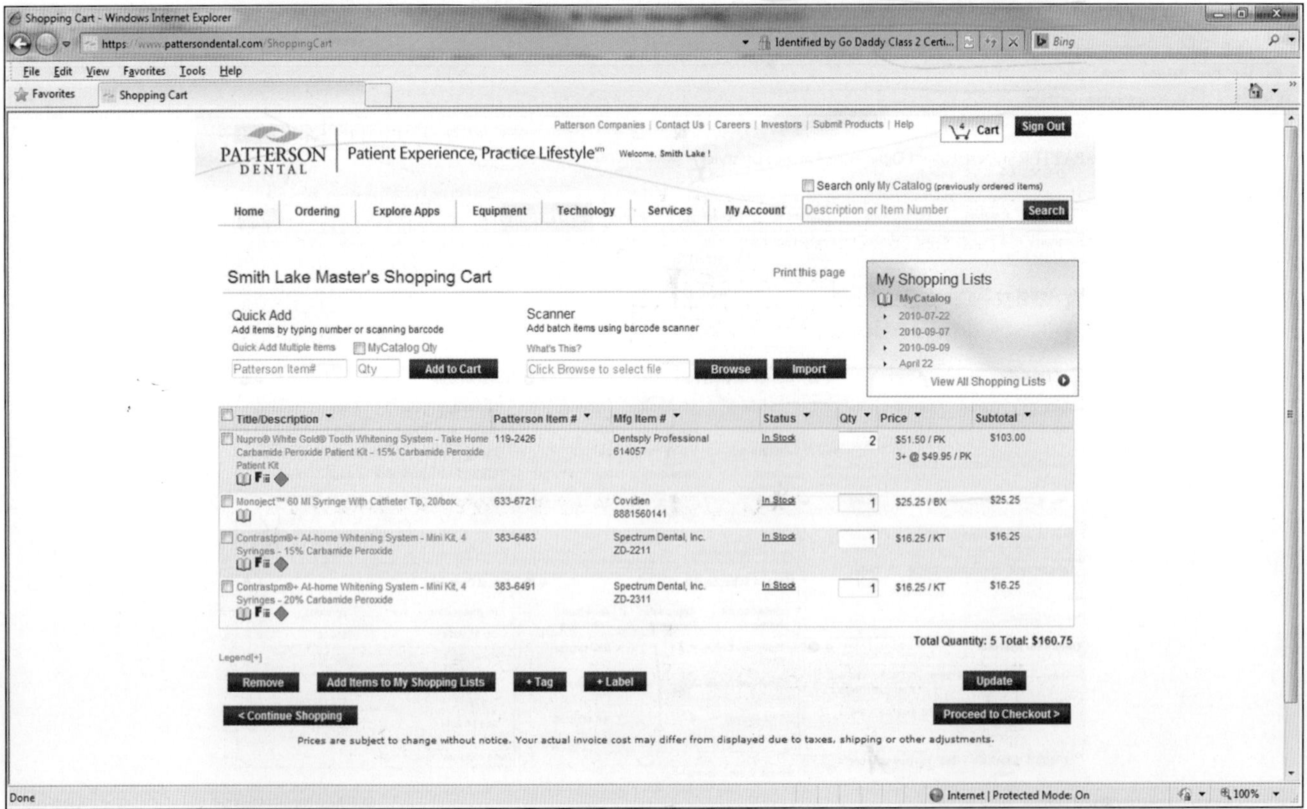

FIGURE 13-5 Screen showing contents of shopping cart. (Courtesy Patterson Dental, St. Paul, Minnesota.)

Reports is an area where the user can view and print purchase summaries for the month or the year as well as comparisons with another year. It is possible to obtain a graph-type report from this area (Figure 13-6).

Another example of an inventory management option is the Cubex system (Figure 13-7). At the end of this chapter is a list of several other inventory management systems. The Cubex system enables users to efficiently manage the ordering, tracking, and costs associated with inventory. The system can be configured to meet the specific needs of each dental practice. Cubex can track operative, hygiene, prosthodontic, endodontic, implant, and other similar supplies.

The Cubex modular system enables shelves and drawers to be intermixed within a single cabinet to accommodate supplies of various sizes. Each cabinet can also be combined with auxiliary cabinets to increase storage capacity. The cabinets house more than 400 items and work much like an ATM machine that dispenses dental supplies. This system is user friendly, and the assistant gains access through manual or badge input. After access is granted, the user simply presses a button to indicate

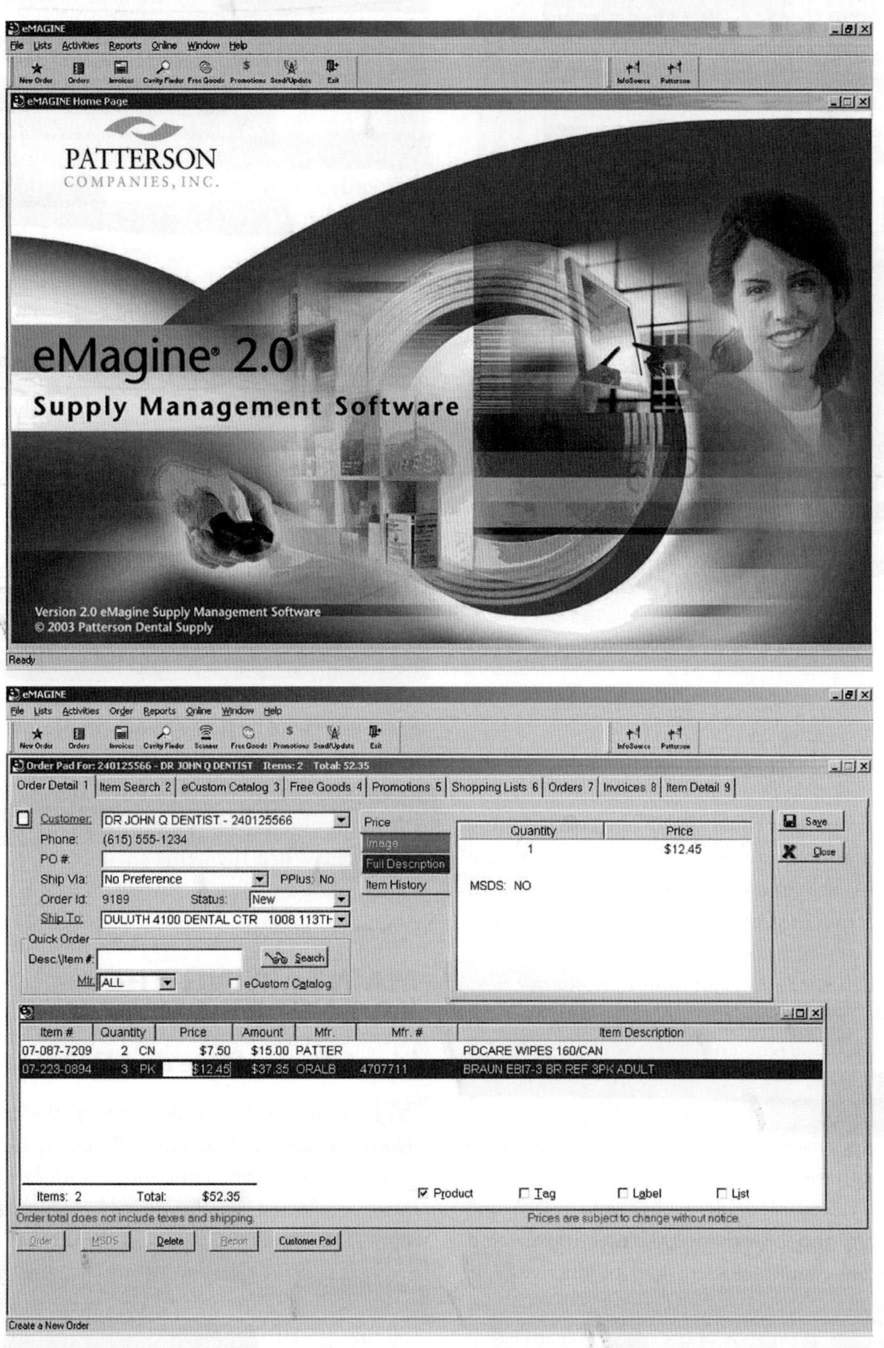

FIGURE 13-6 Inventory system showing a type of report that can be reviewed by the dentist to determine office expenditures. (Courtesy Patterson Dental, St. Paul, Minnesota.)

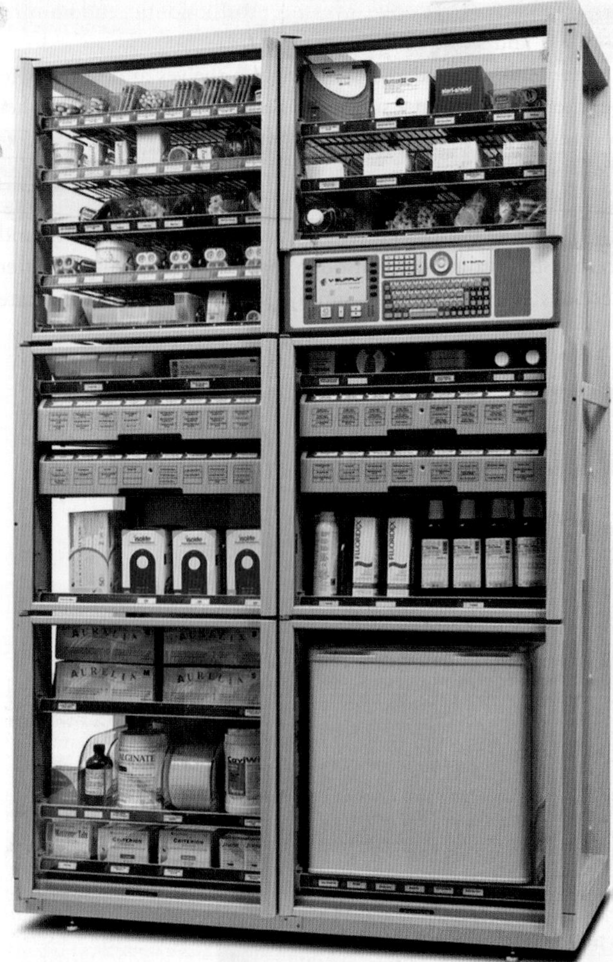

FIGURE 13-7 Cubex inventory system. (Courtesy VSupply, Scottsdale, Arizona.)

the removal of an item. Inventory levels are automatically updated.

Just as ordering supplies on a timely basis can save shipping costs, maintaining an accurate inventory of products can also save money by avoiding the purchase of too many items with short shelf-lives. If too much of certain products is ordered at one time (e.g., certain dental impression materials), not all of that item may be used before the expiration date. Using outdated impression material may result in a poor impression that will need to be discarded and retaken. Inventory management helps to determine the rate of use of items and to identify items that are seldom used any more. This is a good predictor of appropriate quantities to have on hand to avoid wasting materials that exceed their expiration date.

When working in a dental office, it is important to become familiar with the inventory and to work toward better organization to help the dentist become more efficient and productive. The decision regarding whether to use any of these types of automated systems depends on the size and needs of the office. Regardless of the system selected, the inventory manager must determine the desired minimum and maximum stock levels ahead of time.

Manual Inventory Systems

Some dentists still find it difficult to hand over the supply ordering system to automation and may find that a manual system is sufficient. If so, either a card system or an alphabetical list may suffice for an inventory system in some offices.

Card System

The card system requires a separate card for each product. The cards list complete information about each product and its supplier, and they are placed in alphabetical order according to the product name. They are kept in a file drawer or notebook. As it becomes necessary to order an item, the card is placed in a section of the file marked *To be ordered.* Once the item has been ordered, the card is moved to the *On order* section of the file. When the item arrives from the supplier, the card is replaced in its original alphabetical position in the file. If the item is currently out of stock and has been placed on back-order by the supplier, the card is placed in the *On back-order* section of the file.

A modification of this system leaves all of the cards in the alphabetical section at all times; the status of the item is indicated with a colored tag (Figure 13-8). A red label might indicate *To be ordered;* blue, *On order;* and yellow, *On back-order.* This system eliminates the moving of the cards and the chance of misfiling, and it also indicates at a glance the status of the items.

Alphabetical List

Table 13-1 shows an example of an alphabetical list of materials for inventory. This master list includes a code number for each supplier, the name of each product, and columns for the maximum on-hand level and the minimum reorder point. This list is kept in a protective celluloid cover. When the reorder point is reached, the assistant simply places a red check mark in the appropriate space with a wax pencil. When visiting the office, the supply representative can review the list, find all of the items checked off with the supplier's number, and complete the order. When the items are ordered, the red check marks are erased with a tissue.

MAINTAINING THE INVENTORY SYSTEM

Identifying Reorder Points

With an automated dealer system, the rate of use will help to determine the reorder point. If using an in-office data system or a manual system, some form of identifying the reorder point must be selected. An automated system will have some form of reorder point built into the program. For a manual system, colored tape may be used to indicate the reorder point on small items (Figure 13-9), or a tag can be placed on the item (Figure 13-10). For stationery supplies, a paper tab can be inserted into the stack of materials to indicate the reorder point (Figure 13-11).

PRODUCT: Cement, Glass Ionomer

Brand: Shofu

Supplier: Denco Supply Phone: 616.111.1282

Minimum	Maximum	Amount Ordered	Date Ordered	Unit Price

FIGURE 13-8 Colored tag on an inventory card.

TABLE 13-1 Example of a Master Supply List

Supplier Number	Product Name	Manufacturer	Maximum	Minimum Reorder Point
120	Aerosol spray	Regency	12 btls	3 btls
130	Alcohol, isopropyl	Stock	2 gal	1 gal
110	Alginate, Jeltrate Chroma Fast	Dentsply	250 pkgs	100 pkgs
100	Anesthetic, topical ointment	Schein	12 jars	4 jars
110	Anesthetic, lidocaine 2% with epinephrine	Surgimax	50 cans (50)	10 cans (50)
110	Anesthetic, lidocaine 2% without epinephrine	Surgimax	20 cans (50)	5 cans (50)
110	Bite blocks, foam	Strident	500	150
110	Cotton rolls, #2	Richmond	1000	250
111	Esthetx A2-A4-B1-C4	Kerr	6 boxes	2 boxes
111	Gloves, PF Latex Large Accucare	Smart Practice	4 boxes	1 box

Determining Supply Quantity

Several factors help to determine the minimum and maximum amounts of an item to be in stock:

- *Rate of use:* Buying large quantities of infrequently used items is not cost efficient. However, buying bulk quantities of supplies that are used frequently is economical. For example, buying paper products for the dental treatment room in large quantities is a good idea if storage space is available.
- *Shelf-life:* Certain materials, such as medicaments and some impression materials, begin to deteriorate after a certain period. Some manufacturers indicate an expiration date on the box. Do not purchase a large quantity of items that cannot be used before their expiration date.
- *Amount of capital outlay:* In addition to prices, the amount of cash available often determines whether an item is purchased in bulk amounts.
- *Length of delivery time:* This factor affects the minimum quantity desired to have in stock. If several days are required to receive an order for a frequently used item, increase the minimum amount on hand.
- *Amount of storage space:* In some offices, storage space is a crucial factor, and a lack of it prohibits the purchase of large supplies. Consequently, a large storage space is a benefit economically, and it increases efficiency.
- *Manufacturers' special offers:* Manufacturers routinely offer special rates on various materials. However, a special price is not cost efficient if the item stays on the shelf and collects dust.

Receiving Supplies

All incoming materials should be handled and stored safely. Current regulations require that all manufacturers provide an SDS with each hazardous material.

Every order that arrives in the office should have an **invoice**, a packing slip, or both. A **packing slip** is simply an enumeration of the enclosed items. An invoice (Figure 13-12) is a list of the contents of the package, the price of each item enclosed, and the total charge. Some companies use the invoice as a statement

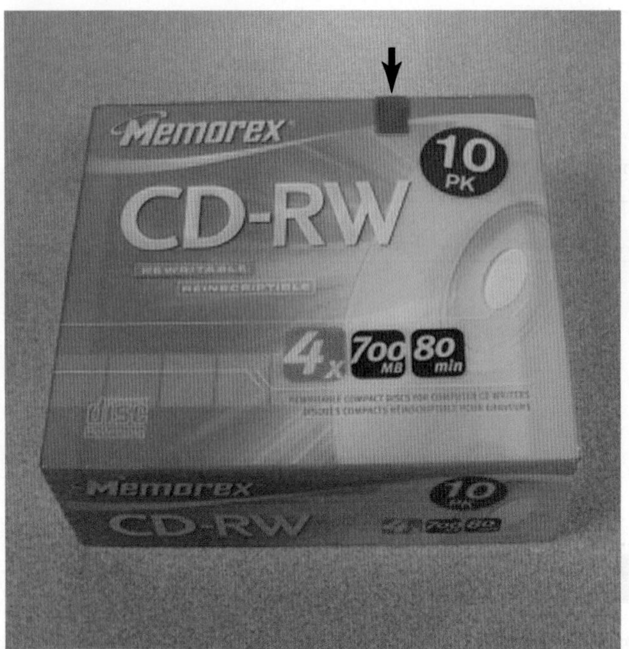

FIGURE 13-9 Colored tape on small items.

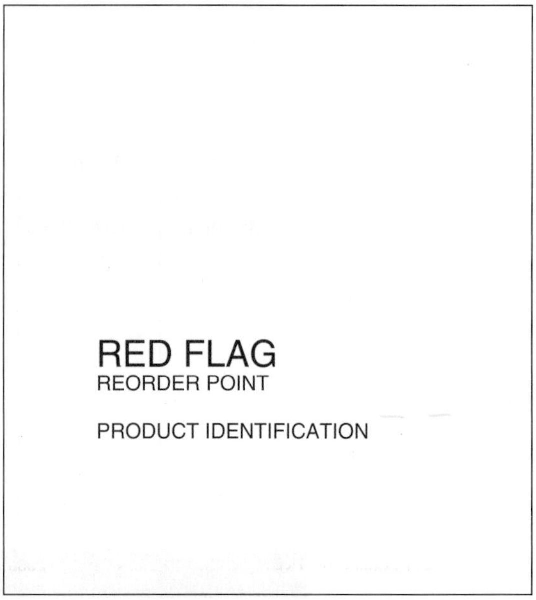

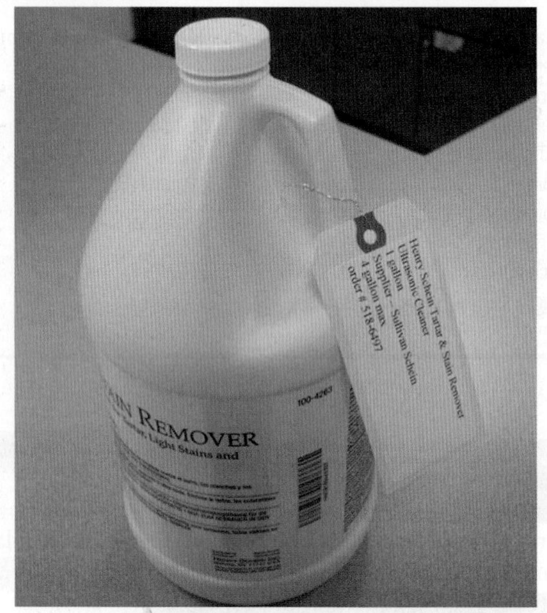

FIGURE 13-10 Tag on a bottle.

and indicate on the form that this is the statement from which the account is to be paid. Make sure that each item listed coincides with the original order, that each item on the invoice is in the package, and that the total amount listed on the invoice is accurate. Then, put the invoice in the *To be paid* file.

At the end of the month, a statement or request for payment will be received from the supplier (Figure 13-13). Each invoice should be checked against the entries on the statement to ensure accuracy before payment is sent.

The check is made payable to the supplier (see Chapter 16). The check number is indicated on the retained portion of the

RED FLAG
REORDER POINT

PRODUCT IDENTIFICATION

FIGURE 13-11 Paper tab.

statement, the invoices are attached, and these documents are filed in the appropriate subject file.

Receiving Credit

Sometimes supplies must be returned for credit. In such cases, the dental supplier sends a credit memo (Figure 13-14), which indicates that the dentist's account has been credited for the cost of the returned item. This amount appears as a credit on the statement at the end of the month.

Back-Ordered Supplies

Sometimes an item ordered is not in stock at the supply house, and a back-order memo is received. The supplier sends notification that the article is back-ordered, or this may be noted directly on the invoice. If the product is needed immediately, attempts should be made to obtain it from another supplier, or an alternative choice may be made.

Purchase Orders

In large institutions, supplies are ordered through a purchasing agent. All items are listed on a requisition, and the order is keyed into a purchase order, which is a standardized order form for supplies. Each purchase order is given a number and sent to the appropriate supplier, who in turn enters this number on all invoices when shipping the supplies.

Storage of Supplies

All supplies should be stored in an organized manner that allows for quick and easy retrieval. Certain materials require a cool, dry, or dark location. In addition, when new materials are

PATTERSON DENTAL

CREDIT MEMO#: 987654321

SHIP TO DENTAL ASSOCIATES, PC
JOSEPH W LAKE, DDS
611 MAIN STREET SE
GRAND RAPIDS MI 49502

Customer #: 555123456

Patterson Plus Level: Gold

SOLD BY PATTERSON DENTAL SUPPLY INC.
MINNESOTA BRANCH
2930 WATERS RD. SUITE 100
EAGAN, MN 55121-1557

Telephone: (651) 555-0000
Representative: 100-70
Order #: 100/1234567
Submitted: 05/11/__ 11:00 AM

Printed: 05/11/__ 11:00 AM

CUSTOMER P.O.: 222-333
Account: REGULAR

Item#	Ordered	Shipped	Pkg	Mfr	MFR Catalog #	Item Description	Unit Price	Amount
07 111-2233	1		1 DZ	ACME	112233A	TOOTHBRUSH CROSS ACTION, 35 SOFT	(18.00)	(18.00)
07 111-4455	1		1 CA	ACME	445566B	TOOTHPASTE CAVT PROTECT .85 OZ	(45.00)	(45.00)
Total	2	2						

CREDIT MEMO

Sample only- Not Valid.

Subtotal		(63.00)
State Tax	6.5%	(4.10)
Total		(67.10)

Payment Terms:
Payment due upon receipt of statement. Overdue balance is subject to service charge not to exceed 1.5% per month. To pay by invoice, send a copy of invoice(s) with remittance to: PATTERSON DENTAL SUPPLY INC., 23254 NETWORK PLACE, CHICAGO, IL 60673-1232

Buy $200 worth of Patterson Private Label bleaching products.
Contact your Patterson representative for details.

Page 1 of 1

FIGURE 13-14 Sample credit memo. (Courtesy Patterson Dental, St. Paul, Minnesota.)

received, they should be stocked behind older supplies so that the older supplies are used first.

The administrative assistant must be aware of the federal Occupational Safety and Health Administration (OSHA) guidelines regarding the use and storage of materials in the dental office. SDSs provided by OSHA should be maintained for any hazardous materials. The information on these sheets (Figure 13-15) includes the manufacturer's name, address, and emergency telephone numbers, as well as specific information about the ingredients of the product. Additional information should include storage instructions, health hazard data, spill or leak procedures, and special safety precautions (e.g., whether the product needs to be stored in a ventilated area). The dentist must make sure that such forms are made available to staff members. If hazardous materials are stored in the office, appropriate labeling must follow the guidelines given in Chapter 17.

When stationery supplies or large boxes are stored, a label describing the contents should be placed on the outside of each box.

BOX 13-1

Questions to Consider During Inventory Evaluation

- Does the system distinguish among expendable, nonexpendable, and capital items?
- Is it user friendly?
- Does everyone understand the system?
- Is the line of responsibility well defined?
- Can you identify different supply sources for various materials?
- Can you determine when an item has been ordered, back-ordered, and received?
- Is stock always current?
- Are supplies stored safely?
- Is the system cost effective?

Inventory Evaluation

Box 13-1 presents some useful questions to help with the evaluation of an inventory system in a dental office.

DENTSPLY/International
DENTSPLY/Caulk
Safety Data Sheet **566398**

1. Identification

Product Name Integrity® Temporary Crown & Bridge Material	SDS Code Number 566398
Substance Identity Integrity® Temporary Crown & Bridge Material	Date of Last Revision 05/17/10
Manufacturer: DENTSPLY Caulk	Address 38 West Clarke Avenue Milford DE 19963-1805 http://www.caulk.com http://www.dentsply.com
Grades or Minor Variant Identities Not Applicable	Information Telephone Number (302) 422-4511 (8:00 AM – 4:30 PM Eastern Time)
Product Use (for Canada) Temporary Crown & Bridge Material	Emergency Telephone Number (302) 422-4511 (8:00 AM – 4:30 PM Eastern Time)

2. Hazard(s) Identification

WARNING
MAY CAUSE AN ALLERGIC SKIN REACTION

Wash hands thoroughly after handling.
Wear protective gloves.

3. Composition/Information on Ingredients

Hazardous Components	C.A.S. Number	Exposure Limits	%
Barium boron alumino silicate glass	65997-17-3	10 mg/m³	< than 50
Hydrophobic Amorphous Fumed Silica	68611-44-9	10 mg/m³	< than 10
Polymerizable dimethacrylate resins	Not Established	Not Established	< than 60

4. First Aid Measures

Routes of Exposure	First Aid Instructions	Immediate Medical Attention	Delayed Effects
Eye	Rinse opened eye for several minutes under running water. If symptoms persist consult physician	Not Applicable	Not Applicable
Skin	Immediately wash with soap and water and rinse thoroughly	Not Applicable	Not Applicable
Inhalation	Not Applicable	Not Applicable	Not Applicable
Ingestion	Not Applicable	Not Applicable	Not Applicable
Mucosa	Rinse tissue for several minutes under running water. If symptoms persist consult physician	Not Applicable	Not Applicable
Note to Physicians (Treating, Testing and Monitoring): Treat symptomatically.			

5. Fire Fighting Measures

Flame Propagation or Burning Rate (for Solids) Not Applicable	Properties Contributing to Fire Intensity Not Applicable	Flammability Classification: Not Applicable	Other: Not Applicable
Extinguishing Media: CO_2, extinguishing powder, foam carbon dioxide or water spray. Fight larger fires with water spray or alcohol resistant foam.		Extinguishing Media to Avoid: Water with full jet.	
Protection and Procedures for Firefighters: Firefighters should wear self-contained respiratory protective devices.			
Unusual Fire and Explosion Hazards: Formation of toxic, irritating gases is possible from the decomposition of the dimethacrylate resins. Product does not present an explosion hazard.			

6. Accidental Release Measures

Containment Techniques: Material is a paste and as such will not flow.		
Spill/Leak Clean-up Procedures and Equipment: Wear protective clothing and scoop up bulk material and place in a labeled plastic or metal container. Avoid gross skin contact to minimize the possibility of contact dermatitis to susceptible persons. Ensure adequate ventilation.		
Evacuation Procedures: Not Applicable	Special Instructions: Not Applicable	Reporting Requirements: Not Applicable

7. Handling and Storage

Handling Practices and Warnings: Product is intended for dental use only. Handling of this product should be by trained dental healthcare professionals only. Observe normal care for working with chemicals.
Storage Practices and Warnings: Store only in the original package. Keep package tightly sealed. Store in a dry area. Protect from exposure to direct light. Store away from food and beverages.

8. Exposure Control / Personal Protection

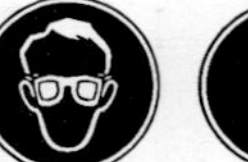
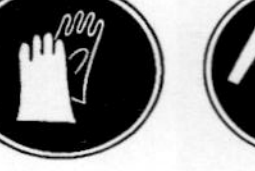
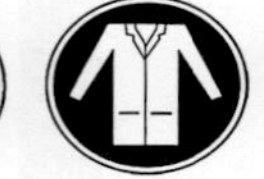

Occupational Exposure Limits: Not Applicable		
Engineering Controls: Not Applicable		
Individual Protection Measures	Personal Protective Equipment for Normal Use	Personal Protective Equipment for Emergencies
Eye/Face	Safety Glasses	Not Applicable
Skin	The glove material has to be impermeable and resistant to the product.	Not Applicable
Inhalation	Not Required	Not Applicable
Body Protection	Protective work clothing	Not Applicable

9. Physical and Chemical Characteristics

Appearance: Creamy white – yellowish paste, with low odor. Multiple shades.		Odor: Characteristic sweet acrylic ester odor.
Normal Physical State: High Viscosity Liquid (Paste)		Melting Point: Not Applicable
Specific Gravity: 1.4 g/cm³	Solubility in Water: Not soluble	pH: Not Applicable
Vapor Pressure (mm Hg): Not Applicable	Vapor Density (AIR=1): Not Applicable	Evaporation Rate (Butyl Acetate =1): Not Applicable
Flashpoint Method: Not Applicable	Flammable (Explosive) Limits in Air LEL: Not Applicable UEL: Not Applicable	Autoignition Temperature: Not Applicable, Product will not autoignite.
Other: Not Applicable		

10. Stability and Reactivity Data

Incompatibility (Materials to Avoid): Strong Oxidizing materials.	
Hazardous Products Produced During Decomposition: No dangerous decomposition products known if used according to Directions for Use.	
Hazardous Polymerization: ☐May Occur ☒May Not Occur	Conditions to Avoid: None known
Stability? ☒Stable ☐Unstable	Conditions to Avoid: None known

11.Toxicological Information

Toxicity Data, Epidemiology Studies, Carcinogenicity, Neurological Effects, Genetic Effects, Reproductive Effects, or Structure Activity Data: Product is an irritant to the skin and mucous membranes. The unpolymerized product may be an irritant to the skin in susceptible persons. On the eye the product has an irritating effect. Sensitization: Repeated or prolonged contact with the unpolymerized material may cause sensitization for persons allergic to acrylates and methacrylates. This product shows the following dangers according to internally approved calculation methods for composite materials: Irritant.

Emergency Overview Material is irritating to eyes, respiratory system and skin.

Routes of Exposure	Signs and Symptoms	Single, Repeated, or Lifetime Exposure	Severity (Mild, Moderate, Severe)	Acute and Chronic Health Effect(s)	Target Organ(s)
Eye	Material can cause irritation.	Single	Moderate	Irritation and possible corneal damage	Not Applicable
Skin	Material may be an irritant	Single & Repeated	Moderate	Irritation or possible allergic response. Severe allergic response may result in breathing difficulties.	Not Applicable
Inhalation	Not Applicable	Not Applicable	Not Applicable	Not Applicable	Not Applicable
Ingestion	Material is not harmful if swallowed using clinically relevant quantities	Not Applicable	Mild	Not Applicable	Not Applicable
Mucosa	Material can cause irritation.	Single	Mild	Inflammation of the mucosa	Not Applicable

Medical Conditions Aggravated by Exposure Open sores and wounds of the skin. Individuals with known sensitivity to methacrylates, acrylates, or urethane dimethacrylate resin used in Dental restorative products.
Carcinogenicity NTP?: Not listed IARC monographs?: Not listed OSHA regulated?: No All components of this product are in compliance with the inventory listing Requirements of the U. S. Toxic Substances Control Act (TSCA) Chemical Substance Inventory.
Potential Environmental Effects Do not allow to enter sewers/ surface or ground water.
NFPA Hazard Classification Ratings (Scale 0-4), Health = 1, Fire = 1, Reactivity = 0

12.Ecological Information

Toxicity Data, Environmental Fate, Physical/Chemical Data, or other Data Supporting Environmental Hazard Statements: Water Hazard class1 (Self-assessment): slightly hazardous for water. Do not allow undiluted product or large quantities of it to reach ground water, water streams or sewage system.

13.Disposal Considerations

Regulations: Must not be disposed of together with household garbage. Do not allow product to reach sewage system.
Dispose of material as solid waste in a closed container. Dispose of in accordance with Federal, State and Local regulations
Properties (Physical/Chemical) Affecting Disposal: Dispose of material as solid waste in a closed container.

FIGURE 13-15 Occupational Safety and Health Administration Safety Data Sheet. (From the Occupational Safety and Health Administration, U.S. Department of Labor, Washington, DC.)

14.Transport Information

Regulated for Shipping: No. Not Regulated	DOT Shipping Name: Not Regulated	Packing Group: Not Applicable
Do Changes in Quantities, packaging, or shipment method change product classification? No	DOT Hazard Class: Not Applicable	UN Number: Not Applicable

15.Regulatory Information

This product has been classified in accordance with the hazard criteria of the Globally Harmonized System of Classification and Labeling of Chemicals and the SDS contains all of the information required by the Canadian Controlled Products Regulations.
U.S. Federal Regulations: CERCLA 103 Reportable Quantity: This product is not subject to CERCLA reporting requirements. Many states have more stringent release reporting requirements. Report spills required under federal, state and local regulations
Section 313 Toxic Chemicals: This product contains the following chemicals subject to Annual Release Reporting Requirements Under SARA Title III, Section 313 (40 CFR 372): None
Section 302 Extremely Hazardous Substances (TPQ): None
EPA Toxic Substances Control Act (TSCA) Status: All of the components of this product are listed on the TSCA inventory.
U.S. State Regulations California Proposition 65: This product does not contain any chemicals, which are on the California Proposition 65 list.
International Regulations: Canadian Environmental Protection Act: This product is a medical device and not subject to chemical notification requirements.
European Community Labeling: Not a dangerous preparation.
European Inventory of New and Existing Chemicals Substances (EINECS): This product is a medical device and not subject to chemical notification requirements.
Other: Not Applicable

16.Other Information

To the best of our knowledge this product does not contain gluten, wheat grains, flaxseed, natural rubber, or natural latex.
All components are synthetically produced; none are derived from animal products.
This information is based on our present knowledge. However, this shall not constitute a guarantee for any specific products features and shall not establish a legally valid contractual relationship.
The attached safety data sheet covers the dangers and measures to be taken when large quantities of material are released, for example due to accidents during transport or storage by the dealer. For quantities of material typically used in clinical practice, information necessary for safe use and storage of the product is given in the DFU.

FIGURE 13-15, cont'd

LEARNING ACTIVITIES

1. Define the following terms: *expendable, nonexpendable, capital items, invoice, statement, credit slip,* and *back-order inventory.*
2. Explain the processing of an item from the time that it is ordered until it is received in the office and the statement is paid.
3. Describe the management of chemicals and hazardous materials in the dental office. What are OSHA guidelines? How do they affect the dental office?

Please refer to the student workbook for additional learning activities.

BIBLIOGRAPHY

Blanks T: An effective system for tracking and ordering inventory developed by a dental assistant. <http://www.dentistryiq.com/articles/2012/04/>.

Massad JJ: An inventory system that can help your practice. <http://www.dentaleconomics.com/article/print/volume-101/issue-11/>.

DENTAL SUPPLIERS

Patterson Office Supplies
3310 N. Duncan Rd.
P.O. Box 9009
Champaign, IL 61822
1-800-843-3676
www.pattersonofficesupplies.com

Henry Schein, Inc.
135 Duryea Rd.
Melville, NY 11747
1-800-772-4346
www.henryschein.com

Smart Practice
(a division of Smart Health, Inc.)
3400 E. McDowell Rd.
Phoenix, AZ 85008-7899
1-800-522-0800
www.SmartPractice.com

Practicon
1112 Sugg Parkway
Greenville, NC 27834
1-800-959-9505
www.practicon.com

Deluxe for Business
3680 Victoria Street North
Shoreview, MN 55126
1-800-865-1913
www.deluxe.com

Medical Arts Press Corporation
P.O. Box 43200
Minneapolis, MN 55443-0200
1-800-328-2119
www.medicalartspress.com

14 Dental Insurance

Rebecca A. Nagy

 http://evolve.elsevier.com/Finkbeiner/practice

LEARNING OUTCOMES

1. Define the key terms for this chapter.
2. Discuss the evolution of dental insurance and the four parties affected by dental benefit plans.
3. Differentiate among the different dental benefit programs.
4. Discuss the preparation of dental claim forms including the use of the current American Dental Association (ADA) Code on Dental Procedures and Nomenclature and the Code of Dental Terminology (CDT) manual.
5. Understand the rules for coordination of benefits.
6. Discuss reviewing the completed claim form, dental claim payments and special programs associated with dental insurance.
7. Understand the guidelines for successful claims administration and identify actions that constitute dental benefits fraud.
8. Explain common dental benefit and claims terminology.

KEY TERMS

Alternative benefit plan A benefit plan other than conventional group dental coverage.

American Dental Association (ADA) A professional association for dentists that promotes the integrity and ethics of the profession; that provides services in education, research, and advocacy; and that develops dental standards.

Approved services Services covered by a benefit plan. Payment for these services may be subject to plan maximums, limitations, and deductibles.

Assignment of benefits Authorization by the enrollee/patient for the dental benefits carrier to issue the claim payment to the treating dentist.

Attending dentist's statement See *claim form*.

Balance billing Requiring the patient to pay the difference between a dentist's actual fee for a service and the amount allowed by the benefits carrier, in addition to any copayment, deductible, or maximum limitation.

Benefits carrier The insurance company, administrator, or other entity that manages eligibility, benefits, claims, and reimbursement for enrollees of a dental benefit contract. See *dental service corporations, insurer,* and *third-party administrator (TPA)*.

Birthday rule A method used to determine the order of liability (e.g., primary, secondary) for dependent children who are covered by more than one dental plan. The primary payer is the benefits carrier/plan of the parent whose birthday (month and day) comes first in a calendar year.

Capitation A benefit delivery system in which a dentist or practice contracts with the program's sponsor or administrator to provide all or most of the dental services covered under the program in return for a fixed monthly or quarterly payment per covered person; also called a *dental health maintenance organization (DHMO)*.

Claim form A paper form used to request payment or predetermination for the treatment costs of patients covered by a dental benefits program. The ADA maintains a standardized form that nearly all dental benefits carriers accept: the *ADA Dental Claim Form*. This is also called an *attending dentist's statement*.

Closed panel system A dental benefits program in which enrollees can receive benefits only when services are provided by dentists who have signed an agreement with the benefits carrier to provide treatment to eligible patients.

COBRA The Consolidated Omnibus Budget Reconciliation Act, which allows a person to temporarily maintain insurance coverage, even if he or she loses his or her job.

Code on Dental Procedures and Nomenclature The dental procedure codes, nomenclature, and descriptors used to report dental services and procedures; this is also called *the Code*. Under the Health Insurance Portability and Accountability Act of 1996, the Code is maintained and regularly updated by the ADA.

Copayment The amount or percentage of the fee for a covered service that the patient is obligated to pay.

Current Dental Terminology (CDT) A reference manual developed by the ADA that includes the *Code on Dental Procedures and Nomenclature* and other instructional tools for reporting dental services to dental benefits plans and administrators.

Customary fee The fee for a service or services determined to be representative of the fees charged by dentists in a specific region or geographic area; this rate may be used by a benefits carrier to establish the maximum payable amount for dental procedures. See also *usual fee* and *reasonable fee.*

Dental benefits carrier A service corporation, insurance company, or other business that contracts with employers or groups of consumers to administer dental benefits coverage.

Dental health maintenance organization (DHMO) A dental capitation plan in which comprehensive care is provided to enrollees through participating providers. The dental provider receives a monthly or quarterly payment for each assigned enrollee, and enrollees are generally required to remain in the program for a specific period. See also *capitation.*

Dental insurance A contract between a licensed insurance company and an employer, organization, or individual that requires the insurance company to make payment toward the costs of covered dental services received by eligible persons.

Dental service corporation A legally constituted, nonprofit organization that contracts with groups, employers, and organizations to administer dental coverage for enrolled individuals.

Dependents Individuals such as a spouse and children who are legally and contractually eligible for benefits under a subscriber's dental benefits contract.

Direct reimbursement An employer's or organization's self-funded program for reimbursing covered individuals based on a percentage of the amount spent for dental care.

Effective date The date an individual and any dependents become eligible for benefits under a dental benefits contract; also called the *eligibility date.*

Eligible person See *enrollee.*

Enrollee A person who is eligible for benefits under a dental benefits contract; also called *covered* or *insured individual, member, participant,* or *beneficiary.*

Exclusions Services or treatments that are not covered by a dental benefits program.

Exclusive provider organization (EPO) plan A dental benefits program in which benefits are provided only if care is rendered by participating providers. Some exceptions may be allowed for emergency and out-of-area services.

Expiration date The date on which the dental benefits contract expires or the date an individual ceases to be eligible for benefits; also called the *termination date.*

Explanation of benefits (EOB) A detailed statement of a processed claim showing the patient, provider, procedure codes, and dates of service as well as the carrier's payment and the patient's copayment. It may also include the maximums used to date and the limitations or exclusions applied to the listed services.

Fee-for-service plan A dental benefits program in which dentists receive payment based on the fee charged for each covered service rendered to an eligible enrollee.

Fee schedule A list of charges established or agreed to by a dentist for specific dental services, which are usually listed by ADA procedure code.

Gender rule A method used to determine the order of liability (e.g., primary, secondary) when dependent children are covered by more than one dental plan. With this method, the primary payer is the carrier or plan that covers the father.

Group The company or organization that contracts with a benefits carrier to administer their dental program. The group determines the program type, benefit levels, maximums, and member eligibility.

Group member See *subscriber.*

Health Insurance Portability and Accountability Act of 1996 (HIPAA) A federal law intended to improve access to health insurance, to limit fraud and abuse, and to control administrative costs. Under the Administration Simplification section of this law, any covered entity that transmits protected health information (PHI) electronically (including dental benefits carriers, clearinghouses, and dental practices) must use a standard format, the ADA procedure codes, and a unique National Provider Identifier (NPI) for all electronic transactions. In addition, covered entities must comply with security and privacy mandates. Paper transactions are not subject to this legislation.

Insured See *enrollee.*

Insurer An organization that bears the financial risk for the cost of defined categories or services for a specific group of policyholders or beneficiaries.

Limitations Restrictions stated in a dental benefits contract that limit the scope of coverage; such restrictions may include age limits for certain procedures, waiting periods before benefits are available, and payment frequency for certain services.

Maximum allowable benefit (MAB) The highest total dollar amount a dental benefits program pays toward the cost of dental care incurred by an individual or family in a specified period, such as a calendar year, a contract year, or a lifetime.

Medicaid A federal assistance program, established as Title XIX under the Social Security Act of 1965, that provides payment for medical and dental care for certain low-income individuals and families. The program is funded jointly by state and federal governments and is administered by each state.

Member See *enrollee.*

National Provider Identifier (NPI) A unique identification number used by a healthcare entity for the electronic transmission of protected personal health information (PHI). The NPI is part of the HIPAA Administrative Simplification provisions.

Nonduplication of benefits A benefit contract provision that limits carrier liability for the coordination of benefits claims. Total reimbursement may not exceed the highest amount payable by either contract rather than the actual fee charged or the maximum allowable amount. This is also called a *carve-out.*

Open panel system A dental benefits program that allows the following: (1) enrollees can receive dental treatment from any licensed dentist; (2) licensed dentists can participate; and (3) benefits are paid to either the enrollee or the dentist. The dentist may accept or refuse any enrollee in accordance with professional rules of conduct.

Point-of-service plan A dental benefits program in which the level of payment is based on the participation status of the dentist rendering treatment. In general, benefit levels are higher and patient copayments lower for services rendered by providers who participate in the enrollee's dental program. Covered services provided by out-of-network providers may be reimbursed on a lower fee scale with higher out-of-pocket costs for the enrollee.

Predetermination A treatment plan submitted to the benefits carrier for the review and estimation of payment before services are rendered. An approved predetermination is not a guarantee of payment; it is subject to eligibility, deductibles, and maximum used to date at the time when services are rendered. Some programs require predetermination for services that are expected to exceed a specific amount, such as $200. This is also called *precertification, preauthorization, pretreatment estimate,* and *prior authorization.*

Preferred provider organization (PPO) plan A dental benefits program in which participating dentists agree to accept payment based on a discounted fee schedule for services rendered to patients enrolled in the program.

Premium The amount charged by a dental benefits carrier for coverage or for the administration of benefits for a specified time.

Primary carrier The benefits carrier that has the initial responsibility for benefit payment when a patient is covered by two or more carriers. The primary carrier processes and pays claims to the full extent of the patient's coverage.

Reasonable and customary (R&C) plan A fee-for-service dental benefits program in which the payment of benefits is based on reasonable and customary fee criteria. See also *customary fee* and *reasonable fee.*

Reasonable fee The fee that is most often charged by the dentist or that is adjusted in consideration of the nature and severity of the condition treated and any medical or dental complications or unusual circumstances that may affect treatment.

Reimbursement Payment made by a benefits carrier or another third-party payer to an enrollee or to a dentist on behalf of the enrollee as repayment for the fees charged for a covered service.

Subscriber The employee or participant who is certified by the company or organization (group) providing the dental program as eligible to receive benefit coverage. If family coverage is offered, the additional people listed on the contract will be designated as spouse or dependent(s). See also *group member.*

Table of allowances plan A dental benefits program that lists an assigned amount payable for each covered service. The payable amount is generally below the average fee charged by dentists; also called a *schedule of allowances.*

Termination date The date on which the dental benefits contract ends or on which the enrollee is no longer eligible for benefits; also called the *expiration date.*

Third-party administrator (TPA) An entity that administers a health benefit plan without assuming any financial risk. The contracting organization reimburses the TPA for the total amount of paid claims plus an administration fee.

Unbundling of procedures The division of a dental procedure into component parts and the assignment of a separate charge for each; the total of these charges is higher than the single fee for the complete procedure.

Usual, customary, and reasonable (UCR) plan A dental benefits program in which payment for covered benefits is based on a formula that considers usual, customary, and reasonable fee data. See also *usual fee, customary fee,* and *reasonable fee.*

Usual fee The fee that a dentist most frequently charges for a given dental service.

OVERVIEW OF DENTAL INSURANCE

Evolution

The emergence of dental insurance and dental benefits programs in the middle of the twentieth century was a major factor in the expansion of general awareness of the importance of oral health and its link to general health and well-being. Dental benefits provided access to care for people who had never considered routine dental treatment. The general perception of dentistry changed as a result of patient education, transforming the dental office from a place best avoided to a familiar and necessary partner in personal healthcare.

As more companies and organizations added dental benefits to their group health coverage, the percentage of people seeking regular preventive services and restorative treatment increased. When oral health improved, patients and healthcare professionals began to notice a trend toward better overall health. By the end of the twentieth century, the connection between oral health and overall general health was clearly established, and certain oral health conditions were found to be warning signs of serious physical illnesses. Dentists can use those oral indicators to help with the detection and early diagnosis of diseases such as diabetes, high blood pressure, oral cancer, anemia, and deficient immune conditions (e.g., acquired immunodeficiency syndrome).

According to the most recent National Health Interview Survey conducted by the Centers for Disease Control and Prevention's National Center for Health Statistics, 73% of the surveyed population had some type of dental coverage. Those who have private dental benefits are much more likely to seek and receive care: nearly 60% of insured people go to the dentist, whereas only approximately 27% of the uninsured seek any dental treatment. Although the percentage of insured patients may vary (e.g., by region, specialty, policy), nearly every dental office offers insurance billing as a service to their patients.

The prompt and efficient insurance billing of dental services can have a direct effect on the profitability of the practice. The majority of dental offices accept the assignment of benefits, which allows the benefit payment to be paid to the dentist or the dental practice. Accepting the assignment of benefits almost always results in accelerated cash flow. For most routine claims (i.e., those with services that do not require a consultant review), insurance companies use automated processing systems that adjudicate and release payment in as little as 24 hours. The dental office almost always receives payment within 2 weeks, which helps with the management of the overall accounts receivable.

Understanding and efficiently using correct billing procedures is the only way to ensure that payment reaches the office as quickly as possible. This job requires organization, perseverance, and strict attention to detail.

Parties Involved

The system of dental insurance involves four parties: the patient, the dentist, the dental benefits carrier, and the group or program sponsor (e.g., employer, union, business association). The dental office administrative assistant works closely with the patient, the dentist, and the benefits carrier to produce the successful adjudication of dental benefit claims.

Patient

The patient is the primary resource for the information needed to submit a claim:

- The name and address of the benefits carrier
- The subscriber's name, address, identification number (Social Security number [SSN] or other assigned number), and date of birth
- The name of the subscriber's group or employer as well as its address and group number

Most patients are not aware of the details of their benefit coverage, and they do not understand most of the dental terminology associated with their treatment and coverage. In some cases, patients may not even have an identification card from their dental benefits carrier. When a patient of record has a change in benefits carrier or when a new patient comes into the office and he or she is uncertain about his or her carrier, the easiest solution is to ask him or her to contact his or her company's human resources department for the name, billing address, and contact information for the carrier. Many companies also have an employee intranet that employees can access to find the carrier's information as well as a breakdown of benefits.

The administrative assistant is usually responsible for explaining dental terms, codes, and benefit details in lay terms. Most dental benefit plans do not pay all costs, and helping patients to understand their treatment options and costs is an essential service. Benefit payment amounts cannot be guaranteed, even when a predetermination has been approved. The administrative assistant should remind patients that any quote for their out-of-pocket costs is an estimate based on information received from the carrier. This interaction empowers patients to be active partners in their dental care and promotes a good relationship between the patients and the practice. *NOTE:* It is important to inform each patient that, even if he or she is covered by a dental benefits program, he or she is ultimately personally liable for all treatment fees.

Dentist

The administrative assistant relies on the dentist to verify the services rendered, to determine the correct procedure codes, and to confirm the fees. Most dental offices work closely with carriers to help their patients make the best use of their benefits; however, the dentist and the patient together make the final decision regarding the best course of treatment. The dentist's primary commitment is to diagnose the patient's oral health status and needs, to discuss and render necessary treatment, to establish and maintain the patient's oral health, and to adhere to the standards of care that prevail in the professional community.

Dental Benefits Carrier

The dental benefits carrier may be an insurer, a third-party administrator (TPA), or a dental service corporation. The benefits carrier administers each plan according to the group contract, which includes maintaining member eligibility, processing claims, and remitting benefit payments to the appropriate party.

Most carriers have customer service representatives or consultants who respond to inquiries from members, group customers, and dental offices. The administrative assistant can contact the carrier to verify the patient's eligibility, the scope and levels of coverage, the claims address, and any other details pertinent to filing claims.

Group or Program Sponsor

The group (i.e., an employer, union, business association, or broker who represents the group) contracts with the benefits carrier and selects the benefit levels, the program type, the maximums, the limitations, and the exclusions for the dental plan. Although communicating with the group is generally the responsibility of the patient—who is also called the *group member* or *subscriber*—occasionally the administrative assistant may contact the group on behalf of the patient when an issue or inquiry cannot be resolved with the benefits carrier.

DENTAL BENEFITS PROGRAMS

The benefits carrier's method of reimbursement depends on the dental plan design. The two basic models of benefits programs are indemnity and capitation, although many variations of each model exist.

Many dental benefits carriers actively recruit dentists to participate in their programs. When a dentist signs a participation contract with a benefits carrier, he or she agrees to certain terms and conditions of payment for services rendered to enrollees. Each carrier has a unique set of terms of participation, which may include the following: accepting the carrier's fee table (no balance billing or unbundling of procedures or fees), receiving assignment of benefits, and filing claims for enrollees. Although the dentist may be required to discount fees to enrollees, participation in one or more programs is proven to do the following:

- *Build the practice.* Carriers encourage enrollees to see participating dentists and provide them with names of local participating dentists. An office can acquire many new patients and families from these referrals.
- *Accelerate cash flow.* Because participating dentists receive payment directly from the carrier, a large percentage of the treatment fees are usually paid within 30 days and sometimes in as few as 2 to 4 days. Maintaining a low accounts receivable is vital for a profitable practice.
- *Improve treatment acceptance.* Patients are much more likely to proceed with high-cost services when half or more of the fee is covered by their benefits plan. Patients without coverage are much more likely to delay treatment or to opt for less expensive services.

Indemnity

Indemnity is compensation for damage, loss, or injury. Dental indemnity plans make reimbursement to insured persons (or to the dentist through the assignment of benefits) for costs incurred through covered dental treatment (approved services).

Indemnity programs are most often referred to as *fee-for-service plans* because the reimbursement is based on the fee applied to each dental service rendered or received. The following list presents types of fee-for-service programs:

- Usual, customary, and reasonable (UCR) plan: Payment for covered benefits is based on a formula that considers usual (the fee most often charged for a service by a dentist), customary (the fee most often charged for a service in a geographic area or in a specialty), and reasonable (the fee that meets the other two criteria or that is adjusted according to the nature or criteria of individual circumstances) fee data.
- Reasonable and customary (R&C) plan: Payment for covered benefits is based on a formula that considers reasonable (the fee most often charged by the dentist or that is adjusted according to the nature or criteria of individual circumstances) and customary (the fee most often charged for a service in a geographic area or in a specialty) fee data.
- Preferred provider organization (PPO) plan: Payment is based on a discounted fee schedule. Dentists who sign an agreement with a carrier agree to accept the discounted fees as the full fee for their patients who are enrolled in the PPO. Any difference between the dentist's usual fee and the discounted fee is not chargeable to these patients. If the treating dentist does not participate with a patient's PPO plan, the patient is responsible for paying any difference between the fee charged and the amount paid by the carrier.
- Exclusive provider organization (EPO) plan: Benefits are payable only when services are rendered by participating providers. Enrollees have no benefit coverage for services received from out-of-network providers. Some exceptions may be allowed for emergency and out-of-area services.
- Point-of-service plan: Fee schedules and benefit levels depend on the dentist's participation status. These plans have a two-tiered payment structure with UCR/R&C and PPO/EPO plan features, and the treating dentist's participation status determines which fee schedule is applied to process claims. These plans often encourage members to seek treatment from PPO/EPO participating dentists by giving them a lower copayment for covered services. For example, members who go to a PPO/EPO participating dentist have coverage at 80% (a 20% copayment), those who see a non-PPO/EPO dentist have 50% coverage (a copayment of 50% of the allowed amount), plus they may have to pay any difference between the dentist's fee and the allowed amount.
- Table of allowances plan: Payment is based on a list of covered services, and each service has a fixed dollar amount for the reimbursement of treatment. This is also called a *schedule of allowances plan.*
- Open panel system: Payment can be made to the patient or the billing dentist, depending on the assignment of benefits guidelines. Panels of participating dentists may be available, and enrollees may choose to receive dental treatment from any licensed dentist. Dentists may accept or refuse any enrollee in accordance with professional rules of conduct.
- Closed panel system: Payment can only be made for services rendered by a participating dentist.

Capitation

Capitation is a benefits delivery system in which a contracting dentist or practice receives a fixed monthly or quarterly payment for providing covered dental services to enrollees who select or who are assigned to a specific office or location. The provider receives the payment regardless of whether services were actually performed. This program type is also called dental health maintenance organization (DHMO), and it is typically a closed panel system. To be covered, enrollees must go to their primary care provider or to a specific location for all of their dental treatment. Most plans allow the primary care dentist to refer enrollees to a participating specialist for qualified services, and exceptions may be allowed for emergency and out-of-area dental care. Enrollees may not have out-of-pocket costs for routine services, although they may have a copayment for high-cost services, such as fixing bridges.

Alternative Benefit Plans

Employers or associations that do not include dental coverage in their benefit package may elect to offer an alternative benefit plan. A variety of options are available, including the following:

- *Group discounts:* Large employers or associations may contract with dentists or dental clinics to deliver dental services to their enrollees at a discounted rate. The enrollee usually pays an annual or monthly membership fee and then pays the dentist directly for services rendered. The dentist does not file claims, and the plan has no exclusions, limitations, or maximums.
- *Discount card:* For an annual fee, purchasers have access to a network of participating dentists who have agreed to charge reduced fees to cardholders. The cardholder pays the dentist directly, and the dentist does not file any claims. This is also called a *dental savings plan* or a *dental savings card.*
- *Health flexible spending account (FSA):* The federal government allows eligible employers to offer their employees a pretax salary savings account for payment assistance with healthcare-related expenses. Contributions to the account are made by payroll deduction, and employees save money because no federal or state taxes are deducted. The employee designates an annual contribution amount, and any amounts not spent by the end of the year are forfeited. Patients with an FSA pay the dentist directly for their out-of-pocket costs and submit receipts to their employer for reimbursement.
- *Health savings account (HSA):* This is a medical savings account available to taxpayers who are enrolled in a high-deductible health plan. The HSA is owned by the eligible person, who can elect to contribute funds to the account through pretax payroll deductions from an employer. These contributions are excluded from gross income and exempt from payroll taxes. Unlike an FSA, the individual does not have to designate an annual contribution amount, and the funds accumulate from year to year if they are not spent. Patients with an HSA withdraw funds for qualified medical expenses and pay the dentist directly.

- *Direct reimbursement:* With direct reimbursement, an employer or organization can set up a self-funded program for reimbursing covered individuals based on a percentage of the amount spent for dental care.
- *Voluntary plans:* These individual dental benefit plans offer many of the same advantages of employer-sponsored plans, including lower rates and comprehensive benefit designs. Eligible persons who elect the coverage pay the full premium, so there is no cost to the employer or organization. Program administration can be assigned or shared among the employer, an insurance broker, and the benefits carrier.

PREPARING DENTAL CLAIM FORMS

Dental claims can be submitted on paper forms or electronically. Both modes require specific and detailed information about the patient or subscriber, the treating dentist, and the services rendered. One small error or omission can cause a claim to be rejected. Rejected claims create more work for the administrative staff and unnecessary delays in payment. The requirements of benefits carriers may vary, and the administrative assistant can streamline the claims process by becoming familiar with or keeping records regarding the specifications and techniques that work best with each carrier.

Some carriers require radiographs or documentation for a limited number of services, such as fixed bridges or miscellaneous procedures. When a carrier receives claims with attachments or documentation, they are automatically routed for review and manual processing, which always involves more time than standard automatic processing. Knowing what services require additional information prevents unnecessary delays in adjudication and payment. The administrative assistant can contact a benefits carrier to verify which procedure codes require special handling, radiographs, or supporting documentation.

Paper Claim Form

The American Dental Association (ADA) claim form (also known as the *attending dentist's statement*) is universally accepted, and it is designed to meet or exceed the informational needs of nearly all dental benefits carriers. The form includes comprehensive completion instructions (Figure 14-1), and it may be purchased from the ADA or from most dental supply vendors. Some dental benefits carriers have a proprietary paper claim form, which may be brought in by the patient or downloaded from the carriers' websites.

Most dental offices use computerized practice management software that generates and prints claim forms in a standard, ADA-compliant format. If the office does not use computers or the carrier requires the use of a specific form, the administrative assistant can legibly print or type the required information on the claim form. The assistant must review the paper claims, attach any required radiographs, and add documentation where needed. Claims are batched by carrier and then mailed out.

NOTE: When radiographs are mailed, they must be placed in a container, such a mount or an envelope. The patient's name, the dental office's name and address, and the tooth number or the area of the mouth shown on the film must be clearly written on the container. Carriers are not required to return radiographs, so any sent with a claim should be duplicates, and the original should be retained in the patient's records.

Electronic Claim Form

Nearly all dental offices have replaced the pegboard and appointment book with computers and sophisticated practice management software. The percentage of dental offices submitting all or part of their claims electronically continues to rise. Some carriers report that they receive more than 70% of dental claims electronically. As compared with the time and expense of preparing and mailing paper claims, electronic claims submission can be faster, less expensive, and more accurate. E-claims can be submitted through a clearinghouse or directly to the carrier through a web-based portal.

Offices that file e-claims must comply with federal laws governing electronic transactions that include personal health information (PHI). Under the Health Insurance Portability and Accountability Act of 1996 (HIPAA), all healthcare providers, health plans, and healthcare clearinghouses that transmit PHI electronically must use a universal language, a standard format, and a government-assigned unique identification number. HIPAA also mandates security and privacy standards for electronic transactions, as discussed in Chapter 7.

- *The Code:* The universal language used for electronic transmission of dental data is the ADA *Code on Dental Procedures and Nomenclature* (also known as *the Code*), which is updated every 2 years (Figure 14-2). *Current Dental Terminology (CDT)* manuals, which are the only official sources for the Code, can be purchased from the ADA; these list the procedure codes with nomenclature and descriptors, changes from the previous code, and other helpful information (Figure 14-3).
- *Electronic data formats:* HIPAA mandates the use of standardized formats for electronic transactions of health information. The standard formats are used for claims, remittance advice (explanation of benefits), eligibility inquiry and response, prior authorization and referral, and claims status inquiry and response. Attachments to the claim form (e.g., radiographs) can also be submitted electronically with the use of specialized software or services that assign a tracking number to match the supporting documentation of the claim. Most carriers prefer digital radiographs because they are easier and more cost-effective to handle and because the possibility of films becoming detached or lost is decreased.
- *Unique identifiers:* Dental offices that submit claims or claims attachments electronically or that use the Internet to look up eligibility, benefits, or claims status are required to have and use a National Provider Identifier (NPI). The NPI is a unique and permanent 10-digit number that identifies the dentist or

ADA American Dental Association® Dental Claim Form

Cigna dental plans are insured and/or administered by:
Cigna Health and Life Insurance Company
Connecticut General Life Insurance Company
Cigna Dental Care®
For mailing address, call Customer Service at the telephone number listed on your Cigna ID card.

Cigna.

HEADER INFORMATION

1. Type of Transaction (Mark all applicable boxes)
■ Statement of Actual Services ☐ Request for Predetermination/Preauthorization
☐ EPSDT / Title XIX

2. Predetermination/Preauthorization Number

INSURANCE COMPANY/DENTAL BENEFIT PLAN INFORMATION

3. Company/Plan Name, Address, City, State, Zip Code
USA Dental Benefits Company
1234 American Boulevard
New York, NY 01432-0001

OTHER COVERAGE (Mark applicable box and complete items 5-11. If none, leave blank.)

4. Dental? ☐ Medical? ☐ (If both, complete 5-11 for dental only.)
5. Name of Policyholder/Subscriber in #4 (Last, First, Middle Initial, Suffix)
6. Date of Birth (MM/DD/CCYY) 7. Gender ☐ M ☐ F 8. Policyholder/Subscriber ID (SSN or ID#)
9. Plan/Group Number 10. Patient's Relationship to Person named in #5 ☐ Self ☐ Spouse ☐ Dependent ☐ Other
11. Other Insurance Company/Dental Benefit Plan Name, Address, City, State, Zip Code

POLICYHOLDER/SUBSCRIBER INFORMATION (For Insurance Company Named in #3)

12. Policyholder/Subscriber Name (Last, First, Middle Initial, Suffix), Address, City, State, Zip Code
Jonathon B. Murphy
30052 Virginia Highway
Dallas, Texas 75150

13. Date of Birth (MM/DD/CCYY) 05/22/1983 14. Gender ■ M ☐ F 15. Policyholder/Subscriber ID (SSN or ID#) 001-23-0567

16. Plan/Group Number 14867-B 17. Employer Name Manufactured Products, Inc.

PATIENT INFORMATION

18. Relationship to Policyholder/Subscriber in #12 Above ☐ Self ■ Spouse ☐ Dependent Child ☐ Other
19. Reserved For Future Use
20. Name (Last, First, Middle Initial, Suffix), Address, City, State, Zip Code
Jessica A. Murphy
30052 Virginia Highway
Dallas, Texas 75150

21. Date of Birth (MM/DD/CCYY) 07/15/1984 22. Gender ☐ M ■ F 23. Patient ID/Account # (Assigned by Dentist)

RECORD OF SERVICES PROVIDED

	24. Procedure Date (MM/DD/CCYY)	25. Area of Oral Cavity	26. Tooth System	27. Tooth Number(s) or Letter(s)	28. Tooth Surface	29. Procedure Code	29a. Diag. Pointer	29b. Qty.	30. Description	31. Fee
1	01/16/20XX		JP	3		D2790			full cast high noble	$900.00
2	01/16/20XX		JP	4		D2750			porcelain fused to high noble	$950.00
3	01/16/20XX		JP	12	MO	D2332			composite - 2 surfaces	$125.00
4	01/16/20XX		JP	14	MOD	D2160			amalgam - three surfaces	$145.00
5										
6										
7										
8										
9										
10										

33. Missing Teeth Information (Place an "X" on each missing tooth.)
1 2 3 4 5 6 7 8 9 10 11 12 13 14 15 16
32 31 30 29 28 27 26 25 24 23 22 21 20 19 18 17

34. Diagnosis Code List Qualifier ☐ (ICD-9 = B; ICD-10 = AB)
34a. Diagnosis Code(s) (Primary diagnosis in "A") A ____ B ____ C ____ D ____

31a. Other Fee(s)
32. Total Fee $0.00

35. Remarks

AUTHORIZATIONS

36. I have been informed of the treatment plan and associated fees. I agree to be responsible for all charges for dental services and materials not paid by my dental benefit plan, unless prohibited by law, or the treating dentist or dental practice has a contractual agreement with my plan prohibiting all or a portion of such charges. To the extent permitted by law, I consent to your use and disclosure of my protected health information to carry out payment activities in connection with this claim.

X Patient/Guardian Signature Date

37. I hereby authorize and direct payment of the dental benefits otherwise payable to me, directly to the below named dentist or dental entity.

X Subscriber Signature Date

ANCILLARY CLAIM/TREATMENT INFORMATION

38. Place of Treatment 11 (e.g. 11=office; 22=O/P Hospital) (Use "Place of Service Codes for Professional Claims")
39. Enclosures (Y or N) Y
40. Is Treatment for Orthodontics? ■ No (Skip 41-42) ☐ Yes (Complete 41-42)
41. Date Appliance Placed (MM/DD/CCYY)
42. Months of Treatment 43. Replacement of Prosthesis ■ No ☐ Yes (Complete 44)
44. Date of Prior Placement (MM/DD/CCYY)
45. Treatment Resulting from ☐ Occupational illness/injury ☐ Auto accident ☐ Other accident
46. Date of Accident (MM/DD/CCYY) 47. Auto Accident State

BILLING DENTIST OR DENTAL ENTITY (Leave blank if dentist or dental entity is not submitting claim on behalf of the patient or insured/subscriber.)

48. Name, Address, City, State, Zip Code
Ashley Lake, D.D.S., PC
22215 Abbot Road Suite 2D
Dallas, Texas 75228

49. NPI 1058910598 50. License Number 24485 TX 51. SSN or TIN 42-485223
52. Phone Number (469) 221-4667 52a. Additional Provider ID

TREATING DENTIST AND TREATMENT LOCATION INFORMATION

53. I hereby certify that the procedures as indicated by date are in progress (for procedures that require multiple visits) or have been completed.

X Signed (Treating Dentist) 01/16/20XX Date

54. NPI 1058910598 55. License Number 24485 TX
56. Address, City, State, Zip Code 22215 Abbot Road Suite 2D Dallas, Texas 75228 56a. Provider Specialty Code 122300000X
57. Phone Number (469) 221-4667 58. Additional Provider ID

Cat. #590154f Rev. 12/2013

ADA American Dental Association®
America's leading advocate for oral health

The following information highlights certain form completion instructions. Comprehensive ADA Dental Claim Form completion instructions are printed in the CDT manual. Any updates to these instructions will be posted on the ADA's web site (ADA.org).

GENERAL INSTRUCTIONS

A. The form is designed so that the name and address (Item 3) of the third-party payer receiving the claim (insurance company/dental benefit plan) is visible in a standard #9 window envelope (window to the left). Please fold the form using the 'tick-marks' printed in the margin.
B. Complete all items unless noted otherwise on the form or in the CDT manual's instructions.
C. Enter the full name of an individual or a full business name, address and zip code when a name and address field is required.
D. All dates must include the four-digit year.
E. If the number of procedures reported exceeds the number of lines available on one claim form, list the remaining procedures on a separate, fully completed claim form.

COORDINATION OF BENEFITS (COB)

When a claim is being submitted to the secondary payer, complete the entire form and attach the primary payer's Explanation of Benefits (EOB) showing the amount paid by the primary payer. You may also note the primary carrier paid amount in the "Remarks" field (Item 35). There are additional detailed completion instructions in the CDT manual.

DIAGNOSIS CODING

The form supports reporting up to four diagnosis codes per dental procedure. This information is required when the diagnosis may affect claim adjudication when specific dental procedures may minimize the risks associated with the connection between the patient's oral and systemic health conditions. Diagnosis codes are linked to procedures using the following fields:

Item 29a – Diagnosis Code Pointer ("A" through "D" as applicable from Item 34a)
Item 34 – Diagnosis Code List Qualifier (B for ICD-9-CM; AB for ICD-10-CM)
Item 34a – Diagnosis Code(s) / A, B, C, D (up to four, with the primary adjacent to the letter "A")

PLACE OF TREATMENT

Enter the 2-digit Place of Service Code for Professional Claims, a HIPAA standard maintained by the Centers for Medicare and Medicaid Services. Frequently used codes are:

11 = Office; 12 = Home; 21 = Inpatient Hospital; 22 = Outpatient Hospital; 31 = Skilled Nursing Facility; 32 = Nursing Facility

The full list is available online at "www.cms.gov/PhysicianFeeSched/Downloads/Website_POS_database.pdf"

PROVIDER SPECIALTY

This code is entered in Item 56a and indicates the type of dental professional who delivered the treatment. The general code listed as "Dentist" may be used instead of any of the other codes.

Category / Description Code	Code
Dentist A dentist is a person qualified by a doctorate in dental surgery (D.D.S.) or dental medicine (D.M.D.) licensed by the state to practice dentistry, and practicing within the scope of that license.	122300000X
General Practice	1223G0001X
Dental Specialty (see following list)	Various
Dental Public Health	1223D0001X
Endodontics	1223E0200X
Orthodontics	1223X0400X
Pediatric Dentistry	1223P0221X
Periodontics	1223P0300X
Prosthodontics	1223P0700X
Oral & Maxillofacial Pathology	1223P0106X
Oral & Maxillofacial Radiology	1223D0008X
Oral & Maxillofacial Surgery	1223S0112X

Provider taxonomy codes listed above are a subset of the full code set that is posted at "www.wpc-edi.com/codes/taxonomy"

FIGURE 14-1 An American Dental Association dental claim form. **A,** Front. **B,** Back (Courtesy American Dental Association, Chicago.)

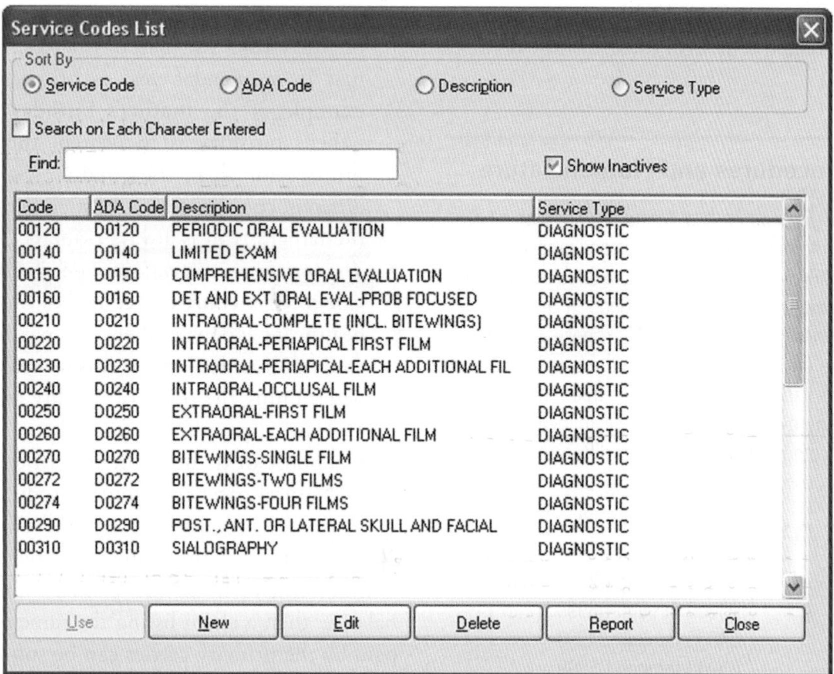

FIGURE 14-2 Pull-down screen of American Dental Association service codes. (Courtesy Patterson Dental, St. Paul, Minnesota.)

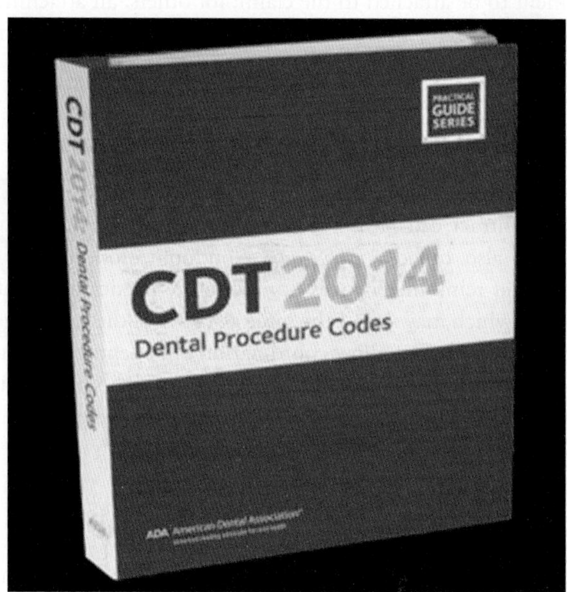

FIGURE 14-3 *Current Dental Terminology* (CDT), the only official source for dental service codes, is published by the American Dental Association and updated every 2 years. (Courtesy American Dental Association, Chicago, Illinois.)

practice and that replaces any other identifiers used in electronic transactions. (It does not replace the tax identification number [TIN] or the treating dentist's state license number, because these are used for purposes other than identification.) To get an NPI, a dentist or a dental practice applies to an agency designated by the federal government.

Via Clearinghouse

A clearinghouse is a company that accepts the transmission of raw data, scans it for errors or missing information, and then transforms it into the appropriate data format for submission to the benefits carrier. The clearinghouse charges either a set amount per claim or a monthly fee for this service.

With the use of practice management software, the dental office administrative assistant collects the patient and treatment information that is ready to be billed to a benefits carrier and transmits it to the clearinghouse. The clearinghouse reformats the data and then transmits any claims with missing or incomplete information back to the dental office for correction. The formatted claims are sorted by benefits carrier or insurance company and mass-transmitted to the carrier for processing. The clearinghouse can also print and mail paper claim forms to the few carriers that are unable to accept electronic claims.

Direct to Carrier

The dental office has to be computerized and connected to the Internet to transmit claims directly to benefits carriers. Most major carriers provide this service free of charge. To submit, the administrative assistant goes online to the carrier's website or portal and enters claim information into an electronic claim form, which can begin processing immediately. Entering claims via the portal eliminates the sorting, scanning, and data entry that a carrier must do with paper claims, so processing time is reduced by an average of 2 to 4 days. In most cases, routine claims are adjudicated and released for payment within 24 hours of entering the carrier's system. The dental practice's transaction history—including payments, rejections, and predeterminations—is maintained in a highly secure system; it can be accessed or downloaded only with the use of the dentist's unique password.

Code on Dental Procedures and Nomenclature

The ADA *Code on Dental Procedures and Nomenclature* (commonly known as *the Code*) is used to report dental services and procedures to dental benefits plans. Per HIPAA, the ADA updates the Code every other year (in odd-numbered years) and publishes the Code in a reference manual called *Current Dental Terminology* (*CDT*). These procedure codes identify and describe each specific dental treatment. The codes and the dentist's fees are used to report and bill treatment to the benefits carrier. Each procedure code starts with a "D" followed by four numerals. The codes are categorized according to different types of treatment:

Diagnostic	D0100 through D0999
Preventive	D1000 through D1999
Restorative	D2000 through D2999
Endodontics	D3000 through D3999
Periodontics	D4000 through D4999
Prosthetics, removable	D5000 through D5899
Maxillofacial prosthetics	D5900 through D5999
Implant services	D6000 through D6199
Prosthodontics, fixed	D6200 through D6999
Oral and maxillofacial surgery	D7000 through D7999
Orthodontics	D8000 through D8999
Adjunctive general services	D9000 through D9999

COORDINATION OF BENEFITS

Coordination of benefits (COB) is the procedure used to determine the order of liability when a person is covered by more than one plan. Dental benefits carriers follow rules established by state law to determine which plan pays first (primary carrier) and the financial obligation of any additional carrier (e.g., secondary, tertiary). The objective is to provide the maximum allowable benefit (MAB) without exceeding the actual fee charged.

Determining the Order of Liability

To identify the primary plan, the administrative assistant needs to know whether the patient is the subscriber or a dependent and whether there are any special COB rules for either plan. The primary carrier must meet at least one of the following criteria:

- *A plan has a no-COB clause.* If the plan does not coordinate benefits, it is the primary plan.
- *The patient is the employee (subscriber).* The plan that covers the patient as an active employee (subscriber) is always primary over a plan that covers the person as a retiree, spouse, dependent, or COBRA-qualified beneficiary. If the patient is the subscriber for both plans, the plan that covers the person as an active employee is primary. If the subscriber is an active employee under both plans, then the plan that has covered the individual the longest is primary.
- *The patient is a dependent child.* Most carriers follow the birthday rule: the plan of the parent whose birthday comes first in a calendar year is primary for the children. For example, if the mother's birthday is in January and the father's birthday is in March, then the mother's plan is primary for all of the children. Some carriers may have a different coordination rule, such as the gender rule, in which the father's plan is always primary.
- *The patient is a dependent child of divorced or legally separated parents.* If a court decree makes one parent responsible for healthcare expenses, then that parent's plan is primary. If a court decree does not mention healthcare, default rules for determining the order of liability are as follows:
  - Natural parent with custody
  - Spouse of natural parent with custody
  - Natural parent without custody
  - Spouse of natural parent without custody

The claim for the primary carrier is always filed first. If reimbursement from the primary carrier leaves an unpaid balance, then a claim listing the same services and the amount paid by the primary carrier can be submitted to the next liable (secondary) carrier. The total amount paid by the primary carrier must be indicated in the field reserved for the primary carrier's payment (if any) or in the "Remarks" section. Some benefits carriers may require a copy of the primary carrier's payment to be attached to the claim; for others, an attachment may actually delay processing. When in doubt, check with the carrier.

Coordination of Benefits Limitations

Some programs limit the scope of benefits coordination. A group contract can have a nonduplication of benefits clause, which is also called a *carve-out*. Nonduplication of benefits means that reimbursement is limited to the maximum payable amount, which may not be the same as 100% of the fee charged. Other groups do not allow coordination of benefits for spouses who are both employees (subscribers) in the same group, although dual coverage may be allowed for their dependents.

REVIEWING THE COMPLETED CLAIM FORM

Figure 14-4 is an example of a correctly completed paper claim form. (*NOTE:* Entering the description is not required.) The completed services and proposed treatment plan are given as follows:

Tooth Number	Treatment	Procedure Number
3	Full cast, high noble	D2790
4	Porcelain fused to high noble	D2750
12MO	Composite—two surfaces	D2332
14MOD	Amalgam—three surfaces	D2160

The administrative assistant must understand the Code and apply it correctly. For example, the number of surfaces and the restorative material used on these fillings determine the procedure code number.

DENTAL CLAIM PAYMENTS

Most carriers provide a voucher that explains the claim payment with a line-by-line breakdown that is commonly called an **explanation of benefits (EOB)**. Depending on a carrier's guidelines for participation or its **assignment of benefits**, payment is sent either to the dentist or to the patient or subscriber.

When the dentist participates with the carrier or when the patient or subscriber assigns benefits to the dentist, the carrier can remit payment to the dental office by mailing a paper check and an EOB (Figure 14-5, *A*) or by performing an electronic funds transfer (EFT) into a designated checking account. Offices that combine e-claims and EFTs can receive payment in their bank accounts within 24 to 48 hours of the transmission of the claim. To use EFT (which is also called *direct deposit*), enrollment forms and authorization must be filed with each carrier. After a dental office has enrolled for this type of payment, most carriers will pay all claims (both electronic and paper) by EFT.

NOTE: Benefits carriers may not send out copies of checks or EOBs for EFT deposits, so the administrative assistant may have to access payment information online from the carrier's secure website or portal.

The administrative assistant should review each voucher to match the billed services with the items on the EOB and to make sure all services were paid correctly. Patients also receive an EOB (see Figure 14-5, *B*) to advise them that the claim is

ADA American Dental Association® Dental Claim Form

HEADER INFORMATION
1. Type of Transaction (Mark all applicable boxes)
[■] Statement of Actual Services [ ] Request for Predetermination/Preauthorization
[ ] EPSDT / Title XIX
2. Predetermination/Preauthorization Number

INSURANCE COMPANY/DENTAL BENEFIT PLAN INFORMATION
3. Company/Plan Name, Address, City, State, Zip Code
USA Dental Benefits Company
1234 American Boulevard
New York, NY 01432-0001

OTHER COVERAGE (Mark applicable box and complete items 5-11. If none, leave blank.)
4. Dental? [ ] Medical? [ ] (If both, complete 5-11 for dental only.)
5. Name of Policyholder/Subscriber in #4 (Last, First, Middle Initial, Suffix)
6. Date of Birth (MM/DD/CCYY)
7. Gender [ ] M [ ] F
8. Policyholder/Subscriber ID (SSN or ID#)
9. Plan/Group Number
10. Patient's Relationship to Person named in #5 [ ] Self [ ] Spouse [ ] Dependent [ ] Other
11. Other Insurance Company/Dental Benefit Plan Name, Address, City, State, Zip Code

POLICYHOLDER/SUBSCRIBER INFORMATION (For Insurance Company Named in #3)
12. Policyholder/Subscriber Name (Last, First, Middle Initial, Suffix), Address, City, State, Zip Code
Jonathon B. Murphy
30052 Virginia Highway
Dallas, Texas 75150
13. Date of Birth (MM/DD/CCYY) 05/22/1983
14. Gender [■] M [ ] F
15. Policyholder/Subscriber ID (SSN or ID#) 001-23-0567
16. Plan/Group Number 14867-B
17. Employer Name Manufactured Products, Inc.

PATIENT INFORMATION
18. Relationship to Policyholder/Subscriber in #12 Above [ ] Self [■] Spouse [ ] Dependent Child [ ] Other
19. Reserved For Future Use
20. Name (Last, First, Middle Initial, Suffix), Address, City, State, Zip Code
Jessica A. Murphy
30052 Virginia Highway
Dallas, Texas 75150
21. Date of Birth (MM/DD/CCYY) 07/15/1984
22. Gender [ ] M [■] F
23. Patient ID/Account # (Assigned by Dentist)

RECORD OF SERVICES PROVIDED

	24. Procedure Date (MM/DD/CCYY)	25. Area of Oral Cavity	26. Tooth System	27. Tooth Number(s) or Letter(s)	28. Tooth Surface	29. Procedure Code	29a. Diag. Pointer	29b. Qty.	30. Description	31. Fee
1	01/16/20XX		JP	3		D2790			full cast high noble	$900.00
2	01/16/20XX		JP	4		D2750			porcelain fused to high noble	$950.00
3	01/16/20XX		JP	12	MO	D2332			composite - 2 surfaces	$125.00
4	01/16/20XX		JP	14	MOD	D2160			amalgam - three surfaces	$145.00
5										
6										
7										
8										
9										
10										

33. Missing Teeth Information (Place an "X" on each missing tooth.)
1 2 3 4 5 6 7 8 9 10 11 12 13 14 15 16
32 31 30 29 28 27 26 25 24 23 22 21 20 19 18 17
34. Diagnosis Code List Qualifier [ ] (ICD-9 = B; ICD-10 = AB)
34a. Diagnosis Code(s) (Primary diagnosis in "A") A ____ B ____ C ____ D ____
31a. Other Fee(s)
32. Total Fee $0.00
35. Remarks

AUTHORIZATIONS
36. I have been informed of the treatment plan and associated fees. I agree to be responsible for all charges for dental services and materials not paid by my dental benefit plan, unless prohibited by law, or the treating dentist or dental practice has a contractual agreement with my plan prohibiting all or a portion of such charges. To the extent permitted by law, I consent to your use and disclosure of my protected health information to carry out payment activities in connection with this claim.
X ____ Patient/Guardian Signature Date
37. I hereby authorize and direct payment of the dental benefits otherwise payable to me, directly to the below named dentist or dental entity.
X ____ Subscriber Signature Date

ANCILLARY CLAIM/TREATMENT INFORMATION
38. Place of Treatment [11] (e.g. 11=office; 22=O/P Hospital) (Use "Place of Service Codes for Professional Claims")
39. Enclosures (Y or N) [Y]
40. Is Treatment for Orthodontics? [■] No (Skip 41-42) [ ] Yes (Complete 41-42)
41. Date Appliance Placed (MM/DD/CCYY)
42. Months of Treatment
43. Replacement of Prosthesis [■] No [ ] Yes (Complete 44)
44. Date of Prior Placement (MM/DD/CCYY)
45. Treatment Resulting from [ ] Occupational illness/injury [ ] Auto accident [ ] Other accident
46. Date of Accident (MM/DD/CCYY)
47. Auto Accident State

BILLING DENTIST OR DENTAL ENTITY (Leave blank if dentist or dental entity is not submitting claim on behalf of the patient or insured/subscriber.)
48. Name, Address, City, State, Zip Code
Ashley Lake, D.D.S., PC
22215 Abbot Road Suite 2D
Dallas, Texas 75228
49. NPI 1058910598
50. License Number 24485 TX
51. SSN or TIN 42-485223
52. Phone Number (469) 221-4667
52a. Additional Provider ID

TREATING DENTIST AND TREATMENT LOCATION INFORMATION
53. I hereby certify that the procedures as indicated by date are in progress (for procedures that require multiple visits) or have been completed.
X ____ Signed (Treating Dentist) 01/16/20XX Date
54. NPI 1058910598
55. License Number 24485 TX
56. Address, City, State, Zip Code
22215 Abbot Road Suite 2D
Dallas, Texas 75228
56a. Provider Specialty Code 122300000X
57. Phone Number (469) 221-4667
58. Additional Provider ID

J430D (Same as ADA Dental Claim Form – J430, J431, J432, J433, J434)
Cat. #590154f Rev. 12/2013

FIGURE 14-4 Sample completed claim form for restorative services. (Courtesy American Dental Association, Chicago, Illinois.)

Explanation of Benefit Payments

(THIS IS NOT A BILL)

Patient Name: CYNTHIA MARTINEZ-JONES
Date of Birth: 10/19/1983
Relationship: SUBSCRIBER
Subscriber: CYNTHIA MARTINEZ-JONES
Subscriber ID: XXX-XX-2065
Patient Acct: 00438300R66889-2727

Business/Dentist: ASHLEY LAKE, D.D.S., P.C.
License No: 24485 /TX (NPI: 1058910598)
Check No: 8027446043
Issue Date: 04/20/20XX
Receipt Date: 04/20/20XX
Claim No: 2804651139940

Pay To: C = Custodial Parent
S = Subscriber
P = Provider

Tooth Code/ Area/Surface	Date of Service	Procedure Code	Submitted Amount	Maximum Approved Fee	Par Dentist Adjustment	Allowed Amount	Deductible/Patient Copay/Office Visits	Copay %	Payment	Patient Payment	Pay To
CLIENT/ID: 11012 ACME MANUFACTURING					PLAN: USA DENTAL BENEFITS COMPANY						
SUBCLIENT: 00044 INTERSTATE DIVISION					PRODUCT: USA DENTAL PPO (POINT OF SERVICE)						
	04/18/XX	D0120	55.00	55.00	0.00	55.00		100%	55.00	0.00	P
	04/18/XX	D0210	122.00	120.00	2.00	120.00		100%	120.00	0.00	P
	04/18/XX	D1110	75.00	71.00	4.00	71.00		100%	75.00	0.00	P
		Total	252.00	246.00	6.00	246.00	0.00		246.00	0.00	

GENERAL MAXIMUM USED TO DATE: 751.60

FOR INQUIRIES: 1-800-555-5555

CLAIMS PROCESSED BY:
USA DENTAL BENEFITS COMPANY
1234 AMERICAN BOULEVARD
NEW YORK, NY 01432-0001

Payment for these services is determined in accordance with the specific terms of the member's dental plan and/or USA Dental Benefit Company's agreements with its participating dentists.

ASHLEY LAKE, D.D.S., P.C.
22215 ABBOT ROAD SUITE 2D
DALLAS, TX 75228

Explanation of Benefit Payments

(THIS IS NOT A BILL)

Patient Name: CYNTHIA MARTINEZ-JONES
Date of Birth: 10/19/1983
Relationship: SUBSCRIBER
Subscriber: CYNTHIA MARTINEZ-JONES
Patient Acct: 00438300R66889-2727

Business/Dentist: ASHLEY LAKE, D.D.S., P.C.
License No: 24485 /TX (NPI: 1058910598)
Check No: 8027446043
Issue Date: 04/20/20XX
Receipt Date: 04/20/20XX
Claim No: 2804651139940

Pay To: C = Custodial Parent
S = Subscriber
P = Provider

Tooth Code/ Area/Surface	Date of Service	Procedure Description	Submitted Amount	Maximum Approved Fee	Par Dentist Savings	Allowed Amount	Deductible/Patient Copay/Office Visits	Copay %	Payment	Patient Payment	Pay To
CLIENT/ID: 11012 ACME MANUFACTURING					PLAN: USA DENTAL BENEFITS COMPANY						
SUBCLIENT: 00044 INTERSTATE DIVISION					PRODUCT: USA DENTAL PPO (POINT OF SERVICE)						
	04/18/XX	ORAL EXAM	55.00	55.00	0.00	55.00		100%	55.00	0.00	P
	04/18/XX	X-RAYS	122.00	120.00	2.00	120.00		100%	120.00	0.00	P
	04/18/XX	CLEANING	75.00	71.00	4.00	71.00		100%	75.00	0.00	P
		Total	252.00	246.00	6.00	246.00	0.00		246.00	0.00	

GENERAL MAXIMUM USED TO DATE: 751.60

FOR INQUIRIES: 1-800-555-5555

CLAIMS PROCESSED BY:
USA DENTAL BENEFITS COMPANY
1234 AMERICAN BOULEVARD
NEW YORK, NY 01432-0001

Payment for these services is determined in accordance with the specific terms of your dental plan and/or USA Dental Benefit Company's agreements with its participating dentists. For inquiries about participating dentist, please call the number listed. USA Dental Benefit Company's decisions do not qualify as dental or medical advice.
If your claim was denied in whole or in part so that you must pay some of the claim, upon written request and free of charge, we will provide you with any internal rule, guideline, or protocol, or if applicable, an explanation of the scientific or clinical judgment relied upon in deciding your claim. If you still believe your claim should have been paid in full, you may ask to have the claim reviewed. Your request for a formal review must be sent within 180 days of your receipt of this EOB at this address. You may submit any additional materials you believe will support your claim. A decision will be made no later than 60 days from the date we receive your request. If your claim is denied in whole or in part after the review, you have the right to seek to have your claim paid by filing a civil action in court within one year from the final denial.

CYNTHIA MARTINEZ-JONES
1156 OAKVIEW TRAIL
DALLAS, TX 75150

FIGURE 14-5 Explanation of benefit (EOB) statements are provided to the provider **(A)** and the patient **(B)**. (Courtesy Delta Dental of Michigan, Ohio, and Indiana, Lansing, Michigan.)

paid and to indicate the amount for which they are responsible for paying the dentist.

Some carriers send payment to the patient even if the assignment of benefits line on the claim form indicates payment to the dentist. When benefit payments are sent to the patient, many carriers do not send a copy of the voucher to the dentist. Patients can easily misplace a check and, even when the patient cashes or deposits the check, the dentist's payment is usually delayed. The simplest solution for both the patient and the dental office is for the administrative assistant to ask the patient to endorse the check and forward it to the office as soon as it is received. If the patient does not get a payment for services billed by the dental office within 30 days, the administrative assistant can contact the carrier to verify that the claim was received, check on the processing status, and ask if a payment has been sent. If the carrier has a web-based portal, claim history may be accessed online, along with patient eligibility and benefit information.

SPECIAL PROGRAMS

Medicaid

Medicaid is a federal assistance program established as Title XIX under the Social Security Act of 1965. It provides payment for healthcare for certain low-income individuals and families. The program is funded jointly by the federal and state governments, and it is administered by each state. Medicaid should not be confused with Medicare, which subsidizes medical expenses for citizens 65 years of age and older.

Eligibility for Medicaid programs is determined by the state, and it is generally for individuals who are receiving public financial assistance. The program provides comprehensive dental benefits to eligible children and adults younger than 21 years, as required by federal law. Dental coverage for adults enrolled in Medicaid may be limited by the state.

Because each state administers its own Medicaid program, rules and regulations governing covered dental services vary. Most programs have the following general conditions:

- Reimbursement is made only to dentists who participate in the Medicaid program. (Medicaid recipients never receive claim payments.)
- The dentist agrees to accept the amount paid by the state (or any carrier designated by the state) as payment in full; there is no patient copayment. (*NOTE:* In states with adult Medicaid dental coverage, adults older than 21 years may have a minimal copayment per visit.)
- Any other third-party payer is primary.
- Reimbursement to the state is required if the patient or dentist receives payment from another third-party source.
- Records must be retained for a specified length of time and may be reviewed by an authorized state or federal official.
- Patients with Medicaid coverage may not be discriminated against for reasons of race, gender, color, creed, or financial status.
- All claims must be submitted within 12 months of the date of treatment.
- Prior authorization is required for certain treatments, as outlined by the state.
- All patient records remain confidential.
- Handwritten forms are not accepted; forms must be typewritten, computer-generated, or submitted electronically.

Medicaid processing centers accept the standard ADA paper claim form and require HIPAA compliance for all electronic submissions. In some states, the Medical Services Administration (MSA) contracts with commercial benefits carriers to partially administer alternative dental programs for children and young adults covered by Medicaid. A national model for expanding access to dental services for low-income individuals who are younger than 21 years, called *Healthy Kids Dental* (HKD) was established in Michigan, and it has replaced Medicaid in 78 Michigan counties. The state maintains enrollee status, and claims, inquiries, eligibility requests, and payments are processed by Delta Dental. Some other states (e.g., Tennessee, Alabama, Connecticut, Vermont) have public-private partnerships set up to improve access to care. More information about how states are working to improve access to oral healthcare for children enrolled in Medicaid and the State Children's Health Insurance Program can be found on the ADA's website at www.ada.org.

U.S. Department of Veterans Affairs

Veterans of the U.S. Armed Forces may be eligible for limited dental benefits. Patients with this coverage receive a claim form from the U.S. Department of Veterans Affairs to give to the attending dentist, and the form includes all information necessary to assess benefits. Prior approval of treatment is usually required.

GUIDELINES FOR SUCCESSFUL CLAIMS ADMINISTRATION

Every team member is vital to the success of the dental office. The administrative assistant takes care of the business end of dentistry, and proper handling of the insurance accounts receivable ensures that the practice meets its financial goals. Claims must be submitted promptly and correctly and records accurately maintained to track claims status and payments. The following are some guidelines and suggestions for controlling claims input and output:

- Keep a record of the subscriber's benefits carrier and scope of coverage. Most practice management software programs have a module that stores information by employer or organization. For offices that keep paper records, a standardized detail sheet for each plan can be kept in a central file, in a notebook, or in the patient's personal record.
- Note any special information or procedures that the carrier requires.
- Require new patients and patients of record who have a change in coverage to provide the new benefits carrier's complete mailing address and telephone number for inquiries.

- Ask patients if they have any changes in coverage at each appointment. If the subscriber has been terminated or laid off, if he or she is on sick leave, or if he or she has changed jobs, dental benefit coverage may be affected. A call to the benefits carrier can to help determine eligibility and effective dates and termination/expiration dates.
- Inform each patient about his or her covered benefits and copayment levels.
- Establish a routine for preparing claim forms, such as setting aside one or two times each day and preparing claims for daily mailings or electronic transmission.
- Keep a current file or computer record of outstanding claims, and review it frequently. Follow up with the benefits carrier on claims that are outstanding for more than 30 days.
- Submit preauthorization for treatment (predetermination) when required by the subscriber's plan or benefits carrier and when requested by the dentist or the patient.
- Regularly verify and update patients' general information.
- If using paper claims, maintain an adequate supply of forms.
- Focus on accuracy and complete all required fields on the claim form. If a field does not apply, leave it blank.
- Add comments only for codes that require documentation, such as miscellaneous codes (e.g., D2999, D6199).
- Always use current CDT codes and refer to the active CDT handbook whenever needed. Attend seminars presented by benefits carriers to stay current with regard to billing practices and to learn new techniques. Many seminars offer CDE credits for licensed or registered dental assistants.

INSURANCE FRAUD

Misrepresenting treatment or inaccurately reporting fees and dates of service to benefits carriers is illegal; accuracy and honesty are not negotiable. Administrative assistants who participate in any way with actions that defraud benefits carriers may be liable to legal prosecution.

The following actions, whether deliberate or unintentional, constitute fraud:

- Billing the benefits carrier for higher fees than the patient is charged
- Billing before the completion of service
- Predating or postdating services on claim forms
- Improperly reporting treatment (e.g., listing a bony extraction instead of a simple extraction)
- Billing for services not rendered

DENTAL INSURANCE TERMINOLOGY

Allowed amount The maximum dollar amount that the benefits carrier sets for a dental procedure. It is not always the same as the approved amount.

Approved amount The amount used by the benefits carrier as the basis of payment for a submitted fee.

Benefits administrator The person or company who manages or directs a dental benefits program on behalf of the program's sponsor.

Benefits plan summary A description or synopsis of employee benefits, which employers are legally required to distribute to employees. This is also called the *summary plan description (SPD).*

Benefit year The 12-month period of the dental contract, which is not always a calendar year. Most patients have a maximum allowable benefit that renews at the beginning of each benefit year.

Cafeteria plan A health coverage system under which employers offer eligible employees a list of options for healthcare benefits and that may include several carriers and levels of coverage. Participants may receive additional taxable cash compensation if they select less expensive benefits.

Claim audit An administrative or professional review of the services reported on a claim to verify information, to determine the appropriateness of treatment, or to propose acceptable alternative treatment.

Claimant A person who files a claim for the reimbursement of covered costs.

Covered charges Charges for services rendered or supplies furnished by a dentist that qualify as covered services and that are paid for in whole or in part by the dental benefits program. These charges may be subject to deductibles, copayments, co-insurance, and annual or lifetime maximums as specified by the terms of the contract.

Covered services A dental service that is payable under the terms of the benefit program.

Deductible The amount of dental expenses a covered person must pay before the dental plan benefits begin. The amount of the deductible may vary and can be applied once or annually or to a specific set of services. Individual deductibles apply to one person; family deductibles are satisfied by combining the expenses of all covered family members. Some services may be exempt from the deductible.

Direct billing Requiring payment in full from the patient or the responsible party for all services rendered.

Extension of benefits An extension of eligibility that covers treatment started before the expiration date. The duration is limited and generally expressed in days.

Individual practice association (IPA) Independent dentists who legally join together as a dental group and contract with a carrier, a business, or an organization to provide services to enrolled populations. Dentists may practice in their own offices and provide care to patients not covered by the contract as well as to IPA patients.

Maximum allowable amount The highest dollar amount payable by a third-party payer for a covered dental treatment. This is also called the *maximum allowable payment.*

Nonparticipating dentist A dentist who does not have a contractual agreement with a dental benefits carrier.

Open enrollment The period during which employees or group members can enroll in healthcare programs.

Overcoding Reporting a more complex or more expensive procedure than was actually performed.

Participating dentist A dentist who has a contractual agreement with a dental benefits carrier.

Peer review A process for reviewing issues that arise from dental treatment. A panel of licensed dentists reviews cases submitted by carriers, patients, and dentists that involve quality of care, appropriateness of treatment, fee disputes, and professionalism. The review panel is typically organized by the state dental association.

Preexisting condition An oral health condition that existed before a person enrolled in a dental program.

Schedule of benefits A list of dental services covered by a dental benefits program.

Waiting period The period between employment or enrollment in a dental program and the date that the enrollee becomes eligible for benefits. This may also be the specific time frame between the date of eligibility and the activation of coverage for some services.

LEARNING ACTIVITIES

1. Identify the four parties affected by dental benefits and the roles of each.
2. Describe the two main types of dental benefits programs.
3. What patient information is needed to complete a standard ADA claim form?
4. Describe the *Code on Dental Procedures and Nomenclature,* and explain how it is used.
5. Differentiate between filing claims on paper and electronically.
6. What is the purpose of the claim payment voucher?
7. Identify five actions that constitute dental benefits fraud.

Please refer to the student workbook for additional learning activities.

BIBLIOGRAPHY

http://www.ada.org/en/publications/cdt/ada-dental-claim-form

American Dental Association: Breaking Down Barriers to Oral Health for All Americans: The Role of Finance, A Statement from the American Dental Association. <http://www.ada.org/~/media/ADA/Public%20Programs/Files/barriers-paper_role-of-finance.ashx/>, 2012.

http://www.treasury.gov/resource-center/faqs/taxes/pages/health-savings-accounts.aspx

http://www.irs.gov/publications/p969/ar02.html

www.hhs.gov/ocr/privacy/hipaa/administrative/

RECOMMENDED WEBSITES

www.ada.org/professional.aspx
www.hhs.gov/ocr/privacy/hipaa/administrative/
www.aetnadental.com/AD/ihtAD/r.WSIHW000/st.35410/t.35410.html
www.anthem.com/dentalproviders/
www.cigna.com/assets/docs/health-care-professionals/forms_dental_claim.pdf
www.deltadental.com/Public/Dentists/Dentists.jsp
www.humanadental.com/tools/
www.metdental.com/prov/execute/Content
http://www.findacode.com/dental-codes/dental-codes-ada-cdt.html

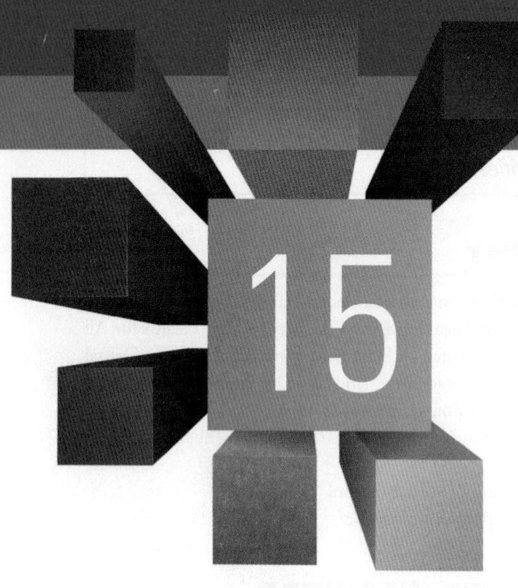

15 Financial Systems: Accounts Receivable

 http://evolve.elsevier.com/Finkbeiner/practice

LEARNING OUTCOMES

1. Define the key terms in this chapter.
2. Explain basic mathematical procedures and how to use decimals and percentages.
3. Describe common bookkeeping systems in dentistry.
4. Identify special bookkeeping situations that can occur in a typical day and identify their solutions.
5. Explain the production of patient statements and discuss identity theft.
6. Discuss the importance of establishing financial arrangements and the functions of a credit bureau.
7. Discuss rules for collecting late payments and the function of a collection agency.

KEY TERMS

Accounting The recording, classifying, and summarizing of financial and business records; this is generally the task of the accountant.

Accounts payable All of the dentist's financial obligations or money that the dentist owes (outgoing money).

Accounts receivable A category that includes all production (incoming money); data are entered for treatment rendered and payments received, and new balances are calculated.

Adjustment The alteration of an account balance as a result of a courtesy discount, the return of a nonsufficient funds (NSF) check, or a payment.

Balance The credit or debit amount on an account.

Bookkeeping The process of the recording of financial transactions.

Credit balance An amount owed to the patient for services for which the dentist has been paid in advance but that have not yet been performed.

Credit bureau An organization that reports specific information about a person's previous payment habits on deferred payment plans.

Creditor An institution or business that sends a bill to a person, agrees to an installment payment plan, accepts insurance payments, or arranges for a loan for payment.

Nonsufficient funds (NSF) check A check returned unpaid to the payee because insufficient funds were available in the payer's account.

Receipt A form given to the payer (patient) that acknowledges payment on an account.

Statement A document that informs patients of their financial status with the dentist; it indicates the charges, payments, and balances on an account for the month just concluded.

As discussed previously in various sections of this textbook, dentistry is a business as well as a healthcare profession. In this chapter, the reader will understand that sound business practices must be integrated into the management of the dental office to maintain a steady cash flow as well as a solvent practice. Whether there is a management company in place or the administrative assistant assumes responsibility for a major portion of the business activities of the dental practice, the person in charge of the accounts receivable must maintain a high degree of efficiency. He or she will become a valuable asset to the practice.

The two financial systems used in a dental business office are accounts receivable and accounts payable. The administrative assistant is responsible for both. The accounts receivable system includes all production; data are entered for treatment rendered, payments received, and account adjustments made, and new balances are calculated. After all computations have been made, the current accounts receivable amount or the amount of money owed to the dentist (incoming money) is determined. **Accounts payable** refers to all of the dentist's financial obligations or money the dentist owes (outgoing money). This chapter discusses accounts receivable; Chapter 16 details accounts payable and other financial systems.

PRACTICE NOTE

The administrative assistant who maintains the business portion of the dental practice with a high degree of efficiency becomes a valuable asset.

As discussed previously, records management is a primary responsibility of the administrative assistant. Financial records are as important as clinical records, but they are maintained separately. They provide the following: (1) protection for both the dentist and the patient; (2) information for tax purposes; and (3) data for business analysis. Inaccurate records result in poor public relations and may create unnecessary litigation with the state or federal government. **Bookkeeping**, or the recording of financial transactions, is the responsibility of the administrative assistant. **Accounting**, which is the recording, classifying, and summarizing of financial and business records, generally is the job of the accountant. Most dentists have an accountant who audits the practice's books and computes a variety of tax reports and financial statements.

UNDERSTANDING BASIC MATHEMATICAL COMPUTATIONS

Before becoming proficient at computing financial activity on various records, review some basic mathematical rules. Because computers are used to produce so many documents, it is often easy to forget how to perform basic calculations or compute percentages on insurance claim forms.

Although a computer can make the necessary calculations, the administrative assistant is responsible for entering the data in the appropriate fields to ensure that the final figures are accurate. The administrative assistant often needs to add and subtract figures with decimals and perform other business-related computations. Most people use manual or electronic calculators for these tasks; however, relying solely on technologic devices without having an understanding of basic computation can result in embarrassment, patient dissatisfaction, and possibly the loss of cash flow when errors are detected. To understand the computations and to be prepared for the day when the electronic functions may fail, it becomes necessary to perform the computations manually. The following descriptions cover the basic mathematical procedures used for routine bookkeeping entries.

DECIMALS

Adding and Subtracting Decimals

Place the numbers to be added or subtracted in a vertical column and align the decimal points before performing the addition or subtraction. To add columns of figures with decimals, add the numbers in each column, beginning with the column farthest to the right and working to the left:

$$\begin{array}{r} 0.5 \\ 2.8 \\ 30.50 \\ 67.945 \\ +750.000 \\ \hline 851.745 \end{array}$$

To subtract, follow the same procedure. Place the numbers to be subtracted in a vertical column, and align the decimal points. Each amount must have the same number of decimals; therefore, it may be necessary to add zeroes before performing this procedure. For example, to subtract 1.75 from 3.876, add one zero at the end of 1.75:

$$\begin{array}{r} 3.876 \\ -1.750 \\ \hline 2.126 \end{array}$$

Multiplying Decimals

To multiply decimals, perform the procedure as for all whole numbers, being sure to place the decimal point correctly in the answer. Count the number of digits to the right of the decimal point in the multiplicand and in the multiplier, count the same number of places from right to left in the product, and then insert the decimal point:

600.75	2 decimals (multiplicand)
× 0.20	2 decimals (multiplier)
120.1500	2 + 2 = 4 decimals

or

$800.50	2 decimals
× 0.75	2 decimals
$600.3750	2 + 2 = 4 decimals

or

$800	0 decimals
× 0.75	2 decimals
$600.00	0 + 2 = 2 decimals

Percentages

Working with percentages is a common function of the routine posting of accounts receivable. For example, when processing insurance claim forms, the administrative assistant may need to determine the subscriber and carrier percentages and any deductible amounts. In an automated system, these figures are calculated, but again, the administrative assistant must understand this process to ensure accuracy. The following are examples of some very basic procedures.

To change a percent to a fraction, drop the percent sign, place the number over 100, and then reduce the fraction to the lowest terms. If the numerator is a decimal, multiply both the numerator and denominator by an appropriate power of 10 to clear the decimal. Consider the following example:

$$5\% = \frac{5}{100} = \frac{1}{20}$$

or

$$7.5\% = \frac{7.5}{100} = \frac{75}{1000} = \frac{3}{40}$$

To change a percent to a decimal, move the decimal point two places to the left, and then drop the percent sign:

$$15\% = 0.15$$
$$2\% = 0.02$$
$$110\% = 1.1$$

To find a certain percent of a number, convert the percent to a decimal, and then multiply by the number. The following computation shows how to calculate 80% of $670:

$$\begin{array}{r} \$670 \\ \times 0.80 \\ \hline \$536.00 \end{array}$$

TYPES OF BOOKKEEPING SYSTEMS

Overview

In the past, dentistry used a variety of bookkeeping systems, including the pegboard or "write it once," system, which was the system most often used in dental offices until the 1990s. With the pegboard system, one notation provided an entry on the daily journal sheet, the ledger card, the receipt and, in some cases, a statement. The system of choice now is a computer software program, which goes beyond the basic transactions of the pegboard system to provide all financial records, insurance claim forms, future appointments, recall management, and documents for practice analysis.

A computerized bookkeeping system can be integrated into total records management. In other words, the administrative assistant can make a clinical entry on a patient record that can then be transferred to a financial record. With the use of designated codes, he or she can transfer this information to a patient statement, and an insurance claim form can be generated from the original data entry. This type of system is more than just a mechanism for bookkeeping.

Components of a Computerized Bookkeeping System

Chapter 5 described the use of dental office management software. One of the major components of these software systems is the accounts receivable program. By entering data for a patient account, one can generate a myriad of reports, forms, and other types of information.

When a dentist purchases a software management system, some type of tutorial is provided, and the administrative assistant probably will be given live or web-based instruction in the use of the software. After the software has been installed in the computer and the training is completed, the administrative assistant can begin entering basic patient clinical and financial data. To generate accounts receivable data, one generally follows specific steps outlined in the software package. The following description is an overview of some of the common steps in basic data entry. Although each software package has its own distinct features, most include these steps. Table 15-1 presents some common commands used in a variety of accounts receivable programs.

Opening the Program

When the administrative assistant opens the program, he or she is commonly required to enter his or her name or username

TABLE 15-1 Common Commands in Accounts Receivable Software

Command	Meaning
Add	Enter additional data; create a new record
Appointment/ Scheduler	Enter data for a patient appointment
Del	Delete; to eliminate part or all of the data entry
Edit	Alter or change data
Enter	Insert data
Esc	Leave the screen
File	Open, close, print, or take action on files
Insurance	Make a data entry or obtain a hard copy of a claim form
List	Provides a screen view or hard copy of lists of patients, accounts, or other data
Locate	Find a patient, an account, or other data
N	No
Patient	Enter a field of patient records
Post	Enter data, financial or otherwise
Print	Produce a hard copy of a document
Recall	Enter data about a patient for recall
Reports	Obtain some form of report programmed into the system
System	Change the system setting, login information, or password
Transaction	Reference to financial activity
View	Changes the format of the screen view
Window	Allows a different configuration of the screen
Word processor	Program that allows letter writing
Y	Yes

and a password. When a password is entered, the characters are generally not displayed on the screen as they are keyed in. Most systems allow for reentry of the password in case an error is made. However, after a specified number of tries, the program may lock the person out.

Locating Account Information

When the administrative assistant wants to select a specific patient, a screen opens from which the chosen patient can be selected (Figure 15-1). If the patient's name does not appear in the list, then he or she can be added as a new patient by clicking on the *New* button and creating a new patient record (Figure 15-2). Certain basic patient information is common to most systems, such as an ID number, the patient's name and address, his or her personal data (e.g., telephone number or numbers, date of birth, gender, age), the name of the person responsible for the patient's charges, the dentist of choice (i.e., the primary provider for the patient if the office has several dentists), the

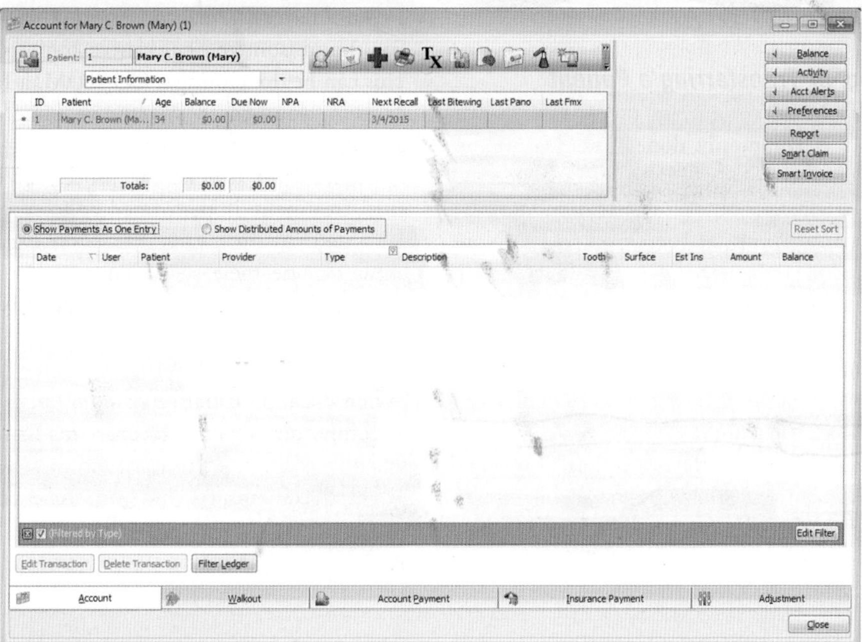

FIGURE 15-1 Account information screen. (Courtesy Patterson Dental, St. Paul, Minnesota.)

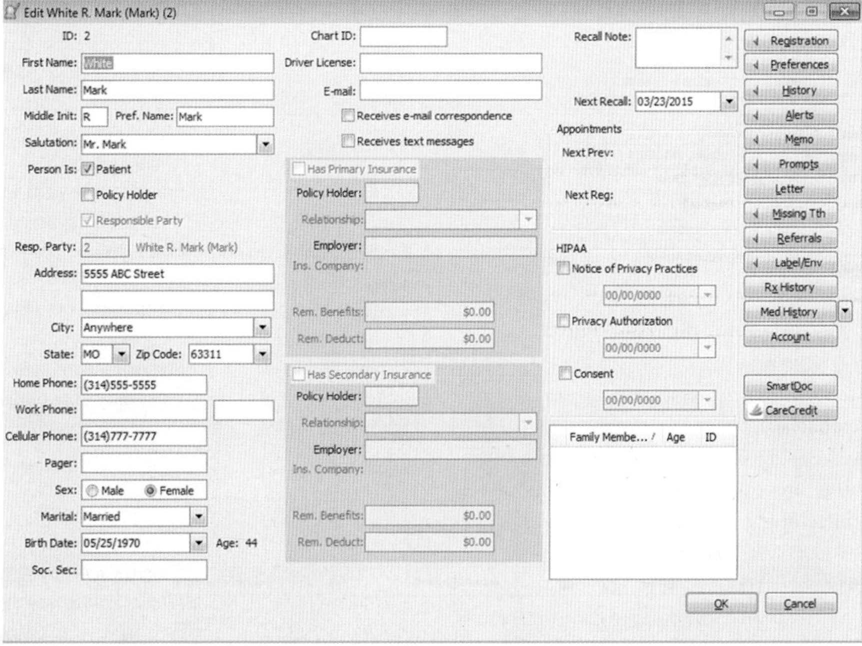

FIGURE 15-2 Patient information screen. (Courtesy Patterson Dental, St. Paul, Minnesota.)

insurance policy holder, relevant insurance numbers, and employer information. Special notes may also be included, such as the patient's preferred pharmacy, the name of the person who referred the patient to the office, and the school that the patient is attending.

Editing Patient Information

At times, one will need to edit patient information, such as when a patient's name or address changes. To do this, enter the *Patient* window, and then select *Edit*. (*Edit* refers to the task of changing existing data.)

Adding, Inactivating, or Transferring a Patient

Patients may be added to an account in the system shown by selecting *New*. This is commonly done to add a spouse or dependent to an account. Inactivating a patient may be necessary as a result of divorce or death. Children may be transferred to their own accounts as they grow older. Note that patient information is rarely deleted but merely inactivated.

Posting Transactions

Perhaps one of the most common daily activities in bookkeeping is entering transaction data. From the *Account* screen (Figure 15-3), most systems are designed to allow the user to enter clinical data about treatment, for which he or she may insert appropriate codes. When the data are entered, the program computes the financial activity and produces an account balance. The data are then saved. There may also be a prompt to complete an insurance claim form or another activity (e.g., recall or appointment scheduling) as part of the walkout process (Figure 15-4).

Backing up Data

As mentioned in Chapter 8, maintaining all of the practice data on a computer's hard drive without a backup is dangerous. Valuable information can be lost as the result of a power surge, a computer crash, or a misdirected *Erase* or *Delete* command. For this reason, the hard drive must be backed up regularly. This can be done using a CD-ROM, a DVD, an external hard drive, a cloud-based system, or some other type of storage device.

Figure 15-5 reviews the process of entering a transaction after treatment is performed. The office procedures manual must describe the backup procedure step by step, and a backup log must be maintained (Figure 15-6).

Today many offices are contracting with offsite backup services and using an existing Internet connection to access an offsite backup provider. The initial step is the installation of the online backup client software. Next, a backup set is created, and important files and records are identified. Finally, a backup schedule is selected. From that point forward, backups generally occur automatically and on schedule, without end-user intervention.

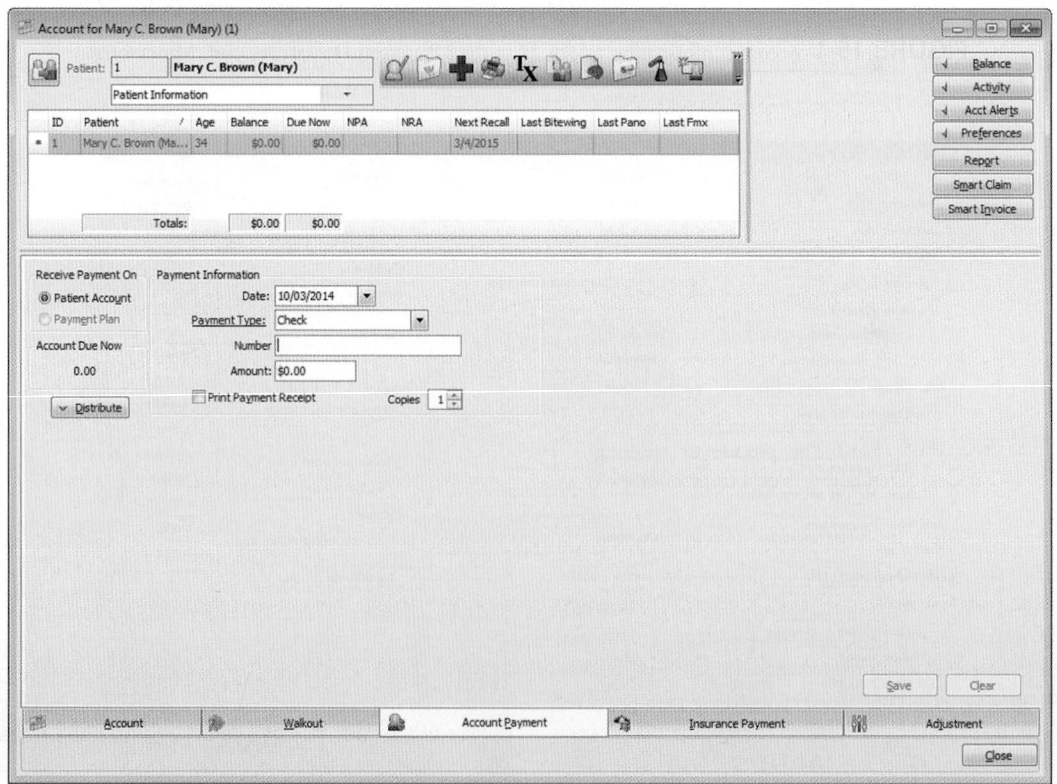

FIGURE 15-3 Transaction screen. (Courtesy Patterson Dental, St. Paul, Minnesota.)

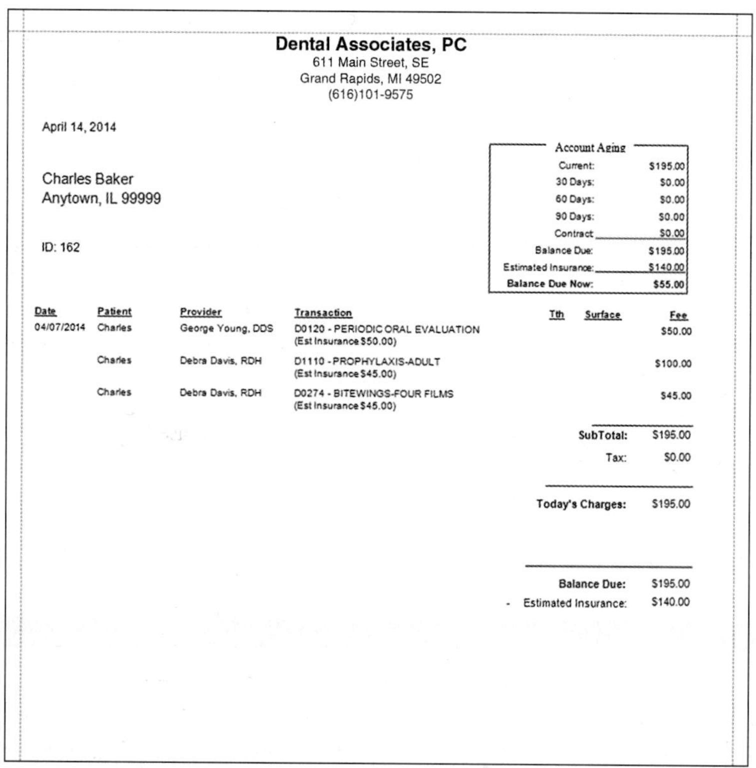

Dental Associates, PC
611 Main Street, SE
Grand Rapids, MI 49502
(616)101-9575

April 14, 2014

Charles Baker
Anytown, IL 99999

ID: 162

Account Aging	
Current:	$195.00
30 Days:	$0.00
60 Days:	$0.00
90 Days:	$0.00
Contract:	$0.00
Balance Due:	$195.00
Estimated Insurance:	$140.00
Balance Due Now:	$55.00

Date	Patient	Provider	Transaction	Tth	Surface	Fee
04/07/2014	Charles	George Young, DDS	D0120 - PERIODIC ORAL EVALUATION (Est Insurance $50.00)			$50.00
	Charles	Debra Davis, RDH	D1110 - PROPHYLAXIS-ADULT (Est Insurance $45.00)			$100.00
	Charles	Debra Davis, RDH	D0274 - BITEWINGS-FOUR FILMS (Est Insurance $45.00)			$45.00

SubTotal: $195.00
Tax: $0.00

Today's Charges: $195.00

Balance Due: $195.00
- Estimated Insurance: $140.00

FIGURE 15-4 Walkout statement. (Courtesy Patterson Dental, St. Paul, Minnesota.)

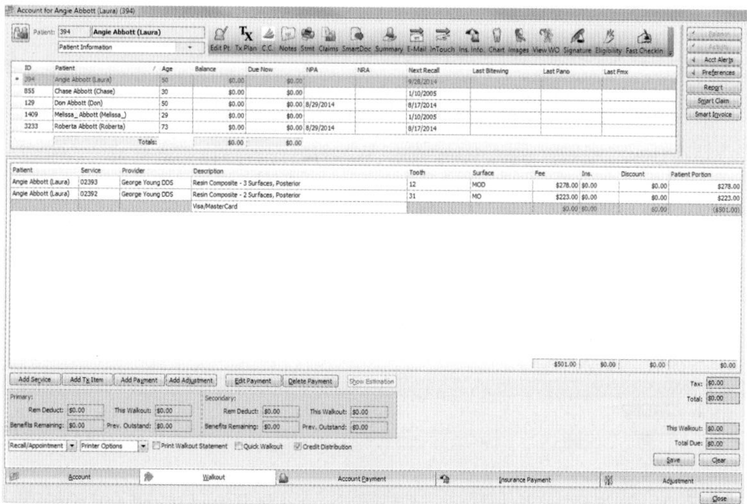

FIGURE 15-5 The process of entering a transaction after treatment is performed. (Courtesy Patterson Dental, St. Paul, Minnesota.)

The backup service transfers encrypted copies of the most critical computer data to a secure, remote storage vault. In the event of data loss, this process is reversed, and missing data are retrieved (restored) from the storage vault and returned to the computer.

Before contracting with such a service, the company must be researched to ensure that it adheres to Health Insurance Portability and Accountability Act of 1996 (HIPAA) standards and that it can be relied on exclusively to provide daily backups. Some offices may use the service as a complement to their local CD or DVD backups.. This better protects the dentist against physical threats such as fire, flood, and theft.

SPECIAL SITUATIONS

A day would not be complete without some unusual activity that cannot be recorded using the procedure exactly as described previously. Several such situations and their solutions are presented in the following discussions.

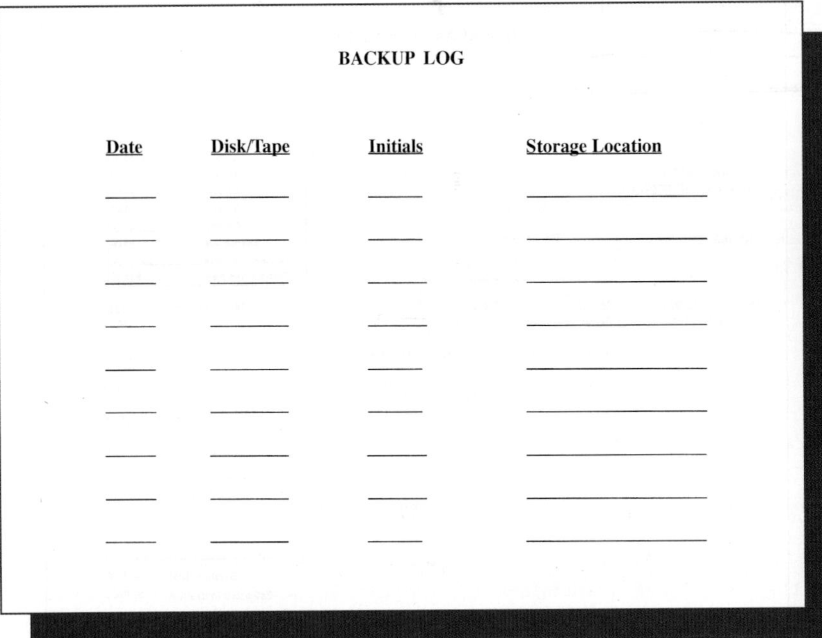

BACKUP LOG

Date	Disk/Tape	Initials	Storage Location

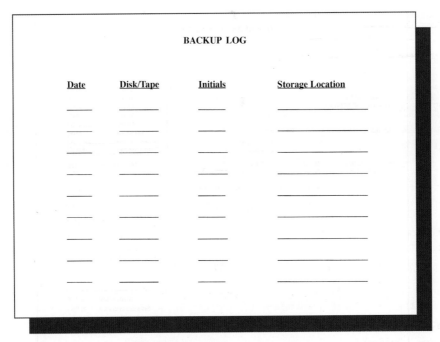

FIGURE 15-6 A manual backup log.

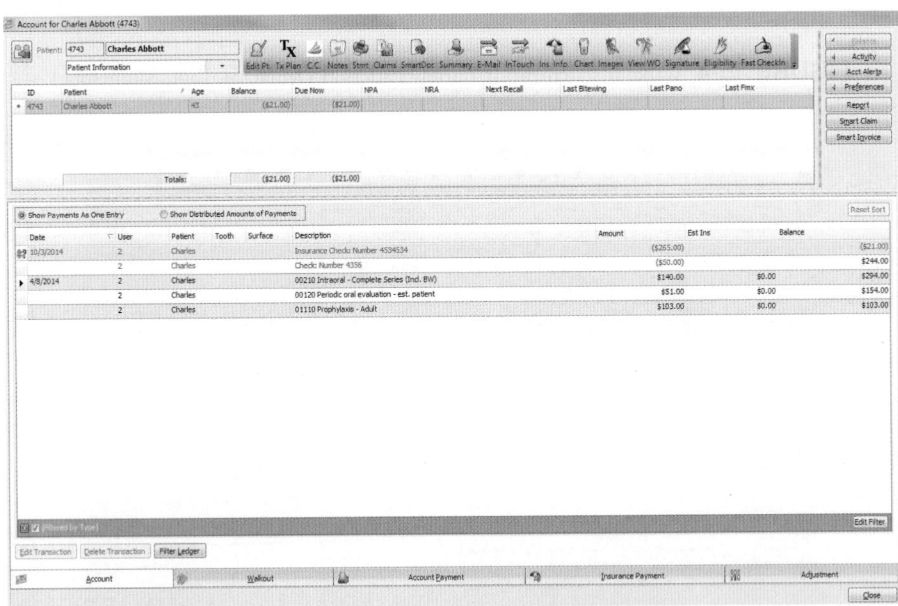

FIGURE 15-7 The current credit balance on the account is indicated in red and parentheses. (Courtesy Patterson Dental, St. Paul, Minnesota.)

Credit Balance

A credit balance often occurs when payment is made in advance, such as when a patient obtains a bank loan to pay for treatment. For example, a credit balance of $50 can be noted in three ways: (1) with the amount preceded by *CR* and shown as *CR$50;* (2) with the amount preceded by a minus sign and shown as *–$50;* and (3) with the amount, in color, enclosed in parentheses and shown as *($50)* (Figure 15-7).

Each time treatment is rendered, charges are made against the credit balance, which reduces the balance. Remember that the credit balance represents what is owed to the patient in services. Note that the credit transaction is also shown when a patient makes a payment on the account (Figure 15-8).

Nonsufficient Funds

Nonsufficient funds (NSF) checks or checks returned to the office for a lack of account funds require some form of adjustment to the account. A person may redeposit the check and not make an entry on the books. However, it may be necessary to charge the account with this returned check. Note that for

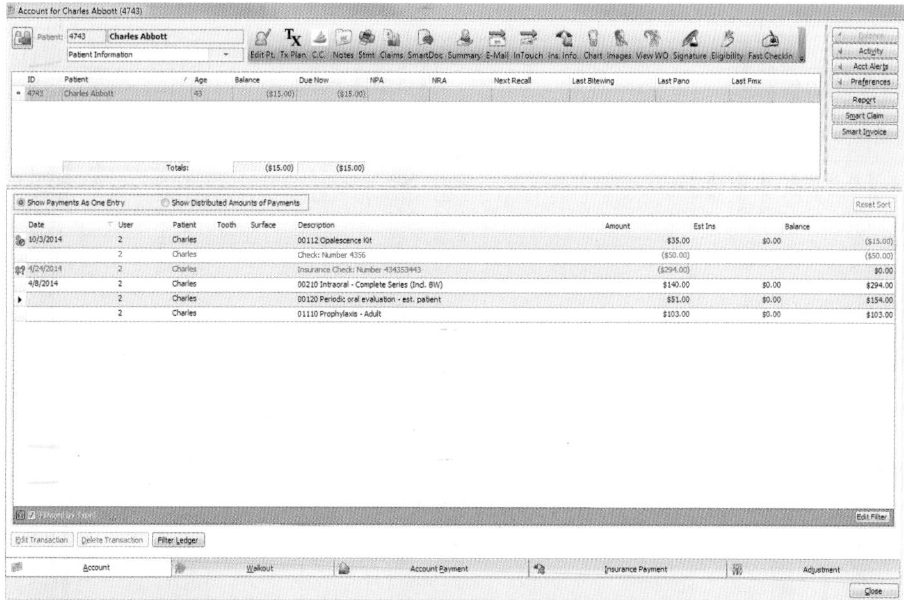

FIGURE 15-8 Credit is adjusted when activity occurs on the account. (Courtesy Patterson Dental, St. Paul, Minnesota.)

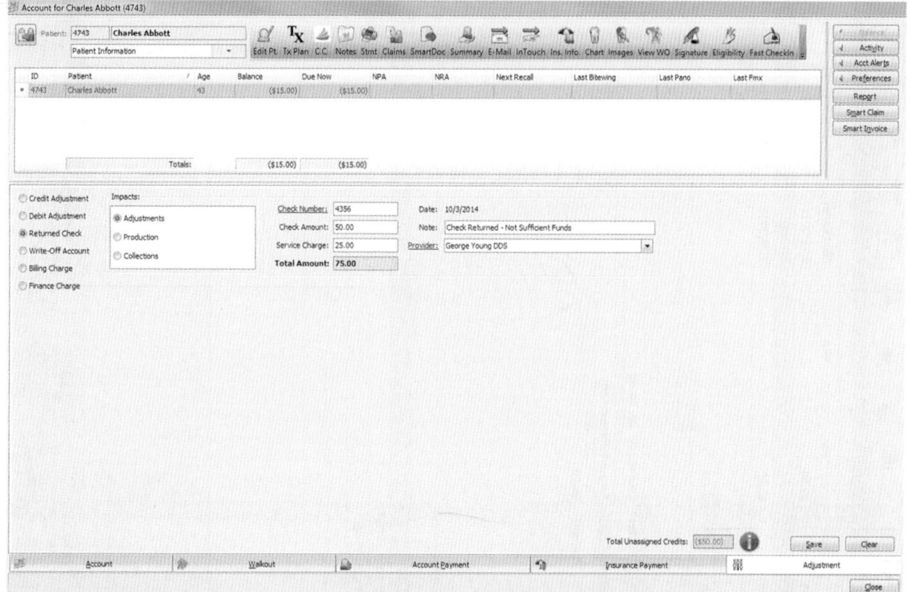

FIGURE 15-9 The account transaction screen indicates a nonsufficient funds (NSF) check with a service charge attached. (Courtesy Patterson Dental, St. Paul, Minnesota.)

the returned check shown in Figure 15-9, an NSF notation has been made, and a service charge of $25 has been assessed against the account. Collection fees are paid to an agency for collecting a delinquent account, and these fees generally are deducted from the payment before it is sent to the dentist.

Courtesy Discount

A courtesy discount is given when the dentist extends a professional courtesy to a patient. The courtesy discount is given at the discretion of the doctor in case of hardship or because the patient is a neighbor, friend, or person associated with a religious organization. In any case, state and federal guidelines must be followed. The courtesy discount is entered in a separate adjustment row (Figure 15-10).

Debit and Credit Cards

When a patient uses a debit or credit card to pay for services, the *Account* window is opened, and the payment is selected as

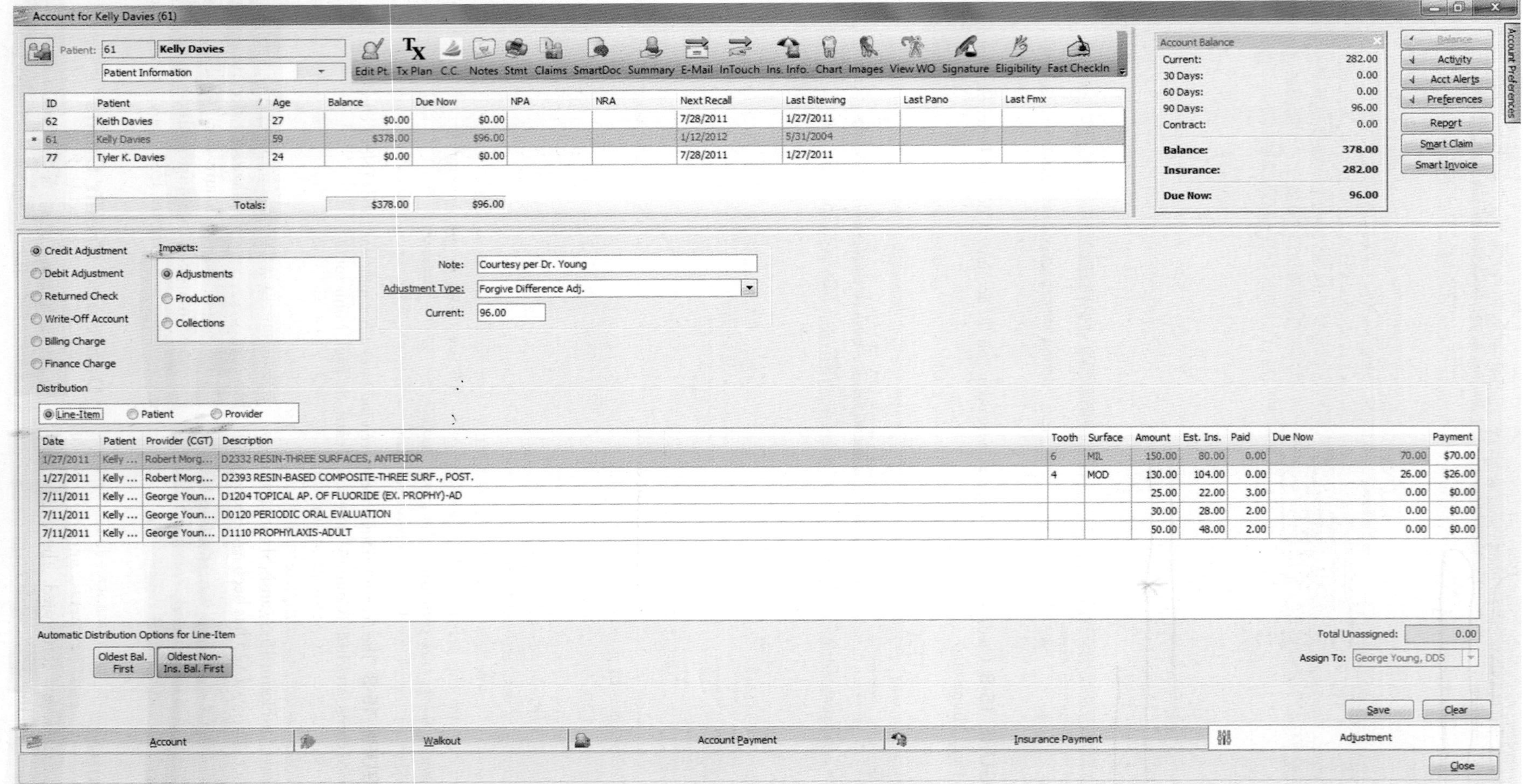

FIGURE 15-10 A courtesy discount is entered as a credit to the account. (Courtesy Patterson Dental, St. Paul, Minnesota.)

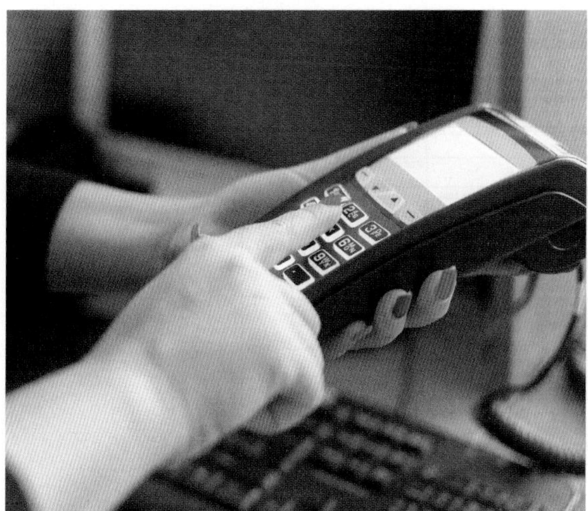

FIGURE 15-11 A patient entering her PIN on a PIN pad for a debit transaction. (Copyright © 2014 Rostislav Sedlacek, BigStock.com.)

a debit or credit card. A terminal to use to perform the debit or credit card transaction is provided either by the software company for the computer system or by the dentist's bank. If the patient pays with a debit card, a field on this same screen will be visible for the patient to enter a personal identification number (PIN). The patient then enters his or her debit card PIN, when prompted, on the PIN pad (Figure 15-11).

Healthcare Credit Cards

Some dental practices accept healthcare credit cards from their patients. These cards are an alternative to consumer credit cards, cash, or checks. This is a benefit for patients who may have used all of their insurance benefits and who want to avoid the use of their major consumer credit cards. A dentist must be a participant in such a plan; CareCredit is one of these plans, and it can be found on the Internet at www.carecredit.com.

Offering a service such as CareCredit removes the accounts receivable responsibilities from the dentist and allows him or her to focus on recommending and providing the best care possible to patients. Many patients may decide to proceed with treatment they otherwise could not have afforded at this time with the use of such a service. The use of the healthcare credit card ensures that the dentist receives payment at the time of service and that the patient is able to complete treatment.

Patient approval is based on information from the credit application and the patient's credit history. This includes information from the primary applicant as well as from any co-applicants.

STATEMENTS

A **statement** informs patients of their financial status with the dentist and indicates the charges, payments, and balances of their accounts for the month just concluded. The statement is also a request for payment. Statements may be sent on the first, 15th, or 30th day of the month or on a staggered basis according to the alphabet or the date of services. The important factor is consistency (i.e., statements should be sent at the same time each month).

A statement can be generated by a computer with an automated bookkeeping system (Figure 15-12). An itemized statement shows the dates of payments and the treatments for each member of the account that occurred during the previous month. With a computerized system, a person can add special messages or aging columns to statements to enhance the collection process.

IDENTITY THEFT

Identity theft occurs in contemporary society when the thief uses a person's personal identifying information to open new accounts or to misuse existing accounts. Try as one might, no small business is immune from identity theft, including the dental office. It is likely that a dental practice may encounter such a situation only once or twice and maybe never, but, in a dental practice, such situations can occur. The administrative assistant should be mindful of potential unknown persons in the practice using stolen credit cards or false information. The American Dental Association provides information for its members about federal regulations that may affect the practice of dentistry. To obtain the latest information about identity theft as it relates to the dental practice, visit www.ada.org and then search for the latest identity theft information.

ESTABLISHING FINANCIAL ARRANGEMENTS

Well-Defined Policies

The old adage, "Inform before you perform," still applies to the management of accounts in the dental office. A well-defined credit policy should be an integral part of the accounts receivable system. This policy must do the following: (1) conform to community standards; (2) reflect the attitude of the dentist toward the patient's welfare; (3) represent sound business concepts; (4) be presented in written form to the patient; (5) provide options for the patient; and (6) be adhered to at all times. Many payment policies exist; therefore, including the financial policy as part of the office policy is a wise move.

Because financial arrangements are generally made by the administrative assistant, he or she must be well acquainted with the office credit policy. Furthermore, he or she must be firm yet polite when adhering to the policy to avoid becoming a victim of any of the following common situations:

- The patient says he or she will take care of the bill in full when treatment has been completed. A patient who is having extensive restorative treatment should not be offended when it is explained that office expenses and laboratory fees require some form of payment before completion of the treatment.
- The patient becomes defensive or angry when asked about payment arrangements. Find out why he or she is irritated; patients with good intentions seldom become defensive when asked about payment.

STATEMENT

Remit To:
PTC & Associates
105 Any Street
P.O. Box 555
Anytown, IL 99999

Page 1 of 1

IF PAYING BY CREDIT CARD, FILL OUT BELOW.

NAME(As it appears on card)	TYPE OF CARD
CARD NUMBER	AMOUNT
SIGNATURE	EXP. DATE

Statement Date:	Balance Due Now:	Acct#:
4/14/2014	$171.50	61

DUE DATE: 5/14/2014	Amount Enclosed:

Kelly Davies
123 Any Street
Anytown, IL 99999

If address has changed, please correct.

For Billing Questions, call: (555)555-5555

TO ENSURE PROPER CREDIT, PLEASE DETACH AND RETURN THIS PORTION OF THE STATEMENT WITH YOUR PAYMENT.

PLEASE RETAIN THIS PORTION OF THE STATEMENT FOR YOUR RECORDS

Date	Patient	Code	Description	Debits	Credits	Balance
			Balance Forward >>>>>>			$378.00
4/14/2014	Kelly		Insurance Claim from April 14, 2014 was Submitted to Prim. Insurance Company: Aetna Life Ins Co, Payer ID: 60054			
4/14/2014	Kelly	D7210	SURGICAL REMOVAL OF ERUPTED TOOTH Tooth 5 Est Insurance $75.50	151.00		529.00

Balance Due:
$529.00

Current	30 Days	60 Days	90 Days	On Contract	Est. Insurance
$75.50	$0.00	$0.00	$96.00	$0.00	$357.50

Your Account Is Now 90 days Overdue, Please Pay Promptly.

PLEASE PAY THIS AMOUNT → $171.50

PTC & Associates
105 Any Street P.O. Box 555 , Anytown, IL 99999

FIGURE 15-12 Computer-generated statement using American Dental Association (ADA) codes. (Courtesy Patterson Dental, St. Paul, Minnesota.)

- The patient says that he or she will pay the bill when his or her income tax refund or another windfall is received. There is no way of knowing whether he or she will actually receive the expected money or use it to pay his dental bills.
- The patient makes promises and does not fulfill them. A consistent follow-up system must be initiated to eliminate such problems. Patients often become lax with regard to their responsibility because the dental staff is not consistent.

Types of Payment Policies

Many payment policies are used in dentistry today, but a few are common to all practices.

Cash-Only System

The cash-only system obviously eliminates much paperwork in the business office, but it may place limitations on the dental practice.

Payment of Statement in Full

Unless other arrangements have been made with the office, the patient is expected to pay in full within 10 days of receipt of the statement. Some form of notice, such as appropriate signage or a written policy statement, must be presented to the patient.

Extended Payment

Regulation 2 of the Truth in Lending Act requires that an agreement exist between the dentist and the patient if payment for services is to be made in more than four installments. Even if no finance charge is involved, the truth-in-lending form (Figure 15-13) must be completed to verify that such a payment agreement has been reached. In some areas, this form has been modified to include an entry for insurance coverage. A payment booklet may be used to help the patient keep track of payments and to identify the payment when the slip is mailed with the check. This system is common in practices such as orthodontics.

FINANCIAL AGREEMENT

DATE ____________

PATIENT NAME ____________

RESPONSIBLE PARTY ____________

ADDRESS ____________

____

HOME PHONE ____________ WORK PHONE ____________

CELL PHONE ____________ E-MAIL ____________

COST OF TOTAL TREATMENT	$______
INITIAL PAYMENT	–______
APPROXIMATE INSURANCE PAYMENTS	–______
BALANCE DUE	=______
INTEREST RATE PERCENTAGE	______
TOTAL AMOUNT OF FINANCE CHARGE	+______
AMOUNT REMAINING TO BE PAID BY PATIENT	=______

AMOUNT DUE TO BE PAID IN____________ MONTHLY PAYMENTS OF $ ____________ STARTING____________. BALANCE TO BE PAID IN FULL BY ____________.

I understand the financial arrangements above and agree to comply with them. I agree that parents are responsible for all fees and services rendered for treatment of a child. I understand that I am responsible for ALL fees regardless of insurance coverage. I also understand that as treatment progresses the above fees may have to be adjusted, but that I will be informed of these adjustments and how they will affect my payment plan. In the event that my payments are not received within 30 days of their due date, I agree to pay all costs of collections, including, but not limited to, reasonable attorney's fees.

____________ Responsible Party Signature ____________ Date

FINANCIAL AGREEMENT

ITEM 07-0513739/9054

FIGURE 15-13 Truth-in-lending form. (Adapted from a form provided courtesy Patterson Office Supplies, Champaign, Ilinois.)

USING A CREDIT BUREAU

Perhaps the best way to define a credit bureau or a consumer reporting agency (CRA) is to explain what it does not do and what it is not: it does not lend money, it does not deny credit, and it is not a collection agency. A credit bureau reports specific information about a person's previous payment habits on deferred payment plans. It reports on accounts placed for collection, and it provides information of public interest, such as that regarding bankruptcies, judgments, and lawsuits.

The Fair Credit Reporting Act (FCRA) was passed in 1992 to promote the accuracy, fairness, and privacy of the information in the files of all CRAs. Most CRAs are credit bureaus that gather and sell information about a person (e.g., whether a person pays bills on time or has filed for bankruptcy) to creditors, employers, landlords, and other businesses. The full text of this legislation is available on the Federal Trade Commission's website (www.ftc.gov). Consumers may have additional rights under state law, and a state or local consumer protection agency or a state attorney general can provide that information.

CRAs charge a nominal fee for supplying information. When seeking information from a credit bureau, complete data should be given about the prospective creditor. This information should include the following details about the individual:

- Full name, including the first and middle names. (Accurate spelling is essential. The spouse's name should be used as a cross-reference for identification purposes only.)
- Address or addresses for the past 3 years
- Place of employment for the past 3 years
- Names of stores and firms where credit has been established
- Name of bank or banks
- Social Security number

After this information has been given to the credit bureau, a credit report for the applicant will be issued. Care must be taken to record the information accurately. The Associated Credit Bureaus of America have designed a common language that incorporates symbols for the reporting of this information (Table 15-2). The symbols should mean the same things throughout the consumer credit industry; these may include *O* for "Open," *R* for "Revolving," and *I* for "Installment."

The dentist decides whether to extend credit to a patient. If the patient is denied credit, the FCRA requires that the patient be informed of the reason for the denial of credit as well as the name of the bureau from which a credit report was obtained. The dental office is not required to report the specific data obtained from the bureau; a patient who wants this information should contact the bureau personally.

TABLE 15-2 Language Used in Consumer Credit Reports

Usual Manner of Payment	Symbol
Open Account, 30-Day Account, or 90-Day Account	0
Too new to rate; approved but not used	0-0
Pays (or paid) within 30 days of billing; pays 90-day accounts as agreed	0-1
Pays (or paid) in more than 30 days but not more than 60 days	0-2
Pays (or paid) in more than 60 days but not more than 90 days	0-3
Pays (or paid) in more than 90 days but not more than 120 days	0-4
Pays (or paid) in 120 days or more	0-5
Bad debt; placed for collection; suit; judgment; bankrupt; skip	0-9
Revolving or Option Account R or R $ ________*	
Too new to rate; approved but not used	R-0
Pays (or paid) according to the terms agreed	R-1
Not paying (or paid) as agreed but not more than one payment past due	R-2
Not paying (or paid) as agreed and two payments past due	R-3
Not paying (or paid) as agreed and three payments past due	R-4
Bad debt; placed for collection; suit; judgment; bankrupt; skip	R-9
Installment Account I or I $ ________*	
Too new to rate; approved but not used	I-0
Pays (or paid) according to terms agreed	I-1
Not paying (or paid) as agreed but not more than one payment past due	I-2
Not paying (or paid) as agreed and two payments past due	I-3
Not paying (or paid) as agreed and three payments or more past due	I-4
Repossession	I-8
Bad debt; placed for collection; suit; judgment; bankrupt; skip	I-9

*When the monthly payment is known, it should be shown (e.g., "R $20" or "I $78").

COLLECTION PROCEDURES

Collecting fees in the dental office is a critical responsibility of the administrative assistant, although sometimes it can be a difficult task. Experience has shown that patients pay their medical and dental bills last. People pay their rent for fear of eviction, their car payments for fear of repossession, and their utility bills for fear of losing service. They even pay off loans before the dental bill because banks generally adhere to a stricter enforcement of collection procedures than the dentist does. Fortunately, only about 5% of patients become "uncollectable," but this 5% can be exasperating.

Aging Accounts

Before sending out statements, the administrative assistant should make sure that the accounts receivable has been appropriately aged. With a computer, this may be automatic, or it may require the administrative assistant to initiate the process of aging of the accounts. The dentist must determine a policy for aging accounts, and the administrative assistant must follow through with this policy routinely so that statements reflect the days since a charge was incurred and so that delinquent accounts do not become a drain on the practice.

Fair Debt Collection Practices Act

Collection procedures are regulated by the Fair Debt Collection Practices Act of 1996. This act was passed to protect the public from unethical collection procedures. The activities outlined specifically in the law are listed in Box 15-1.

Because these regulations generally apply to collection agencies, it is important that an agency verify its stringent adherence to them. These same regulations should be considered by the administrative assistant when performing collection procedures in the office.

Collection Letters

Letters may be sent at the discretion of the dentist. In offices that use a computer, a reminder notice can be included on the statement, and the first collection letter (Figure 15-14) is

BOX 15-1

Provisions of the Fair Debt Collection Practices Act

- Debtors may not be subjected to harassment, oppressive tactics, or abusive treatment. The law prohibits the collector from making any false statements to a debtor, such as claiming to be an attorney or a government agency.
- Debtors may not be called at work if the employer or debtor objects and requests no calls.
- Debtors may not be called at inconvenient places or times, such as before 9 AM or after 9 PM.
- No one except the debtors themselves may be told they are behind on their bills.

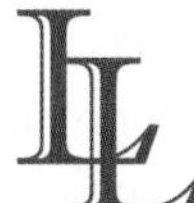

Dental Associates, PC
611 Main Street, SE
Grand Rapids, MI 49502
Phone: 616.101.9575 Fax: 616.101.9999
E-mail: office@dapc.com or Visit us at: www.Lakedental.com

Joseph W. Lake, DDS Ashley M. Lake, DDS

November 5, 20__

Mr. Marvin Beattie
1407 Colorado Street N.W.
Grand Rapids, MI 49505

Dear Mr. Beattie:

Your account of $565.00 is over 90 days past due. If you are unable to pay this account in full, perhaps we can help you in making arrangements to take care of this account.

Please contact us before November 15, 20__ at 5:00 p.m.

Sincerely,

Jennifer Ellis, RDA
Administrative Assistant

FIGURE 15-14 Sample first collection letter.

automatically generated when an account becomes past due. The administrative assistant may use a series of computer-generated reminder notices automatically sent at specified intervals (e.g., 30, 60, and 90 days past due) before assigning an account to a collector. Be responsible, however, when reviewing the list of delinquent accounts. One of these accounts might be a patient of long standing who, as a result of extenuating circumstances, was unable to pay the account. It is not wise to risk the loss of a well-established patient relationship by adding a message or sending an account to a collector without first checking to see if a reason exists for the oversight.

Generally, the collection process should have four stages: reminder, inquiry/discussion, urgency, and ultimatum. The previous discussion concerned the first stage (reminder), which is accomplished through a notice on the statement. During the second stage (inquiry/discussion), the patient is personally contacted to determine the problem. The third stage (urgency) can be completed with letters. The letter of urgency must be more persuasive and urgent (Figure 15-15). An urgent phone call may be used as a follow up as long as it does not result in harassment. In either case, be courteous, considerate, helpful, and firm.

The final stage (ultimatum) arrives when a patient has failed to respond to all messages sent thus far. Confront the patient with the ultimatum. Refrain from referring directly to lawsuits, attorneys, or collection agencies unless the intention is to follow through. Send only one ultimatum letter with a deadline date (Figure 15-16). Send this letter by certified mail with a return receipt requested to prove that the debtor has received the letter. If payment is not received by the designated date, the account must be turned over immediately to an attorney or a collection agency.

The following rules can guide the composition of collection letters:

1. Keep the letter brief.
2. Make sure that data regarding the account are complete and accurate.
3. Use simple words and uncomplicated sentences.
4. Use phrases that will motivate the patient, such as "cooperation" and "maintenance of a good credit rating."
5. Do not make statements about actions that the practice has no intention of carrying out. If the patient is told that the account will be sent to a collection agency in 10 days, give a specific date, and then follow through, if necessary.
6. Set a specific date by which payment is expected, rather than saying "by the end of the month" or "in 10 days."
7. Be firm and polite.

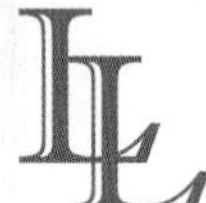

Dental Associates, PC
611 Main Street, SE
Grand Rapids, MI 49502
Phone: 616.101.9575 Fax: 616.101.9999
E-mail: office@dapc.com or Visit us at: www.Lakedental.com

Joseph W. Lake, DDS **Ashley M. Lake, DDS**

November 26, 20__

REGISTERED

Mr. Marvin Beattie
1407 Colorado Street N.W.
Grand Rapids, MI 49505

Dear Mr. Beattie:

Since we have not heard from you regarding your account of $565.00 from June 1, 20__, please be informed that it will be necessary to transfer this account to a collection agency.

This account must be paid in full by Friday, December 1, 20__ to avoid such legal action.

Sincerely,

Jennifer Ellis, RDA
Administrative Assistant

FIGURE 15-15 Sample urgent collection letter.

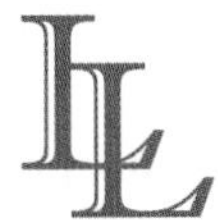

Dental Associates, PC
611 Main Street, SE
Grand Rapids, MI 49502
Phone: 616.101.9575 Fax: 616.101.9999
E-mail: office@dapc.com or Visit us at: www.Lakedental.com

Joseph W. Lake, DDS — Ashley M. Lake, DDS

December 1, 20__

REGISTERED

Mr. Marvin Beattie
1407 Colorado Street N.W.
Grand Rapids, MI 49505

Dear Mr. Beattie:

Please be informed that your account of $565.00 from June 1, 20__, has been transferred to the Dunhill Collection Agency for collection.

Sincerely,

Ashley M. Lake, DDS

je

FIGURE 15-16 Sample final collection letter.

8. Include a "thank you" in the letter closing. This can be an important part of the collection procedure, and it is a valuable aid to public relations.

Telephone as a Collection Instrument

Many assistants find it difficult to use the telephone during the collection process for delinquent accounts. Experience should instill confidence in the assistant, but, if not, another method of collection should be pursued. The telephone allows for more personal contact with a patient. Direct contact after a payment deadline is missed is most effective. When a patient who normally pays his or her account on time becomes delinquent, a phone call seems less formal than a letter and helps to maintain a friendly relationship.

The biggest mistake that most small business owners make is to wait too long to follow up. The probability of collecting a delinquent account diminishes dramatically each month after the due date, from 83% after 2 months to 52% after 6 months, according to the Commercial Collection Agency Association. If an account is outstanding after 12 months, the possibility of collection drops to less than 25%.

Specific rules should be followed when using the telephone for collections:

1. Do not call before 9 AM or after 9 PM.
2. Verify that you are speaking to the person whose account is overdue. Ask, "Is this Mr. Johnson?"
3. Identify yourself: "This is Miss Ellis, from Dr. Lake's office."
4. Ask whether it is a convenient time to talk. If not, ask when you may call back, or find out when the patient will be able to call you. Do not give details to a third party or leave detailed messages on an answering machine or voicemail system.
5. State the purpose of your call. Be friendly, and display a helping attitude.

6. Be positive. Don't say, "I'm sorry to call you." Act as though you know the patient intends to pay, and you are simply determining the arrangements for such a payment.
7. Have all of the information about the account in front of you.
8. Attempt to obtain a definite commitment that includes the date and amount of the payment. Follow up with written confirmation of the telephone discussion.
9. Make calls in a private area that is out of the hearing range of anyone in the reception room.
10. Do not threaten the patient.
11. Follow up on the promises that the patient makes. If the new due date arrives and a check is nowhere to be found, the broken promise indicates that the client is likely not trustworthy.
12. Do not ever discuss the account with anyone else. If you call the patient at work and the person cannot talk with you, leave a message to "Call Miss Ellis at 101-9575." Do not leave the dentist's name, because the patient may not return the call.
13. Do not leave a message on an answering machine that includes the reason for the call; simply leave a message to "Call Miss Ellis at 101-9575."

Collection Agency

After every attempt has been made to collect payment on an account, it may be necessary to engage the services of a collection agency. These services are required when the patient fails to respond to a final collection letter or can no longer be located and becomes a "skip."

Delay in sending the account to a collection agency results in less chance of recovering a portion of the fee. Although the agency's fee reduces the portion recovered, continued unsuccessful attempts by the office are even less rewarding.

A collection agency that maintains high standards of professionalism should be selected. Investigate the agency thoroughly to determine its ethics and reliability.

1. Check the ownership of the agency through a banker, the local Chamber of Commerce, or the Better Business Bureau.
2. Contact the local dental society, the National Retail Credit Association, or the Associated Credit Bureaus of America for information about the agency.
3. Find out whether the agency has contacts out of town to help with the collection of accounts.
4. Make sure that the agency will not start legal action without the dentist's consent.
5. Make sure that the agency understands the patient's needs and that a report is wanted regarding its activities.

After the dentist has sought the services of an agency, the office should use these services routinely. To allow action to be taken promptly, complete data about each case should be given to the agency, including the following:

- Debtor's full name
- Debtor's last known address and phone number
- Total amount of account
- Date of last entry on account (credit or debit)
- Debtor's occupation
- Debtor's business address and phone number
- Any other pertinent information

When an account is turned over to a collection agency, the administrative assistant no longer pursues collection procedures on it. However, the dental office staff must cooperate with the agency. The staff should do the following:

- Send the debtor no more statements.
- Indicate the transfer to the collection agency on the patient's financial record, including the date of transfer.
- Refer the patient to the agency if the person contacts the office.
- Report the amount to the agency when payment is received in the office.
- Rely on the agency staff members to do the job (i.e., do not pester them with inquiries about the account).

From the time that the patient enters the office until the final collection of the fee, the administrative assistant has many important duties for the management of the accounts receivable. The importance of accuracy in each aspect cannot be overemphasized. If the administrative assistant can carry out this responsibility, his or her value to the office becomes immeasurable.

LEARNING ACTIVITIES

1. Explain the differences between accounting and bookkeeping.
2. List common types of bookkeeping systems used in dentistry.
3. List and explain the function of the components of a pegboard system.
4. List and explain the function of the components of a computer bookkeeping system.

Please refer to the student workbook for additional learning activities.

BIBLIOGRAPHY

Blaes J: Pearls for Your Practice, *Dental Economics* 20:37, 2014.

McDonough D: Dental administrator alert: "new red flags" requirements for financial in situations and creditors to help fight identity theft, *ADAA Business Beat* 1, Spring 2009.

Mehta M: Five rules for collecting late payments, *Bus Week* August 31, 2010. Available at http://www.businessweek.com/smallbiz/content/aug2010/sb20100831_006151.htm.

RECOMMENDED WEBSITES

www.ada.org
www.dentalassistant.org
www.drbackup.com

16 Other Financial Systems

 http://evolve.elsevier.com/Finkbeiner/practice

LEARNING OUTCOMES

1. Define the key terms in this chapter.
2. Discuss the advantages of using of financial management software.
3. Explain the function of a budget.
4. Discuss the use of electronic banking and the steps in accessing an online bank account.
5. Discuss the process of establishing a checking account and identify various types of checks.
6. Describe how to prepare checks for deposit with correct endorsements and how to complete a deposit slip.
7. Discuss how to reconcile bank statements and how to record business expenses.
8. Identify the purpose of payroll records and the importance of having every employee complete an Employee's Withholding Allowance Certificate (Form W-4).
9. Discuss employee's earnings records, including:
   - Discuss calculating gross and net wages.
   - Explain how withheld income tax and Social Security taxes are deposited.
   - Describe how federal unemployment taxes are deposited.
   - Describe how to complete a Form W-2.
   - Discuss the importance of retaining payroll records.
   - Discuss the employer's responsibility for tax information.

KEY TERMS

American Bankers Association (ABA) A national organization of banks and holding companies of all sizes that deals with issues of importance to national institutions.

Automatic teller machine (ATM) A computer workstation that electronically prompts the user through most routine banking activities.

Bank deposit The accumulation of money received for a single day or longer period that is deposited into the office bank account.

Bank draft A check drawn by the cashier of one bank on another bank in which the first bank has available funds on deposit or credit.

Bank statement A printed statement from the bank showing the balance of the account at the beginning of the month, deposits made during the month, checks drawn against the account, corrections or charges against the account (e.g., service charges, stop-payment charges), and the bank balance at the end of the month.

Budget A financial plan of operation for a given period, usually 1 year.

Cashier's check A bank's own order to make payment from its own funds.

Certified check A check for which a guarantee exists and for which funds have been set aside to cover.

Check A means of ordering the bank to pay cash from a bank customer's account.

Employee's Withholding Allowance Certificate (Form W-4) The federal form used to determine the status of each employee for income tax deductions from wages.

Employer identification number (EIN) A nine-digit number assigned to sole proprietors or corporations for filing and reporting payroll information.

Endorsement The signature or stamp of the payee.

Expenditures The amount of money spent to operate a business or practice.

Federal Insurance Contributions Act (FICA) A law that requires deductions for Social Security and Medicare taxes.

Form SS-4 The application form used to obtain an employer identification number.

Gross wages The total amount of earnings before deductions.

Money order A means of transferring money without using cash or a personal check.

Net pay The total amount of earnings after deductions.

PIN Personal identification number code that permits authorized individuals to access an account.

Petty cash A small amount of cash kept on hand in the office to pay for small expenses.

Revenue The amount of income received by a business or practice.

Traveler's check A payment device purchased through a bank or another agency that serves as cash for a person who is away from home.

Voucher check A check that provides a detachable stub that can be used as an accounting record for itemizing the payment of invoices or for any type of itemization that the payer would like as a reference.

**Wage and Tax Statement (Form W-2)** A wage and tax statement for a calendar year must be provided for each employee no later than January 31 of the following year.

Withholding The amount of money withheld for federal and state taxes.

All dental practices, regardless of size, have financial matters that need to be addressed by either internal or external accounting staff. The administrative assistant can expect to perform many tasks in addition to the accounts receivable activities highlighted in the previous chapter. These tasks may include receiving and organizing statements, paying for materials and supplies, processing payroll or tax forms, recording and analyzing expenses, and other responsibilities. In a group practice or a larger organization, the administrative assistant may collect the data for these activities and support accounting personnel in the preparation of financial documents, or he or she may be responsible for entering data in a software package such as QuickBooks (Figure 16-1).

Although some offices may still perform these tasks manually, the use of computer software will provide the practice with the benefits shown in Box 16-1. The administrative assistant must have a basic understanding of the software system involved. All financial activities can be performed online via the Internet in most modern practices.

When processing financial documents, accuracy is essential. The verification of data and attention to detail are necessary to ensure that the processed information is accurate. Incorrect data can mean improper cash flow analysis, inaccurate accounts receivable, erroneous claim form preparation, and inaccurate budget and expense figures. All of these can have very serious repercussions for the entire business.

As the administrative assistant becomes more skilled in the business office, his or her responsibilities will probably include completing many monthly and annual forms vital to the dental practice. This chapter presents the major types of financial systems and the data that must be processed and managed in a modern dental practice. The chapter shows how technology is applied to the financial operations of a practice to make it more productive. In addition, it discusses the resources available

> **PRACTICE NOTE**
> When processing financial documents, accuracy is essential. The verification of data and attention to detail are necessary to ensure that the processed information is accurate.

BOX 16-1

Advantages of Using Financial Software

- Organize the office finances all in one place.
- Be ready at tax time with complete and accurate reports.
- Be aware of whether a profit is being made.
- Easily create specific cost analysis reports.
- Generate forecasts and business plans.
- Track invoices and back orders.
- Generate checks, track payments, and manage expenses.
- Manage payroll activity.
- Access finances from anywhere, anytime.
- Keep data backed up and secure automatically.
- Obtain support and upgrades.
- Provide a seamless transition from accounts receivable dental software.

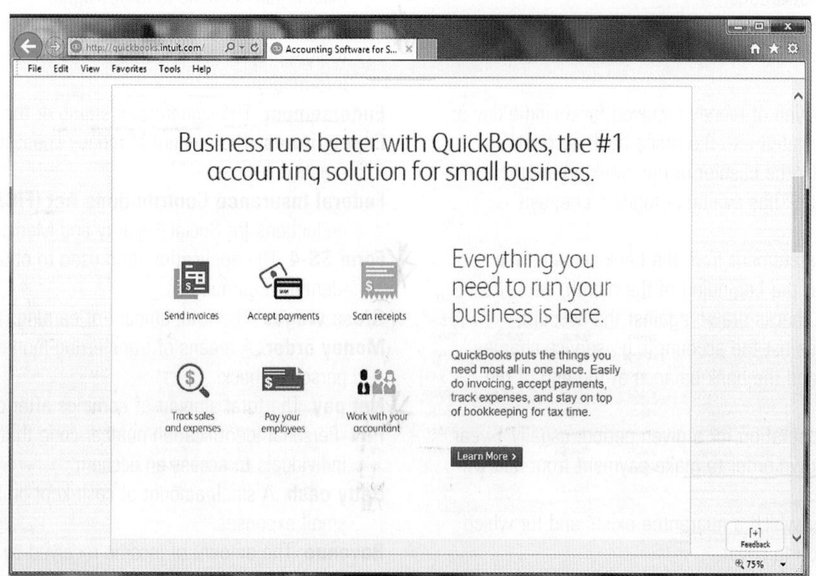

FIGURE 16-1 QuickBooks software web page. (Screenshot © Intuit, Inc. All rights reserved.)

through the Internet that can act as guides for procuring and filling out many of the financial forms needed by the practice.

DETERMINING A BUDGET

A budget is a dental practice's financial plan of operation for a given period, usually 1 year. The purpose of the budget is to establish the practice's financial goals. To achieve an acceptable level of profit, expenditures (the amount of money spent to operate the practice) must be kept in balance with revenue (the amount of income received by the practice). Dentists can use spreadsheet software to develop a budget so that they can plan more thoroughly and in less time than with paper-and-pencil methods. Spreadsheets allow planners to see how a change in one calculation affects all of the related calculations. A template of a business budget created in QuickBooks software for a dental practice is shown in Figure 16-2.

BANK ACCOUNTS

One of the daily routine functions of the dental office administrative assistant is the control of the *cash flow,* which is the amount of money received and the amount disbursed. Although this is being accomplished electronically in most practices today, a good understanding of banking technology and procedures is necessary. Some of the administrative assistant's banking responsibilities are check writing, accepting checks from patients for the payment of services, endorsing and depositing checks, keeping an accurate bank balance, and reconciling the bank statement; these may be done manually or electronically.

PRACTICE NOTE

One of the daily routine functions of the dental office administrative assistant is the control of the cash flow, which is the amount of money received and the amount disbursed.

ONLINE BANKING

For many dental offices, electronic or online banking means 24-hour access to cash through an automated teller machine or the direct deposit of paychecks and accounts receivable into a checking or savings account. Electronic banking now involves many different types of transactions. For example, the federal government is even moving toward the direct deposit or transfer of funds for employment taxes as well as for the many other government forms required to conduct business.

Online banking makes use of a computing or mobile device and electronic technology as a substitute for checks and other paper transactions. Electronic fund transfers (EFTs) are initiated through devices such as cards or with codes that let the dentist or those authorized by the dentist access an account. Many financial institutions use automatic teller machines (ATMs) or debit cards and personal identification numbers (PINs) for this purpose. Other institutions use devices such as debit cards or a signature or scan to access to an account. The federal Electronic Fund Transfer Act (EFT Act) covers some electronic consumer transactions.

ATMs or 24-hour tellers are electronic devices that allow banking to occur at almost any time. To withdraw money, make deposits, or transfer funds between accounts, an ATM card is inserted, and a PIN number is entered. Generally, ATMs must

Dental Associates, PC - QuickBooks Pro 2014

File Edit View Lists Favorites Company Customers Vendors Employees Banking Reports Window Help

Budget

FY20__ - Profit & Loss by Account

Create New Budget

ACCOUNT	ANNUAL TOTAL	JAN14	FEB14	MAR14	APR14	MAY14	JUN14	JUL14	AUG14	SEP14	OCT14	NOV14	DEC14
Capitation Fees	19,800.00	1,650.00	1,650.00	1,650.00	1,650.00	1,650.00	1,650.00	1,650.00	1,650.00	1,650.00	1,650.00	1,650.00	1,650.00
Fee for Service Income	1,020,000.00	85,000.00	85,000.00	85,000.00	85,000.00	85,000.00	85,000.00	85,000.00	85,000.00	85,000.00	85,000.00	85,000.00	85,000.00
Nonmedical Income	8,400.00	700.00	700.00	700.00	700.00	700.00	700.00	700.00	700.00	700.00	700.00	700.00	700.00
Refunds	3,600.00	300.00	300.00	300.00	300.00	300.00	300.00	300.00	300.00	300.00	300.00	300.00	300.00
Advertising and Promotion	39,600.00	3,300.00	3,300.00	3,300.00	3,300.00	3,300.00	3,300.00	3,300.00	3,300.00	3,300.00	3,300.00	3,300.00	3,300.00
Automobile Expense	9,600.00	800.00	800.00	800.00	800.00	800.00	800.00	800.00	800.00	800.00	800.00	800.00	800.00
Bank Service Charges	1,800.00	150.00	150.00	150.00	150.00	150.00	150.00	150.00	150.00	150.00	150.00	150.00	150.00
Business Licenses and Perm...	525.00	325.00	0.00	0.00	150.00	0.00	0.00	0.00	50.00	0.00	0.00	0.00	0.00
Computer and Internet Expen...	4,200.00	350.00	350.00	350.00	350.00	350.00	350.00	350.00	350.00	350.00	350.00	350.00	350.00
Continuing Education	1,150.00	0.00	0.00	0.00	0.00	0.00	500.00	0.00	0.00	0.00	0.00	0.00	650.00
Dental Supplies	24,000.00	2,000.00	2,000.00	2,000.00	2,000.00	2,000.00	2,000.00	2,000.00	2,000.00	2,000.00	2,000.00	2,000.00	2,000.00
Depreciation Expense	7,200.00	600.00	600.00	600.00	600.00	600.00	600.00	600.00	600.00	600.00	600.00	600.00	600.00
Dues and Subscriptions	2,400.00	200.00	200.00	200.00	200.00	200.00	200.00	200.00	200.00	200.00	200.00	200.00	200.00
Equipment Rental	17,400.00	1,450.00	1,450.00	1,450.00	1,450.00	1,450.00	1,450.00	1,450.00	1,450.00	1,450.00	1,450.00	1,450.00	1,450.00
Insurance Expense		0.00	0.00	0.00	0.00	0.00	0.00	0.00	0.00	0.00	0.00	0.00	0.00
General Liability Insurance	3,600.00	300.00	300.00	300.00	300.00	300.00	300.00	300.00	300.00	300.00	300.00	300.00	300.00
Health Insurance	6,000.00	500.00	500.00	500.00	500.00	500.00	500.00	500.00	500.00	500.00	500.00	500.00	500.00
Life and Disability Insurance	600.00	50.00	50.00	50.00	50.00	50.00	50.00	50.00	50.00	50.00	50.00	50.00	50.00
Malpractice Insurance	7,200.00	600.00	600.00	600.00	600.00	600.00	600.00	600.00	600.00	600.00	600.00	600.00	600.00
Worker's Compensation	1,800.00	150.00	150.00	150.00	150.00	150.00	150.00	150.00	150.00	150.00	150.00	150.00	150.00
Interest Expense	1,800.00	150.00	150.00	150.00	150.00	150.00	150.00	150.00	150.00	150.00	150.00	150.00	150.00

Copy Across Adjust Row Amounts Clear Save OK Cancel Help

FIGURE 16-2 Business budget modified for a dental practice with the use of QuickBooks software.

indicate if a fee will be charged and then provide the amount of the fee on or at the display screen before the transaction is completed.

Direct deposit enables a person to make a deposit to an account on a regular basis. With this system, the dentist may preauthorize recurring bills to be paid automatically; such bills may include insurance premiums, mortgages, and utility bills.

Online banking allows the account to be accessed from a remote location, such as the office or a personal computer. The account holder can view the account balance, request transfers between accounts, and pay bills electronically.

The use of electronic transfers should be monitored carefully. The dentist and any other person responsible for electronic banking must read the documents that are received from the financial institution that issued the access device. No one should know the PIN except the responsible person or persons. The steps that are common to accessing an account are illustrated in Figure 16-3. Each bank will set up some form of security system to verify that an authorized person is accessing the account.

Before any electronic transfer system is used, the institution must provide the following information, which should be filed:

- A summary of the practice's liability for unauthorized transfers
- The telephone number or contact information of the person to be notified if an unauthorized transfer has been or may have been made, a statement of the institution's business days, and the number of days allowed to report suspected unauthorized transfers
- The type of transfers that can be made, the fees for transfers, and any limits on the frequency and amount of transfers
- A summary of the right to receive documentation of transfers and to stop payment on a preauthorized transfer as well as the procedures for stopping payment
- A summary of the institution's liability
- Privacy assurance

If problems arise in the use of online banking, a complaint can be filed through the website for the state member banks of the Federal Reserve System at www.federalreserve.gov.

ESTABLISHING A CHECKING ACCOUNT

As a rule, the checking account for the dental practice will have been opened before the administrative assistant begins working for the practice. However, when opening the account, the dentist had to decide what type of an account would be used: either a traditional manual account or an account with online access. The dentist also signed a signature card (Figure 16-4) that permitted him or her to write checks against the account. If another person is permitted to process transactions against the account, that person's signature must also appear on a signature card for the account or on the same signature card that the dentist signed. However, if the administrative assistant is allowed to sign the checks, the bank may require that the assistant be given power of attorney (Figure 16-5).

Checks

Checks are a means of ordering the bank to pay cash from the bank customer's account. In the past, checks accounted for a majority of all financial transactions in the United States.

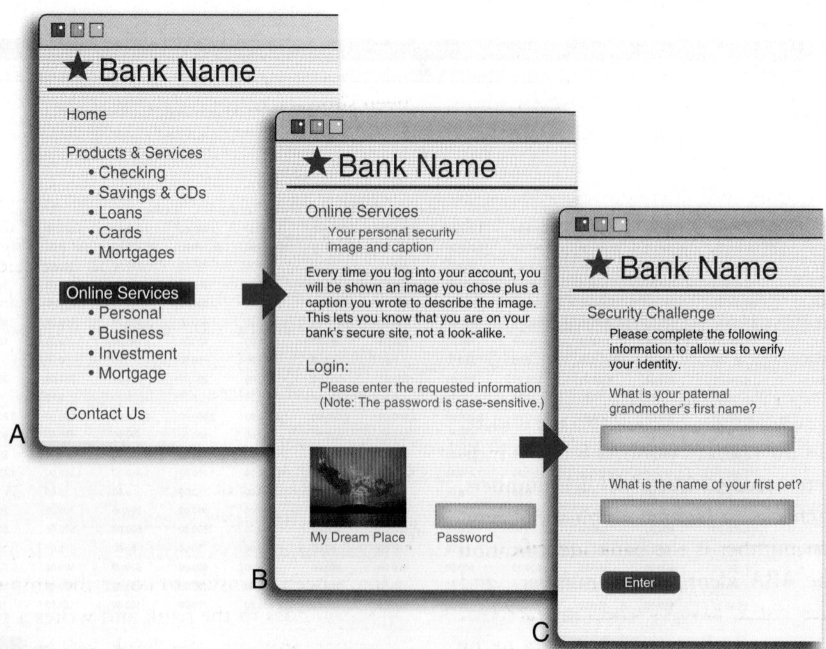

FIGURE 16-3 Basic security steps built into online banking account access. **A,** Home page with menu. **B,** Login screen. **C,** Security check.

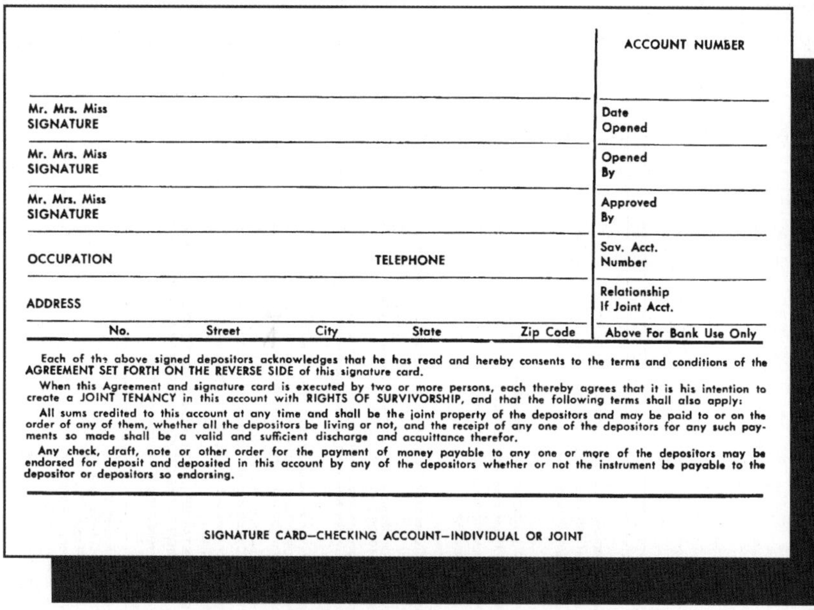

ACCOUNT NUMBER

Mr. Mrs. Miss
SIGNATURE

Date
Opened

Mr. Mrs. Miss
SIGNATURE

Opened
By

Mr. Mrs. Miss
SIGNATURE

Approved
By

OCCUPATION TELEPHONE

Sav. Acct.
Number

ADDRESS

Relationship
If Joint Acct.

No. Street City State Zip Code

Above For Bank Use Only

Each of the above signed depositors acknowledges that he has read and hereby consents to the terms and conditions of the AGREEMENT SET FORTH ON THE REVERSE SIDE of this signature card.

When this Agreement and signature card is executed by two or more persons, each thereby agrees that it is his intention to create a JOINT TENANCY in this account with RIGHTS OF SURVIVORSHIP, and that the following terms shall also apply:

All sums credited to this account at any time and shall be the joint property of the depositors and may be paid to or on the order of any of them, whether all the depositors be living or not, and the receipt of any one of the depositors for any such payments so made shall be a valid and sufficient discharge and acquittance therefor.

Any check, draft, note or other order for the payment of money payable to any one or more of the depositors may be endorsed for deposit and deposited in this account by any of the depositors whether or not the instrument be payable to the depositor or depositors so endorsing.

SIGNATURE CARD—CHECKING ACCOUNT—INDIVIDUAL OR JOINT

FIGURE 16-4 Signature card.

However, the use of online banking and debit cards has risen dramatically. Patients increasingly will use debit and credit cards rather than cash or checks to pay their bills. However, checks still constitute a significant portion of the receipts for the dental practice.

PRACTICE NOTE

Debit cards and electronic transactions have decreased the percentage of financial transactions in this country done by check.

Many parts of a check are self-explanatory; however, some parts need additional explanation. In Figure 16-6, the number 3 indicates the American Bankers Association (ABA) bank identification number. With this coding system, every bank is given its own number, which constitutes a numeric name for the bank. This number aids the sorting of checks for distribution to their proper destination. The ABA number is a fraction, and it is usually printed in the upper right corner of the check or slightly to the left of the check number. The number 4 in the figure indicates the *payee,* which is the individual or company that will receive the money. The number 7 indicates the *drawee,* which is the bank that pays the check. Numbers 8 and 9 indicate magnetic ink character recognition (MICR) numbers. These are encoded on all checks to facilitate high-speed handling by machine. The first number is the bank identification number (also found in the ABA identification number), and the second number is the check writer's checking account number. These numbers can easily be read by people or by machine. The number 10 indicates the signature of the *drawer* or check writer, which is the person who orders the bank to pay cash from the account.

Preparing Checks

In the past, the administrative assistant prepared checks manually. Today, with the use of financial management software, the assistant can set aside some time during the working day as the schedule permits to prepare the checks with the use of the selected software. If a manual system is used, the following steps are taken when writing the check. The check stub or checkbook register should be completed before the check is written or printed. The stub or register provides a record of the following: (1) the check number; (2) the date; (3) the payee; (4) the amount of the check; (5) the purpose of the check; and (6) the new balance brought forward after the amount of the check has been subtracted. It also provides the new balance if a deposit is to be added to the previous balance, as shown in the manual system (Figure 16-7).

Figure 16-8 presents a step-by-step procedure for manually writing a check. A check produced by a software system such as QuickBooks requires that the user select the icon for check writing from the main screen (Figure 16-9) and then follow through with the data entry as requested on each screen. A check written to a dental supplier includes information important about the check and the account (Figure 16-10).

Types of Checks

The following list describes a few of the types of checks that the administrative assistant may receive:

- *Certified check:* A certified check is a guarantee that funds have been set aside to cover the amount of the check. The person goes to the bank and writes a personal check for the proper amount; the bank sets aside that amount from the customer's account by placing it in a special account and then stamps the word *Certified* across the face of the check. Usually a nominal fee is charged for certifying a check.

Form **2848** (Rev. March 2012) Department of the Treasury Internal Revenue Service

Power of Attorney and Declaration of Representative

▶ Type or print. ▶ See the separate instructions.

OMB No. 1545-0150

For IRS Use Only
Received by:
Name
Telephone
Function
Date / /

Part I Power of Attorney

Caution: *A separate Form 2848 should be completed for each taxpayer. Form 2848 will not be honored for any purpose other than representation before the IRS.*

1 **Taxpayer information.** Taxpayer must sign and date this form on page 2, line 7.

Taxpayer name and address	Taxpayer identification number(s)	
	Daytime telephone number	Plan number (if applicable)

hereby appoints the following representative(s) as attorney(s)-in-fact:

2 **Representative(s)** must sign and date this form on page 2, Part II.

Name and address — CAF No. / PTIN / Telephone No. / Fax No.
Check if to be sent notices and communications ☐ Check if new: Address ☐ Telephone No. ☐ Fax No. ☐

Name and address — CAF No. / PTIN / Telephone No. / Fax No.
Check if to be sent notices and communications ☐ Check if new: Address ☐ Telephone No. ☐ Fax No. ☐

Name and address — CAF No. / PTIN / Telephone No. / Fax No.
Check if new: Address ☐ Telephone No. ☐ Fax No. ☐

to represent the taxpayer before the Internal Revenue Service for the following matters:

3 **Matters**

Description of Matter (Income, Employment, Payroll, Excise, Estate, Gift, Whistleblower, Practitioner Discipline, PLR, FOIA, Civil Penalty, etc.) (see instructions for line 3)	Tax Form Number (1040, 941, 720, etc.) (if applicable)	Year(s) or Period(s) (if applicable) (see instructions for line 3)

4 **Specific use not recorded on Centralized Authorization File (CAF).** If the power of attorney is for a specific use not recorded on CAF, check this box. See the instructions for Line 4. **Specific Uses Not Recorded on CAF** . . . . ▶ ☐

5 **Acts authorized.** Unless otherwise provided below, the representatives generally are authorized to receive and inspect confidential tax information and to perform any and all acts that I can perform with respect to the tax matters described on line 3, for example, the authority to sign any agreements, consents, or other documents. The representative(s), however, is (are) not authorized to receive or negotiate any amounts paid to the client in connection with this representation (including refunds by either electronic means or paper checks). Additionally, unless the appropriate box(es) below are checked, the representative(s) is (are) not authorized to execute a request for disclosure of tax returns or return information to a third party, substitute another representative or add additional representatives, or sign certain tax returns.

☐ Disclosure to third parties; ☐ Substitute or add representative(s); ☐ Signing a return;

☐ Other acts authorized: (see instructions for more information)

Exceptions. An unenrolled return preparer cannot sign any document for a taxpayer and may only represent taxpayers in limited situations. An enrolled actuary may only represent taxpayers to the extent provided in section 10.3(d) of Treasury Department Circular No. 230 (Circular 230). An enrolled retirement plan agent may only represent taxpayers to the extent provided in section 10.3(e) of Circular 230. A registered tax return preparer may only represent taxpayers to the extent provided in section 10.3(f) of Circular 230. See the line 5 instructions for restrictions on tax matters partners. In most cases, the student practitioner's (level k) authority is limited (for example, they may only practice under the supervision of another practitioner).

List any specific deletions to the acts otherwise authorized in this power of attorney:

For Privacy Act and Paperwork Reduction Act Notice, see the instructions. Cat. No. 11980J Form **2848** (Rev. 3-2012)

Form 2848 (Rev. 3-2012) Page **2**

6 **Retention/revocation of prior power(s) of attorney.** The filing of this power of attorney automatically revokes all earlier power(s) of attorney on file with the Internal Revenue Service for the same matters and years or periods covered by this document. If you **do not** want to revoke a prior power of attorney, check here . . . . ▶ ☐
YOU MUST ATTACH A COPY OF ANY POWER OF ATTORNEY YOU WANT TO REMAIN IN EFFECT.

7 **Signature of taxpayer.** If a tax matter concerns a year in which a joint return was filed, the husband and wife must each file a separate power of attorney even if the same representative(s) is (are) being appointed. If signed by a corporate officer, partner, guardian, tax matters partner, executor, receiver, administrator, or trustee on behalf of the taxpayer, I certify that I have the authority to execute this form on behalf of the taxpayer.

▶ IF NOT SIGNED AND DATED, THIS POWER OF ATTORNEY WILL BE RETURNED TO THE TAXPAYER.

Signature Date Title (if applicable)

Print Name PIN Number Print name of taxpayer from line 1 if other than individual

Part II Declaration of Representative

Under penalties of perjury, I declare that:

- I am not currently under suspension or disbarment from practice before the Internal Revenue Service;
- I am aware of regulations contained in Circular 230 (31 CFR, Part 10), as amended, concerning practice before the Internal Revenue Service;
- I am authorized to represent the taxpayer identified in Part I for the matter(s) specified there; and
- I am one of the following:

a Attorney—a member in good standing of the bar of the highest court of the jurisdiction shown below.
b Certified Public Accountant—duly qualified to practice as a certified public accountant in the jurisdiction shown below.
c Enrolled Agent—enrolled as an agent under the requirements of Circular 230.
d Officer—a bona fide officer of the taxpayer's organization.
e Full-Time Employee—a full-time employee of the taxpayer.
f Family Member—a member of the taxpayer's immediate family (for example, spouse, parent, child, grandparent, grandchild, step-parent, step-child, brother, or sister).
g Enrolled Actuary—enrolled as an actuary by the Joint Board for the Enrollment of Actuaries under 29 U.S.C. 1242 (the authority to practice before the Internal Revenue Service is limited by section 10.3(d) of Circular 230).
h Unenrolled Return Preparer—Your authority to practice before the Internal Revenue Service is limited. You must have been eligible to sign the return under examination and have signed the return. **See Notice 2011-6 and Special rules for registered tax return preparers and unenrolled return preparers in the instructions.**
i Registered Tax Return Preparer—registered as a tax return preparer under the requirements of section 10.4 of Circular 230. Your authority to practice before the Internal Revenue Service is limited. You must have been eligible to sign the return under examination and have signed the return. **See Notice 2011-6 and Special rules for registered tax return preparers and unenrolled return preparers in the instructions.**
k Student Attorney or CPA—receives permission to practice before the IRS by virtue of his/her status as a law, business, or accounting student working in LITC or STCP under section 10.7(d) of Circular 230. See instructions for Part II for additional information and requirements.
r Enrolled Retirement Plan Agent—enrolled as a retirement plan agent under the requirements of Circular 230 (the authority to practice before the Internal Revenue Service is limited by section 10.3(e)).

▶ IF THIS DECLARATION OF REPRESENTATIVE IS NOT SIGNED AND DATED, THE POWER OF ATTORNEY WILL BE RETURNED. REPRESENTATIVES MUST SIGN IN THE ORDER LISTED IN LINE 2 ABOVE. See the instructions for Part II.

Note: For designations d-f, enter your title, position, or relationship to the taxpayer in the "Licensing jurisdiction" column. See the instructions for Part II for more information.

Designation—Insert above letter **(a–r)**	Licensing jurisdiction (state) or other licensing authority (if applicable)	Bar, license, certification, registration, or enrollment number (if applicable). See instructions for Part II for more information.	Signature	Date

Form **2848** (Rev. 3-2012)

FIGURE 16-5 Power of attorney (Form 2848). (From Internal Revenue Service, Department of the Treasury, Washington, DC.)

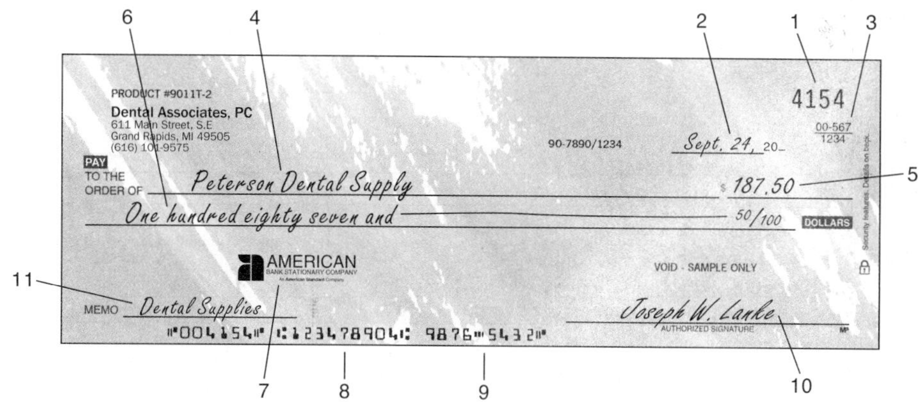

FIGURE 16-6 Parts of a check. **1,** Check number. **2,** Date of check. **3,** American Bankers Association (ABA) bank identification number. **4,** Payee (the person or company to be paid). **5,** Amount of check in figures. **6,** Amount of check in words. **7,** Drawee (the bank on which the check is drawn). **8,** Bank identification number magnetically printed for electronic processing. **9,** Customer account number magnetically printed for electronic processing. **10,** Signature of drawer. **11,** Reason check was written.

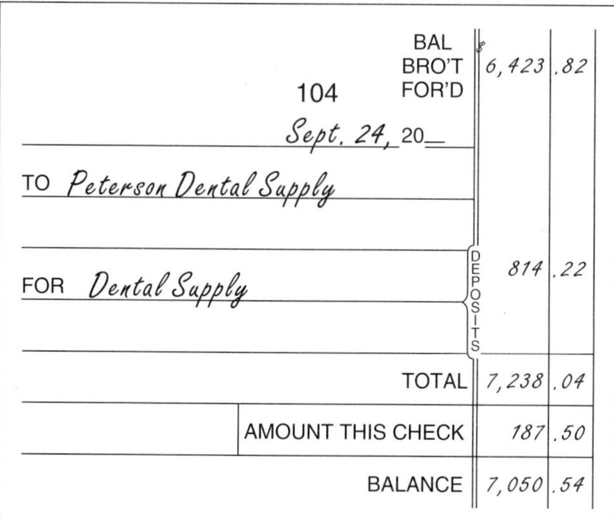

104	BAL BRO'T FOR'D	6,423	.82
Sept. 24, 20__			
TO Peterson Dental Supply			
FOR Dental Supply	DEPOSITS	814	.22
	TOTAL	7,238	.04
	AMOUNT THIS CHECK	187	.50
	BALANCE	7,050	.54

FIGURE 16-7 Sample check stub.

- *Cashier's check:* A cashier's check is the bank's own order to make payment out of its own funds. When a cashier's check is purchased, the person specifies to whom the bank makes the check payable and receives a carbon or stub of the check as a record. A fee is usually charged for this type of check.
- *Money order:* A money order is a means of transferring money without using cash or a personal check. People who do not maintain a personal checking account often use money orders to pay their creditors. The money order may be purchased in the form of a bank money order, a postal money order, or an express money order. The money order shows the name of the purchaser and the person who is to receive the payment (the payee). A fee is charged for this service.
- *Traveler's check:* Although the traveler's check is designed as a payment device for a person who is away from home, it is uncommon to receive a traveler's check in payment for dental services. Traveler's checks are purchased through a bank, the American Express Company, or the Railway Express Agency. The checks are preprinted in various denominations, usually $10, $20, $50, and $100. A small fee, which is determined by the amount purchased, is charged. When the checks are purchased, the individual signs his or her name in a designated place on each check. When the checks are used for payment or are cashed, they are *countersigned*; that is, the purchaser signs them again in the presence of the individual who cashes the check or accepts it for payment. Fewer traveler's checks are being used today, but they are still in existence in some countries.
- *Bank draft:* A bank draft is a check drawn by the cashier of one bank on another bank where the first bank has available funds on deposit or credit. A bank draft is used if a person or company wants to send a sum of money and a personal check is not acceptable.
- *Voucher check:* A voucher check provides a detachable stub that serves as an excellent accounting record for itemizing the payment of invoices or any other type of itemization that the payer would like as a reference.

Accepting and Cashing Checks

Many different types of checks may be used as payment for services. When a check is accepted, make sure that it has the following characteristics: (1) it is legibly written in ink or typewritten; (2) it is currently dated; (3) it has been signed by the check writer; (4) it is drawn on a US bank; (5) it has been made payable for a certain sum of money (the amount in figures and the amount in words should agree); and (6) it has been made payable to a payee or bearer.

At times, the administrative assistant may be asked to accept a check for more than the charges. This may present a problem. For example, if the individual owes $100 and wants to pay $50 but writes a check for $100 and asks for $50 to be returned, a

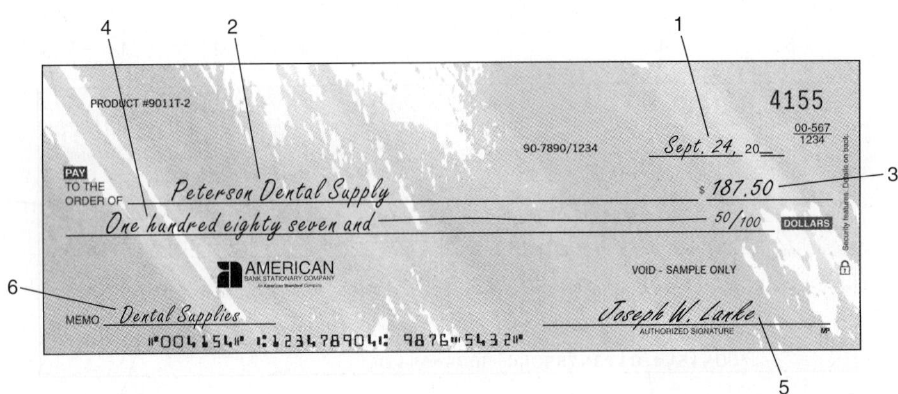

FIGURE 16-8 How to write a check. **1,** Date the check. **2,** Key or write the name of the person or firm to whom the check will be payable. **3,** Enter the amount of the check in figures opposite the dollar sign. **4,** Write the amount of the check in words under the "Pay to the order of" line. Start as far to the left margin as possible. **5,** The name on the signature line should be signed as it appears on the bank signature card. **6,** On the memo line, record the purpose of the payment.

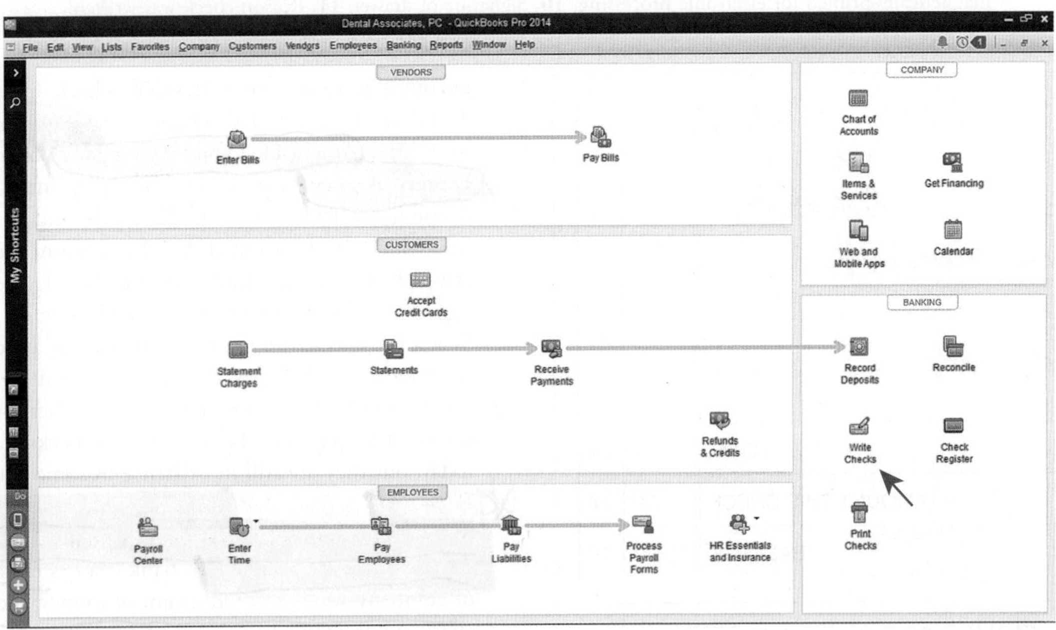

FIGURE 16-9 The main screen of QuickBooks contains icons that represent various accounting options, including one for check writing. (Screenshot © Intuit, Inc. All rights reserved.)

question may arise at a later date if the patient tries to use the canceled check as a receipt for full payment of the account. Another problem that may be encountered is the acceptance of payment for more than the balance and the return of the difference in cash to the patient. If the bank returns the patient's check for insufficient funds, cash has been paid out from the business, and the patient has the cash. To avoid problems of this nature, it is better to establish a firm policy of not accepting checks for more than the amount owed. This policy should be established by the dentist and enforced at all times.

Other Forms of Payment

As mentioned previously, credit and debit cards (e.g., MasterCard, VISA, Discover, American Express) are increasingly being used to pay professional fees. The dentist makes arrangements through a bank—usually the one in which the business account has been established—to use this banking service. The bank charges a fee for this service, and this is generally 1% to 5% of the amount of the transactions handled. A merchant's service company provides the terminal with a scanner and a PIN pad.

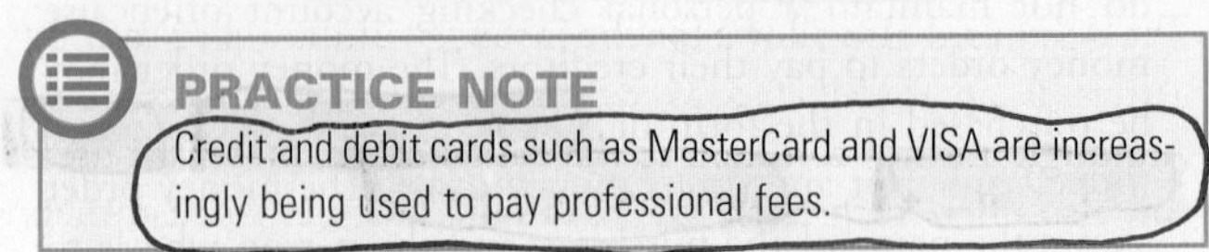

PRACTICE NOTE

Credit and debit cards such as MasterCard and VISA are increasingly being used to pay professional fees.

The debit card (also known as a *bank card* or *check card*) is a plastic card that provides a method other than cash for the making of payments. In reality, the card is essentially an

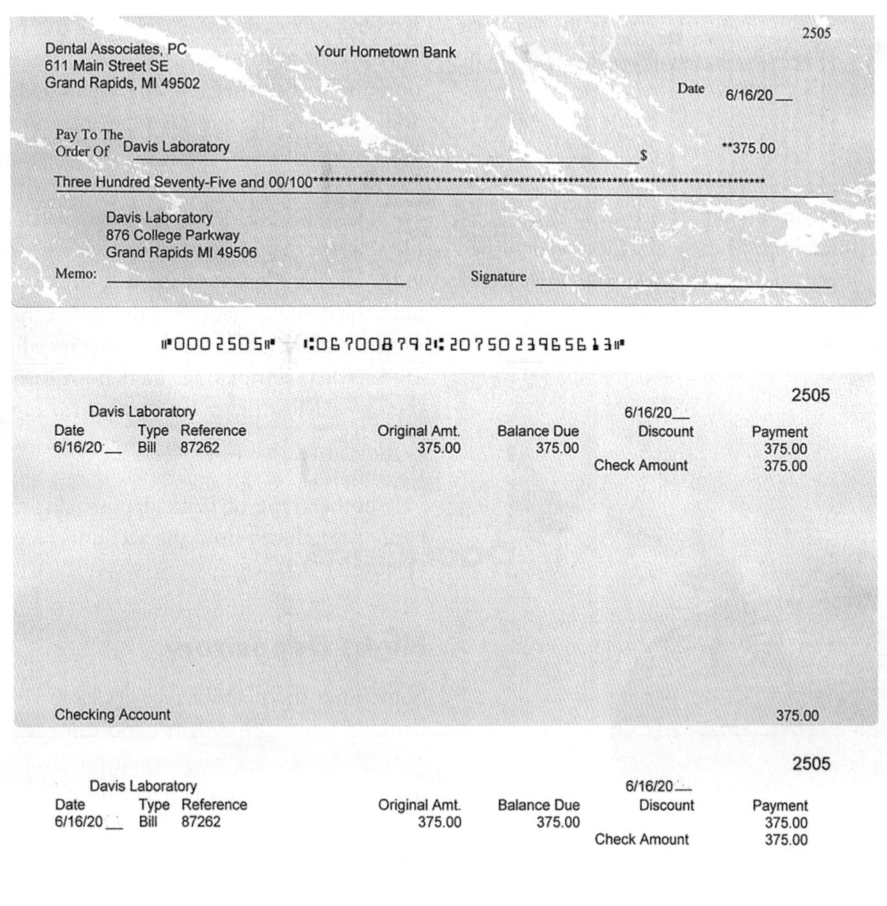

Dental Associates, PC
611 Main Street SE
Grand Rapids, MI 49502

Your Hometown Bank

2505

Date 6/16/20__

Pay To The Order Of Davis Laboratory $ **375.00

Three Hundred Seventy-Five and 00/100***

Davis Laboratory
876 College Parkway
Grand Rapids MI 49506

Memo: ______ Signature ______

0002505 067008792 2075023965613

2505

Davis Laboratory 6/16/20__

Date	Type	Reference	Original Amt.	Balance Due	Discount	Payment
6/16/20__	Bill	87262	375.00	375.00		375.00
					Check Amount	375.00

Checking Account 375.00

2505

Davis Laboratory 6/16/20__

Date	Type	Reference	Original Amt.	Balance Due	Discount	Payment
6/16/20__	Bill	87262	375.00	375.00		375.00
					Check Amount	375.00

Checking Account 375.00

FIGURE 16-10 A sample check produced on the QuickBooks system for a payment for dental supplies. (Software © Intuit, Inc. All rights reserved.)

electronic check; the funds are withdrawn directly from either the bank account (often referred to as a *check card*) or from the remaining balance on a prepaid debit card.

When a patient presents a debit card, it is entered as payment, and a request is made to have the PIN entered by the patient. The administrative assistant has the patient enter the PIN on the PIN pad (Figure 16-11), and the transaction is then completed. Debit cards for the office may be used by the dentist and other authorized persons to make purchases for the office. The debit card also allows for the instant withdrawal of cash by acting as an ATM card as well as a check guarantee card. Although it is not common to the dental office, merchant users can also offer "cash back" or "cash out" facilities to customers so that customers can withdraw cash along with their payment or purchase.

At the end of the day, when the administrative assistant prints out a collection reconciliation sheet of the day's financial activities from the dental software program, the sheet will indicate which payments were made with cash and which were made by debit or credit cards (Figure 16-12).

A few precautions are necessary when patients use credit or debit cards for payment. Be sure to check the card's expiration date and the signature on the back of the card to ensure that it matches the patient's signature of the patient. Occasionally a person may opt not to sign the back of the card for security reasons. It is then necessary to ask for another form of photo identification with a signature to ensure proper identification. Sometimes a card may be rejected for payment; the administrative assistant then must ask for an alternate form of payment. Do not discuss the card rejection, because this is the patient's private business.

Because some patients pay their accounts with cash, some cash must be kept in the office. However, large amounts of cash should not be routinely kept in the office, because it may end up being counted as part of the total cash receipts for the day. A separate cash balance can be maintained for petty cash, which will be discussed later in this chapter.

DEPOSITS

Checks received by the practice are either manually deposited or scanned for online processing. The checks that need to be deposited should have been endorsed as soon as they were received to ensure safekeeping in the office. A stamp can be obtained from most office supply stores with the vital information about the office and the account. Figure 16-13 illustrates and describes the various types of **endorsements**. Depositing money into the practice's checking account is usually a daily routine, but it may vary according to the office's schedule. A **bank deposit** represents the accumulation of money received for a single day or possibly for a longer period. The bank provides checking account deposit slips for a nominal fee; these have the dental practice's name and account number imprinted on them. Follow the step-by-step procedure presented in Figure 16-14 when completing the deposit form. A duplicate copy of the deposit form may be retained for office use for verification with the check register and the bank statement at the end of the month.

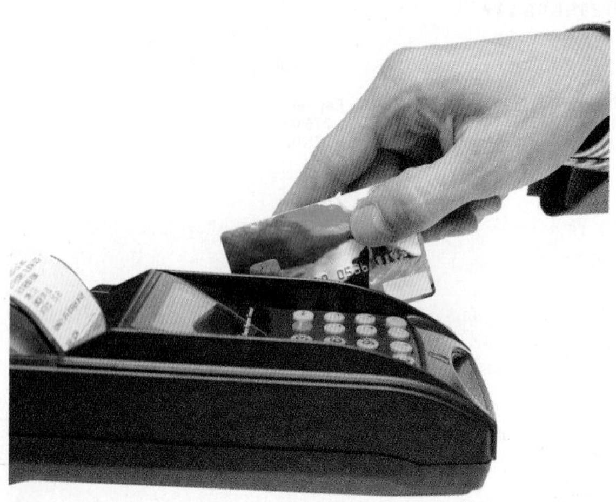

FIGURE 16-11 A credit or debit machine contains a card reader to allow the office to swipe the card and a PIN pad for the patient to enter the PIN for payment. (Copyright © 2014, Kokhanchikov, BigStock.com.)

Another type of bank deposit slip that may be generated easily is produced from the accounts receivable software system (Figure 16-15).

Night Depository

Sometimes the practice receives large amounts of money after banking hours. The night depository is a means of depositing money in the bank vault when the bank is closed. Usually the deposit is completed the next business day by a bank teller; the depositor must go to the bank to pick up the deposit bag and receipt. However, if the depositor prefers, the deposit bag can remain locked until the person arrives at the bank to make the deposit personally.

TIME 4:24 PM George Young, D.D.S. DATE 7/28/2009

PAYMENT RECONCILIATION
Today
All Providers

Patient Name	Date	User	Payment	Amount
Check Payments				
3446 - Abbott, Charles K	7/28/2009	BAB	Acct Pymt Check Number: 123456	$4,756.00
1120 - Allen, Cathy	7/28/2009	BAB	Acct Pymt Check Number: 4562	$80.00
2815 - Campbell, Chris	7/28/2009	BAB	Acct Pymt Check Number: 1232123	$30.25
2815 - Campbell, Chris	7/28/2009	BAB	Acct Pymt Check Number: 1232123	$33.00
			Total Check	$4,899.25
Visa Payments				
868 - Lange, Jack	7/28/2009	BAB	Acct Pymt Visa Number: Credit card payment	$78.00
			Total Visa	$78.00
Discover Payments				
463 - Farkas, Paul	7/28/2009	BAB	Acct Pymt Discover Number: Credit card payment	$397.50
			Total Discover	$397.50
Insurance Ck Payments				
8 - Abbott, Angie A	7/28/2009	BAB		$16.28
3446 - Abbott, Charles K	7/28/2009	BAB		$807.60
3432 - Abbott, Mark	7/28/2009	BAB		$20.00
2517 - Macphee, Christy	7/28/2009	BAB		$48.50
2517 - Macphee, Christy	7/28/2009	BAB		$21.50
			Total Insurance Ck	$913.88
			TOTAL PAYMENTS:	$6,288.63

FIGURE 16-12 Payment reconciliations indicating debit and credit card use for the day. (Courtesy Patterson Dental, St. Paul, Minnesota.)

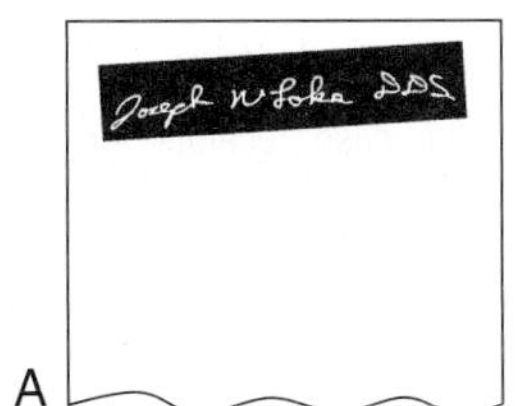

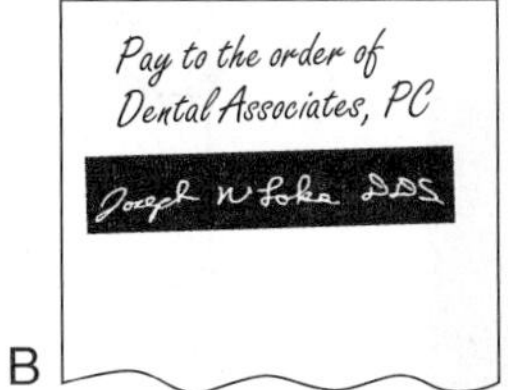

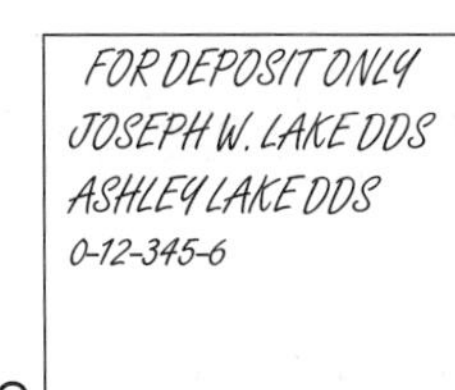

FIGURE 16-13 Check endorsements. **A,** *Blank endorsement,* which is an endorsement that consists of the signature of the payee. A blank endorsement makes the check payable to any holder. **B,** *Endorsement in full,* which is an endorsement that states to whom the check is to be paid and which includes the signature of the payee. This endorsement specifies that the check can be cashed or transferred only on the order of the person, bank, or company named in the endorsement. **C,** *Restrictive endorsement,* which is an endorsement that includes special conditions or which limits the receiver of the check with regard to the uses that can be made of it. This type of endorsement commonly is used when checks are prepared for deposit.

Automatic Teller Machine

As mentioned previously, in conjunction with a checking account, financial institutions offer special access cards that can be used to perform banking transactions virtually 24 hours a day, 7 days a week. The cards can be used at ATMs, which are computer workstations that electronically prompt the user through most routine banking activities. Deposits or withdrawals can be made, and funds can be transferred between accounts. However, some precautions must be taken when using an ATM (Box 16-2).

> **BOX 16-2**
>
> **Important Points to Remember When Using an ATM**
>
> - Never use an ATM to deposit cash or other items that can be used by unauthorized personnel.
> - Only receipts of deposit are received; no copies of deposit slips are given.
> - Multiple checks can be deposited in most systems, with copies of checks commonly provided.
> - Use an ATM only to deposit checks with restrictive endorsements.
> - Notify the bank immediately of any discrepancies between its records and the transactions on the bank statement.
> - Notify the bank immediately if the office's ATM access card is lost or stolen.

RECONCILING THE BANK STATEMENT

Basic Steps

Although procedures may differ, most banks send a bank statement (Figure 16-16) to the depositor each month, or the statement may be obtained online with appropriate identification. The bank statement shows the balance of the account at the beginning of the month, the deposits made during the month, the checks drawn against the account, any corrections or charges against the account (e.g., service charges, stop-payment charges), and the bank balance at the end of the month. To maintain an accurate record of the checking account, reconcile the bank statement as soon as the records are received from the bank. An online bank statement is available after the close of business on the last day of each month. This can be printed or reconciled online, thereby helping to create a paperless office.

Use the following procedure to reconcile the bank statement:

1. Verify the amount of the canceled checks with the amounts shown on the bank statement. (The canceled checks are usually returned in the order listed on the statement.)
2. Arrange the canceled checks numerically.
3. Compare the amounts on the canceled checks and the deposits with the amounts written in the checkbook register. Check off all canceled checks and deposits in the checkbook register.
4. List the *outstanding checks* (checks not yet returned to the bank), including the check number and the amount.
5. Total the outstanding checks. If a deposit has been made but does not appear on the bank statement, the deposit must be added to the bank statement balance before the outstanding checks are subtracted.
6. Look for charges other than checks that have been deducted from the account, such as service charges (SCs), debit memos (DMs), and overdrafts (ODs). These charges must be subtracted from the checkbook register.

In Figure 16-17, a reconciliation of the bank statement has been prepared for the practice of Dental Associates, PC.

Petty Cash

Although the cash receipts are deposited in the bank and invoices and miscellaneous items are paid by check, a small amount of cash should be kept on hand in the office. This should be established as a petty cash fund and controlled with the same accuracy as the checking account.

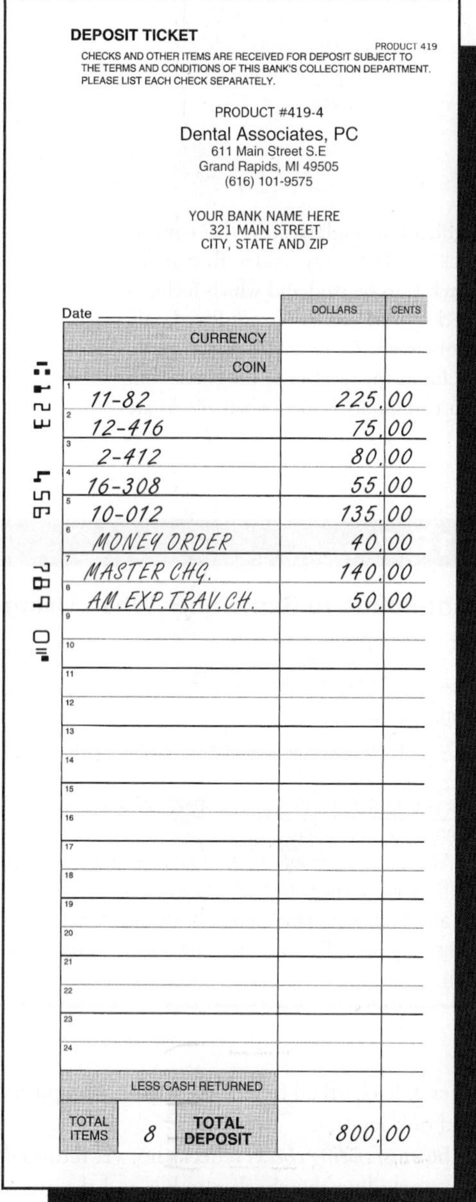

DEPOSIT TICKET

PRODUCT 419

CHECKS AND OTHER ITEMS ARE RECEIVED FOR DEPOSIT SUBJECT TO THE TERMS AND CONDITIONS OF THIS BANK'S COLLECTION DEPARTMENT. PLEASE LIST EACH CHECK SEPARATELY.

PRODUCT #419-4

Dental Associates, PC
611 Main Street S.E
Grand Rapids, MI 49505
(616) 101-9575

YOUR BANK NAME HERE
321 MAIN STREET
CITY, STATE AND ZIP

Date

		DOLLARS	CENTS
	CURRENCY		
	COIN		
1	11-82	225	00
2	12-416	75	00
3	2-412	80	00
4	16-308	55	00
5	10-012	135	00
6	MONEY ORDER	40	00
7	MASTER CHQ.	140	00
8	AM.EXP.TRAV.CH.	50	00
9			
10			
11			
12			
13			
14			
15			
16			
17			
18			
19			
20			
21			
22			
23			
24			
	LESS CASH RETURNED		
TOTAL ITEMS 8	TOTAL DEPOSIT	800	00

⑈0 789 4567 123⑈

FIGURE 16-14 Deposit slip. **1,** Write or type the date on the front side. **2,** List the currency and coins to be deposited. **3,** Identify the checks to be deposited individually; if there are more than three, use the back side of the deposit slip. Checks should be listed on the deposit slip by their ABA numbers. However, the administrative assistant may prefer to list checks with the patient's name and number. If it is a money order, traveler's check, or MasterCard or VISA charge receipt, the total amount of money and the name of the item should be listed. **4,** Enter the total from the back side of the slip on the front side of the deposit slip. **5,** Total the entire deposit (net deposit). **6,** Optional: some deposit slips provide a line in case the depositor wants part of the deposit back in cash. The amount desired is entered on this line and subtracted from the total line above it; the net deposit then is entered as in 5.

PRACTICE NOTE

Although the cash receipts are deposited in the bank and invoices and miscellaneous items are paid by check, a small amount of cash should be kept on hand in the office.

When it has been determined how much cash will be placed in the petty cash account, a check is written against the business account and cashed, and the cash is returned to the office and kept in a separate fund. To help eliminate errors in disbursements from the fund, one person in the office should have control over the petty cash. A voucher is completed each time money is taken from the fund. The voucher shows the date, the voucher number, the amount of payment, what the payment was for, to whom the payment was made, and the name of the person who approved the payment (Figure 16-18).

After the voucher is completed, it is placed in the drawer as a reminder of the amount of cash taken from the fund. The vouchers and cash together should equal the original balance of petty cash.

A formal record of petty cash disbursements may also be used. This record shows all of the disbursements in chronological order as well as the voucher number, and special columns are used for each expense item disbursed from the fund. It also provides a complete summary of how the money was disbursed. At the end of the month, the fund must be replenished. This involves writing another check for cash purposes and charging the various expense accounts for the amount used from the petty cash fund.

RECORDING BUSINESS EXPENSES

As invoices are processed, the expenditures represented on them need to be analyzed and verified for payment. If using a financial management software system, this information is listed in the accounts payable file. A check is then made out to each supplier for the payment of these statements. The payments are automatically entered in an expense category. A monthly income and expense register provides a list of all of the expenditures for the month, including the date of payment, the company to which the payment was made, the category of deduction, and the amount of payment. These totals are transferred to the annual summary. When using a system like QuickBooks, the entries are made, the categories of expenses are updated automatically (Figure 16-19), and checks can then be produced, as illustrated in Figure 16-10. QuickBooks also allows users to convert the entered bills into paid bills via electronic funds transfer.

MAINTAINING PAYROLL RECORDS

Various federal and state laws require that most businesses keep records to provide information about wages paid and to help with the preparation of required tax reports. Therefore, the administrative assistant must have a good working knowledge of payroll and tax records.

October 24, 20__ at 3:05p　　　　Page 1

DEPOSIT SLIP
PRACTICE
Dates Included: 10/24/__ to 10/24/__

Dental Associates, PC
611 Main Street S.E
Grand Rapids, MI 49505
(616) 101-9575

Account Number:

Code	Bank No.	Check No.	Amount	Reference (ID, Name)
3	87/44323	634	206.00	(7301) Gable, Catherine M
3	55/980	978	380.00	(12202) Page, Michael W
3	90/4532	709	326.00	(26901) Glass, Steven
3	77/345-0	4793	148.00	(48201) Nair, Ernest
3	445/0983	345	513.00	(50101) O'brien, Armando
3	12-9855	746	121.00	(234101) Jackewitz, Jerry

TOTAL

6 Checks Total	1694.00
Total Cash	211.00
Total Deposit	1905.00

FIGURE 16-15 Sample computer-generated deposit slip.

Previous Statement Transactions on CHECKING ACCOUNT 0-12-345-6 - $35019.27 as of June 01, 20__

Date	Check Number	Description	Debit	Credit	Balance
5/4		MERCHANT SERVICE MERCH DEP 731668000667		870.50	40,698.57
5/5		MERCHANT SERVICE MERCH DEP 731668000667		684.00	41,382.57
5/6	1789	CHK	104.18		41,278.39
5/6	1794	CHK	600.00		40,678.39
5/6	1793	CHK	89.60		40,588.79
5/6	1792	CHK	175.19		40,413.60
5/6	1790	CHK	165.00		40,248.60
5/6	1791	CHK	15.00		40,233.60
5/6	1788	CHK	95.00		40,138.60
5/6	1787	CHK	706.13		39,432.47
5/6	1786	CHK	52.83		39,379.64
5/6	1785	CHK	49.51		39,330.13
5/6	1784	CHK	161.96		39,168.17
5/7		DEPOSIT		438.00	39,606.17
5/11	1795	CHK	36.10		39,570.07
5/11		MERCHANT SERVICE MERCH DEP 731668000667		787.75	40,357.82
5/12		MERCHANT SERVICE MERCH DEP 731668000667		543.50	40,901.32
5/14		MERCHANT SERVICE MERCH DEP 731668000667		658.00	41,559.32
5/14	1796	CHK	52.50		41,506.82
5/14		DEPOSIT		579.51	42,086.33
5/14	1797	CHK	10,336.00		31,750.33
5/14	1799	CHK	451.00		31,299.33
5/18		MERCHANT SERVICE MERCH DEP 731668000667		594.00	31,893.33
5/19		MERCHANT SERVICE MERCH DEP 731668000667		471.75	32,365.08
5/21		MERCHANT SERVICE MERCH DEP 731668000667		511.00	32,876.08
5/21		DEPOSIT		870.00	33,746.08
5/21		PROOF CORRECTION CREDIT		9.00	33,755.08
5/21	1801	CHK	110.00		33,645.08
5/21	1802	CHK	37.50		33,607.58
5/21	1800	CHK	11.76		33,595.82
5/25		MERCHANT SERVICE MERCH DEP 731668000667		658.75	34,254.57
5/27		MERCHANT SERVICE MERCH DEP 731668000667		261.00	34,515.57
5/28		MERCHANT SERVICE MERCH DEP 731668000667		465.00	34,980.57
5/28		DEPOSIT		369.00	35,349.57
5/31		MERCHANT SERVICE MERCH FEE 731668000667	333.16		35,016.41
5/31		INTEREST		2.86	35,019.27

FIGURE 16-16 Sample bank statement.

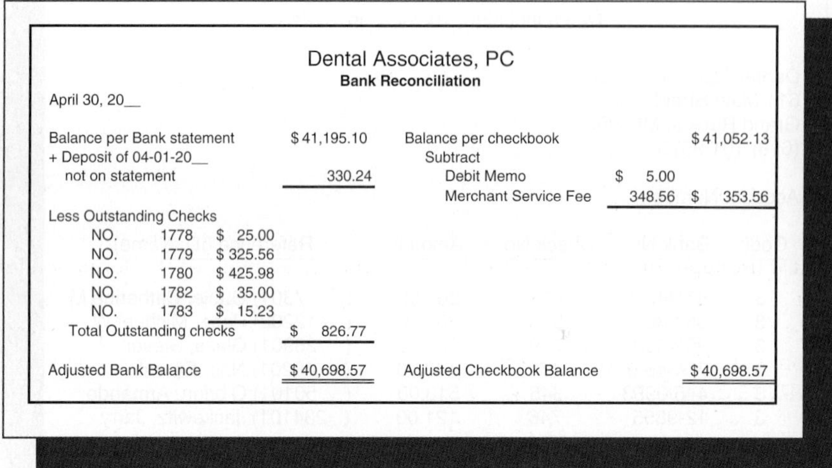

Dental Associates, PC

Bank Reconciliation

April 30, 20__

Balance per Bank statement	$ 41,195.10	Balance per checkbook			$ 41,052.13
+ Deposit of 04-01-20__		Subtract			
not on statement	330.24	Debit Memo	$ 5.00		
		Merchant Service Fee	348.56	$	353.56
Less Outstanding Checks					
NO. 1778 $ 25.00					
NO. 1779 $ 325.56					
NO. 1780 $ 425.98					
NO. 1782 $ 35.00					
NO. 1783 $ 15.23					
Total Outstanding checks	$ 826.77				
Adjusted Bank Balance	$ 40,698.57	Adjusted Checkbook Balance			$ 40,698.57

FIGURE 16-17 Sample bank reconciliation.

Petty Cash Voucher

No.________ Date________

Paid to________________________________ Amount

For________________________________ ________

Charge to____________________________

_____________________ _____________________

Approved by Payment received

FIGURE 16-18 Petty cash voucher.

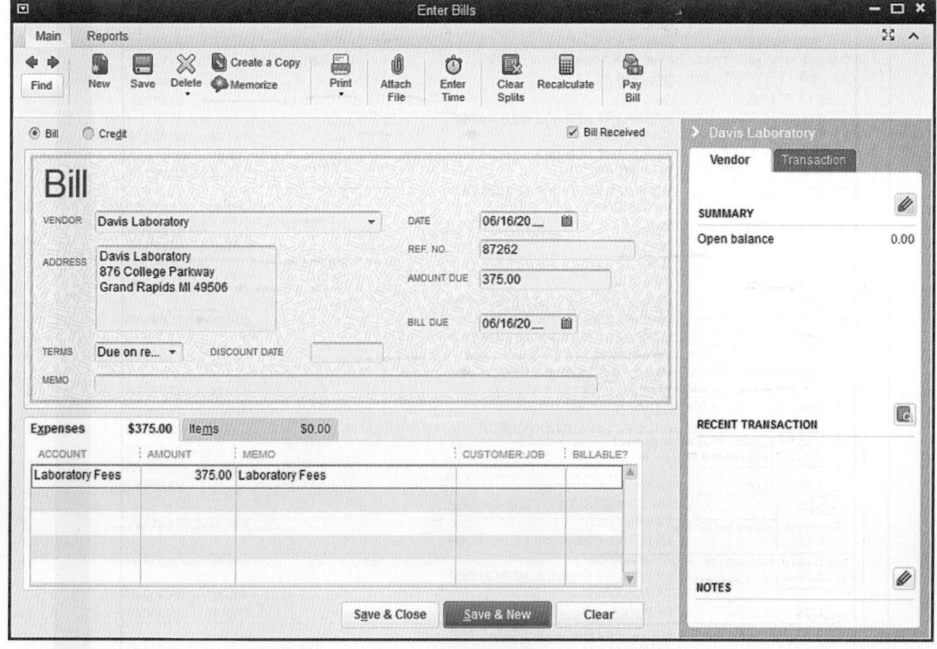

FIGURE 16-19 Sample of a bill entered into QuickBooks. The *Enter Bills* function allows a user to keep a record of expenditures and also to pay those bills electronically if the office is set up for that functionality. (Screenshot © Intuit, Inc. All rights reserved.)

PRACTICE NOTE

Various federal and state laws require that most businesses keep records to provide information about wages paid and to help with the preparation of required tax reports.

INITIAL PAYROLL RECORDS

As an employer, the dentist must apply for an employer identification number; this is a nine-digit number assigned to sole proprietors or corporations for filing and reporting payroll information. The application, Form SS-4, is available from the Internal Revenue Service (IRS; Figure 16-20). Some states also require a state employer identification number. Visit www.irs.gov for the current rules for the SS-4 because the Paperwork Reduction Act is moving some of these processes online.

The employer is required to have every employee complete an Employee's Withholding Allowance Certificate (Form W-4) (Figure 16-21). This form is needed to determine the status of each employee for income tax deductions from wages. Employees are required to complete a new Form W-4 when they change the number of withholding exemptions claimed.

EMPLOYEE EARNINGS RECORDS

The employer must maintain employees' earnings records, including a summary of information for each employee (Figure 16-22). If the record has been properly designed, it provides the information needed for quarterly and annual reports. The employee's earnings record should contain the following information, which is used for various state and federal reports:

- Name, address, Social Security number, rate of pay, withholding exemptions claimed, marital status, and special deductions (e.g., credit union account, bonds)
- The number of pay periods in a quarter and the date on which each pay period ends

Form **SS-4** (Rev. January 2010) Department of the Treasury Internal Revenue Service

Application for Employer Identification Number

(For use by employers, corporations, partnerships, trusts, estates, churches, government agencies, Indian tribal entities, certain individuals, and others.)

► See separate instructions for each line. ► Keep a copy for your records.

OMB No. 1545-0003

EIN

Type or print clearly.

1 Legal name of entity (or individual) for whom the EIN is being requested

2 Trade name of business (if different from name on line 1)
3 Executor, administrator, trustee, "care of" name

4a Mailing address (room, apt., suite no. and street, or P.O. box)
5a Street address (if different) (Do not enter a P.O. box.)

4b City, state, and ZIP code (if foreign, see instructions)
5b City, state, and ZIP code (if foreign, see instructions)

6 County and state where principal business is located

7a Name of responsible party
7b SSN, ITIN, or EIN

8a Is this application for a limited liability company (LLC) (or a foreign equivalent)? . . . . ☐ Yes ☐ No
8b If 8a is "Yes," enter the number of LLC members . . . . ►

8c If 8a is "Yes," was the LLC organized in the United States? . . . . ☐ Yes ☐ No

9a **Type of entity** (check only one box). **Caution.** If 8a is "Yes," see the instructions for the correct box to check.

☐ Sole proprietor (SSN)
☐ Partnership
☐ Corporation (enter form number to be filed) ►
☐ Personal service corporation
☐ Church or church-controlled organization
☐ Other nonprofit organization (specify) ►
☐ Other (specify) ►
☐ Estate (SSN of decedent)
☐ Plan administrator (TIN)
☐ Trust (TIN of grantor)
☐ National Guard ☐ State/local government
☐ Farmers' cooperative ☐ Federal government/military
☐ REMIC ☐ Indian tribal governments/enterprises
Group Exemption Number (GEN) if any ►

9b If a corporation, name the state or foreign country (if applicable) where incorporated | State | Foreign country

10 **Reason for applying** (check only one box)
☐ Started new business (specify type) ►
☐ Hired employees (Check the box and see line 13.)
☐ Compliance with IRS withholding regulations
☐ Other (specify) ►
☐ Banking purpose (specify purpose) ►
☐ Changed type of organization (specify new type) ►
☐ Purchased going business
☐ Created a trust (specify type) ►
☐ Created a pension plan (specify type) ►

11 Date business started or acquired (month, day, year). See instructions.
12 Closing month of accounting year

13 Highest number of employees expected in the next 12 months (enter -0- if none). If no employees expected, skip line 14.

Agricultural	Household	Other

14 If you expect your employment tax liability to be $1,000 or less in a full calendar year **and** want to file Form 944 annually instead of Forms 941 quarterly, check here. (Your employment tax liability generally will be $1,000 or less if you expect to pay $4,000 or less in total wages.) If you do not check this box, you must file Form 941 for every quarter. ☐

15 First date wages or annuities were paid (month, day, year). **Note.** If applicant is a withholding agent, enter date income will first be paid to nonresident alien (month, day, year) . . . . ►

16 Check **one** box that best describes the principal activity of your business. ☐ Health care & social assistance ☐ Wholesale-agent/broker
☐ Construction ☐ Rental & leasing ☐ Transportation & warehousing ☐ Accommodation & food service ☐ Wholesale-other ☐ Retail
☐ Real estate ☐ Manufacturing ☐ Finance & insurance ☐ Other (specify)

17 Indicate principal line of merchandise sold, specific construction work done, products produced, or services provided.

18 Has the applicant entity shown on line 1 ever applied for and received an EIN? ☐ Yes ☐ No
If "Yes," write previous EIN here ►

Third Party Designee
Complete this section **only** if you want to authorize the named individual to receive the entity's EIN and answer questions about the completion of this form.
Designee's name | Designee's telephone number (include area code) ( )
Address and ZIP code | Designee's fax number (include area code) ( )

Under penalties of perjury, I declare that I have examined this application, and to the best of my knowledge and belief, it is true, correct, and complete. | Applicant's telephone number (include area code) ( )
Name and title (type or print clearly) ► | Applicant's fax number (include area code) ( )
Signature ► Date ►

For Privacy Act and Paperwork Reduction Act Notice, see separate instructions. Cat. No. 16055N Form **SS-4** (Rev. 1-2010)

FIGURE 16-20 Application for Employer Identification Number (Form SS-4). (From Internal Revenue Service, Department of the Treasury, Washington, DC.)

Separate here and give Form W-4 to your employer. Keep the top part for your records.

Form **W-4**
Department of the Treasury
Internal Revenue Service

Employee's Withholding Allowance Certificate

▶ **Whether you are entitled to claim a certain number of allowances or exemption from withholding is subject to review by the IRS. Your employer may be required to send a copy of this form to the IRS.**

OMB No. 1545-0074
2014

1 Your first name and middle initial | Last name | 2 **Your social security number**

Home address (number and street or rural route) | 3 ☐ Single ☐ Married ☐ Married, but withhold at higher Single rate.
Note. If married, but legally separated, or spouse is a nonresident alien, check the "Single" box.

City or town, state, and ZIP code | 4 **If your last name differs from that shown on your social security card, check here. You must call 1-800-772-1213 for a replacement card.** ▶ ☐

5 Total number of allowances you are claiming (from line **H** above **or** from the applicable worksheet on page 2) 5
6 Additional amount, if any, you want withheld from each paycheck . . . . 6 $
7 I claim exemption from withholding for 2014, and I certify that I meet **both** of the following conditions for exemption.
• Last year I had a right to a refund of **all** federal income tax withheld because I had **no** tax liability, **and**
• This year I expect a refund of **all** federal income tax withheld because I expect to have **no** tax liability.
If you meet both conditions, write "Exempt" here . . . . ▶ 7

Under penalties of perjury, I declare that I have examined this certificate and, to the best of my knowledge and belief, it is true, correct, and complete.

Employee's signature
(This form is not valid unless you sign it.) ▶ **Date** ▶

8 Employer's name and address (Employer: Complete lines 8 and 10 only if sending to the IRS.) | 9 Office code (optional) | 10 Employer identification number (EIN)

For Privacy Act and Paperwork Reduction Act Notice, see page 2. Cat. No. 10220Q Form **W-4** (2014)

Form W-4 (2014) Page **2**

Deductions and Adjustments Worksheet

Note. Use this worksheet *only* if you plan to itemize deductions or claim certain credits or adjustments to income.

1 Enter an estimate of your 2014 itemized deductions. These include qualifying home mortgage interest, charitable contributions, state and local taxes, medical expenses in excess of 10% (7.5% if either you or your spouse was born before January 2, 1950) of your income, and miscellaneous deductions. For 2014, you may have to reduce your itemized deductions if your income is over $305,050 and you are married filing jointly or are a qualifying widow(er); $279,650 if you are head of household; $254,200 if you are single and not head of household or a qualifying widow(er); or $152,525 if you are married filing separately. See Pub. 505 for details . . . . 1 $

2 Enter: { $12,400 if married filing jointly or qualifying widow(er); $9,100 if head of household; $6,200 if single or married filing separately } . . . . 2 $

3 **Subtract** line 2 from line 1. If zero or less, enter "-0-" . . . . 3 $

4 Enter an estimate of your 2014 adjustments to income and any additional standard deduction (see Pub. 505) 4 $

5 **Add** lines 3 and 4 and enter the total. (Include any amount for credits from the *Converting Credits to Withholding Allowances for 2014 Form W-4* worksheet in Pub. 505.) . . . . 5 $

6 Enter an estimate of your 2014 nonwage income (such as dividends or interest) . . . . 6 $

7 **Subtract** line 6 from line 5. If zero or less, enter "-0-" . . . . 7 $

8 **Divide** the amount on line 7 by $3,950 and enter the result here. Drop any fraction 8

9 Enter the number from the **Personal Allowances Worksheet,** line H, page 1 9

10 **Add** lines 8 and 9 and enter the total here. If you plan to use the **Two-Earners/Multiple Jobs Worksheet,** also enter this total on line 1 below. Otherwise, **stop here** and enter this total on Form W-4, line 5, page 1 10

Two-Earners/Multiple Jobs Worksheet (See *Two earners or multiple jobs* on page 1.)

Note. Use this worksheet *only* if the instructions under line H on page 1 direct you here.

1 Enter the number from line H, page 1 (or from line 10 above if you used the **Deductions and Adjustments Worksheet**) 1

2 Find the number in **Table 1** below that applies to the **LOWEST** paying job and enter it here. **However,** if you are married filing jointly and wages from the highest paying job are $65,000 or less, do not enter more than "3" 2

3 If line 1 is **more than or equal to** line 2, subtract line 2 from line 1. Enter the result here (if zero, enter "-0-") and on Form W-4, line 5, page 1. **Do not** use the rest of this worksheet 3

Note. If line 1 is **less than** line 2, enter "-0-" on Form W-4, line 5, page 1. Complete lines 4 through 9 below to figure the additional withholding amount necessary to avoid a year-end tax bill.

4 Enter the number from line 2 of this worksheet 4

5 Enter the number from line 1 of this worksheet 5

6 **Subtract** line 5 from line 4 6

7 Find the amount in **Table 2** below that applies to the **HIGHEST** paying job and enter it here . . . . 7 $

8 **Multiply** line 7 by line 6 and enter the result here. This is the additional annual withholding needed . . 8 $

9 Divide line 8 by the number of pay periods remaining in 2014. For example, divide by 25 if you are paid every two weeks and you complete this form on a date in January when there are 25 pay periods remaining in 2014. Enter the result here and on Form W-4, line 6, page 1. This is the additional amount to be withheld from each paycheck 9 $

Table 1				Table 2			
Married Filing Jointly		All Others		Married Filing Jointly		All Others	
If wages from **LOWEST** paying job are—	Enter on line 2 above	If wages from **LOWEST** paying job are—	Enter on line 2 above	If wages from **HIGHEST** paying job are—	Enter on line 7 above	If wages from **HIGHEST** paying job are—	Enter on line 7 above
$0 - $6,000	0	$0 - $6,000	0	$0 - $74,000	$590	$0 - $37,000	$590
6,001 - 13,000	1	6,001 - 16,000	1	74,001 - 130,000	990	37,001 - 80,000	990
13,001 - 24,000	2	16,001 - 25,000	2	130,001 - 200,000	1,110	80,001 - 175,000	1,110
24,001 - 26,000	3	25,001 - 34,000	3	200,001 - 355,000	1,300	175,001 - 385,000	1,300
26,001 - 33,000	4	34,001 - 43,000	4	355,001 - 400,000	1,380	385,001 and over	1,560
33,001 - 43,000	5	43,001 - 70,000	5	400,001 and over	1,560		
43,001 - 49,000	6	70,001 - 85,000	6				
49,001 - 60,000	7	85,001 - 110,000	7				
60,001 - 75,000	8	110,001 - 125,000	8				
75,001 - 80,000	9	125,001 - 140,000	9				
80,001 - 100,000	10	140,001 and over	10				
100,001 - 115,000	11						
115,001 - 130,000	12						
130,001 - 140,000	13						
140,001 - 150,000	14						
150,001 and over	15						

Privacy Act and Paperwork Reduction Act Notice. We ask for the information on this form to carry out the Internal Revenue laws of the United States. Internal Revenue Code sections 3402(f)(2) and 6109 and their regulations require you to provide this information; your employer uses it to determine your federal income tax withholding. Failure to provide a properly completed form will result in your being treated as a single person who claims no withholding allowances; providing fraudulent information may subject you to penalties. Routine uses of this information include giving it to the Department of Justice for civil and criminal litigation; to cities, states, the District of Columbia, and U.S. commonwealths and possessions for use in administering their tax laws; and to the Department of Health and Human Services for use in the National Directory of New Hires. We may also disclose this information to other countries under a tax treaty, to federal and state agencies to enforce federal nontax criminal laws, or to federal law enforcement and intelligence agencies to combat terrorism.

You are not required to provide the information requested on a form that is subject to the Paperwork Reduction Act unless the form displays a valid OMB control number. Books or records relating to a form or its instructions must be retained as long as their contents may become material in the administration of any Internal Revenue law. Generally, tax returns and return information are confidential, as required by Code section 6103.

The average time and expenses required to complete and file this form will vary depending on individual circumstances. For estimated averages, see the instructions for your income tax return.

If you have suggestions for making this form simpler, we would be happy to hear from you. See the instructions for your income tax return.

FIGURE 16-21 Employee's Withholding Allowance Certificate (Form W-4). (From Internal Revenue Service, Department of the Treasury, Washington, DC.)

EMPLOYEE'S EARNINGS RECORD

Exemptions ______ Name ______
Date of Birth ______ Address ______
Date Employed ______
Phone ______ Soc. Sec. No. ______
In Emergency Notify ______

REMARKS	DATE	CHECK NO.	GROSS SALARY	FEDERAL W.H. TAX	F.I.C.A.	STATE W.H. TAX	OTHER	OTHER	NET CHECK
THIRD QUARTER									
FOURTH QUARTER									
YEAR'S TOTALS									

FIGURE 16-22 Employee's earnings record.

- Columns for regular earnings, overtime earnings, and total earnings

Earnings records are available that provide columns for the rate of pay and the hours or days worked during a specific pay period.

- A column for each deduction and for the total deductions
- A column for entering the net amount (net pay) received

Net pay is the difference between total earnings and deductions.

- A column for recording accumulated taxable earnings

This column provides the employer with information for taxable earnings, Federal Insurance Contributions Act (FICA) deductions (see the next section), and taxable wages for unemployment taxes.

- Columns for quarterly and annual totals

Determining Employee Wages

The dentist and the employee must reach an agreement regarding an acceptable wage. This may be determined as an hourly rate, a weekly rate, or a monthly amount. After this rate has been established, the procedure must be decided for determining the employee's **net pay**. The administrative assistant is often responsible for figuring the payroll and preparing the checks for the dentist's signature, as follows:

PRACTICE NOTE

The dentist and the employee must reach an agreement regarding an acceptable wage.

1. The administrative assistant's hourly wage is $32 per hour.

2. If the work week is based on 36 hours per week, the gross wages (i.e., the amount earned before deductions) are $1152 (36 hours × $32 per hour = $1152).
3. Deductions are made from the wages as follows:
   a. *FICA deduction (Social Security and Medicare taxes):* The amount to be withheld is determined by calculating at the combined 2014 rate (7.65% [or 0.0765] × $ = $88.13). This tax rate is divided into two parts: (1) the Social Security part, which is 6.2% on the first $117,000 earned in 2014; and (2) the Medicare part, which is 1.45% on all earnings, with no ceiling. These tax rates are subject to change by Congress. The employer must keep track of such changes and make deductions according to the current rate. *Publication 15 (Circular E), Employer's Tax Guide,* which is available from the IRS, can be used to check the current tax rates.
   b. ***Withholding** (income tax deductions):* The amount withheld depends on the number of exemptions indicated on Form W-4. The tax amount withheld is determined from a table in *Publication 15 (Circular E), Employer's Tax Guide.* According to the table shown in Figure 16-23, the withholding tax on $1152 for a single person claiming one exemption is $178.
   c. *Local income tax:* Some cities and states have personal income taxes that must be deducted. Again, the employer must be familiar with the state and local laws regarding these taxes.
   d. *Other deductions:* In addition to the standard deductions, the administrative assistant may have a weekly deduction of $60 for the credit union. (This is noted on the earnings record.)
4. The net pay (take-home pay)—and the amount for which the paycheck is written—is $824.88. The check is generated by financial software (e.g., QuickBooks), as shown in Figure 16-24.

Gross Wages	Minus Deductions	Deductions Total	Net Pay
$1152	FICA: $71.42 Medicare: $16.70 Withholding tax: $179 Credit union: $60	$327.12	$824.88

The net pay for each member of the office staff must be calculated. After the amounts have been determined, the paychecks are written, the information is entered on each employee's earnings record, and a record is made on the expense sheet.

SINGLE Persons—**WEEKLY** Payroll Period
(For Wages Paid Through December 2014)

If the wages are–		And the number of withholding allowances claimed is—										
At least	But less than	0	1	2	3	4	5	6	7	8	9	10
		The amount of income tax to be withheld is—										
$780	$790	$103	$85	$73	$62	$52	$41	$31	$20	$10	$2	$0
790	800	105	88	74	64	53	43	32	22	11	3	0
800	810	108	90	76	65	55	44	34	23	13	4	0
810	820	110	93	77	67	56	46	35	25	14	5	0
820	830	113	95	79	68	58	47	37	26	16	6	0
830	840	115	98	80	70	59	49	38	28	17	7	0
840	850	118	100	83	71	61	50	40	29	19	8	1
850	860	120	103	85	73	62	52	41	31	20	10	2
860	870	123	105	88	74	64	53	43	32	22	11	3
870	880	125	108	90	76	65	55	44	34	23	13	4
880	890	128	110	93	77	67	56	46	35	25	14	5
890	900	130	113	95	79	68	58	47	37	26	16	6
900	910	133	115	98	80	70	59	49	38	28	17	7
910	920	135	118	100	83	71	61	50	40	29	19	8
920	930	138	120	103	85	73	62	52	41	31	20	10
930	940	140	123	105	88	74	64	53	43	32	22	11
940	950	143	125	108	90	76	65	55	44	34	23	13
950	960	145	128	110	93	77	67	56	46	35	25	14
960	970	148	130	113	95	79	68	58	47	37	26	16
970	980	150	133	115	98	80	70	59	49	38	28	17
980	990	153	135	118	100	83	71	61	50	40	29	19
990	1,000	155	138	120	103	85	73	62	52	41	31	20
1,000	1,010	158	140	123	105	88	74	64	53	43	32	22
1,010	1,020	160	143	125	108	90	76	65	55	44	34	23
1,020	1,030	163	145	128	110	93	77	67	56	46	35	25
1,030	1,040	165	148	130	113	95	79	68	58	47	37	26
1,040	1,050	168	150	133	115	98	80	70	59	49	38	28
1,050	1,060	170	153	135	118	100	83	71	61	50	40	29
1,060	1,070	173	155	138	120	103	85	73	62	52	41	31
1,070	1,080	175	158	140	123	105	88	74	64	53	43	32
1,080	1,090	178	160	143	125	108	90	76	65	55	44	34
1,090	1,100	180	163	145	128	110	93	77	67	56	46	35
1,100	1,110	183	165	148	130	113	95	79	68	58	47	37
1,110	1,120	185	168	150	133	115	98	80	70	59	49	38
1,120	1,130	188	170	153	135	118	100	83	71	61	50	40
1,130	1,140	190	173	155	138	120	103	85	73	62	52	41
1,140	1,150	193	175	158	140	123	105	88	74	64	53	43
1,150	1,160	195	178	160	143	125	108	90	76	65	55	44
1,160	1,170	198	180	163	145	128	110	93	77	67	56	46
1,170	1,180	200	183	165	148	130	113	95	79	68	58	47
1,180	1,190	203	185	168	150	133	115	98	80	70	59	49
1,190	1,200	205	188	170	153	135	118	100	82	71	61	50
1,200	1,210	208	190	173	155	138	120	103	85	73	62	52
1,210	1,220	210	193	175	158	140	123	105	87	74	64	53
1,220	1,230	213	195	178	160	143	125	108	90	76	65	55
1,230	1,240	215	198	180	163	145	128	110	92	77	67	56
1,240	1,250	218	200	183	165	148	130	113	95	79	68	58
$1,250 and over		Use Table 1(a) for a **SINGLE person** on page 5. Also see the instructions on page 3.										

FIGURE 16-23 Tax withholding table. (From Internal Revenue Service, Department of the Treasury, Washington, DC.)

TO VERIFY AUTHENTICITY, SEE REVERSE SIDE FOR DESCRIPTION OF THE 11 SECURITY FEATURES

2506

Dental Associates, PC
611 Main Street SE
Grand Rapids, MI 49502

Your Hometown Bank

Date 6/16/20__

Pay To The Order Of Jennifer M Ellis $ **782.13

Seven Hundred Eighty-Two and 13/100***

Jennifer M Ellis

Memo: Signature

Pay Period: 05/25/20__ - 05/31/20__

⑈0002506⑈ ⑆067008792⑆ 207502396561 3⑈

2506

Employee					SSN	Status (Fed/State)	Allowances/Extra
Jennifer M Ellis					***-**-6789	Single	Fed-1/0
					Pay Period: 05/25/20__ - 05/31/20__		Pay Date: 06/16/20__

Earnings and Hours	Hours	Rate	Current	YTD Amount
Hourly Rate	36:00	29.00	1,044.00	1,044.00

Taxes	Current	YTD Amount
Medicare Employee Addl Tax	0.00	
Federal Withholding	-152.00	-152.00
Social Security Employee	-64.73	-64.73
Medicare Employee	-15.14	-15.14
	-231.87	-231.87

Adjustments to Net Pay	Current	YTD Amount
Credit Union Deduction	-30.00	-30.00
Net Pay	782.13	782.13

Dental Associates, PC, 611 Main Street SE, Grand Rapids, MI 49502

2506

Employee					SSN	Status (Fed/State)	Allowances/Extra
Jennifer M Ellis					***-**-6789	Single	Fed-1/0
					Pay Period: 05/25/20__ - 05/31/20__		Pay Date: 06/16/20__

Earnings and Hours	Hours	Rate	Current	YTD Amount
Hourly Rate	36:00	29.00	1,044.00	1,044.00

Taxes	Current	YTD Amount
Medicare Employee Addl Tax	0.00	
Federal Withholding	-152.00	-152.00
Social Security Employee	-64.73	-64.73
Medicare Employee	-15.14	-15.14
	-231.87	-231.87

Adjustments to Net Pay	Current	YTD Amount
Credit Union Deduction	-30.00	-30.00
Net Pay	782.13	782.13

Dental Associates, PC, 611 Main Street SE, Grand Rapids, MI 49502

FIGURE 16-24 QuickBooks-generated payroll check for a single person claiming one withholding allowance. (Software © Intuit, Inc. All rights reserved.)

Electronically Depositing Withheld Income Tax and Social Security Taxes

You must deposit employment taxes, including Form 94X taxes, via electronic funds transfer.

Electronic Deposit Requirement

You must use electronic funds transfer to make all federal tax deposits (e.g., employment tax, excise tax, corporate income tax). Generally, electronic fund transfers are made using the Electronic Federal Tax Payment System (EFTPS). If you do not want to use EFTPS, you can arrange for your tax professional, financial institution, payroll service, or other trusted third party to make electronic deposits on your behalf. EFTPS is a free service provided by the Department of the Treasury. To get more information or to enroll in EFTPS, call 1-800-555-4477 or 1-800-733-4829 (TDD). You can also visit the EFTPS website at www.eftps.gov. Additional information about EFTPS is also available in Publication 966.

Generally the employer must deposit withheld income tax, Social Security, and Medicare taxes in an authorized commercial bank or a Federal Reserve Bank. Electronic coupon forms used for depositing taxes are created online at the EFTPS website using Form 941 (Figure 16-25).

The amount of taxes determines the frequency of deposits. These taxes are owed when the employer pays the wages (or makes the payments from which the taxes are withheld) rather than when the payroll period ends. To determine when the taxes are due and the amount on which they are based, the administrative assistant should check the instructions in *Publication 15 (Circular E), Employer's Tax Guide*, which is available at www.irs.gov.

There are two deposit schedules—monthly and semiweekly—for determining when to deposit Social Security, Medicare, and withheld income taxes. These schedules tell employers when a deposit is due after a tax liability arises (e.g., when there is a payday). Before the beginning of each calendar year, it must be

▼ Detach Here and Mail With Your Payment and Form 941. ▼

Form **941-V**
Department of the Treasury
Internal Revenue Service

Payment Voucher

▶ Do not staple this voucher or your payment to Form 941.

OMB No. 1545-0029
2014

1 Enter your employer identification number (EIN).	2 **Enter the amount of your payment.** ▶ Make your check or money order payable to "United States Treasury"	Dollars	Cents
3 Tax Period	4 Enter your business name (individual name if sole proprietor).		
○ 1st Quarter ○ 3rd Quarter	Enter your address.		
○ 2nd Quarter ○ 4th Quarter	Enter your city, state, and ZIP code or your city, foreign country name, foreign province/county, and foreign postal code.		

Form **941 for 2014: Employer's QUARTERLY Federal Tax Return** 950114
(Rev. January 2014) Department of the Treasury — Internal Revenue Service OMB No. 1545-0029

Employer identification number (EIN) ☐☐ – ☐☐☐☐☐☐☐

Name *(not your trade name)*

Trade name *(if any)*

Address
Number Street Suite or room number
City State ZIP code
Foreign country name Foreign province/county Foreign postal code

Report for this Quarter of 2014
(Check one.)
☐ **1:** January, February, March
☐ **2:** April, May, June
☐ **3:** July, August, September
☐ **4:** October, November, December
Instructions and prior year forms are available at *www.irs.gov/form941.*

Read the separate instructions before you complete Form 941. Type or print within the boxes.

Part 1: **Answer these questions for this quarter.**

1	**Number of employees who received wages, tips, or other compensation for the pay period including:** *Mar. 12* (Quarter 1), *June 12* (Quarter 2), *Sept. 12* (Quarter 3), or *Dec. 12* (Quarter 4)			1	
2	**Wages, tips, and other compensation**			2	.
3	**Federal income tax withheld from wages, tips, and other compensation**			3	.
4	**If no wages, tips, and other compensation are subject to social security or Medicare tax**				☐ Check and go to line 6.
		Column 1	**Column 2**		
5a	**Taxable social security wages**	.	× .124 = .		
5b	**Taxable social security tips**	.	× .124 = .		
5c	**Taxable Medicare wages & tips.**	.	× .029 = .		
5d	**Taxable wages & tips subject to Additional Medicare Tax withholding**	.	× .009 = .		
5e	**Add Column 2 from lines 5a, 5b, 5c, and 5d**			5e	.
5f	**Section 3121(q) Notice and Demand—Tax due on unreported tips** (see instructions)			5f	.
6	**Total taxes before adjustments.** Add lines 3, 5e, and 5f			6	.
7	**Current quarter's adjustment for fractions of cents**			7	.
8	**Current quarter's adjustment for sick pay**			8	.
9	**Current quarter's adjustments for tips and group-term life insurance**			9	.
10	**Total taxes after adjustments.** Combine lines 6 through 9			10	.
11	**Total deposits for this quarter, including overpayment applied from a prior quarter and overpayments applied from Form 941-X, 941-X (PR), 944-X, 944-X (PR), or 944-X (SP) filed in the current quarter**			11	.
12	**Balance due.** If line 10 is more than line 11, enter the difference and see instructions			12	.
13	**Overpayment.** If line 11 is more than line 10, enter the difference	.	Check one: ☐ Apply to next return. ☐ Send a refund.		

▶ **You MUST complete both pages of Form 941 and SIGN it.** **Next ▶**

For Privacy Act and Paperwork Reduction Act Notice, see the back of the Payment Voucher. Cat. No. 17001Z Form **941** (Rev. 1-2014)

FIGURE 16-25 Employer's Payment Voucher (Form 941-V) and Quarterly Federal Tax Return (Form 941). (From Internal Revenue Service, Department of the Treasury, Washington, DC.)

determined which of the two deposit schedules is required. The deposit schedule used is based on the total tax liability reported on Form 941 during a lookback period, which is discussed in the next section. The deposit schedule is not determined by how often the employees are paid or when deposits are made.

Lookback Period

If the employer is a Form 941 filer, the deposit schedule for a calendar year is determined from the total taxes reported on Form 941, line 10, for a four-quarter lookback period. The lookback period begins July 1 and ends June 30, as shown in the table below. If the employer reported $50,000 or less in taxes for the lookback period, he or she is a monthly schedule

Lookback Period for Calendar Year 2014			
July 1, 2012, through Sept. 30, 2012	Oct. 1, 2012, through Dec. 31, 2012	Jan. 1, 2013, through Mar. 31, 2013	Apr. 1, 2013, through June 30, 2013

950214

Name (not your trade name) | Employer identification number (EIN)

Part 2: Tell us about your deposit schedule and tax liability for this quarter.

If you are unsure about whether you are a monthly schedule depositor or a semiweekly schedule depositor, see Pub. 15 (Circular E), section 11.

14 Check one: ☐ **Line 10 on this return is less than $2,500 or line 10 on the return for the prior quarter was less than $2,500, and you did not incur a $100,000 next-day deposit obligation during the current quarter.** If line 10 for the prior quarter was less than $2,500 but line 10 on this return is $100,000 or more, you must provide a record of your federal tax liability. If you are a monthly schedule depositor, complete the deposit schedule below; if you are a semiweekly schedule depositor, attach Schedule B (Form 941). Go to Part 3.

☐ **You were a monthly schedule depositor for the entire quarter.** Enter your tax liability for each month and total liability for the quarter, then go to Part 3.

Tax liability: Month 1 ______ .

Month 2 ______ .

Month 3 ______ .

Total liability for quarter ______ . **Total must equal line 10.**

☐ **You were a semiweekly schedule depositor for any part of this quarter.** Complete Schedule B (Form 941), Report of Tax Liability for Semiweekly Schedule Depositors, and attach it to Form 941.

Part 3: Tell us about your business. If a question does NOT apply to your business, leave it blank.

15 **If your business has closed or you stopped paying wages** . . . . . ☐ Check here, and

enter the final date you paid wages ___ / ___ / ___ .

16 **If you are a seasonal employer and you do not have to file a return for every quarter of the year** . . ☐ Check here.

Part 4: May we speak with your third-party designee?

Do you want to allow an employee, a paid tax preparer, or another person to discuss this return with the IRS? See the instructions for details.

☐ Yes. Designee's name and phone number ______ ______

Select a 5-digit Personal Identification Number (PIN) to use when talking to the IRS. ☐☐☐☐☐

☐ No.

Part 5: Sign here. You MUST complete both pages of Form 941 and SIGN it.

Under penalties of perjury, I declare that I have examined this return, including accompanying schedules and statements, and to the best of my knowledge and belief, it is true, correct, and complete. Declaration of preparer (other than taxpayer) is based on all information of which preparer has any knowledge.

✗ **Sign your name here** ______ Print your name here ______ Print your title here ______

Date ___ / ___ / ___ Best daytime phone ______

Paid Preparer Use Only Check if you are self-employed . . . ☐

Preparer's name ______ PTIN ______

Preparer's signature ______ Date ___ / ___ / ___

Firm's name (or yours if self-employed) ______ EIN ______

Address ______ Phone ______

City ______ State ______ ZIP code ______

Page **2** Form **941** (Rev. 1-2014)

FIGURE 16-25, cont'd

depositor; if he or she reported more than $50,000, then he or she is a semiweekly schedule depositor.

Federal Unemployment Tax

The employer is subject to a federal unemployment tax under the provisions of the Federal Unemployment Tax Act (FUTA). This tax is 6% of the wages paid, and it applies to the first $7000 of wages paid during the calendar year. Generally a credit may be taken against the federal unemployment tax for contributions to be paid into state unemployment funds. The federal unemployment tax is imposed on employers and must not be deducted from employees' wages. On or before January 31, the employer must file an unemployment tax return (Employers' Annual Federal Unemployment [FUTA] Tax Return [Form 940]) (Figure 16-26) and deposit or pay the balance of the tax in full. For deposit purposes, the employer must compute the federal unemployment tax on a quarterly basis. The deposit must be made on or before the last day of the first month after the close of the quarter.

When to Deposit FUTA Taxes

Quarter	Ending	Due Date
Jan.-Feb.-Mar.	Mar. 31	Apr. 30
Apr.-May-June	June 30	July 31
July-Aug.-Sept.	Sept. 30	Oct. 31
Oct.-Nov.-Dec.	Dec. 31	Jan. 31

To determine whether the employer must make a deposit for any of the first three quarters in a year, compute the total tax as follows:

1. Multiply the first $7000 of each employee's annual wages paid during the quarter by 0.006.
2. If the amount subject to deposit (plus the amount subject to deposit but not deposited for any prior quarter) is more than $100, a deposit should be made during the first month after the quarter ends.

▼ Detach Here and Mail With Your Payment and Form 940. ▼

Form **940-V** Department of the Treasury Internal Revenue Service

Payment Voucher

► Do not staple or attach this voucher to your payment.

OMB No. 1545-0028 **2013**

1 Enter your employer identification number (EIN).

2 **Enter the amount of your payment. ►** Make your check or money order payable to "United States Treasury" | Dollars | Cents

3 Enter your business name (individual name if sole proprietor).

Enter your address.

Enter your city, state, and ZIP code or your city, foreign country name, foreign province/county, and foreign postal code.

Form **940 for 2013: Employer's Annual Federal Unemployment (FUTA) Tax Return** 850113

Department of the Treasury — Internal Revenue Service OMB No. 1545-0028

Employer identification number (EIN)

Name (not your trade name)

Trade name (if any)

Address Number Street Suite or room number

City State ZIP code

Foreign country name Foreign province/county Foreign postal code

Type of Return (Check all that apply.)
- a. Amended
- b. Successor employer
- c. No payments to employees in 2013
- d. Final: Business closed or stopped paying wages

Instructions and prior-year forms are available at *www.irs.gov/form940.*

Read the separate instructions before you complete this form. Please type or print within the boxes.

Part 1: Tell us about your return. If any line does NOT apply, leave it blank.

1a **If you had to pay state unemployment tax in one state only, enter the state abbreviation** . 1a

1b **If you had to pay state unemployment tax in more than one state, you are a multi-state employer** . . . . 1b Check here. Complete Schedule A (Form 940).

2 **If you paid wages in a state that is subject to CREDIT REDUCTION** . . . . 2 Check here. Complete Schedule A (Form 940).

Part 2: Determine your FUTA tax before adjustments for 2013. If any line does NOT apply, leave it blank.

3 **Total payments to all employees** 3

4 **Payments exempt from FUTA tax** 4

Check all that apply: 4a Fringe benefits 4b Group-term life insurance 4c Retirement/Pension 4d Dependent care 4e Other

5 **Total of payments made to each employee in excess of $7,000** 5

6 **Subtotal** (line 4 + line 5 = line 6) 6

7 **Total taxable FUTA wages** (line 3 – line 6 = line 7) (see instructions) 7

8 **FUTA tax before adjustments** (line 7 x .006 = line 8) 8

Part 3: Determine your adjustments. If any line does NOT apply, leave it blank.

9 **If ALL of the taxable FUTA wages you paid were excluded from state unemployment tax, multiply line 7 by .054** (line 7 × .054 = line 9). Go to line 12 9

10 **If SOME of the taxable FUTA wages you paid were excluded from state unemployment tax, OR you paid ANY state unemployment tax late** (after the due date for filing Form 940), complete the worksheet in the instructions. Enter the amount from line 7 of the worksheet . . 10

11 **If credit reduction applies,** enter the total from Schedule A (Form 940) 11

Part 4: Determine your FUTA tax and balance due or overpayment for 2013. If any line does NOT apply, leave it blank.

12 **Total FUTA tax after adjustments** (lines 8 + 9 + 10 + 11 = line 12) 12

13 **FUTA tax deposited for the year, including any overpayment applied from a prior year** . 13

14 **Balance due** (If line 12 is more than line 13, enter the excess on line 14.)
- If line 14 is more than $500, you must deposit your tax.
- If line 14 is $500 or less, you may pay with this return. (see instructions) 14

15 **Overpayment** (If line 13 is more than line 12, enter the excess on line 15 and check a box below.) 15

► You **MUST** complete both pages of this form and **SIGN** it. Check one: Apply to next return. Send a refund.

Next ►

For Privacy Act and Paperwork Reduction Act Notice, see the back of Form 940-V, Payment Voucher. Cat. No. 11234O Form **940** (2013)

FIGURE 16-26 Employer's Payment Voucher (Form 940-V) and Annual Federal Unemployment (FUTA) Tax Return (Form 940). (From Internal Revenue Service, Department of the Treasury, Washington, DC.)

Wage and Tax Statement (Form W-2)

A federal Wage and Tax Statement (Form W-2) for a calendar year must be provided for each employee no later than January 31 of the following year (Figure 16-27). The W-2 form is prepared in six parts and distributed in the following manner: one copy for IRS use; one copy to state, city, or local tax departments; three copies to the employee (one for filing federal tax returns, one for state or local tax purposes, and one for the employee's files); and one copy retained by the employer.

Form W-2 includes the following information:

- Employer's identification number, name, and address
- Employee's Social Security number, name, and address
- Federal income tax withheld

850212

Name (not your trade name) | Employer identification number (EIN)

Part 5: **Report your FUTA tax liability by quarter only if line 12 is more than $500. If not, go to Part 6.**

16 **Report the amount of your FUTA tax liability for each quarter; do NOT enter the amount you deposited. If you had no liability for a quarter, leave the line blank.**

16a **1st quarter** (January 1 – March 31) . . . . 16a .

16b **2nd quarter** (April 1 – June 30) . . . . 16b .

16c **3rd quarter** (July 1 – September 30) . . . . 16c .

16d **4th quarter** (October 1 – December 31) . . . . 16d .

17 **Total tax liability for the year** (lines 16a + 16b + 16c + 16d = line 17) 17 . **Total must equal line 12.**

Part 6: **May we speak with your third-party designee?**

Do you want to allow an employee, a paid tax preparer, or another person to discuss this return with the IRS? See the instructions for details.

☐ **Yes.** Designee's name and phone number

Select a 5-digit Personal Identification Number (PIN) to use when talking to IRS

☐ **No.**

Part 7: **Sign here. You MUST complete both pages of this form and SIGN it.**

Under penalties of perjury, I declare that I have examined this return, including accompanying schedules and statements, and to the best of my knowledge and belief, it is true, correct, and complete, and that no part of any payment made to a state unemployment fund claimed as a credit was, or is to be, deducted from the payments made to employees. Declaration of preparer (other than taxpayer) is based on all information of which preparer has any knowledge.

✗ **Sign your name here**

Print your name here

Print your title here

Date / /

Best daytime phone

Paid Preparer Use Only

Check if you are self-employed . ☐

Preparer's name | PTIN

Preparer's signature | Date / /

Firm's name (or yours if self-employed) | EIN

Address | Phone

City | State | ZIP code

Page **2** | Form **940** (2013)

FIGURE 16-26, cont'd

22222 | a Employee's social security number | OMB No. 1545-0008

b Employer identification number (EIN) | 1 Wages, tips, other compensation | 2 Federal income tax withheld

c Employer's name, address, and ZIP code | 3 Social security wages | 4 Social security tax withheld

5 Medicare wages and tips | 6 Medicare tax withheld

7 Social security tips | 8 Allocated tips

d Control number | 9 | 10 Dependent care benefits

e Employee's first name and initial | Last name | Suff. | 11 Nonqualified plans | 12a Code

13 Statutory employee ☐ | Retirement plan ☐ | Third-party sick pay ☐ | 12b Code

14 Other | 12c Code

12d Code

f Employee's address and ZIP code

15 State | Employer's state ID number | 16 State wages, tips, etc. | 17 State income tax | 18 Local wages, tips, etc. | 19 Local income tax | 20 Locality name

Form **W-2** **Wage and Tax Statement** 2014 | Department of the Treasury—Internal Revenue Service

Copy 1—For State, City, or Local Tax Department

FIGURE 16-27 Wage and Tax Statement (Form W-2). (From Internal Revenue Service, Department of the Treasury, Washington, DC.)

- Total sum of wages paid to the employee
- Total FICA employee tax withheld (Social Security and Medicare)
- Total wages paid that are subject to FICA
- State and local taxes withheld, when applicable

To correct a W-2 form after one has been issued to an employee, a corrected statement must be issued. The corrected statement must completely replace the original statement and be clearly marked as "CORRECTED RETURN" in capital letters directly above the title, "Wage and Tax Statement." If a W-2 form is lost or destroyed, the substitute copy issued to the employee is marked as "Reissued Return."

Report of Withheld Income Tax (Form W-3)

On or before February 28 of the current year, copy A of all W-2 forms issued for the previous year and Form W-3, Transmittal of Wage and Tax Statements (Figure 16-28), must be sent to the IRS.

Retention of Payroll and Tax Records

The employer must keep all records that pertain to employment taxes available for inspection by the IRS. Although no form has been devised for such records, the employer must be able to supply the following information:

- Amounts and dates of all wages paid
- Names, addresses, and occupations of employees
- Periods of employees' employment
- Periods for which employees were paid while absent because of sickness
- Employees' Social Security numbers
- Employees' income tax withholding allowance certificates
- Employer's identification number
- Duplicate copies of returns filed and the dates and amounts of deposits made

PRACTICE NOTE

The employer must keep all records that pertain to employment taxes available for inspection by the IRS.

These tax records should be kept for at least 4 years after the date on which the taxes to which they apply become due.

Employer's Responsibility for Tax Information

Publication 15 (Circular E), Employer's Tax Guide, which was mentioned previously, summarizes the employer's responsibilities for withholding, depositing, paying, and reporting federal income taxes, Social Security taxes, and federal unemployment taxes. The circular is available to all employers, and it may be obtained from a local IRS office. Because tax rates increase so often, the administrative assistant would be wise to check with the IRS to make sure that the most up-to-date forms and percentages are used for tax calculations. A document entitled Quick and Easy Access to IRS Tax Products and Tax Help is shown in Figure 16-29. Additional information and help are available at the American Payroll Association website, www.americanpayroll.org.

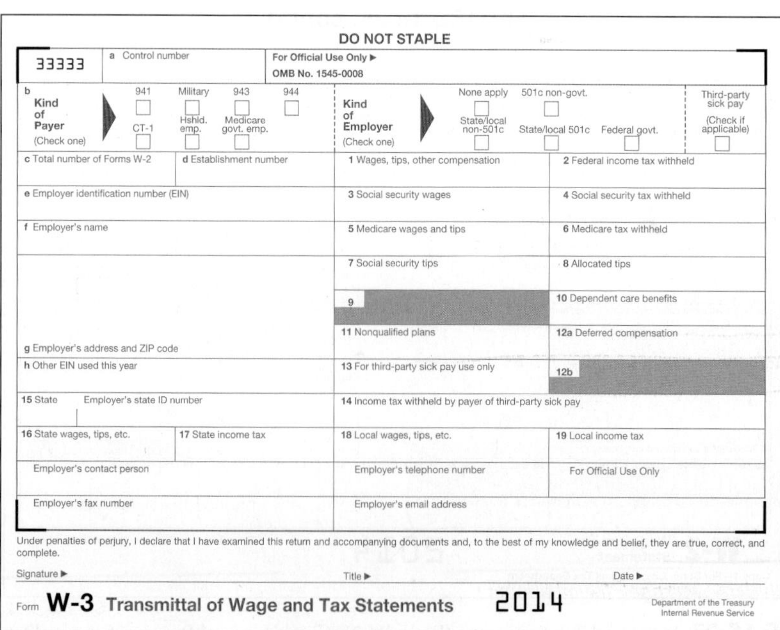

DO NOT STAPLE

33333 | a Control number | For Official Use Only ► OMB No. 1545-0008

b Kind of Payer (Check one): 941, Military, 943, 944, CT-1, Hshld. emp., Medicare govt. emp.

Kind of Employer (Check one): None apply, 501c non-govt., State/local non-501c, State/local 501c, Federal govt.

Third-party sick pay (Check if applicable)

c Total number of Forms W-2	d Establishment number
1 Wages, tips, other compensation	2 Federal income tax withheld
e Employer identification number (EIN)	
3 Social security wages	4 Social security tax withheld
f Employer's name	
5 Medicare wages and tips	6 Medicare tax withheld
7 Social security tips	8 Allocated tips
9	10 Dependent care benefits
11 Nonqualified plans	12a Deferred compensation
g Employer's address and ZIP code	
h Other EIN used this year	
13 For third-party sick pay use only	12b
15 State	Employer's state ID number
14 Income tax withheld by payer of third-party sick pay	
16 State wages, tips, etc.	17 State income tax
18 Local wages, tips, etc.	19 Local income tax
Employer's contact person	Employer's telephone number
For Official Use Only	
Employer's fax number	Employer's email address

Under penalties of perjury, I declare that I have examined this return and accompanying documents and, to the best of my knowledge and belief, they are true, correct, and complete.

Signature ► Title ► Date ►

Form **W-3** Transmittal of Wage and Tax Statements 2014 Department of the Treasury Internal Revenue Service

FIGURE 16-28 Transmittal of Wage and Tax Statements (Form W-3). *NOTE:* This form is provided for informational purposes only. Employers should not file this red copy (downloaded from www.irs.gov) but should instead call and order an official form from 1-800-TAX-FORM (1-800-829-3676). (From Internal Revenue Service, Department of the Treasury, Washington, DC.)

Quick and Easy Access to IRS Tax Products and Tax Help

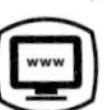

Internet

The Internet is the quickest way to access and obtain current and prior year IRS tax products. Visit *www.irs.gov/Forms-&-Pubs* for available tax products.

View & Download Products

Visit the IRS website at www.irs.gov and select Forms and Pubs, or simply type www.irs.gov/Forms-&-Pubs in your Internet search window to view or download Current and Prior Year Tax Products, and Accessible Forms & Pubs.

Online Ordering of Products

To order Tax Products delivered by mail, go to www.irs.gov/Forms-&-Pubs, then select "Order Forms & Pubs"

- For current year products, select "Forms and Publications by Mail"
- For Employer Products (e.g. W-4, Pub. 15) and Information Returns (e.g. W-2, W-3, 1099 series), select "Employer and Information Returns"

Online Tools & Services

Access the IRS website 24 hours a day, 7 days a week at www.irs.gov to obtain information on:

- **Free File:** Prepare and file your federal income taxes online—it's easy and it's free!
- **Order a Return or Account Transcript:** Order A Tax Return or Account Transcript Application
- **Where's My Refund:** Your refund status anytime from anywhere
- **Where's My Amended Return?** Track the status of your amended return after it has been filed.
- **Online Payment Agreement (OPA) Application:** Online agreements
- **Electronic Federal Tax Payment System:** Pay your federal taxes on-line or by phone through EFTPS, a free tax payment system.
- **IRS Withholding Calculator:** Estimate the amount that should be withheld from your paycheck for federal income tax purposes.

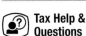

Tax Help & Questions

Individuals: 1-800-829-1040

Business & Specialty Tax: 1-800-829-4933

Deaf/Hard of Hearing/Speech Disability TDD/TTY: 1-800-829-4059

TeleTax 24 hour tax Information: 1-800-829-4477

See instructions 1040, 1040A, or 1040EZ for topic numbers and details.

Refund Hotline: 1-800-829-1954

National Taxpayer Advocate Helpline: 1-877-777-4778

Federal Relay Service: Deaf and hard of hearing individuals may also obtain access through relay services such as the Federal Relay Service at www.gsa.gov/fedrelay.

IRS

Publication 2053-A (Rev. 01-2014) Catalog Number 23267Z
Department of the Treasury **Internal Revenue Service** www.irs.gov

Other Ways to Obtain IRS Tax Products

Community Locations

You can pick up or photocopy some of the most requested forms, instructions, and publications at many IRS offices, libraries, post offices, and some state and local government offices.

Some locations include tax product availability information on their websites.

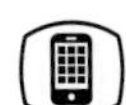

Telephone

Tax Forms & Publications

1-800-829-3676

Call to order current and prior year forms, instructions, and publications.

Mail

Do not send your tax return or payments to the address shown here. Instead, see the tax form instructions.

Send written request to:
Internal Revenue Service
1201 N. Mitsubishi Motorway
Bloomington, IL 61705-6613

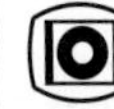

IRS Social Media

Connect with the IRS

The IRS uses social media tools to share the latest information on tax changes, initiatives, products and services:

IRS2Go

Download the free IRS2Go Mobile App.

YouTube

Tune in to the IRS YouTube channels. Watch short, informative videos in English, American Sign Language and other languages.

Twitter

IRS tweets include various tax-related announcements and news.

Tumblr

The IRS Tumblr blog provides current tax information.

FIGURE 16-29 Quick and Easy Access to IRS Tax Products and Tax Help. (From Internal Revenue Service, Department of the Treasury, Washington, DC.)

LEARNING ACTIVITIES

1. Name and define the parts of a check.
2. List the necessary steps for writing a check.
3. Explain how a certified check and a cashier's check are different.
4. Describe the procedure for making a bank deposit.
5. Define the following:
   a. Blank endorsement
   b. Endorsement in full

Please refer to the student workbook for additional learning activities.

BIBLIOGRAPHY

Fulton-Calkins PJ, Rankin DS, Shumack KA: The administrative professional, ed 14, Mason, OH, 2011, Thomson South-Western.

Internal Revenue Service: Publication 15 (Circular E), Employer's Tax Guide (revised), Washington, DC, 2014, US Department of the Treasury.

RECOMMENDED WEBSITES

www.ftc.gov
www.americanbankassociation.com
www.federalreserve.gov
www.fdic.gov
www.irs.gov/publications
www.quickbooks.com/support (Additional terms and conditions may apply.)
www.intuit.com

Infection Control Systems

Mary Govoni

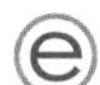 http://evolve.elsevier.com/Finkbeiner/practice

LEARNING OUTCOMES

1. Define the key terms in this chapter.
2. Identify the importance to the administrative assistant of an understanding of disease transmission.
3. Identify the routes of disease transmission.
4. Discuss infection control in the dental office, including:
   - Discuss the occupational health protection program for the dental staff.
   - Identify the various regulatory agencies that impact the dental office.
   - Identify the various records required by the Occupational Safety and Health Administration that must be maintained in the business office.
   - Discuss the safety equipment for hazardous situations the administrative assistant may be responsible for ordering.
5. Describe basic infection control procedures.
6. Discuss the importance of educating patients about infection control programs.
7. Discuss waste disposal in the dental office.

KEY TERMS

Acquired immunodeficiency syndrome (AIDS) A disease caused by a retrovirus known as the *human immunodeficiency virus type 1* (HIV-1). A related but distinct retrovirus (HIV-2) has recently appeared in a limited number of patients in the United States.

Antiseptic An antimicrobial agent that can be applied to a body surface, usually the skin or the raw mucosa, to try to prevent or minimize infection in the area of application.

Autogenous infection Self-produced infection, originating within the body.

Barrier techniques Protocols used in infection control to prevent cross-contamination between a healthcare worker and a patient or between patients.

Bioburden Any substance that interferes with the sterilization process.

Blood-borne pathogens Organisms transmitted through blood or blood products that can cause infectious diseases, such as human immunodeficiency virus (HIV) infection, acquired immunodeficiency syndrome (AIDS), and hepatitis B virus (HBV) infection.

Centers for Disease Control and Prevention (CDC) A federal agency responsible for investigating the incidence of disease, monitoring diseases throughout the world, and conducting research directed toward controlling and preventing disease. The CDC also establishes standards of care for patient safety in healthcare settings, such as dentistry.

Communicable disease A disease that may be transmitted directly or indirectly from one individual to another.

Cross-contamination The transfer of impurities, infection, or disease from one source to another.

Dental healthcare personnel (DHCP) A dental professional who provides care to patients or who has some contact with dental patients in the office.

Disease transmission The spread of disease-causing organisms from one person to another.

Disinfectant Chemicals used to destroy some forms of pathogenic microorganisms.

Disinfection The process of destroying some pathogenic microorganisms.

Environmental Protection Agency (EPA) A federal agency that regulates the use and disposal of hazardous materials. The workplace management of hazardous materials falls under the jurisdiction of OSHA.

Eyewash An OSHA-required device used to flush the eyes with water when exposure to unnatural contaminants has occurred.

Hazardous waste Materials identified as being hazardous to human health; local, state, and federal regulations require the special handling of such materials.

Hepatitis B virus (HBV) Virus that causes a form of hepatitis B that is transmitted in contaminated serum in blood transfusions, via the passing of contaminated fluids, or by the use of contaminated needles and instruments. Caution: Any DHCP who comes in contact with blood, body fluids, or body tissues has an increased risk of developing this type of hepatitis. A DHCP who does not have protection against the HBV antigen should be immunized with a hepatitis B vaccine.

Hepatitis C virus (HCV) Virus that causes a form of hepatitis C that is transmitted by contact with blood that contains the hepatitis C surface antigen. There is no vaccine for HCV.

Human immunodeficiency virus (HIV) See *Acquired immunodeficiency virus (AIDS).*

Infection The invasion of body tissues by disease-producing microorganisms and the reaction of the tissues to these microorganisms, their toxins, or both.

Infectious waste Blood and blood products, contaminated sharps, pathologic wastes, and microbiological wastes.

Occupational Safety and Health Administration (OSHA) A federal agency that establishes guidelines and regulations for worker safety. These guidelines include the storage and disposal of toxic chemicals and hazardous materials and the safe and proper use of clinical and office equipment.

Personal protective equipment (PPE) Materials used to protect the employee when occupational exposure is possible. Such equipment includes but is not limited to disposable gloves, disposable surgical masks and gowns, laboratory coats and scrubs, and face shields or eye protection with side shields.

Sanitization The act of making something sanitary or clean and free of dirt.

Sepsis A pathologic state characterized by the presence of pathogens.

Sharps containers Enclosed containers from which an article cannot be retrieved. They are used for the disposal of sharp items that may cause punctures or cuts when handled, such as broken medical glassware, needles, scalpel blades, and suture needles.

Sterilization The process of rendering an item free of germs; dental sterilization commonly is achieved by steam under pressure, dry heat, or chemical vapor.

Standard precautions Protocols used to maintain an aseptic field and to prevent cross-contamination and cross-infection between healthcare providers, between healthcare providers and patients, and between patients. Such measures, which were formerly called *universal precautions,* include but are not limited to the sterilization of instruments and other equipment; the isolation and disinfection of the immediate clinical environment; the use of sterile disposables; scrubbing; the use of personal protective equipment (e.g., mask, gown, protective eyewear, gloves); and the proper disposal of contaminated wastes.

The administrative assistant generally has no direct patient contact. Nevertheless, he or she must understand both the risks and management of occupational exposures to blood-borne pathogens. Although his or her primary duties are in the business office, the administrative assistant may be called on to perform some clinical task that could cause exposure to such a risk. The assigned job, therefore, does not make it impossible to contract a communicable disease. The role of the administrative assistant in infection control is vital, because it involves the following responsibilities:

- Acquiring a thorough understanding of the routes of disease transmission
- Maintaining an adequate inventory of acceptable disinfectants, chemical sterilants, personal protective equipment (PPE), and barrier covers
- Maintaining records verifying compliance with the requirements of the Occupational Safety and Health Administration (OSHA)
- Transmitting spore samples to the appropriate monitoring agencies for the determination of sterilizer effectiveness
- Participating in training sessions
- Verifying employee compliance with OSHA regulations and Centers for Disease Control and Prevention (CDC) guidelines
- Maintaining employee records for training, vaccinations, and exposure incidents
- Scheduling continuing education courses for the staff
- Verifying quality assurance for infection control protocols
- Maintaining all Safety Data Sheets (SDSs)
- Arranging for the disposal of hazardous and biohazardous waste
- Providing infection control training and other safety training for new employees within 10 days of the start of employment
- Interacting with outside agencies

A variety of diseases can be transmitted by means of routine dental care. Fortunately for the dental profession, the American Dental Association (ADA), the Organization for Safety and Asepsis Procedures (OSAP), and the CDC have worked vigorously to establish infection control and safety procedures for dental healthcare personnel (DHCP) to prevent the transmission of disease.

The CDC report entitled *Guidelines for Infection Control in Dental Health-Care Settings* was revised in 2003. Every dental office should have direct access to these guidelines through a link on the ADA's website (www.ada.org) or the CDC's website (www.cdc.gov). This report consolidates previous recommendations and adds new ones for infection control in dental settings. It provides recommendations regarding the following: (1) educating and protecting dental healthcare personnel; (2) preventing the transmission of blood-borne pathogens; (3) hand hygiene; (4) PPE; (5) contact dermatitis and latex hypersensitivity; (6) sterilization and disinfection of patient care items; (7) environmental infection control; (8) dental unit water lines, biofilm, and water quality; and (9) special considerations (e.g., dental handpieces and other devices, radiology, parenteral medications, oral surgical procedures, dental laboratories). These recommendations were developed in collaboration with and after review by authorities on infection control from the CDC and other public agencies, academia, and private and professional organizations.

DISEASE TRANSMISSION

Dental treatment involves a number of sources whereby infectious diseases can be transmitted, including blood, saliva, nasal discharge, dust, hands, clothing, and hair. Any of these media can transmit a microbial or viral infection. Table 17-1 presents a list of several communicable diseases and their routes of transfer.

PRACTICE NOTE

Infectious diseases can be transmitted by a number of media during dental treatment, including blood, saliva, nasal discharge, dust, hands, clothing, and hair.

TABLE 17-1 Common Communicable Diseases and Routes of Transmission

Disease	Medium of Transmission	Route of Transmission
Acquired immunodeficiency syndrome (AIDS)	Blood, semen, and other body fluids, including breast milk	Inoculation by use of contaminated needles or by direct contact so that infected body fluids can enter the body
Gonococcal disease	Lesions; discharge from infected mucous membranes	Direct contact, such as sexual intercourse; towels, bathtubs, and toilets; hands of infected individuals soiled with their own discharges; through breaks in the skin of the hands
Hepatitis B, viral	Blood and serum-derived fluids, including semen and vaginal fluids	Contact with blood and body fluids
Herpes	Cold sores; genital sores	Direct skin-to-skin contact as through kissing or sexual intercourse
Measles (rubella)	Discharges from nose and throat	Direct contact, hands of healthcare worker, and articles used by and for the patient
Mumps	Discharges from infected glands and throat	Direct contact with the affected person
Pneumonia	Sputum; discharges from nose and throat	Direct contact, hands of healthcare worker, and articles used by and for the patient
Rubeola	Secretions from nose and throat	Through the mouth and nose
Streptococcal sore throat	Discharges from nose and throat; skin lesions	Through the mouth and nose
Syphilis	Infected tissues; lesions and blood; transfer though placenta to fetus	Direct contact as through kissing or sexual intercourse, contaminated needles and syringes
Tuberculosis	Saliva, lesions, and feces	Direct contact, droplet infection from a person coughing with the mouth uncovered, saliva transferred from the mouth to the fingers and then to food and other articles

Types of Infections

Infections common to dental treatment generally can be divided into two categories: autogenous infections and cross-infections. Autogenous infections are infections for which the patient is the source. For example, a patient who undergoes dental treatment, such as an extensive scaling procedure, may subsequently develop endocarditis; this condition can result from the introduction of virulent organisms (e.g., staphylococci, pneumococci) that live in the mouth into the bloodstream during the scaling procedure.

PRACTICE NOTE
With autogenous infections, the patient is the source of the infection.

Cross-infections are transferred from one patient or person to another. For example, when a child has an infection and coughs or sneezes, the caregiver may contract the infection through airborne or droplet transmission.

PRACTICE NOTE
Cross-infections are transferred from one patient or person to another.

Routes of Infection Transmission

Microbial transmission through dental-related secretions and exudates occurs by three general routes: (1) direct contact with a lesion, organisms, or debris during an intraoral procedure; (2) indirect contact through contaminated dental instruments, equipment, or records; and (3) the inhalation of microorganisms aerosolized from a patient's blood or saliva during the use of high-speed or ultrasonic equipment, such as a high-speed handpiece or an ultrasonic scaler.

In many dental practices, treatment providers may not realize the dissemination potential of saliva and blood by these routes. Potential dangers often are missed because much of the spatter from the patient's mouth is not readily noticeable. For example, bioburden (i.e., blood, saliva, and exudate) may be transparent; it may dry as a clear film on contaminated surfaces. Consequently, the administrative assistant must understand the potential risk of handling contaminated items and touching contaminated surfaces.

INFECTION CONTROL IN THE DENTAL OFFICE

Because patient care actually begins in the business office, it is important to identify the role of the administrative assistant as it relates to infection control in the clinical area. Every dental healthcare worker is responsible for breaking the cycle of disease transmission (Figure 17-1). Safe practice is based on the following principles:

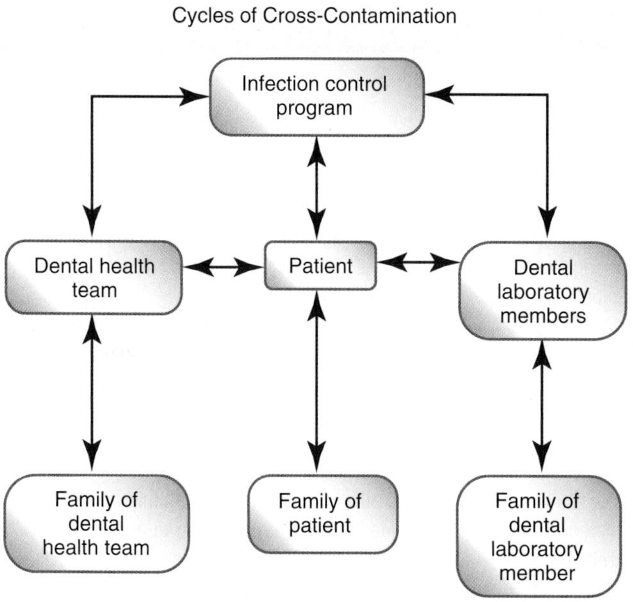

Cycles of Cross-Contamination

FIGURE 17-1 Cycle of disease transmission.

- A complete and accurate patient history must be obtained, and screening must be done.
- Aseptic techniques must be observed during the use of PPE.
- Healthcare workers must strictly adhere to acceptable disinfection and sterilization procedures.
- Equipment asepsis and dental laboratory asepsis must be practiced.

The administrative assistant is responsible for the first step in safe practice: obtaining complete and detailed information about the patient. The records discussed in Chapter 7 must be completed, dated, signed, and reviewed thoroughly by the dentist. During treatment procedures, the administrative assistant must make sure that protocols are followed and that the necessary barrier materials are available for use. Finally, the administrative assistant ensures that the records used during the treatment procedure are transferred safely from the clinical site to the business office without cross-contamination.

PRACTICE NOTE

Every dental healthcare worker is responsible for breaking the cycle of disease transmission.

Table 17-2 presents several situations that the administrative assistant may encounter when attempting to maintain safe practice in the office. The administrative assistant must be able to distinguish between right actions and wrong actions, and he or she must understand the consequences of a wrong action in infection control. Box 17-1 presents a self-assessing list of points that the administrative assistant should live by when working in the dental office to make sure that disease transmission is not being promoted.

BOX 17-1

Self-Assessment for the Administrative Assistant

If the administrative assistant can agree with each of the following statements, he or she can probably perform the duties safely and free of potential risks. If the administrative assistant cannot agree with one of these statements, then that person may jeopardize his or her own health and the safety of others with whom he or she has had contact.

1. I completely understand the Occupational Safety and Health Administration (OSHA) concepts and the need to perform my duties safely.
2. I understand the need for immunizations.
3. I am sure that the pencils, pens, and records with which I come in contact regularly are free of contamination.
4. I am never in contact with exposed surfaces, body fluids, or contaminated areas or involved with sterilization processes.
5. I never receive materials from the hands of a dental healthcare worker (DHCP) who is wearing contaminated examination gloves.
6. I never retrieve dental floss or toothbrushes that were used in a patient education treatment room.
7. I never subject myself to the potential for disease transmission by performing simple tasks such as removing armamentaria from a treatment room.
8. I will never be required to provide emergency care to patients or others without protective personal barriers.
9. I never come in contact with infectious waste or patient laboratory cases.
10. I have never encountered my colleagues wearing their clinical attire into a public area.
11. I never assume that because the patient is a family member or personal friend that he or she is not potentially contagious.

If the administrative assistant answers "no" to any of the preceding points, he or she must do so only if he or she strictly adheres to the appropriate barriers and protocols provided by the Centers for Disease Control and Prevention (CDC), OSHA, or the American Dental Association (ADA).

Occupational Health Protection Program for the Dental Staff

The administrative assistant plays a role in maintaining the health and safety of the patients and healthcare workers in the office. Although he or she is not usually assigned the task of infection control coordinator, he or she should be familiar with the aspects of this process. After all, the administrative assistant is responsible for managing the office and thus must be able to access all records.

The office's personnel policy must include a health service program for the staff that covers the following:

- Education and training
- Immunizations
- Exposure prevention and postexposure management
- Medical conditions, work-related illnesses, and work restrictions
- Allergies or sensitivities to work-related materials (e.g., latex)
- Records maintenance, data management, and confidentiality issues

TABLE 17-2 Recognizing Wrong from Right in Infection Control

Wrong	Effect	Right
Shaking hands while wearing contaminated gloves	Disease transmission may occur via cross-contamination.	Remove gloves and wash hands before leaving examination gloves in treatment room; nod and greet the individual.
Pulling mask on and off	Contact with the face with contaminated gloves can expose unprotected tissues to disease; if the mask is contaminated, contact with gloved or ungloved hands will also allow disease transmission.	Always leave mask in place; if movement for repositioning is necessary, do it with clean gloves; slight readjustment may be made by using the upper arm or shoulder.
Wearing the same mask for more than one patient	Masks become moist fields, which allow for the penetration of particles through the mask.	Always change masks between patients; use more than one mask if the treatment procedure is lengthy.
Reusing the same gloves	Most gloves have microscopic openings that allow for the penetration of microbes; washing gloves increases the potential for disease transmission.	Gloves are always changed between patients; gloves may need to be changed during a lengthy treatment procedure.
Placing patient records in the treatment room	Records may become exposed to aerosols or through handling; these records are transferred to the business office after treatment, thereby exposing the business personnel to the potential for disease.	Records other than radiographs should be kept outside of the treatment room to avoid contamination; if the records must be in the treatment room, they should be kept out of reach of aerosols and handled with clean hands or with overgloves rather than examination gloves.
Storing instruments in trays or drawers instead of sealed bags in treatment rooms	Instruments that are not individually bagged (if not part of a tray setup) may be exposed to aerosols or other contact during treatment and may become contaminated.	All instruments processed through sterilization should be bagged to ensure their sterility when they are used; even in closed drawers, instruments may not remain sterile.
Eating in the laboratory or in another contaminated site	Surfaces can become contaminated from instruments or materials exposed to patient aerosols or handling.	A staff lounge or eating area must be available in a site away from potentially contaminated materials.
Wearing a V-neck laboratory coat	Garments worn under the lab coat can become contaminated; if wearing a V-neck shirt underneath such a coat, the skin will be exposed.	Always wear high-neck lab coats when working with patients or in the laboratory; these coats should be removed before leaving the workplace.
Wearing dangling earrings, piercings, necklaces, bracelets, or ties	These items can become contaminated; they may hang in the patient's face or catch on something.	Minimize jewelry; only wear wedding bands and small post earrings in the workplace.

- A referral arrangement with a physician or medical facility for the treatment of staff members after emergencies and exposure incidents and for the quick and appropriate performance of medical evaluation and treatment
- Confidential, up-to-date medical records for all workers, including the documentation of immunizations and antibody titer tests

The administrative assistant and the dentist must work together to maintain the safety of all staff members and patients. Attention to records maintenance and continual education and training can ensure safe practice.

Government Regulations

All dental professionals are expected to comply with the current guidelines and regulations that govern infection control, hazard communication, and medical waste disposal. Several agencies are responsible for providing the dental professional with the current regulations that affect each of these areas. The employer is primarily responsible for maintaining current copies of all state and federal regulations that relate to the dental office. These guidelines must be reviewed, and their implementation in the office must be documented.

OSHA established guidelines to protect workers from occupational exposure to blood-borne diseases. Regulations now require that employees who come in direct contact with blood or infectious materials and substances are required to use standard precautions. In other words, all patients must be treated as if they are potentially infectious with the human immunodeficiency virus (HIV), the hepatitis B virus (HBV), the hepatitis C virus (HCV), and other infectious organisms. An overview of the latest required OSHA standards is presented in Box 17-2.

PRACTICE NOTE

All dental professionals are expected to comply with current guidelines and regulations that govern infection control, hazard communication, and medical waste disposal.

BOX 17-2

Overview of Standards Established by the Occupational Safety and Health Administration (OSHA)

- Employers must identify and train workers "reasonably anticipated" to be at risk of exposure. They also must reduce or eliminate exposure and offer medical care and counseling if exposure occurs.
- Employers must have written exposure control plans identifying workers with occupational exposure to blood and other infectious materials and specifying ways to protect and train those workers.
- Employers must have a plan that includes protocols for **barrier techniques**, sterilization, disinfection, hepatitis B vaccination, and the handling of office accidents, including exposure to infectious materials. They must also have plans to protect and train employees; these plans must be reviewed and updated annually and must be available to employees at all times.
- The use of puncture-resistant containers, handwashing as gloves are changed, and proper personal protective equipment are required.
- Employers must provide laundering of protective clothing. Laundering of protective clothing at home is prohibited.
- Sharps must be recapped with a one-handed technique or a mechanical recapping device.
- Employees must wear gowns and gloves when a risk exists of exposure to or skin contact with blood, body fluids, or saliva.
- General work clothes are not considered protection against exposure to blood, body fluids, or saliva.
- Employees must wear masks, eyewear, or a face shield during exposure to splashes, spray, spatter, droplets of blood, body tissue, or saliva.
- Eyewear must have fixed side shields.
- Employers must provide personal protective equipment to be worn by all employees (gowns, gloves, masks, and eyewear) at no expense to employees.
- **Sharps containers** must be labeled and easily accessible to areas where sharps are used.
- Hepatitis B vaccinations must be offered to employees at no cost after training is completed but within 10 days of placement in a position that involves occupational exposure.
- If a worker declines the hepatitis B vaccination, access is still required if the employee changes his or her mind.
- Employers must have provided a training program during working hours for all employees in occupational exposure positions by June 4, 1992, and annually in subsequent years.
- Training records must be kept for 3 years after the training sessions.
- The following must be handled as infectious waste (placed in special labeled containers): pathologic waste sharps; blood and body fluid items that release blood, body fluid, or saliva when compressed; and items caked with dried blood, body fluid, or saliva if such contaminants can be released from the materials during handling.

Adapted from the Occupational Safety and Health Administration: CP2–2.69: Exposure procedures for occupational exposure to bloodborne pathogens, Washington, DC, 2001, U.S. Department of Labor.

When standard precautions are used, additional procedures are not necessary for treating a patient who is known to have an infectious disease. Under standard precautions, each workplace must meet the following goals:

- Strive for a hazard-free environment.
- Provide personal protective clothing and PPE.
- Maintain employee training and health records.

PRACTICE NOTE

When standard precautions are used, additional procedures are not necessary for treating a patient who is known to have an infectious disease.

The Environmental Protection Agency (EPA), a federal regulatory agency, developed a program for overseeing the handling, tracking, transportation, and disposal of medical waste after it leaves the dental office.

The CDC, a division of the US Public Health Service, also provides recommendations for healthcare workers. It is responsible for investigating and controlling various diseases, such as dental caries, hepatitis, and tuberculosis, which is currently on the rise.

Maintaining Regulatory Records

The dentist may assign the administrative assistant the job of maintaining the myriad records required to meet the various standards and regulations. To aid this process, many companies and organizations have provided brochures and manuals, such as the ADA's *Regulatory Compliance Manual* (Figure 17-2). An implementation control form (Figure 17-3) can help to ensure that all records are kept as required. Examples of all records should be included in the office procedures manual or the *Regulatory Compliance Manual.*

These records should be kept confidential and should include the following:

- Exposure determination forms (Figure 17-4), which describe the office's infection control program and procedures
- Employee training records (Figure 17-5), which describe HBV vaccination availability, requirements, and implementation
- Employee medical records (Figure 17-6)
- Informed refusal or declination statement for HBV vaccination (Figure 17-7)
- Postexposure evaluation and follow-up training and protocols
- Employee-informed refusal of postexposure medical evaluation (Figure 17-8)
- Incident report of exposure to occupational illness (Figure 17-9)

Hazard Communication Program

OSHA's hazard communication standards require all dental professionals to develop and implement a program that involves

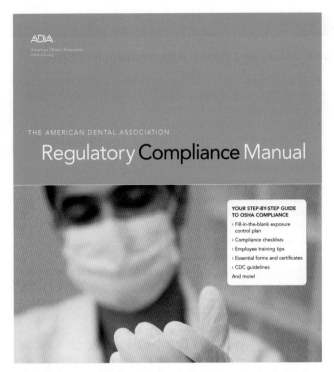

FIGURE 17-2 The American Dental Association's *Regulatory Compliance Manual* is a good resource to help the administrative assistant ensure that the dental office is complying with the necessary standards and regulations related to infection control. (Courtesy of American Dental Association, Chicago, Illinois.)

employee training, the compilation of a list of hazardous chemicals, the maintenance of SDSs, and the proper labeling of all chemicals in the office. This program must apply to all activities during which an individual may be exposed to hazardous chemicals under normal working conditions or during an emergency. In 2013, OSHA and the World Health Organization introduced the Globally Harmonized System (GHS) of classifying and labeling hazardous chemicals in the workplace. Among the changes adopted with this system were changing the name of *Material Safety Data Sheets* to *Safety Data Sheets* (SDSs). In addition, OSHA introduced pictograms (Figure 17-10) to identify specific hazard classes and warning statements. OSHA also introduced a sample of a new label for use with the required safety information (Figure 17-11). Additional information regarding the new SDS format is illustrated in Figure 17-12. Employers are required to provide training related to these new requirements, which take effect in 2016.

One individual—often the administrative assistant—is designated as the hazard communication program coordinator. This person is responsible for the following:

- Disseminating information about the program
- Recognizing the hazardous properties of chemicals found in the workplace
- Keeping up to date regarding the procedures for the safe handling of chemicals
- Implementing measures for protecting the office staff from hazardous chemicals

Safety Data Sheets

If assigned the job of hazard communication program coordinator, the administrative assistant should make and maintain a list of all products in the office that contain hazardous chemicals (Figure 17-13). SDSs, which are government-approved or equivalent forms that provide specific information about chemicals purchased for use in the workplace, are an important part of the records. SDSs for all products with hazardous potential are compiled and kept updated in a master list that is available to all individuals. An SDS must include the manufacturer's name and address, the product name, and the additional information listed in Figure 17-14.

Labeling of Hazardous Materials

The hazard communication program coordinator is also responsible for properly labeling hazardous chemicals and substances. Products that remain in the manufacturer's original container do not need additional labeling in the dental facility. However, products that are dispensed into secondary containers (e.g., chemical sterilants) must be labeled with hazardous chemical labels to identify the product and the hazards associated with it.

Safety Equipment for Hazardous Situations

The administrative assistant may be responsible for ordering equipment and training office staff members in the use of a variety of materials during a hazardous situation. Spills of chemicals, gypsum products, mercury, and flammable materials may produce different reactions, depending on the hazardous chemicals involved. Again, although the administrative assistant may not work directly with hazardous materials, it becomes his or her responsibility to ensure that safe practice is implemented, to understand how to prevent accidents, and to know how to react in the event of an accident.

The following equipment should be kept readily available for use in preventing or dealing with a hazardous spill:

- Fire extinguisher
- Eyewash stations
- Mercury spill kit
- Masks approved by the National Institute for Occupational Safety and Health (NIOSH)
- Protective clothing (with long sleeves and a high neck and made of fluid-impervious fabric)
- Kitty litter and a broom and dustpan
- Protective nitrile gloves and glasses
- Bags in which to seal spilled materials and contaminated objects
- Well-ventilated areas for work (which allow the ventilation to be turned off if an accident occurs)
- Scavenging system (for use with nitrous oxide)
- Safety shields on model trimmers and laboratory lathes

INFECTION CONTROL TECHNIQUES

During the course of dental treatment, some bioburden contamination of equipment, surfaces, instruments, and other

Text continued on p. 319

Implementation Records of OSHA Requirements

SECTION	DATE
Exposure determination	____________
Infection control program	____________
HBV vaccination	____________
Postexposure evaluation and follow-up	____________
Training	____________
Recordkeeping	____________

FIGURE 17-3 An implementation control form can help to ensure that the necessary infection control records are kept in order.

Exposure determination form

All employees holding the following positions in my office have occupational exposure.

Position	Names
1.	1.
2.	2.
3.	3.

Some employees holding the following positions in my office have occupational exposure. That is, they are occasionally called upon to perform tasks that may result in occupational exposure.

Position	Names
1.	1.
2.	2.
3.	3.

This table contains tasks and procedures that might result in occupational exposure to employees in job classifications in which only some employees have occupational exposure.

Position	Name	Tasks that may result in exposure
1.	1.	1.
2.	2.	2.

Positions listed below have no occupational exposure

Position	Names
1.	1.
2.	2.

The office of ____________________

located at ____________________

____

FIGURE 17-4 Sample exposure determination form.

Hazard Communication Training Record

This office facility has conducted a training session for individuals incorporating OSHA Hazard Communication Standard.

Name of Employer ______________________________

Office Address ______________________________

Date ______________________________

Conducted by ______________________________

Signature ______________________________

Attended by ______________________________

Signatures ______________________________

A

FIGURE 17-5 **A,** Sample employee training record.

Continued

Employee Comment Form

Please provide your view of the training program to the program coordinator.

Name of Employer__________

Office Address __________

Date of training session __________

What items did you find useful? __________

What items would you like to be covered in more detail? __________

What suggestions can you offer for improvement in the training program? __________

B

FIGURE 17-5, cont'd B, Sample employee evaluation form for training session.

Confidential employee medical record

Employee medical record

Employee name____________________

Employee address____________________

Employee social security number____________________

Employee starting date____________________

Employee termination date (if any)____________________

History of HBV vaccination (date received, or, if not received, a brief explanation of why not)____________________

History of other immunizations____________________

History of exposure incident(s) (dates, brief explanation, attachments)____________________

Results of medical exams and follow-up procedures regarding exposure incident or hepatitis B immunity, including written opinion of healthcare professional
(dates, brief explanation, attachments)

Information provided to the healthcare professional regarding hepatitis B vaccination and/or exposure incident(s)
(dates, brief explanation, attachments)

Attach pre-employment health records to this document.
Note: maintain the record for duration of employment plus 30 years

FIGURE 17-6 Sample employee medical record.

Informed Refusal for Hepatitis B Vaccination

I, ______________________ am employed as a dentist/dental assistant/ dental hygienist/laboratory technician in the office of ____________. I have been provided training regarding the hepatitis B vaccine. I understand the effectiveness of the vaccine, the risks of contracting hepatitis B in the dental office, and the importance of taking active steps to reduce the risk.

However, I, of my own free will and volition, and despite the urging of Dr. ____________, have elected not to be vaccinated against hepatitis B. I have personal reasons for making the decision not to be vaccinated.

Signature

Witness

Name

Address

City State Zip Code

Date

FIGURE 17-7 Sample form for informed refusal of hepatitis B vaccination.

Employee Informed Refusal of Postexposure Medical Evaluation

I, ________________________, am employed by ____________________ as a dentist, dental assistant, dental hygienist, or laboratory technician. Dr. __________ has provided training for me regarding infection control and the risk of disease transmission in this dental facility.

On ________________________, 20__, I was involved in an exposure incident when I

____

____

____

____

(describe details of needlestick, etc.) I have been offered follow-up medical evaluation in order to ensure that I have full knowledge of whether I have been exposed to or contracted an infectious disease from this incident.

However, I, of my own free will and volition, and despite Dr. _______________'s offer, have elected not to have a medical evaluation. I have personal reasons for making this decision.

____
Signature

_______________________ Witness

____
Name

____
Address

____
City State Zip Code

____
Date

FIGURE 17-8 Sample employee form for informed refusal of postexposure medical evaluation.

Bureau of Statistics
Supplementary Record of
Occupational Injuries and Illnesses

U.S. Department of Labor

This form is required by Public Law 91-596 and must be kept in the establishment for 5 years. Failure to maintain can result in the issuance of citations and assessment of penalties.	Case or File No.	Form approved O.M.B. No. 1220-0029

Employer

1. Name

2. Mail address *(No. and street, city or town, State, and zip code)*

3. Location, if different from mail address

Injured or Ill Employee

4. Name *(First, middle, and last)* — Social Security No.

5. Home address *(No. and street, city or town, State, and zip code)*

6. Age — 7. Sex: *(Check one)* Male ☐ Female ☐

8. Occupation *(Enter regular job title,* not *the specific activity he was performing at the time of injury.)*

9. Department *(Enter name of department or division in which the injured person is regularly employed, even though he may have been temporarily working in another department at the time of injury.)*

The Accident or Exposure to Occupational Illness

If accident or exposure occurred on employer's premises, give address of plant or establishment in which it occurred. Do not indicate department or division within the plant or establishment. If accident occurred outside employer's premises at an identifiable address, give that address. If it occurred on a public highway or at any other place which cannot be identified by number and street, please provide place references locating the place of injury as accurately as possible.

10. Place of accident or exposure (*No. and street, city or town, State, and zip code*)

11. Was place of accident or exposure on employer's premises? Yes ☐ No ☐

12. What was the employee doing when injured? *(Be specific. If he was using tools or equipment or handling material, name them and tell what he was doing with them.)*

13. How did the accident occur? *(Describe fully the events which resulted in the injury or occupational illness. Tell what happened and how it happened. Name any objects or substances involved and tell how they were involved. Give full details on all factors which led or contributed to the accident. Use separate sheet for additional space.)*

Occupational Injury or Occupational Illness

14. Describe the injury or illness in detail and indicate the part of body affected. *(E.g., amputation of right index finger at second joint; fracture of ribs; lead poisoning; dermatitis of left hand, etc.)*

15. Name the object or substance which directly injured the employee. *(For example, the machine or thing he struck against or which struck him; the vapor or poison he inhaled or swallowed; the chemical or radiation which irritated his skin; or in cases of strains, hernias, etc., the thing he was lifting, pulling, etc.)*

16. Date of injury or initial diagnosis of occupational illness — 17. Did employee die? *(Check one)* Yes ☐ No ☐

Other

18. Name and address of physician

19. If hospitalized, name and address of hospital

Date of report	Prepared by	Official position

OSHA No. 101 (Feb. 1981)

FIGURE 17-9 Sample incident report of exposure to occupational illness. (From Bureau of Statistics, Department of Labor, Washington, DC.)

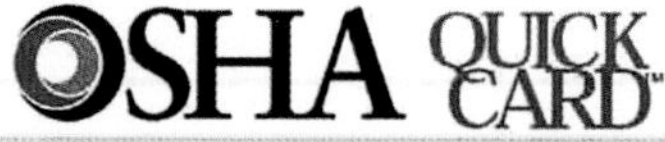

Hazard Communication Standard Pictogram

As of June 1, 2015, the Hazard Communication Standard (HCS) will require pictograms on labels to alert users of the chemical hazards to which they may be exposed. Each pictogram consists of a symbol on a white background framed within a red border and represents a distinct hazard(s). The pictogram on the label is determined by the chemical hazard classification.

HCS Pictograms and Hazards

Health Hazard	Flame	Exclamation Mark
▪ Carcinogen ▪ Mutagenicity ▪ Reproductive Toxicity ▪ Respiratory Sensitizer ▪ Target Organ Toxicity ▪ Aspiration Toxicity	▪ Flammables ▪ Pyrophorics ▪ Self-Heating ▪ Emits Flammable Gas ▪ Self-Reactives ▪ Organic Peroxides	▪ Irritant (skin and eye) ▪ Skin Sensitizer ▪ Acute Toxicity ▪ Narcotic Effects ▪ Respiratory Tract Irritant ▪ Hazardous to Ozone Layer (Non-Mandatory)
Gas Cylinder	**Corrosion**	**Exploding Bomb**
▪ Gases Under Pressure	▪ Skin Corrosion/Burns ▪ Eye Damage ▪ Corrosive to Metals	▪ Explosives ▪ Self-Reactives ▪ Organic Peroxides
Flame Over Circle	**Environment** (Non-Mandatory)	**Skull and Crossbones**
▪ Oxidizers	▪ Aquatic Toxicity	▪ Acute Toxicity (fatal or toxic)

For more information:

OSHA® Occupational Safety and Health Administration

U.S. Department of Labor

www.osha.gov (800) 321-OSHA (6742)

OSHA 3491-02 2012

FIGURE 17-10 OSHA Hazard Communication Standard Pictograms. (Courtesy Occupational Safety and Health Administration, www.osha.gov.)

OSHA (800) 321-OSHA (6742)

SAMPLE LABEL

PRODUCT IDENTIFIER

CODE ________________

Product Name ________________

SUPPLIER IDENTIFICATION

Company Name ________________

Street Address ________________

City ________________ State ______

Postal Code ________ Country ______

Emergency Phone Number ________

PRECAUTIONARY STATEMENTS

Keep container tightly closed. Store in cool, well ventilated place that is locked.

Keep away from heat/sparks/open flame. No smoking.

Only use non-sparking tools.

Use explosion-proof electrical equipment.

Take precautionary measure against static discharge.

Ground and bond container and receiving equipment.

Do not breathe vapors.

Wear Protective gloves.

Do not eat, drink or smoke when using this product.

Wash hands thoroughly after handling.

Dispose of in accordance with local, regional, national, international regulations as specified.

In Case of Fire: use dry chemical (BC) or Carbon dioxide (CO_2) fire extinguisher to extinguish.

First Aid

If exposed call Poison Center.

If on skin (on hair): Take off immediately any contaminated clothing. Rinse skin with water.

HAZARD PICTOGRAMS

SIGNAL WORD

Danger

HAZARD STATEMENT

Highly flammable liquid and vapor.

May cause liver and kidney damage.

SUPPLEMENTAL INFORMATION

Directions for use

____

____

____

Fill weight: ________ Lot Number ______

Gross weight: ________ Fill Date: ______

Expiration Date: ________

FIGURE 17-11 OSHA Sample Label. (Courtesy Occupational Safety and Health Administration, www.osha.gov.)

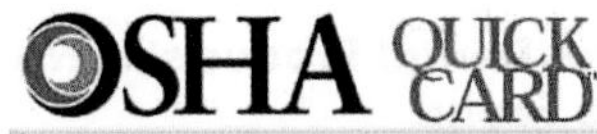

Hazard Communication Safety Data Sheets

The Hazard Communication Standard (HCS) requires chemical manufacturers, distributors, or importers to provide Safety Data Sheets (SDSs) (formerly known as Material Safety Data Sheets or MSDSs) to communicate the hazards of hazardous chemical products. As of June 1, 2015, the HCS will require new SDSs to be in a uniform format, and include the section numbers, the headings, and associated information under the headings below:

Section 1, Identification includes product identifier; manufacturer or distributor name, address, phone number; emergency phone number; recommended use; restrictions on use.

Section 2, Hazard(s) identification includes all hazards regarding the chemical; required label elements.

Section 3, Composition/information on ingredients includes information on chemical ingredients; trade secret claims.

Section 4, First-aid measures includes important symptoms/ effects, acute, delayed; required treatment.

Section 5, Fire-fighting measures lists suitable extinguishing techniques, equipment; chemical hazards from fire.

Section 6, Accidental release measures lists emergency procedures; protective equipment; proper methods of containment and cleanup.

Section 7, Handling and storage lists precautions for safe handling and storage, including incompatibilities.

Section 8, Exposure controls/personal protection lists OSHA's Permissible Exposure Limits (PELs); Threshold Limit Values (TLVs); appropriate engineering controls; personal protective equipment (PPE).

Section 9, Physical and chemical properties lists the chemical's characteristics.

Section 10, Stability and reactivity lists chemical stability and possibility of hazardous reactions.

Section 11, Toxicological information includes routes of exposure; related symptoms, acute and chronic effects; numerical measures of toxicity.

Section 12, Ecological information*

Section 13, Disposal considerations*

Section 14, Transport information*

Section 15, Regulatory information*

Section 16, Other information, includes the date of preparation or last revision.

*Note: Since other Agencies regulate this information, OSHA will not be enforcing Sections 12 through 15 (29 CFR 1910.1200(g)(2)).

Employers must ensure that SDSs are readily accessible to employees.
See Appendix D of 1910.1200 for a detailed description of SDS contents.

For more information: www.osha.gov

OSHA (800) 321-OSHA (6742)

U.S. Department of Labor

FIGURE 17-12 Sample medical waste tracking form. (Courtesy Occupational Safety and Health Administration, www.osha.gov.)

Hazardous Chemicals and the Dental Products in Which They Are Found

CHEMICAL NAME	MAY BE FOUND IN:
acetic acid	photographic solutions
acetone	solvents
aluminum oxide	polishing disks
aluminum soluble salts	astringent agents
asbestos	some cast ring liners
benzoyl peroxide	resin systems, denture resins
beryllium	nickle based casting alloys
calcium carbonate	polishing agents
carbon tetrachloride	solvents
chloroform	solvents
chromium	casting alloys
cobalt	casting alloys
copper	amalgam, casting alloys
cresol, all isomers	endodontic materials
cyanide as CN	plating solutions
dibutylphthalate	impression materials
ethyl acetate	solvents
ethyl acrylate	resins
ethyl alcohol	solvents, sterilizing agents
ethyl chloride	solvents, topical refrigerants
ethyl silicate	silicate investments, impression materials (condensation silicones)
ethylene oxide	sterilizing agents
fluoride dust	fluoride-containing composites
formaldehyde	sterilizing agents
glutaraldehyde	sterilizing agents
hydrochloric acid	pickling solutions, bleaching agents
hydrogen fluoride	etching agents for porcelain
hydroquinone	methacrylate and denture base resins, photographic solutions
iodine	iodophor disinfectants and antimicrobial hand cleansers
isopropyl alcohol	solvents, wiping agents
lead/inorganic lead compounds	impression materials (some polysulfides)
LPG (liquid petroleum gas)	burners
mercury	amalgam
mercury/organic	topical antiseptics
methyl acetate	solvents
methyl alcohol	denatured alcohol
methyl methacrylate	denture base resins
methylene chloride	solvents
molybdenum, insoluble compounds	casting alloys (chromium-cobalt alloys, stainless steel)

CHEMICAL NAME	MAY BE FOUND IN:
nickel (metal and soluble compounds)	nickel-based casting alloys, stainless steel orthodontic appliances
nitric acid	pickling solutions, some bleaching solutions
nitrous oxide	nitrous oxide
oil mist, mineral	handpiece lubricants
petroleum distillates	solvents, waxes, jellies
phenol	disinfectants
phosphoric acid	etching agents, phosphate cements
phthalic anhydride	resins
picric acid	pickling agents
platinum soluble salts	impression materials (addition silicones)
platinum	casting alloys
propane	burners
rouge	polishing agents
silica, amorphous including natural diatomaceous earth	composite resins, materials
silica, crystalline (quartz)	composite resins, porcelain, investments
silicon carbide	polishing disks, cutting wheels
silver (metal and soluble compounds)	amalgam, endodontic points, casting alloys, photographic solutions
sulfuric acid	etchant for alloys, copper plating solutions
talc, nonasbestos form	gloves
tantalum	nickel-chromium-cobalt alloys
tin, inorganic compounds	amalgam, polishing pastes
tin, organic compounds	impression material (condensation silicones)
titanium dioxide	porcelain, impression materials
toluene	solvents
trichloroethane	solvents
uranium, insoluble compounds	porcelain
vinyl chloride	maxillofacial plastics, mouth guard trays
xylene	solvents
zirconium compounds	porcelain, polishing pastes

FIGURE 17-13 List of common chemicals found in a dental office. (From Finkbeiner BL, Johnson CS: *Mosby's comprehensive dental assisting*, St. Louis, 1995, Mosby.)

DENTSPLY/International
DENTSPLY/Caulk
Safety Data Sheet **578617**

1. Product and Company Identification

Product Name Aquasil	SDS Code Number 578617
Substance Identity Aquasil, Aquasil Ultra, Aquasil Ultra Xtra, Smart Wetting® Impression Material Vinyl Polysiloxane Impression Material Aquasil Ultra Cordless Tissue Managing Wash Impression Material, Aquasil Ultra Cordless Tissue Managing Tray Impression Material	Date of Last Revision 09/24/13
Manufacturer: DENTSPLY Caulk	Address 38 West Clarke Avenue Milford DE 19963-1805 http://www.caulk.com, http://www.dentsply.com
Grades or Minor Variant Identities AQUASIL MONOPHASE, AQUASIL RIGID, AQUASIL LV, AQUASIL Easy Mix PUTTY, Smart Wetting® Impression Material, AQUASIL ULTRA MONOPHASE, AQUASIL ULTRA RIGID, AQUASIL ULTRA XLV, AQUASIL ULTRA LV, AQUASIL ULTRA HEAVY – Smart Wetting® Impression Material Super Fast Set, Fast Setting and Regular Setting – Including AQUASIL ULTRA DECA™ Smart Wetting® Impression Material for Dynamic Mixing Machines and digit® Targeted Delivery Systems. AQUASIL ULTRA Xtra – Wash, Tray and DECA Tray. Aquasil Ultra Cordless Tissue Managing Wash Impression Material and Aquasil Ultra Cordless Tissue Managing Tray Impression Material	Information Telephone Number (302) 422-4511 (8:00 AM – 4:30 PM Eastern Time)
Product Use (for Canada) Dental Impression Material	Emergency Telephone Number (302) 422-4511 (8:00 AM – 4:30 PM Eastern Time)

2. Hazard(s) Identification

WARNING
CAUSES SKIN IRRITATION

WASH HANDS THOROUGHLY AFTER HANDLING
WEAR PROTECTIVE GLOVES
IF ON SKIN: WASH WITH PLENTY OF SOAP AND WATER.
IF SKIN IRRITATION OCCURS: GET MEDICAL ADVICE / ATTENTION
TAKE OFF CONTAMINATED CLOTHING AND WASH BEFORE REUSE

3. Composition/Information on Ingredients

Hazardous Components	C.A.S. Number	Exposure Limits	%
Silicon Dioxide -Crystalline	14464-46-1	0.05 mg/m^3	< than 30
Silicon Dioxide - Amorphous	68855-54-9	1.20 mg/m^3	< than 30
Hydrophobic Amorphous Fumed Silica	68909-20-6	10 mg/m^3	< than 10
Titanium Dioxide	13463-67-7	10 mg/m^3	< than 10

Colorant Information: The base pastes may contain fluorescent organic dyes and/or ultramarine pigments and/or inorganic iron oxides. The base pastes may also contain a red pigment known as a Red 2B Toner or a Calcium salt of a beta oxynaphthoate. The Chemical structure of all Ultramarine pigments, regardless of color, is Sodium Aluminosulfosilicate.
Odorant Information: This product contains Peppermint oil which may cause irritation to skin or mucosa or other allergic responses in susceptible persons.

4. First Aid Measures

Routes of Exposure	First Aid Instructions	Immediate Medical Attention	Delayed Effects
Eye	Rinse opened eye for several minutes under running water. If symptoms persist consult physician	Not Applicable	Not Applicable

FIGURE 17-14 Safety Data Sheet form. (Courtesy Dentsply International).

Continued

Skin	Immediately wash with soap and water and rinse thoroughly	Not Applicable	Not Applicable
Inhalation	Supply fresh air, consult physician if symptoms persist	Not Applicable	Not Applicable
Ingestion	If symptoms persist consult physician	Not Applicable	Low order of toxicity is expected when large amounts of material are ingested. Acute toxicology study in rats LD_{50} >2,000mg/kg.
Other	Not Applicable	Not Applicable	Not Applicable
Note to Physicians (Treating, Testing and Monitoring): Treat symptomatically.			

5. Fire Fighting Measures

Flame Propagation or Burning Rate (for Solids): Not Applicable	Properties Contributing to Fire Intensity: Not Applicable	Flammability Classification: Not Applicable	Other: Not Applicable
Extinguishing Media: CO_2, extinguishing powder, foam carbon dioxide or water spray. Fight larger fires with water spray or alcohol resistant foam.		Extinguishing Media to Avoid: Water with full jet.	
Protection and Procedures for Firefighters: Firefighters should wear self-contained respiratory protective devices.			
Unusual Fire and Explosion Hazards: No dangerous decomposition products known. - Product does not present an explosion hazard.			

6. Accidental Release Measures

Containment Techniques: Material is a paste and as such will not flow.		
Spill/Leak Clean-up Procedures and Equipment: Wear protective clothing and scoop up bulk material and place in a labeled plastic or metal container. Avoid gross skin contact to minimize the possibility of contact dermatitis to susceptible persons. Ensure adequate ventilation.		
Evacuation Procedures: Not Applicable	Special Instructions: Not Applicable	Reporting Requirements: Not Applicable

7. Handling and Storage

Handling Practices and Warnings: Product is intended for dental use only. Handling of this product should be by trained dental healthcare professionals only. Observe normal care for working with chemicals.
Storage Practices and Warnings: Store only in the original package. Keep package tightly sealed. Store in a dry area. Protect from exposure to direct light. Store away from food and beverages.

8. Exposure Control / Personal Protection

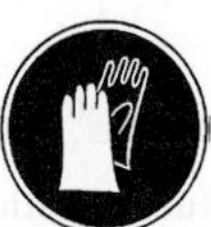

Individual Protection Measures	Personal Protective Equipment for Normal Use	Personal Protective Equipment for Emergencies
Eye/Face	Safety Glasses	Not Applicable
Skin	The glove material has to be impermeable and resistant to the product.	Not Applicable
Inhalation	Not Required	Not Applicable
Body Protection	Protective work clothing	Not Applicable
Occupational Exposure Limits: Not Applicable		Engineering Controls: Not Applicable

9. Physical and Chemical Characteristics

Appearance: Various colored pastes, may be high viscosity paste or runny. Catalyst is white to grey-colored.		Odor: Peppermint odor.
Normal Physical State: Material is available in several viscosities. It varies from a very high viscosity liquid (Paste) to a more runny material.		Melting Point: Not Applicable
Specific Gravity: Varies from 1.1 g/cm^3 to 1.5 g/cm^3	Solubility in Water: Not soluble	pH: Not Applicable
Vapor Pressure (mm Hg): Not Applicable	Vapor Density (AIR=1): Not Applicable	Evaporation Rate (Butyl Acetate =1): N A
Flashpoint Method: Not Applicable	Flammable (Explosive) Limits in Air LEL: Not Applicable UEL: Not Applicable	Autoignition Temperature: Not Applicable, Product will not autoignite.
Other: Not Applicable		

10. Stability and Reactivity Data

Incompatibility (Materials to Avoid): Strong oxidizing materials.	
Hazardous Products Produced During Decomposition: No dangerous decomposition products known if used according to Directions for Use.	
Hazardous Polymerization: ☐May Occur ☒May Not Occur	Conditions to Avoid: None known
Stability? ☒Stable ☐Unstable	Conditions to Avoid: None known

11.Toxicological Information

Toxicity Data, Epidemiology Studies, Carcinogenicity, Neurological Effects, Genetic Effects, Reproductive Effects, or Structure Activity Data: Product may irritate the skin and mucous membranes. The unpolymerized product may cause irritation to the skin in susceptible persons. On the eye the product has an irritating effect. Sensitization: No sensitizing effects known.

Emergency Overview: Material may be mildly irritating to eyes.

Routes of Exposure	Signs and Symptoms	Single, Repeated, or Lifetime Exposure	Severity (Mild, Moderate, Severe)	Acute and Chronic Health Effect(s)	Target Organ(s)
Eye	Material can cause irritation.	Single	Moderate	Irritation and possible corneal damage	Not Applicable
Skin	Material may be an irritant	Single & Repeated	Moderate	Irritation or possible allergic response.	Not Applicable
Inhalation	Not Applicable	Not Applicable	Not Applicable	Not Applicable	Not Applicable

FIGURE 17-14, cont'd

Ingestion	Material is probably not harmful if swallowed	Not Applicable	Mild	Low order of toxicity is expected when large amounts of material are ingested. Acute toxicology study in rats LD_{50} >2,000mg/kg.	Not Applicable
Other	Not Applicable	Not Applicable	Not Applicable	Not Applicable	Not Applicable
Medical Conditions Aggravated by Exposure Open sores and wounds of the skin.					
Carcinogenicity NTP?: Not listed IARC monographs?: Not listed OSHA regulated?: No All components of this product are in compliance with the inventory listing Requirements of the U. S. Toxic Substances Control Act (TSCA) Chemical Substance Inventory.					
Potential Environmental Effects Do not allow to enter sewers/ surface or ground water.					
NFPA Hazard Classification Ratings (Scale 0-4), Health = 0, Fire = 1, Reactivity = 0					

12.Ecological Information

Toxicity Data, Environmental Fate, Physical/Chemical Data, or other Data Supporting Environmental Hazard Statements: Water Hazard class1 (Self-assessment): slightly hazardous for water. Do not allow undiluted product or large quantities of it to reach ground water, water streams or sewage system.

13.Disposal Considerations

Regulations: Must not be disposed of together with household garbage. Do not allow product to reach sewage system. Dispose of material as solid waste in a closed container. Dispose of in accordance with Federal, State and Local regulations
Properties (Physical/Chemical) Affecting Disposal: Dispose of material as solid waste in a closed container.

14.Transport Information

Regulated for Shipping: No. Not Regulated	DOT Shipping Name: Not Regulated	Packing Group: Not Applicable
Do Changes in Quantities, packaging, or shipment method change product classification? No	DOT Hazard Class: Not Applicable	UN Number: Not Applicable

15.Regulatory Information

This product has been classified in accordance with the hazard criteria of the Globally Harmonized System of Classification and Labeling of Chemicals and the SDS contains all of the information required by the Canadian Controlled Products Regulations.
U.S. Federal Regulations: CERCLA 103 Reportable Quantity: This product is not subject to CERCLA reporting requirements. Many states have more stringent release reporting requirements. Report spills required under federal, state and local regulations
Section 313 Toxic Chemicals: This product contains the following chemicals subject to Annual Release Reporting Requirements Under SARA Title III, Section 313 (40 CFR 372): None
Section 302 Extremely Hazardous Substances (TPQ): None
EPA Toxic Substances Control Act (TSCA) Status: All of the components of this product are listed on the TSCA inventory.
U.S. State Regulations California Proposition 65: This product does not contain any chemicals, which are on the California Proposition 65 list.
International Regulations: Canadian Environmental Protection Act: This product is a medical device and not subject to chemical notification requirements.
European Community Labeling: Not a dangerous preparation.
European Inventory of New and Existing Chemicals Substances (EINECS): This product is a medical device and not subject to chemical notification requirements.
Other: Not Applicable

16.Other Information

To the best of our knowledge this product does not contain gluten, wheat grains, flaxseed, natural rubber, or natural latex. All components are synthetically produced; none are derived from animal products. This information is based on our present knowledge. However, this shall not constitute a guarantee for any specific products features and shall not establish a legally valid contractual relationship. The attached safety data sheet covers the dangers and measures to be taken when large quantities of material are released, for example due to accidents during transport or storage by the dealer. For quantities of material typically used in clinical practice, information necessary for safe use and storage of the product is given in the DFU.

FIGURE 17-14, cont'd

devices occurs; sometimes these items and areas simply are not clean. The goal of any infection control program must be to maintain aseptic techniques to prevent cross-infection.

Aseptic Technique

The term *aseptic technique* or *asepsis* refers to procedures that break the circle of infection (the term *sepsis* indicates the presence of pathogens) and that ideally eliminate cross-contamination. With cross-contamination, a previously sterile environment is exposed to harmful agents. In some situations (e.g., during hand scrubbing), an antiseptic—an antimicrobial agent that can be applied to a body surface, usually skin or raw mucosa, to try to prevent or minimize infection in the area of application—is used.

Procedures that are commonly used to maintain asepsis and prevent cross-contamination include the following:

- Barrier coverings are used on surfaces that cannot be disinfected easily or without damage to the surface or equipment.
- Exposed surfaces are cleaned and disinfected.
- Sterile disposable items are used whenever possible.
- All contaminated reusable items are cleaned and sterilized, either by heat sterilization or with liquid chemical steriliants.
- Contaminated gloved hands are not allowed to touch protective eyewear, masks, or the hair.
- Patients are asked to use a pretreatment antimicrobial mouth rinse.
- The hands are washed regularly throughout the day with an antimicrobial cleanser (soap and water or a waterless hand sanitizer), such as before and after lunch and just before and immediately after the treatment of each patient. This is the single most important way to prevent cross-contamination.
- A complete and comprehensive health history is obtained for every patient.

All patients should be treated in the same manner: as potentially infectious for HBV, HCV, HIV, or other blood-borne pathogens or infectious diseases, regardless of what information is contained in their medical history form. Consistent adherence to these standard precautions is a primary professional standard of care that reduces the guesswork of determining a patient's infection status.

The following sections describe techniques that can be used to minimize contamination during treatment procedures (Box 17-3).

BOX 17-3

Flowchart for Management of Occupational Exposures to Blood-Borne Pathogens

Before an Exposure Occurs

Dental Worker

- Receives training in risks of occupational exposures, immediate reporting of injuries/exposures, and reporting procedures within the practice setting

Employer/Infection Control Coordinator

- Establishes referral arrangements and protocol for employees to follow in the event of exposures to blood or saliva via puncture injury, mucous membrane, or non-intact skin
- Trains occupationally exposed employees in postexposure protocols
- Makes available and pays for hepatitis B vaccine for workers at occupational risk

Qualified Healthcare Provider

- Contracts with dentist-employer to provide medical evaluation, counseling, and follow-up care to dental office employees exposed to blood or other potentially infectious materials
- Keeps current on public health guidelines for managing occupational exposure incidents and is aware of evaluating healthcare provider's responsibilities ethically and by law

When an Exposure Incident Occurs

Dental Worker

1. Performs first aid
2. Reports injury to employer
3. Reports to the designated healthcare professional for medical evaluation and follow-up care, as indicated
4. Receives copy of Written Opinion ←

Employer/Infection Control Coordinator

1. Documents events in the practice setting
2. Immediately directs employee to evaluating healthcare professional
3. Sends to evaluating healthcare professional:
   - Copy of standard job description of employee
   - Exposure report
   - Source patient's identity and bloodborne infection status (if known)
   - Employee's HBV status and other relevant medical information
   - Copy of the Occupational Safety and Health Administration (OSHA) Bloodborne Pathogen Standard
4. Arranges for source patient testing if the source patient is known and has consented
5. Pays for postexposure evaluation and, if indicated, prophylaxis
6. Receives Written Opinion from evaluating healthcare professional
   - Files copy of Written Opinion in employee's confidential medical record (if maintained by the dentist employer)
   - Provides copy of Written Opinion to exposed employee

Qualified Healthcare Provider

1. Evaluates exposure incident, worker, and source patient for HBV, HCV, and HIV, maintaining confidentiality
   - Arranges for collection and testing (with consent) of exposed worker and source patient as soon as feasible (if serostatus is not already known)
   - In the event that consent is not obtained for HIV testing, arranges for blood sample to be preserved for up to 90 days (to allow time for the exposed worker to consent to HIV testing)
   - Arranges for additional collection and testing as recommended by the U.S. Public Health Service/CDC
   - Notifies worker of results of all testing and of the need for strict confidentiality with regard to source patient results
   - Provides counseling
   - Provides postexposure prophylaxis, if medically indicated
2. Assesses reported illnesses/side effects.
3. ← Within 15 days of evaluation sends to the employer a Written Opinion, which contains (only) the following:*
   - Documentation that the employee was informed of evaluation results and the need for any further follow-up
   - Whether HBV vaccine was indicated and if it was received

*All other findings or diagnoses remain confidential and are not included in the written report.

Courtesy Organization for Safety and Asepsis Procedures (OSAP): CDC guidelines: from policy to practice, Annapolis, Maryland, 2007, OSAP.

Personal Protection

Personal protection involves two basic considerations: immunologic protection (immunization) and barrier protection.

Immunization

Immunization is the process whereby resistance to an infectious disease is induced or augmented. The human body can produce immunity to particular diseases or conditions. When no natural immunity exists for a disease, immunization may be provided through certain vaccinations.

Immunization to prevent and control cross-infection is an important aspect of healthcare for dental professionals. For example, the HBV vaccine is effective and widely available. However, several other diseases may also pose a threat to the health and well-being of dental personnel and potentially to patients. It is important to note that the HBV vaccine is the only immunization that is addressed by OSHA for the protection of healthcare workers. OSHA requires employers to provide the vaccine to employees who are at risk of exposure to HBV (typically clinical team members) at no charge to the employees. Employees can refuse the vaccine for various reasons; if that occurs, the employee must sign a declination form that states that they have been afforded the opportunity to be vaccinated but choose not to do so at the present time.

DHCPs should receive the appropriate vaccines to prevent the onset of clinical or subclinical infection when symptoms of the disease are not apparent. The occupational risks for HBV, measles, rubella, influenza, and certain other microbial infections can be minimized considerably via the stimulation of artificial active immunity. Approved vaccines are available for each of these conditions, and individuals who provide patient care should receive them.

Common childhood immunizations may be given for several diseases, including diphtheria, tetanus, pertussis, polio, and rubella. Other vaccinations help to prevent rubella, mumps, and influenza. The tuberculin Mantoux test, which is not a vaccine, can determine whether an individual has been exposed to or has tuberculosis. This test is extremely important because tuberculosis, which was once thought to be almost nonexistent in North America, is on the rise. DHCPs should have this test done annually, although it is not mandated in all areas of the country or in all dental settings.

Barrier Protection

Although vaccines are effective at minimizing the transmission of certain infections, they are not sufficient protection against the wide variety of potential pathogens encountered during patient treatment. Physical barriers are a fundamental component of an infection control program. Disposable examination gloves, overgloves, and utility gloves should be used, and, during treatment, face masks and protective clinic attire and eyewear should be worn. The administrative assistant should maintain an adequate inventory of all necessary barrier equipment. A variety of barrier covers can be used during treatment (Box 17-4).

BOX 17-4

Commonly Used Barrier Covers

Barriers coverings may be used on a variety of surfaces to lessen the need for surface disinfection.

Treatment Room

- Light handle covers
- On/off switch on operating light
- Plastic bag over dental chair and adjustment buttons
- Paper towel folded to cover working end of thumb forceps used to retrieve instruments from the mobile cabinetry
- Plastic tubing over hoses of unit (when accessible)
- Plastic bag attached to mobile cabinetry for debris
- Overgloves to retrieve armamentaria and charts

Radiography Treatment Room

- Plastic bag over radiographic head and Position Indicating Device
- Plastic covering over on/off switch
- Plastic covering over touch/control panel
- Plastic bag over dental chair
- Barrier-type film packets
- Covering over area from which each dental film is retrieved (If the film is laid out on a surface before exposure, a covering placed under the film before use eliminates disinfection of the surface.)

Instrument Sterilization

Sterilization is the process of rendering an item free of germs; dental sterilization is commonly achieved with the use of steam under pressure, dry heat, or unsaturated chemical vapor. The processing of dental instruments and armamentarium is the primary responsibility of the clinical assistant and requires the use of utility gloves. To maintain sterility, the CDC guidelines recommend that all instruments be packaged or wrapped before sterilization. Typically, loose instruments are placed in sterilization pouches or bags, and cassettes are wrapped with specialized paper. Color-coded indicators signify whether an instrument package has reached the sterilizing temperature. In addition, the CDC recommends that process integrators be placed in sterilization pouches or inside wrapped cassettes to measure additional parameters for sterilization, such as time and steam penetration.

The administrative assistant may assume a major role in monitoring the efficiency of the sterilization systems. Several factors may diminish the effectiveness of the various sterilizers that are used in the office. Frequent problems include the improper wrapping of instruments; the prevention of adequate penetration to the instrument surface; human error in timing the cycle; defective control gauges that do not reflect actual conditions inside the sterilizer; and sterilizer malfunction.

Although chemically treated tapes are available to determine color changes or biologic controls as a means of checking for proper sterilizer function, the use of calibrated biologic controls remains the gold standard of sterilization. A test strip called a *biologic monitor* or *indicator* that contains harmless active spores is placed in the sterilization chamber with a normal load of instruments. The test strip is returned to the manufacturer or a monitoring agency for verification that sterilization has occurred. The office receives written documentation that is maintained as a record. Biologic monitoring of a sterilizer can also be accomplished in the dental facility with the use of vials of spores that are processed in the sterilizer and then incubated in the office. The results are recorded in a logbook that comes with the sterilizer monitoring kit.

Disposables

Disposable items are manufactured and identified for single use only. These items—which may include needles, saliva ejectors, prophylaxis cups, sealant, and composite brushes—should not be reused. Disposables are becoming even more widely available as manufacturers, distributors, and office personnel recognize their usefulness. Examples of recently marketed items include disposable prophylaxis angles, rag wheels, evacuation line traps, and high-volume evacuator tips. These products pose less of a risk of cross-contamination because they do not undergo recleaning and recycling; however, they must be disposed of properly.

Laboratory Asepsis

Special handling is required when impressions, prosthetic devices, and other materials are transferred from the dental office to a commercial dental laboratory. These items, which are contaminated with the patient's saliva, blood, and other substances, can be a source of disease transmission. The ADA's Councils on Dental Therapeutics and Prosthetic Services and Dental Laboratory Relations updated the guidelines for infection control in dental laboratories in 1988. The ADA and the CDC recommend that impressions, appliances, and other items removed from a patient's mouth be cleaned and disinfected before they are sent to the laboratory. Items received from the laboratory for delivery to a patient should be cleaned and disinfected before placement. All items must be disinfected according to product directions. Because the administrative assistant often prepares cases for and receives them from the dental laboratory, this person should have a clear understanding of the recommended guidelines.

The disinfection of dental impressions and prostheses must be done carefully to avoid the distortion of impressions or damage to the metal, porcelain, or acrylic surfaces of prostheses. The administrative assistant should always consult the dentist or the dental laboratory before disinfecting any material.

EDUCATING PATIENTS ABOUT INFECTION CONTROL PROGRAMS

Effective infection control must become a routine component of professional activity. The use of standard precautions for the treatment of all patients greatly minimizes occupational exposure to microbial pathogens because it addresses the reality that most potentially infectious individuals are asymptomatic and therefore undiagnosed.

PRACTICE NOTE

Effective infection control must become a routine component of professional activity.

Procedures aimed at preventing the spread of infectious disease during dental treatment are constantly evaluated by the profession as well as by consumer agencies. Therefore, the best course of action is to educate the staff and patients about the importance of safe practice and the use of standard precautions for all patients. The dental professional should be willing to freely discuss infection control with patients using valid data. Remember, the two best ways to avoid potential litigation and OSHA inspections are prevention and good documentation.

The dental profession has done much during the past 40 years to encourage the clinical application of infection control techniques and procedures. The implementation of appropriate recommendations by many dental professionals and government organizations continues to have a major impact on the way dental treatment is practiced in the twenty-first century. It is important for dental professionals to keep up with developments and to incorporate new technology into their practices as it becomes available. Membership in OSAP is most beneficial for the practice. This organization is dedicated to promoting infection control and safety policies as well as practices supported by science and research to the global dental community. OSAP provides a method of remaining on the cutting edge in these areas. To obtain information about this organization, visit www.osap.org.

WASTE DISPOSAL IN THE DENTAL OFFICE

Two basic types of waste are found in the dental office: regulated waste and nonregulated waste. Nonregulated waste refers to the total discarded solid waste that is generated from patient diagnosis, treatment, and other management areas. This includes items such as gloves and face masks but not sharps or other infectious or hazardous waste. According to OSHA, "Infectious or regulated waste means blood and blood products, contaminated sharps, pathological wastes, and microbiological wastes." In the past, differences among federal agencies with regard to the definition of infectious medical waste have narrowed. Some states and local jurisdictions may supersede these definitions, but no state or local agency can mandate a regulation that does not first encompass all federal rules.

In general, all **infectious waste** destined for disposal should be placed in closable, leak-proof containers or bags that are color-coded or labeled appropriately while in the dental facility. In the book *Infection Control and Management of Hazardous Materials for the Dental Team*, 4th edition, Miller and Palenik state that "the prevailing view is that no epidemiologic evidence suggests that most medical waste is any more infective than residential waste. Also, no epidemiologic evidence indicates that current medical/dental waste handling and disposal procedures have caused disease in the community. Therefore identifying wastes for which special precautions are necessary is largely a matter of judgment concerning the relative risk of disease transmission."

The primary factor in defining regulated medical waste is determined by the presence of blood or other potentially infectious material (OPIM). In dentistry, OPIM is mainly saliva. Most of the regulated waste in dental offices consists of contaminated sharps and extracted teeth. Some offices involved with surgeries may also generate a small amount of nonsharp solid medical waste, such as 2 × 2 gauze or cotton rolls that are saturated or caked with blood or saliva.

Warning labels should be affixed to containers of infectious waste. The labels required by OSHA should be used in the office. These labels should be fluorescent orange, orange-red, or predominantly so and should have lettering or symbols in a contrasting color.

Although the administrative assistant is not directly responsible for the preparation of the waste, this person should ensure that all infectious material is disposed of in accordance with federal, state, and local regulations and that appropriate forms are maintained. A medical waste tracking form (Figure 17-15) is completed for medical waste disposal, if required by a particular state, and a shipment log (Figure 17-16) is used to verify the mode of transport and other vital information.

Sharp contaminated items should be disposed of in a specialized sharps container, which must be disposed of according to local and state regulations. Amalgam waste, such as used capsules and disposable suction traps, may not be placed in trash containers; it must be recycled according to best practices for amalgam waste disposal. The ADA has prepared a brochure for dental practices that details these practices and can be found at www.ada.org.

MEDICAL WASTE TRACKING FORM

GENERATOR

1. Generator's Name and Mailing Address
2. Tracking Form Number
4. State Permit or ID No.
3. Telephone Number ( )
5. Transporter's Name and Mailing Address
6. Telephone Number ( )
7. State Transporter Permit or ID No.
EPA Med. Waste ID No.
8. Destination Facility Name and Address
9. Telephone Number ( )
10. State Permit or ID No.

11. US EPA Waste Description	12. Total No. Containers	13. Total Weight or Volume
a. Regulated Medical Waste (Untreated)		
b. Regulated Medical Waste (Treated)		
c. State Regulated Medical Waste		

14. Special Handling Instructions and Additional Information

15. Generator's Certification:
Under penalty of criminal and civil prosecution for the making or submission of false statements, representations, or omissions, I declare, on behalf of the generator ______, that the contents of this consignment are fully and accurately described above and are classified, packaged, marked, and labeled in accordance with all applicable State and Federal regulations, and that I have been authorized, in writing, to make such declarations by the person in charge of the generator's operation.

Printed/Typed name Signature Date

INSTRUCTIONS

INSTRUCTIONS FOR COMPLETING MEDICAL WASTE TRACKING FORM

Copy 1 — GENERATOR COPY: Mailed by Destination Facility to Generator
Copy 2 — DESTINATION FACILITY COPY: Retained by Destination Facility
Copy 3 — TRANSPORTER COPY: Retained by Transporter
Copy 4 — GENERATOR COPY: Retained by Generator
As required under 40 CFR Part 259:
1. This multicopy (4-page) shipping document must accompany each shipment of regulated medical waste generated in a Covered State.
2. Items numbered 1-14 must be completed before the generator can sign the certification. Items 4, 7, 10, 11c, & 19 are optional unless required by the State. Item 22 must be completed by the destination facility.

For assistance in completing this form, contact your nearest State office or Regional EPA office, or call (800) 424-9346.

TRANSPORTER

16. Transporter 1 (Certification of Receipt of Medical Waste as described in items 11, 12, & 13)
Printed/Typed name Signature Date
17. Transporter 2 or Intermediate Handler (name and address)
18. Telephone Number ( )
19. State Transporter Permit or ID No.
EPA Med. Waste ID No.
20. Transporter 2 or Intermediate Handler (Certification of Receipt of Medical Waste as described in items 11, 12, &13)
Printed/Typed name Signature Date
21. New Tracking Form Number (for consolidated or remanifested waste)

DESTINATION

22. Destination facility (Certification of Receipt of Medical Waste as described in items 11, 12, & 13)
☐ Received in accordance with items 11, 12, &13
Printed/Typed name Signature Date
(If other than destination facility, indicate address, phone, and permit or ID no. in box 14.)
23. Discrepancy Box (Any discrepancies should be noted by item number and initials)

FIGURE 17-15 Sample medical waste tracking form.

Transporter Name and Address	Transporter State Permit or ID Number	Quantity and Category of Waste Transported: Containers	Pounds	Date of Shipment	Signature of Representative Accepting Waste for Transport
		Untreated		__/__/__	
		Treated			
		Untreated		__/__/__	
		Treated			
		Untreated		__/__/__	
		Treated			
		Untreated		__/__/__	
		Treated			
		Untreated		__/__/__	
		Treated			
		Untreated		__/__/__	
		Treated			
		Untreated		__/__/__	
		Treated			

FIGURE 17-16 Sample generator shipment log.

LEARNING ACTIVITIES

1. Explain why it is important that each member of the dental team understand the concepts of infection control and the need for immunization.
2. Identify common barrier materials and explain their use.
3. Explain what is meant by *standard* (formerly *universal*) *precautions*.
4. Describe the role that the administrative assistant plays in infection control.
5. Review various office situations, and identify incidents that might require special attention to prevent the transmission of disease-causing organisms from the treatment room or dental laboratory to the business office.

Please refer to the student workbook for additional learning activities.

BIBLIOGRAPHY

American Dental Association: ADA regulatory compliance manual, Chicago, 2014, American Dental Association.

Centers for Disease Control and Prevention: 2005 guidelines for preventing *M. tuberculosis* in health care settings, Washington, DC, 2005, Centers for Disease Control and Prevention.

Kohn WG, Collins AS, Cleveland JL; Centers for Disease Control and Prevention: Guidelines for infection control in dental health-care settings—2003, MMWR Recomm Rep 52(RR-17):1–61, 2003.

Miller CH, Palenik CJ: Infection control and management of hazardous materials for the dental team, ed 5, St Louis, 2013, Mosby.

Molinari JA: Infection control: its evolution to the current standard precautions, J Am Dent Assoc 134(5):569–574, 2003.

Molinari JA, Harte JA, editors: Cottone's practical infection control in dentistry, ed 3, Philadelphia, 2009, Lippincott Williams & Wilkins.

RECOMMENDED WEBSITES

www.cdc.gov/handhygiene
www.ada.org
www.needlestick.com
www.cdcresources.org
www.osha.gov/fso/osp/index.html
www.osap.org
www.hepfi.org/hepinfo/fact5201-99.htm

Planning and Managing Your Career Path

http://evolve.elsevier.com/Finkbeiner/practice

LEARNING OUTCOMES

1. Define the key terms in this chapter.
2. Discuss preparing for a job search and five important questions you should ask yourself.
3. Identify your personal assets and liabilities for a job.
4. Discuss methods of marketing your skills.
5. Identify personal priorities for a potential job.
6. Identify potential areas of employment.
7. Discuss places to find employment opportunities.
8. Prepare employment data for job applications.
9. Discuss the steps that can help you prepare for a job interview and how to follow-up after the interview.
10. List hints for success in a job on the dental team and discuss the best way to ask for a raise.
11. Describe how to terminate a job and the importance of a good attitude for continued success.

KEY TERMS

Blind ad An advertisement that does not show the person or organization that placed the ad.

Chronological résumé A résumé that includes education and experience information in chronological order.

Functional résumé A résumé that will list your skills first and then your work experience.

Job application A form with a series of questions that request comprehensive data about the applicant, including educational background and work and professional experience.

Letter of application The letter that accompanies a personal résumé; it introduces the applicant and tries to arouse interest to prompt an interview with the prospective employer; also called a *cover letter.*

Portfolio A compilation of samples of the applicant's work; it may include letters, spreadsheets, reports, PowerPoint slides, or other items.

Professional summary An element of a résumé that may also be referred to as an *objective.* It is a succinct listing of personal data, qualifications, experience, education, and the goal of seeking a job.

Résumé A listing of all the applicant's vital data, as well as information about the person's education and career experiences.

PREPARING FOR THE JOB SEARCH

Planning and Organizing

At this juncture in reading this text, you have mastered a variety of skills. It is now time to begin a job search. The emphasis in this text has been placed on the administrative assistant and the business office. However, this chapter is designed to apply to all members of the dental health team looking to secure a position as a healthcare provider.

As a clinical or administrative assistant, you may have completed a formal educational program or course of study, or you may already have passed a certification examination or another credentialing examination. Similarly, as a dental hygienist, you will have completed an accredited formal education program and have obtained or be in the process of obtaining a license for a specific state. Now you are ready to begin the job search. A successful job search requires organization and effort. You cannot simply walk out the door and wander around asking about jobs, and you cannot look for work only when you feel like it or when it is convenient. Planning and organizing are critical to job search success. This chapter will help you to plan and organize yourself to begin the most important career task of your working life.

When you apply for various jobs, your prospective employers will assume that you have completed your studies and obtained your credentials as a Certified Dental Assistant, a Registered Dental Assistant, or a Registered Dental Hygienist or that you have some form of business specialty credentials. This chapter emphasizes the tasks necessary to market your skills as a highly educated healthcare provider with special training in business office management, clinical dental assisting, or dental hygiene.

You sometimes may feel nervous about the prospect of taking a credentialing examination or finding a job. Even after attending formal classes or studying for a specific job, your self-confidence may falter. However, cultivating positive attitudes and taking time to reflect on career goals often help a person to get on track when seeking a job. This is the time in your career when you must reflect on all of the skills you have acquired. The top nine *hard skills* sought by dentist employers are as follows:

1. Interpersonal skills
2. Teamwork skills
3. Verbal communication skills
4. Critical thinking skills
5. Technical skills
6. Computer skills
7. Written communication skills
8. Leadership skills
9. Clinical skills for the specific job

PRACTICE NOTE

Cultivating positive attitudes and taking time to reflect on career goals often help a person get on track when seeking a job.

In addition to hard skills, you have gained *soft skills*, such as value clarification, self-discipline, ethical behavior, positive attitudes, creativity, and anger and stress management. As you reflect on your skills, both hard and soft, you should analyze what they mean to your career path.

Five Important Questions

Before you venture into the job market as a dental healthcare provider, you must identify your career goals. Obviously you are interested in a facet of dentistry (either clinical or the business office) because you have spent considerable time studying this field. Therefore, you should explore ways your career can develop in this area in the future. A career path is based on careful planning and preparation, but it can be altered by unexpected opportunities and luck. To begin preparation, you should ask yourself the series of questions shown in the job preparation ladder (Figure 18-1). Prospective employers will put your résumé on the top of the job application pile if you spend some time reflecting on each of these questions: Where have I been? Where am I now? Where am I going? How am I going to get there? How will I know when I have arrived?

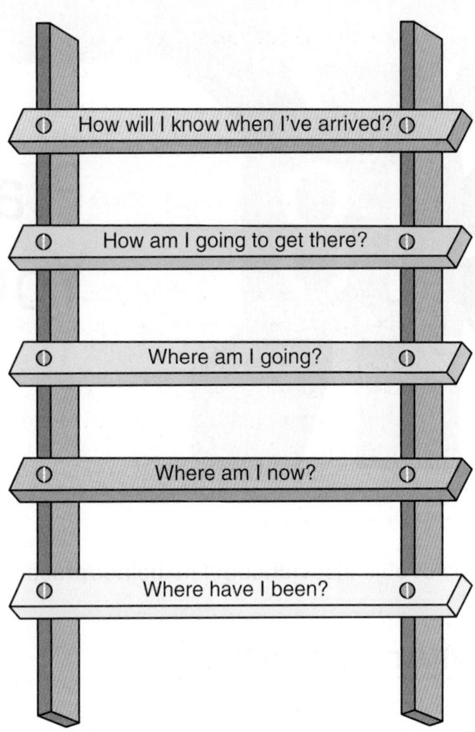

FIGURE 18-1 Job preparation ladder. Questions to ask yourself when preparing for a job search.

Before going to any job interviews, you should share your thoughts about these questions with peers or spend some time alone reflecting on them. This sharing and introspection can help you to build confidence in your plans and goals for a career.

Where Have I Been?

This question helps you to review your past and identify some of the reasons you arrived where you are. It is your origin and thus forms the foundation of your preparation ladder. Some individuals may find looking at the past depressing, whereas others may yearn for the comfort of the past. Regardless of the impact of your past, reflection is worthwhile. Some personal information is confidential, and certain types of questions may not be asked during a job interview; however, it is wise to be prepared for questions about your past employment. For example, if you have worked at several jobs in the past, you may be asked about your reasons for having changed jobs frequently. You should explain your job history honestly.

Where Am I Now?

This question seems obvious, yet you need to reassure yourself about where you are in your career path. You have just completed a course of study, you are secure or insecure in a personal or family relationship, and you are looking forward to finding a job soon or sometime in the future. Knowing where you are at the present time enables you to continue on your career path.

Where Am I Going?

This is a goal-oriented question that requires you to identify what you want to do. As you progress up the preparation ladder, you must stop to think about what you want in both the near future and the distant future. For some individuals, getting a job and gaining independence are their primary goals. For others, the job may be the means to a future goal. Obtaining a job now, gaining experience, and continuing with one's education may be several short-range goals that are needed to reach the ultimate goal of teaching, obtaining a business degree, or even going to dental school. Regardless of your goals, you must realize that they may change; remaining flexible in your goals enables you to accept challenges along the way.

How Am I Going to Get There?

This question identifies the route or steps that must be taken to achieve your goals. For some, a job means independence or a sense of security and self-worth. For others, who are pursuing additional education, a short-term job supports a return to school for another degree.

How Will I Know When I Have Arrived?

This is the top rung of the ladder. To answer this question, you must define what success means to you. For some people, the definition of success is always changing. Money, material goods, or a feeling of security and satisfaction can represent success. No one answer is correct for this question. It is an individual response that only you can give.

Taking time to prepare yourself for your future career can influence a job interview. When a dentist or office manager asks you to describe yourself, your background, and your career goals, you will be prepared. If you simply say something like, "Oh, I don't know, there isn't much to tell," this indicates that you have not given your career much thought, and a potential employer might think you feel the same about employment.

SELF-ASSESSMENT

Critical Analysis

As you begin the job search, ask yourself, "What skills and characteristics can I bring to a job and a prospective employer?" Take the time to write down your skills, strengths, and weaknesses with a prospective job in mind.

PRACTICE NOTE

Take the time to write down your skills, strengths, and weaknesses with a prospective job in mind.

As you begin this exercise, you may find that you seem to concentrate on your weaknesses. This is not uncommon. Parents, teachers, and associates share criticism willingly, thinking that it improves a person, but sincere praise might not be given as freely. Criticism may be so common that, when praise is offered, it might be difficult to accept. Learn to accept praise, identify your positive characteristics, and develop your assets.

This is also a time to be optimistic. Remember earlier in the text when the term *locus of control* was discussed? The "internal locus of control" was related to outcomes that are within your control. Good outcomes can result from positive attitudes, and optimism is an attitude that helps people to succeed and bounce back from hardship. There are many benefits from being an optimistic person, as shown in Box 18-1.

Identifying Personal Assets and Liabilities

How do you begin to do this? First, identify your positive characteristics and your skills. Next, identify your liabilities, but analyze how these weaknesses can be overcome. For example, if you are prompt and seldom absent and if you pay attention to details, you have characteristics that employers seek in a new employee (Box 18-2). You may find it difficult to use a specific type of software, or you may have a problem remembering all

BOX 18-1

Benefits of Optimism

- It enables you to generate an alternative, more hopeful explanation for difficulties experienced.
- It reduces your level of stress.
- It increases longevity.
- It promotes happiness.
- It forges persistence, which is an essential trait required for achieving success.
- It creates a sense of fulfillment and satisfaction.
- It promotes healthy living.
- It creates a positive anticipation of the future.
- It allows you to deal with failure and mistakes constructively.
- It makes you proactive.
- It enables you to deal with the constant negative thoughts that arise.
- If increases the likelihood of effective problem solving.
- It creates a positive attitude.
- It increases your level of motivation.
- It promotes laughter.
- It welcomes any form of constructive change.
- It creates positive expectations.
- It sets your mood for the day.
- It promotes positive relationships.
- It builds resilience in the face of adversity.
- It promotes self-confidence and boosts self-esteem.
- It improves your social life.
- It increases your spiritual development and awakening.
- It increases your mental flexibility.
- It is therapeutic.

From Job readiness for health professionals, St. Louis, 2013, Elsevier.

BOX 18-2

Desirable Characteristics of a New Employee

- Promptness
- Initiative
- Dependability
- Creativity
- Flexibility
- Self-motivation
- Enthusiasm
- Honesty
- Sense of humor
- Good general health
- Willingness to accept change
- Good listener
- Willingness to work with a team
- Effective organizational skills
- Knowledge of automated equipment
- Use of proper language skills in verbal and written communications
- Attention to detail

of the American Dental Association (ADA) insurance codes; however, these skill deficiencies can be improved with experience. If a prospective employer asks about any weaknesses, you could explain that, although you have had difficulty using a specific type of software, you would like to improve this skill and are willing to spend some extra time on your own to do so. This is a positive attitude that shows an interest in improving yourself rather than demonstrating an attitude of not caring.

Likewise, a person in the clinical arena of the office may find using a specific type of instrument intraorally quite difficult. Again, a willingness to overcome this weaker skill will illustrate an eagerness for improvement.

MARKETING YOUR SKILLS

A well-educated and experienced dental healthcare provider with the appropriate credentials has valuable bargaining power for obtaining a job that requires the desired skills and provides adequate compensation. Stating that you are a graduate of a dental assistant, hygiene, or business program is a credible assertion; however, supporting this claim with valid data that demonstrate the positive effect you can have on the practice is likely to win you the job.

As you discuss your skills either in the interview or in the letter of application, use action words that end in "-ed," such as *implemented, applied,* or *educated.* These words describe activities or actions that you have taken. Terms like *go-getter* and *people person* are vague and do not really mean anything.

Supporting Your Skills in Marketing

Administrative Assistant

Often a dentist will claim that he or she cannot afford a well-educated administrative assistant. Your response might be, "I don't believe that you can afford *not* to have a well-educated administrative assistant." Consider the following rebuttals to the dentist's reluctance:

- Credentialed administrative assistants have proved by some form of study and perhaps by a test given by a valid national dental or business board that they have a basic understanding of dental knowledge and business procedures. Delegating business functions to an inexperienced person with no formal knowledge of business principles or the standards required by the Occupational Safety and Health Administration (OSHA) is opening the door to potential penalties and litigation.
- Losses caused by errors in records management, claim form management, appointment scheduling, payroll, accounts receivable, banking, accounts payable, or patient communication can be significantly reduced if a qualified educated administrative assistant is put in charge of those elements of the practice. Although an initial orientation period is necessary in any office, an educated administrative assistant is already aware of the procedures and terminology used in business and dentistry.

Clinical Assistant

A similar situation can occur when the dentist makes this claim to a clinical assistant who is a graduate of an accredited program and who has met the state licensure requirements for advanced functions. This assistant should explain how she or he can increase productivity. Studies in the past have indicated that a skilled clinical assistant at chairside can increase productivity by more than 30%. An assistant credentialed in advanced functions can increase productivity even more, because this allows the dentist to proceed to another patient while the expanded-function dental assistant performs specific intraoral duties.

Dental Hygienist

The dental hygienist needs to promote himself or herself by indicating that he or she is able to perform the basic skills allowed in the state as well as additional skills that can be legally performed. These include the use of computer software, an intraoral camera, and digital radiography; the making of bleaching trays; the placement of antimicrobial agents; and, if certified in that state, the administration of local anesthesia and nitrous oxide. These tasks all become great time savers for the dentist.

Other factors that might be considered when a hygienist is marketing himself or herself include the following:

- An educated person remains in the profession longer than an inexperienced person because the former has made a commitment to the profession through the educational process.
- Mature students who return to school from other careers, such as homemaking, teaching, and nursing, can bring with them many life experiences that are valuable assets to any one of the healthcare provider positions.

You must develop a caring, positive attitude about your ability to become an asset to the dental office. It is your responsibility, however, to live up to the claims you make. Your skills, knowledge of dentistry, investment in your education, and credentials are all tools that can be used to achieve compensation commensurate with that of other allied health or business professionals with similar backgrounds and responsibilities.

PRACTICE NOTE

You must develop a caring, positive attitude about your ability to become an asset to the dental office.

JOB PRIORITIES

Each person dreams of his or her ideal job. However, many people are so excited to be given an interview that they take the first job offered without considering their goals, needs, and priorities. Before applying for a job or preparing for a job interview, decide what you need and want in a job and what your basic philosophy is about your career.

Determining Your Career Philosophy

As mentioned previously, before seeking employment, you should determine your needs, clarify your life goals, and then develop a philosophy that is consistent with them. Unfortunately, a dental healthcare provider may accept the first job offered with little consideration given to how his or her philosophy coincides with the philosophy of the prospective employer. Carefully evaluate yourself, establish some realistic goals, and then ask yourself the following questions: Are my professional, moral, and social values compatible with those of my prospective employer? With what type of work environment do I want to be associated: a solo practice or a large group practice? Which of my skills in dentistry or business do I want to use to the greatest extent? What are my strengths? What are my weaknesses? How can I compensate for my weaknesses? What do I want to be doing in 5 years and in 10 years? How important are salary, hours, and location?

Once you have written down your philosophy of life and enumerated your goals, remind yourself that these goals will be ever changing. You will undoubtedly reevaluate your philosophy as you gain confidence from your new experiences.

After you have reviewed the various factors involved in job selection, determine your top five priorities for a job, and then rate each job offer. A decision-making grid such as the one shown in Table 18-1 may be helpful for this purpose. The job offers are listed in the left vertical column, and the priorities are listed across the top. Starting on the left, the priorities are given a point value based on your personal needs. Each job is evaluated, and the points are totaled. If a tie occurs, other characteristics may be considered.

Remember, you may need to do more than one or two interviews to find the job that satisfies your goals, needs, and priorities. Remain steadfast in your job search.

Determining Your Worth to a Practice

Although many elements may be considered important when deciding whether to accept a job offer, salary and benefits are the primary factors in job selection for most people. The difficulty often arises when a dentist asks you during an interview what salary you expect. You need to prepare yourself for this question and not simply say, "Oh, I don't know, what have you paid your other assistants or hygienists?" You need to have a firm understanding of the cost of living in your area, the comparable salaries for similar responsibilities and educational attainment, the local and national salary data available for reference, and what you are really worth in terms of your skills and knowledge. The following discussion provides ideas for formulating a benefits and salary package that could reasonably be suggested to a prospective employer. Box 18-3 lists several benefits that are commonly offered to employees.

Salary is often a difficult subject to bring up, yet it must be discussed openly before you accept a job. You need to know the beginning salary, how salary increases are obtained, and when salary increases are awarded. An employer must expect to pay a fair salary that is based on education, experience, credentials, and merit performance. The salary should be competitive with

BOX 18-3

Potential Job Benefits

- Dress/uniform allowance
- Retirement plan
- Health insurance
- Vision insurance
- Dental care/insurance (for self and family)
- Profit sharing
- Child care
- Membership in professional organizations
- Travel and expenses for professional meetings
- Special bonuses for holidays or production achievement

TABLE 18-1 Job Decision-Making Grid

	Practice Environment	Salary	Benefits	Location	Challenge	Hours	Total
Point value	6	5	4	3	2	1	
Job offer 1		√	√	√	√	√	15
Job offer 2	√		√	√			13
Job offer 3	√	√		√			14

other allied health professionals who have equal responsibilities, yet it should also be cost-effective.

PRACTICE NOTE

An employer must expect to pay a fair salary that is based on education, experience, credentials, and merit performance.

The economics of dentistry vary widely across the country, depending on the specific position, its responsibilities, and the geographical location of the practice. Salary data may be obtained from the American Dental Association (ADA) website (www.ada.org), the American Dental Hygienist's Association website (www.adha.org), and the American Dental Assistant's Association website (www.dentalassistant.org). The Dental Assistant National Board website (www.danb.org) also has information for dental assistants about studies completed regarding salaries in various areas of the country. Information may also be found in the *Occupational Outlook Handbook* produced by the U.S. Department of Labor.

Realize that these studies often present a median national hourly salary with no benefits included. It is sometimes stated that some dental healthcare providers make higher hourly salaries than others. When salaries are discussed, care must be taken to determine that all factors related to the salaries being compared are the same. Some dollar value must be given to each of the benefits to determine the total salary and benefits package. Determine whether the job responsibilities are equitable. Education, experience, credentials, and performance evaluations are factored into the salary. Some value must also be placed on the job environment. It is possible that a person could take a job because its salary was so much better than another offer. However, this person may soon find out that the environment is hostile and not friendly and thus realize that perhaps a dollar amount should have been placed on the environment. Maybe this person should have accepted the job that paid a dollar less an hour but that included a more pleasant work environment.

Remember, no skilled administrative assistant, clinical assistant, or dental hygienist in today's market should be making a salary that does not reflect an honest respect for the individual's productivity. It is wise to ask for a contract or an employment agreement that verifies in writing the conditions of employment. These conditions might include the salary scale, an explanation of the merit performance evaluation, the required probationary period, and how the benefits package is to be administered.

POTENTIAL AREAS OF EMPLOYMENT

For the dental healthcare worker, there is a myriad of opportunities for potential employment. These can range from a small solo practice to a large clinic. They can also include the public or the private sector, practice management consulting firms, dental manufacturers, job placement, and teaching.

Private Practice

One may seek employment in a private practitioner's office, a group practice, or a clinic with several dentists. The practice may be a general dental practice, which means that all phases of dental treatment are rendered for a patient, or it may be limited to one of the dental specialties recognized by the ADA (e.g., endodontics, orthodontics and dentofacial orthopedics, oral and maxillofacial surgery, oral and maxillofacial pathology, pediatric dentistry, periodontics, prosthodontics, oral and maxillofacial radiology, and dental public health).

In private practice, the administrative or clinical assistant may find a position that is limited specifically to clinical assisting, office management, or laboratory duties, or it may involve a combination of all of these responsibilities. Private practice affords many opportunities to work closely with the dentist and the patients as well as the diversification of duties, individuality, and considerable personal responsibility. As the value of a highly skilled dental assistant continues to increase, compensation and benefits in this area will continue to rise.

A similar situation may be available for the dental hygienist. In some situations, a hygienist may find that, to work a full-time load, it may be necessary to work in two different practices. This takes special skill in that the hygienist must learn policies from both offices and maintain confidentiality for both practices.

Institutional Dentistry

As federal, state, and local governments demonstrate increased interest in the delivery of dental care, more facilities are being established to provide more dental services for the public. One institution that should be considered as a source of employment is a dental school. Schools offer many areas of potential employment, such as working with undergraduate or graduate dental students at chairside, supervising clinical activities, and managing business functions. Other institutions are a part of the civil service programs and offer employment in prisons, public clinics, and Veterans Administration hospitals. Additionally, hospitals—some of which are associated closely with dental schools—offer employment in various departments. The dental healthcare provider working in an institution has the opportunity to work with a larger staff than is possible in private dental practice. Diversification of duties, participation in newly developed techniques, potential advancement to several levels of supervision, and possibly more liberal vacations (in learning institutions, vacations are often coordinated with school calendars) may be available in this setting.

Insurance Offices

Work in insurance offices is especially appealing to the person who aspires to perform various business tasks and become involved in management. With the increase in dental insurance coverage, more companies are seeking highly qualified dental healthcare providers to work in management positions because a broad knowledge of dentistry is an asset to their business. A position in insurance may also involve public speaking activities and travel.

Research

Hospitals and dental schools hire many dental healthcare providers to work in research laboratories. Individuals who enjoy working with data, mathematical computations, and details and who enjoy being independent often seek positions in research.

Dental Manufacturers

An area of potential employment that should not be overlooked is with dental manufacturers, which employ dental assistants and hygienists for sales and teaching. Such employment would limit contact with dentistry to a specific type or line of products, but it also offers a great opportunity to travel throughout the country and meet people.

A form of manufacturing would also include software and business system companies. These companies offer the same opportunities as those mentioned previously, and they also offer a special opportunity for the person who is interested in the business component of the dental office.

Management Consulting Firms

Experienced dental assistants and hygienists with a broad knowledge of clinical and business concepts are turning their interests into profitable businesses. Many highly qualified administrative assistants have joined management consulting firms or created their own companies to assist dental practices with increasing their productivity through more efficient practices and marketing.

Teaching

Numerous colleges and universities have developed occupational education programs that include dental assisting and dental hygiene. A graduate of a dental assistant or hygiene program who is a Certified Dental Assistant (CDA), a Registered Dental Assistant (RDA), or a Registered Dental Hygienist (RDH) may transfer into a baccalaureate degree program. Anyone who has broad experience in dental assisting or hygiene, who is highly motivated to teach, and who is patient and objective should perhaps contact a college or university about entering its program. Other sources of information include the American Dental Assistants Association (www.dentalassistant.org) and the American Dental Hygienist Association (www.adha.org).

WHERE DO YOU BEGIN TO FIND EMPLOYMENT OPPORTUNITIES?

After surveying some of these potential areas of employment, where do you begin looking for the right job? Many prospects are available, and several different avenues may be used.

School Placement

The school placement office and its faculty members are often notified regarding job opportunities in the area. Instructors frequently know employers who are interested in hiring new graduates, and they also know their students' qualifications and abilities. Most schools spend considerable time and effort obtaining information about potential job opportunities, and they take a great deal of pride in placing their graduates.

Often a dental assistant finds a job opportunity during a clinical rotation or an externship. This is ideal in that the assistant will have completed a clinical rotation in the office, so he or she will be familiar with the staff and how the office functions; the staff will also have gained some relationship with the student during the externship experience.

Newspaper Advertisements

Both local and out-of-area newspapers have classified sections that list available jobs. Advertisements in the classified section state the qualifications required and other details about the job, including whether it is for an administrative or clinical assistant (Figure 18-2). However, in some cases, the employer does not give the name of the practice or the telephone number but instead places a blind ad asking the applicant to submit a résumé (Figure 18-3). This type of ad should not be overlooked, because it becomes the employer's first means of screening applicants.

When composing a letter of application and a résumé, always remember that although first impressions are not necessarily the most accurate, they often are the most influential. A little more initiative is required of the applicant to construct a résumé than to pick up the telephone and call for an interview. The letter of application and the résumé give the prospective employer an opportunity to evaluate the applicant's keyboarding skills, communication skills, and neatness.

Employment Agencies

Both free and private employment agencies are available. Most states provide an employment service, and applicants may register with this service at no charge.

Private employment agencies, which are service enterprises, provide many good job opportunities, but they do charge a fee. Before registering with an employment agency, always check its reputation. This can be done locally or through the National Employment Association in Washington, DC. In many states, dental healthcare providers have begun their own employment agencies; this type of firm is more likely to work with applicants with a dental background as determined by the agency's screening processes. After selecting a reputable agency, the applicant should find out about testing and placement procedures.

Professional Organizations and Journals

Local dental societies and dental assistant organizations frequently maintain employment placement services. By checking

Clinical Dental Assistant needed to join a large team-oriented practice. Must have credentials for advanced functions in this state and experience in periodontics. Challenging opportunity for a skilled, ambitious professional assistant. Many benefits included. Salary commensurate to education and credentials. Send résumé to: Joseph W. Lake, 611 Main St., SE, Grand Rapids, MI 49502

A

Dental Administrative Assistant needed for a busy orthodontic office. This position requires an energetic, ambitious person who has a broad knowledge of dentistry and business applications. For a person who enjoys a fast pace, this office provides a challenging career opportunity in practice management utilizing modern electronic business systems. Current practice management education preferred. Write to: Ashley M. Lake, DDS, 611 Main St., SE, Grand Rapids, MI 49502

B

Our established dental office staff is looking for an experienced Dental Hygienist. Must be a motivated self-starter! Applicants must be friendly, possess excellent communication skills and have the ability to deliver exceptional patient service. Bilingual a plus. Dentrix knowledge helpful. Compensation: based on experience. Write to Box 1334 Grand Rapids Press, 228 Fulton St., E., Grand Rapids, MI 49502

C

FIGURE 18-2 **A,** Job advertisement for a clinical chairside assistant. **B,** Advertisement for an administrative assistant describing the position and the type of dental practice. **C,** A job application for a dental hygienist with specific skill requirements listed.

Dental Administrative Assistant: Interested in an exciting position in a small, professional office? A group dental practice is expanding its clinical facilities. Position demands strong supervisory skills; ability to work effectively under pressure, use good judgment, and accept responsibility; and a working knowledge of OSHA standards. Forward your résumé to: 228 Fulton St., E., Grand Rapids News, Grand Rapids, MI 49502

FIGURE 18-3 A sample blind advertisement.

your local telephone directory or the Internet, you can quickly establish contact with one of these organizations. State and national professional journals generally have a classified section devoted to job offerings for dental assistants. Many of these jobs offer unique opportunities and possibly even relocation. State and local dental associations often allow new graduates to publish their contact information in the association's newsletter or journal free of charge.

Internet and World Wide Web

The Internet is a group of computers connected all over the world that allows people to communicate with each other. For example, on the Internet, you can obtain information about companies and dental offices worldwide.

If you are interested in working with a large dental manufacturing company or a dental school, you can use the Internet and the computer files of the World Wide Web to find information about them. Many major companies and dental schools post company profiles and employment opportunities on the Internet. More dental practices are using this method to seek potential employees. Many websites are available (e.g., www.craigslist.com, www.monster.com, www.careerbuilder.com) that can provide information for your job search or allow you to post your résumé.

Personal Networks

Networking is the process of identifying and establishing a group of acquaintances, friends, and relatives who can assist you in the job search process. This approach is one of the best strategies for finding a job. In fact, some studies have shown that as many as 80% of jobs are obtained through some form of networking. Friends, relatives, business associates, local dental assistant societies, dental associations, dental supply houses, and dental schools all offer myriad contacts; these contacts can then provide potential contacts in the profession, which may lead to a job opportunity. If a friend is leaving a job and knows that you are interested in the same area of dentistry and available to work, a good recommendation from him or her is always welcome.

How do you go about networking? If you have a part-time job or had a clinical rotation in an office or clinic while you were a student, let the dentist or other staff members know that you are ready for a full-time position. If these individuals know you are interested in a full-time job, they can talk with friends in the community about your skills and often can serve as an excellent reference for you. You may want to consider a social networking website such as Facebook, MySpace, Twitter, and others that provide an opportunity to interact with a network of friends, personal profiles, groups, and other professionals worldwide.

PREPARING EMPLOYMENT DATA

Several steps must be taken between the time you determine your goals and choice of employment and the time you actually begin work. These steps, in addition to career preparation planning, include searching for job information, writing the letter of application, creating a personal résumé, preparing for the interview, completing a job application, participating in the interview, touring the facility and meeting the staff, and following up on the interview (Figure 18-4).

Preparing a Letter of Application

The letter of application or *cover letter* has three basic goals: to arouse interest, to describe your abilities, and to request an interview. The letter of application should be kept to a single page that includes the date and the closing signature. Every effort must be made to customize this letter and to express your philosophy, motivations, and character in a less formal format than the résumé. In fact, this letter may very well be the most important business letter you ever write.

Arouse Interest

In the opening of the letter, indicate how you located the job opportunity, and then introduce yourself to the prospective employer. Include a brief description of your personal qualifications. This opening essentially gives you the opportunity to promote yourself. The letter should make the reader interested enough in your skills and abilities to grant you an interview.

Example 1: "The position you have advertised in the *Grand Rapids News* sounds challenging. My certificate in dental assisting and my credential as a certified dental practice management assistant have provided me the skills necessary to perform the job well. You will find that I have the necessary talents to become an asset to your practice."

Example 2: "Your employment announcement posted on my school bulletin board calls for a clinical chairside assistant who is interested in applying the latest concepts of four-handed dentistry. My education at Grand Rapids Community College has provided me with the skills necessary to be an asset to your office while increasing your productivity."

Example 3: "Your employment announcement calls for an administrative assistant who is interested in learning the latest technology and who has good computer skills. My education at Grand Rapids Community College for the past 2 years has provided me with these skills, and I am ready to become a valuable member of your dental team."

Example 4: "Your advertisement for an experienced dental hygienist piqued my interest. My experience in both a general practice and a periodontal practice as well as teaching part time have provided me with the wealth of experience that you are seeking in a dental hygienist. I am certain that you will find me to be an asset to your staff."

In each of these cases, the applicant lets the prospective employer know that she or he is interested in the position and believes that she or he has the skills needed for the job. Note that each paragraph is oriented toward the reader.

Describe Your Skills and Abilities

The second paragraph of the letter should describe your skills in more detail. It should also call attention to your enclosed résumé, curriculum vitae, or data sheet; these are explained in the next section.

Example: "In August of this year, I will graduate from Grand Rapids Community College. I will have completed courses in business office procedures, clinical procedures, laboratory and radiographic procedures, and dental specialties, and I also have 300 hours of clinical practice in the local community. I had taken courses in accounting, management, business

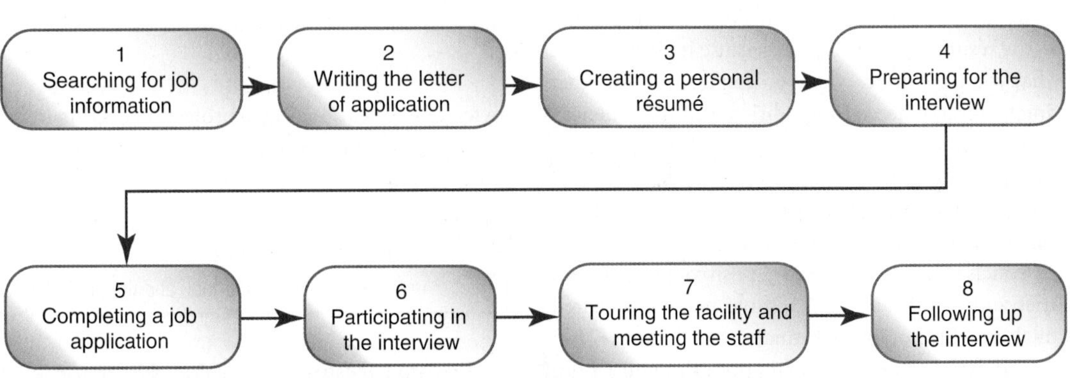

FIGURE 18-4 The career planning process.

communications, and computers before entering the dental assisting program. While in school, I worked part time as a clinical dental assistant in a local dental office."

This brief description includes an overview of basic skills. Further details about the skills and the dates of education and work experience are included in the attached résumé.

Request an Interview

Because the purpose of a cover letter is to obtain an interview, you should ask for the interview directly.

Example: "I would appreciate an opportunity to discuss my qualifications with you. My telephone number is 616-999-2041."
or
"I look forward to an appointment with you so we can discuss how I can become an asset to your dental team."

Box 18-4 presents a list of action verbs that can be used to describe your activities. General guidelines for creating a cover letter are provided in Box 18-5.

Figures 18-5 through 18-8 show letters of application submitted by three applicants with varying backgrounds.

Contacting an Office by Telephone

If you have been informed of a job opening by an instructor or a friend, time may not allow you to write a letter of application; in such cases, a telephone call is required. This situation requires a different approach. First, place a call to the office, and indicate to the individual receiving your call who you are and why you are calling. Second, explain how you learned about the position. Finally, if the job is available, ask for an interview.

Whether you plan to send a letter of application or decide to contact the office by telephone, you must prepare a résumé that you can either enclose with the letter or take with you to the office.

Creating a Résumé

A **résumé**, personal data sheet, or personal history should be prepared to accompany the letter of application or to take with you to the interview. A résumé is a marketing tool, and the product is you. The objective is to capture the attention of the reader and maintain that person's interest. From the employer's point of view, the résumé is a time saver, because it gives a quick account of what you have done, what you can do, and for what you are striving. A résumé needs to be a brief, well-documented account of your qualifications. A simple résumé is best suited for those who are entering the job market or who have limited work experience. Remember, your objective is to be granted an interview; therefore, you want to impress the reader with a résumé that is concise and that presents a positive presentation of your abilities and qualifications. A résumé may be prepared in a functional or chronological format. (See Figures 18-5 through 18-8 to determine which format appeals to you.) Both are acceptable formats, but sometimes the person who has more extensive educational and professional skills may prefer to use the chronological résumé because it lists these categories more succinctly.

BOX 18-4

Action Verbs for Use in Résumés and Cover Letters

- Accomplished
- Achieved
- Active in
- Assisted
- Attained
- Attended
- Brought about
- Communicated
- Completed
- Conducted
- Contributed
- Cooperated
- Coordinated
- Counseled
- Created
- Demonstrated
- Designed
- Formed
- Founded
- Generated
- Graduated
- Headed
- Implemented
- Improved
- Increased
- Initiated
- Installed
- Instructed
- Interviewed
- Kept
- Lectured
- Led
- Maintained
- Managed
- Mediated
- Motivated
- Observed
- Obtained
- Operated
- Ordered
- Organized
- Originated
- Overcame
- Participated
- Perfected
- Performed
- Persuaded
- Placed
- Planned
- Prepared
- Presented
- Printed
- Processed
- Produced
- Programmed
- Proposed
- Proved
- Provided
- Publicized
- Realized
- Received
- Recognized
- Recommended
- Recruited
- Reevaluated
- Refined
- Regulated
- Represented
- Restored
- Reviewed
- Scheduled
- Secured
- Served
- Set up
- Simplified
- Sold
- Spearheaded
- Staffed
- Streamlined
- Substituted
- Trained
- Transformed
- Updated
- Validated

PRACTICE NOTE
A résumé is a marketing tool, and the product is you.

Prepare a customized résumé. Never use a one-size-fits-all document. If you are in an educational program, avoid copying

BOX 18-5

Guidelines for Writing a Letter of Application

1. Create a professional letterhead that includes vital data: your full name, address, telephone number (home, cell, and fax), and e-mail address.
2. Use a standard business letter format.
3. Use personal stationery made of quality bond paper; do not use your current employer's stationery.
4. Make sure your spelling, grammar, punctuation, and capitalization are correct. If you are composing your letter on a computer, always use the spell checker, but remember to have someone else look over the letter, because the spell checker is not always correct.
5. Avoid opening with "My name is. . . ." Your name is on the letterhead and in the closing signature line.
6. Keep the letter short and around three to four paragraphs. Put details in the résumé.
7. Limit the letter to one page.
8. Address the letter to a specific person. Never address an application letter "To whom it may concern." Take time to find out the name of the employer. If it is not available, use "Dear Doctor," or, if the letter is going to a larger organization, "Dear Human Resources Manager."
9. Put the employer's needs first by making the letter "you" oriented; avoid using "I."
10. Send an original letter for each application. Do not send photocopies.
11. Do not copy a letter of application from a book. Make your letter representative of your personal characteristics.
12. Consider mailing your letter and résumé in a large envelope so that it will stand out from the more commonly used no. 10 envelopes on the employer's desk.

a sample from this or any textbook because others in your class may do the same thing. Remember, you want to make your résumé stand out and grab the attention of the reader.

Customize the résumé to fit the position for which you are applying. It is best to create the document in a word processing program on the computer and then save it for future reference. Most software provides several optional templates that allow you to create a professional personal letterhead and a matching résumé. Other suggested templates are available at a variety of websites geared toward job searches. You want to get the attention of the prospective employer when he or she reads the letter, so take time to create an attractive professional image through your stationery. After the letter has been completed, create an original copy on résumé-quality paper, and remember to never send a copied résumé. If this is not possible, try to obtain the finest quality copy possible from a commercial printer. You should also keep a copy for yourself to take with you when going to an office for an interview.

In general, your résumé should be designed with the following suggestions in mind:

- Put yourself in the position of your prospective employer. Try to determine the qualities that the person may be seeking, and emphasize these qualifications.
- Be as impressive as possible, but do not deviate from the truth. This is not the time to be shy and modest. You must tell the reader what you can do, because no one else will do it for you. You are in the position to sell yourself, and you must be positive without being overly assertive.
- Review the material carefully to make sure that you did not forget anything. An overlooked item may be just what the employer is seeking. Box 18-6 presents some hints for writing a résumé.

Every résumé should contain certain information. This includes a professional summary or objective, personal data, qualifications, experience, and education. Optional areas may include objectives, affiliations, and references. The arrangement of and headings for this information can vary, depending on the person's work experience, education, and general goals. It is wise to select a standard format and to emphasize sections in which you have the greatest assets. Regardless of the format selected, there are dos and don'ts for creating an effective résumé; these are presented in Box 18-7.

Personal Data

Personal data include the following:

- Full name
- Address
- Telephone number (home and cell, if available)
- Fax number and e-mail address (if you have these)

Professional Summary

The professional summary section lets the reader know instantly in two or three sentences what you offer and what you seek. Avoid using generic or vague phrases such as "looking for a position at a well-known practice with room to grow." Instead, use this section to promote specific goals and accomplishments, and tout your desire to work in a specific field or area of a dental practice.

> *Example*: "Professional summary: Administrative assistant with 5 years of exceptional dental practice management experience. Extensive knowledge of practice management software, insurance management, and staff supervision. Seeking management role that will use my technology, dental, and human relations skills."

Notice that this summary did not specify what type of dental practice but rather emphasized the person's interest in an office management position. You may also want to list your long-term goals. In that case, the summary might be concluded with the following statement:

> *Example*: "Professional summary: A position as an administrative assistant in a dental office, with a long-range goal of supervisory management."

Education

Be sure to include relevant information about your educational background. List all colleges and universities attended and the date you graduated. The most recent schools should be listed first. List diplomas or degrees as well as awards and scholarships

Text continued on p. 343

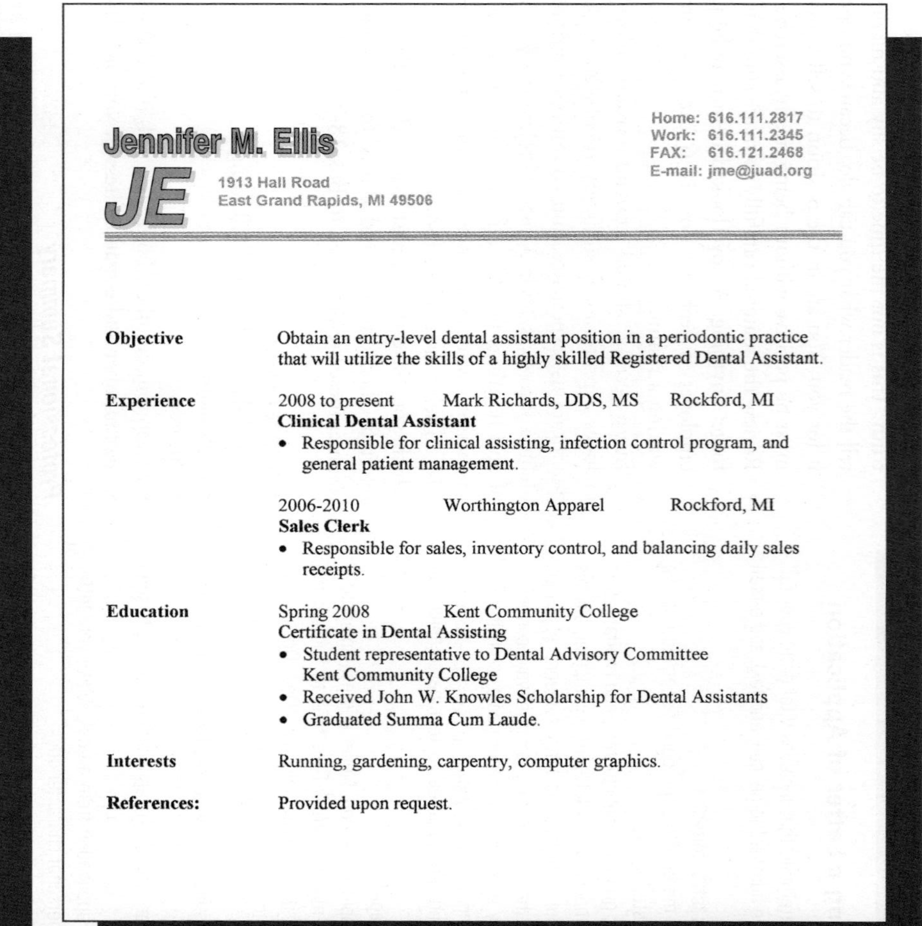

A

Jennifer M. Ellis
JE
1913 Hall Road
East Grand Rapids, MI 49506

Home: 616.111.2817
Work: 616.111.2345
FAX: 616.121.2468
E-mail: jme@juad.org

November 17, 20..

Joseph W. Lake, DDS
611 Main Street SE
Grand Rapids, MI 49502

Dear Dr. Lake:

This letter is in response to your advertisement in the Grand Rapids News, November, 12, 20... You asked for a dental assistant who is skilled in advanced functions, is ambitious, and has experience in Periodontics. I wish to be an applicant for this job and am forwarding my résumé to you. I believe I possess the qualifications you desire.

You will see from the enclosed résumé that I have taken courses at Kent Community College in Grand Rapids, Michigan, to prepare me as a Registered Dental Assistant. I have successfully completed courses in dental assisting that will be valuable to your practice and have had considerable clinical and business office experience. For the past three months I have been working part-time in a periodontic practice while an assistant has been on maternity leave.

You may contact me at 616.111.2817 after 3:00 P.M. any day of the week. I am available for an interview at your convenience.

Sincerely,

Jennifer M. Ellis, RDA

Enclosure

B

Jennifer M. Ellis
JE
1913 Hall Road
East Grand Rapids, MI 49506

Home: 616.111.2817
Work: 616.111.2345
FAX: 616.121.2468
E-mail: jme@juad.org

Objective Obtain an entry-level dental assistant position in a periodontic practice that will utilize the skills of a highly skilled Registered Dental Assistant.

Experience 2008 to present Mark Richards, DDS, MS Rockford, MI
Clinical Dental Assistant
- Responsible for clinical assisting, infection control program, and general patient management.

2006-2010 Worthington Apparel Rockford, MI
Sales Clerk
- Responsible for sales, inventory control, and balancing daily sales receipts.

Education Spring 2008 Kent Community College
Certificate in Dental Assisting
- Student representative to Dental Advisory Committee Kent Community College
- Received John W. Knowles Scholarship for Dental Assistants
- Graduated Summa Cum Laude.

Interests Running, gardening, carpentry, computer graphics.

References: Provided upon request.

FIGURE 18-5 **A,** Letter of application for an entry-level position as a clinical assistant. **B,** Personal résumé to accompany the letter applying for an entry-level position as a clinical assistant.

1847 Sheffield
Ann Arbor, MI 48105
Home: 734.673.1235
Work: 734.768.2800
E-Mail: amy@hotmail.com

From the Desk of Amy S. March

February 5, 20—

Ashley M. Lake, DDS
611 Main St., SE
Grand Rapids, MI 49502

Dear Dr. Lake:

You will find enclosed a resumé I am sending in response to your advertisement in the *Grand Rapids News* for an administrative assistant in your busy orthodontic practice. I believe, after you review this resumé, you will find that I have the qualifications needed to fill this position.

Over the past two years, I have gained a great deal of experience in a large orthodontic practice in Ann Arbor, Michigan. During the second year, I was in charge of insurance management and appointment scheduling. I have attended seminars sponsored by noted insurance companies and had an opportunity recently to attend a practice management course in Chicago on automated claim forms management.

My spouse has recently accepted a position with a law firm in the Grand Rapids area. Since our families both reside in nearby communities, we are delighted to be returning to Grand Rapids. In fact, we will be in the area looking for housing during the next thirty days, so I would welcome a call for an interview.

You may reach me at 734.673.1235 after 6 p.m. or you may leave a message on our answering machine and I will return the call as soon as possible.

Sincerely,

Amy S. March, RDA

Enclosure

A

FIGURE 18-6 A, Letter of application for an office manager in a specialty practice.

Continued

1847 Sheffield
Ann Arbor, MI 48105
Home: 734.673.1235
Work: 734.768.2800
E-Mail: amym@hotmail.com

From the Desk of Amy S. March

PROFESSIONAL SUMMARY

I am seeking a position that needs a highly conscientious, detail-minded professional with education and clinical experience in orthodontics. Accustomed to working with a diverse patient clientele. Excellent communication and motivational skills with an interest in a challenging career in dental assisting.

EXPERIENCE

2009-Present	Orthodontic Associates Ann Arbor, MI *Business office manager*
2006-2009	Gerald Wilson, DDS, MS Ann Arbor, MI *Clinical dental assistant*
2002-2006	University of Michigan School of Dentistry Ann Arbor, MI ♦ Operative Dentistry Department ♦ Oral Diagnosis Department

EDUCATION

June 2004	Delta Midwest Insurance Lansing, MI ♦ Processing claim forms seminar
June 2002	Washtenaw Community College Ann Arbor, MI ♦ Certificate, Dental Assisting ♦ WCC Dental Departmental Scholarship

CREDENTIALS

December 2002	Michigan Board of Dentistry Licensure RDA
August 2002	Dental Assisting National Board CDA

REFERENCES

Provided upon request.

B

FIGURE 18-6, cont'd **B,** Personal résumé, chronological style, to accompany the letter applying for the position of office manager in a specialty office.

Amy S. March
1847 Sheffield
Ann Arbor, MI 48105
Home: 734-673-1235
Cell phone: 734.768.1111
E-mail: amym@hotmail.com

CAREER OBJECTIVE

Highly conscientious, detailed minded with great ability to multitask and able to work with a diverse clientele. Excellent communication and motivational skills and am seeking an opportunity in a challenging orthodontic practice.

PROFESSIONAL SKILLS

EXCEPTIONAL PATIENT SERVICE: Strong communication skills to understand patient needs and provide exceptional results. Track record of successfully managing difficult patients.

ADAPTABLE TO TECHNOLOGY: Proficient in several types of dental software, Microsoft Office including Word, Excel, and PowerPoint and able to operate all major office equipment.

INDEPENDENT AND TEAM PLAYER: Enjoy collaborating with colleagues, patients as well as completing tasks independently. Eager to motivate and inspire others to deliver their best.

LANGUAGE SKILLS: Conversant in Spanish.

PROFESSIONAL (AND/OR VOLUNTEER) EXPERIENCE

2009-Present	Orthodontic Associates Ann Arbor, MI *Business office manager*
2006-2009	Gerald Wilson, DDS, MS Ann Arbor, MI *Clinical dental assistant*
2002-2006	University of Michigan School of Dentistry Ann Arbor, MI ♦ Operative Denstistry Department ♦ Oral Diagnosis Department

EDUCATION

June 2004	Delta Midwest Insurance Lansing, MI ♦ Processing claim forms seminar
June 2002	Washtenaw Community College Anna Arbor, MI ♦ Certificate, Dental Assisting ♦ WCC Dental Departmental Scholarship

CREDENTIALS

December 2002	Michigan Board of Dentistry Licensure RDA
August 2002	Dental Assisting National Board CDA

REFERENCES

Provided upon request.

C

FIGURE 18-6, cont'd C, Personal résumé, functional style, to accompany the letter applying for the position of office manager in a specialty office.

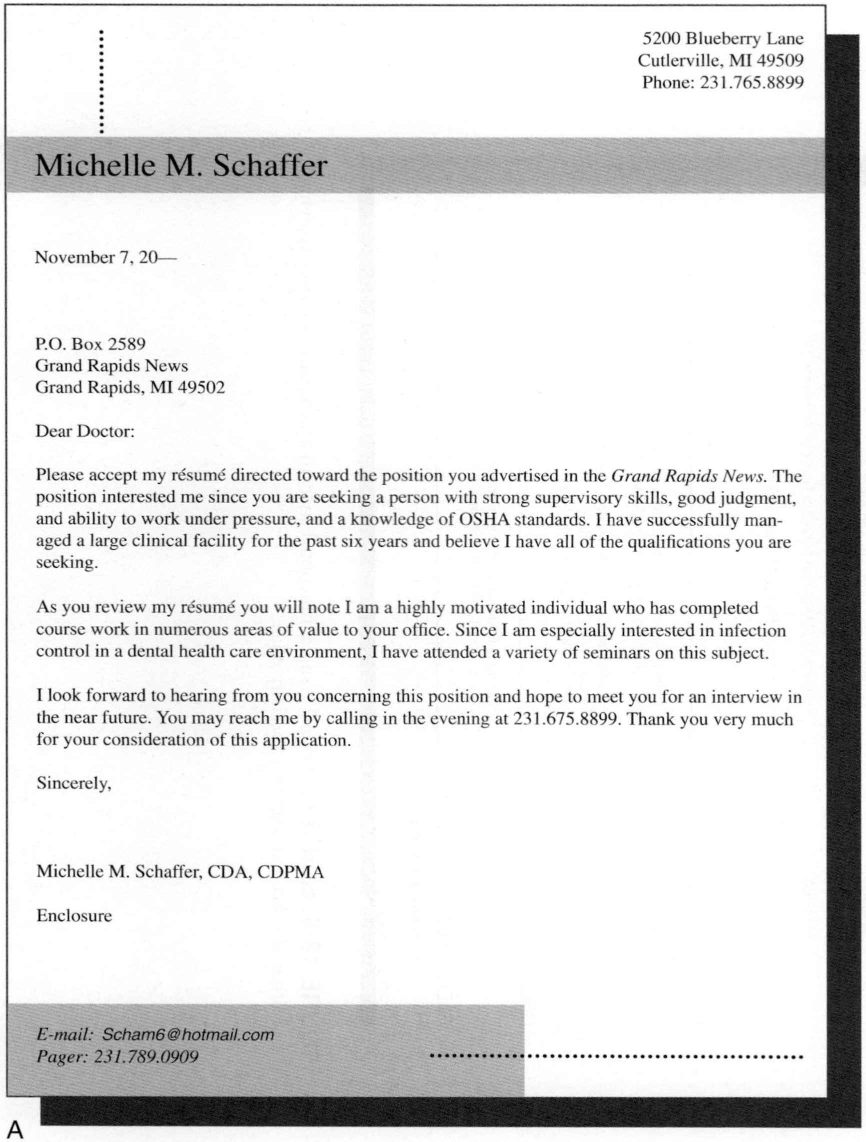

5200 Blueberry Lane
Cutlerville, MI 49509
Phone: 231.765.8899

Michelle M. Schaffer

November 7, 20—

P.O. Box 2589
Grand Rapids News
Grand Rapids, MI 49502

Dear Doctor:

Please accept my résumé directed toward the position you advertised in the *Grand Rapids News*. The position interested me since you are seeking a person with strong supervisory skills, good judgment, and ability to work under pressure, and a knowledge of OSHA standards. I have successfully managed a large clinical facility for the past six years and believe I have all of the qualifications you are seeking.

As you review my résumé you will note I am a highly motivated individual who has completed course work in numerous areas of value to your office. Since I am especially interested in infection control in a dental health care environment, I have attended a variety of seminars on this subject.

I look forward to hearing from you concerning this position and hope to meet you for an interview in the near future. You may reach me by calling in the evening at 231.675.8899. Thank you very much for your consideration of this application.

Sincerely,

Michelle M. Schaffer, CDA, CDPMA

Enclosure

E-mail: Scham6@hotmail.com
Pager: 231.789.0909

A

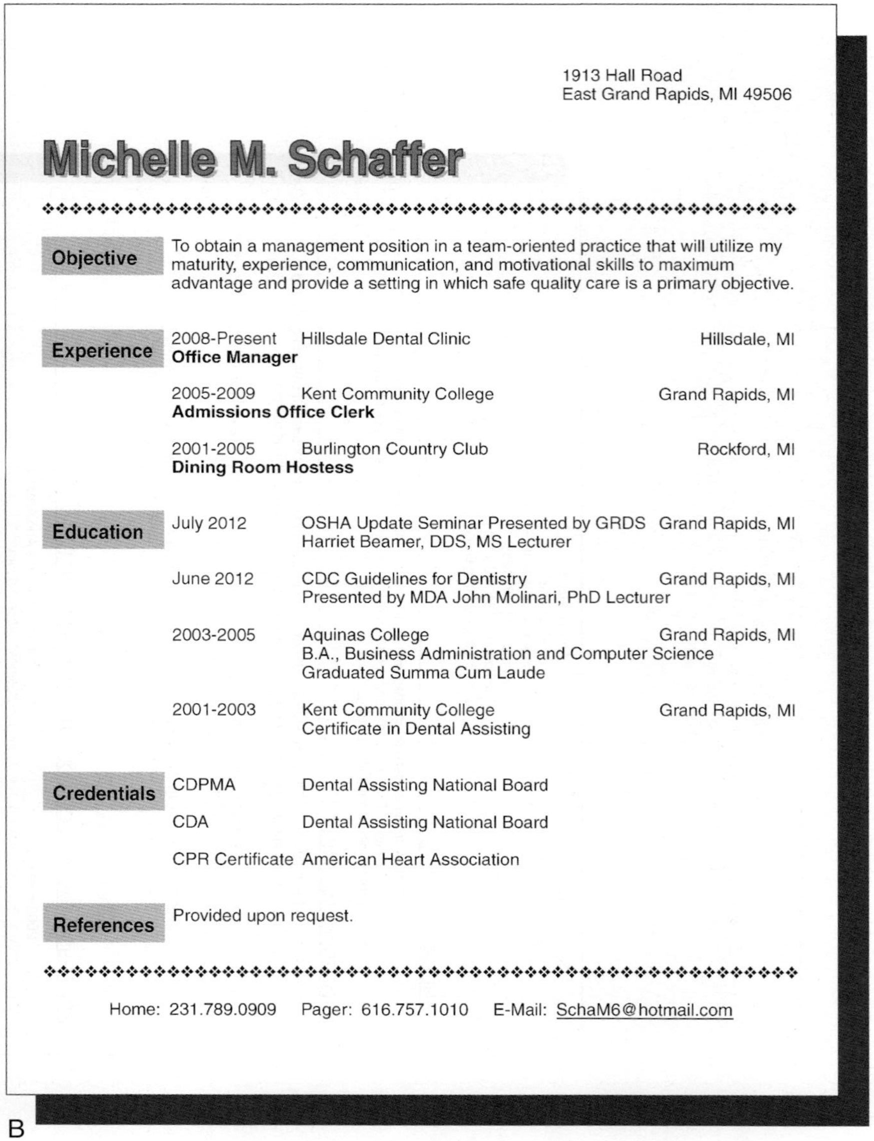

1913 Hall Road
East Grand Rapids, MI 49506

Michelle M. Schaffer

Objective To obtain a management position in a team-oriented practice that will utilize my maturity, experience, communication, and motivational skills to maximum advantage and provide a setting in which safe quality care is a primary objective.

Experience

2008-Present Hillsdale Dental Clinic Hillsdale, MI
Office Manager

2005-2009 Kent Community College Grand Rapids, MI
Admissions Office Clerk

2001-2005 Burlington Country Club Rockford, MI
Dining Room Hostess

Education

July 2012 OSHA Update Seminar Presented by GRDS Grand Rapids, MI
Harriet Beamer, DDS, MS Lecturer

June 2012 CDC Guidelines for Dentistry Grand Rapids, MI
Presented by MDA John Molinari, PhD Lecturer

2003-2005 Aquinas College Grand Rapids, MI
B.A., Business Administration and Computer Science
Graduated Summa Cum Laude

2001-2003 Kent Community College Grand Rapids, MI
Certificate in Dental Assisting

Credentials

CDPMA Dental Assisting National Board

CDA Dental Assisting National Board

CPR Certificate American Heart Association

References Provided upon request.

Home: 231.789.0909 Pager: 616.757.1010 E-Mail: SchaM6@hotmail.com

B

FIGURE 18-7 **A,** Letter of application in response to a blind advertisement for an office manager. **B,** Personal résumé to accompany the letter applying for the office manager position.

CAROL WOODALL

122 SOUTHWICK DR., LEXINGTON, MI 49507

4/12/2020

Grand Rapids Press
Box 321
Grand Rapids, MI 49502

Dear Doctor:

In response to the advertisement placed in the Grand Rapids Press, I am most interested in the part time position as a Registered Dental Hygienist in your office. I am moving to Grand Rapids with my husband who has received a promotion in Hopkins Pharmaceutical. I am currently a part time Clinical Coordinator in the Dental Hygiene Program at Kalamazoo Valley Community College and work part time in a local dental office.

Enclosed you will find my resume and I am certain you will find that I have the qualifications for which you are looking. In addition to my clinical skills I am fluent in both English and Spanish. I know that there is a large Spanish Community now on the northern side of your city. I have also had extensive experience with both Eaglesoft and Dentrix dental software in various projects where I have worked.

I welcome a personal interview and am available any time and any day except on Monday. You may contact me at 616-777-7777 or on my email at caw777@vintagemail.com. I look forward to meeting you and your staff in the very near future.

Sincerely,

Carol Woodall

A

FIGURE 18-8 **A,** Letter of application in response to an advertisement for a dental hygienist.

Continued

Carol A. Woodall CDA RDA RDH MS
caw777@vintagemail.com
616-777-7777

Education

Master of Science — April 2008
Health Science/Health Professions Education
Florida Gulf Coast University
Fort Myers, FL 33965

Bachelor of Science — December 2006
Health Science
Florida Gulf Coast University
Fort Myers, FL 33965

Associate of Applied Science — June 1998
Dental Hygiene/Dental Assisting
Kalamazoo Valley Community College
Kalamazoo, MI 498071

Experience:

Clinical Coordinator — January 2002 – Present
Kalamazoo Community College
8900 College Pkwy
Kalamazoo, MI 48071

Clinical Responsibilities:
Train/evaluate Dental Hygiene I and II students in instrumentation
Train/evaluate Dental Hygiene I students in radiology techniques

Didactic Responsibilities:
Teach Dental Hygiene II – Practice of Dental Hygiene

Dental Hygienist
Peter Parks, DDS (retired) — 1999-2010
1550 Matthew Drive
Kalamazoo, Michigan 48070

George Kazakos DMD (periodontist) — 2010-present
6323 Corporate Court Suite B
Kalamazoo, Michigan 48069

Other
Elsevier, Inc. — January 2013 - present
11011 Richmond Avenue Suite 450
Houston, TX 77042
• Contracted Item Writer/Content Expert for Dental Assisting and Dental Hygiene
Anatomy of Orofacial Structures 8th Ed — 2013
• Contributor/Developed Power Points
Elsevier
Periodontology for the Dental Hygienist 4th Ed — 2012
Elsevier
• Contributor/Developed Power Points

Licensure/Certification:
• Registered Dental Hygienist
State of Michigan
State of Colorado
• Certified in Local Anesthesia
• Certified Dental Assistant
• Registered Dental Assistant
State of Michigan

Professional Affiliations:
• American Dental Hygiene Association

B

FIGURE 18-8, cont'd B, Personal résumé to accompany the letter applying for a position as a dental hygienist using the chronological style.

BOX 18-6

Hints for Preparing a Résumé

- Use all of the layout, formatting, and finishing techniques available to you.
- Use headings that allow the reader to find information easily.
- Be succinct.
- Use a spell checker, and have the résumé reviewed by a competent person.
- Make the résumé easy to read (e.g., print size, font styles, and arrangement of information).
- Put your education and experience information in chronological order unless using a functional format.
- Leave sufficient white space to avoid a cluttered look.

BOX 18-7

Dos and Don'ts for Creating an Effective Résumé

Do

- Emphasize your qualities and experience.
- Substantiate your educational and experience qualifications to justify the abilities you claim.
- Be clear and concise in your descriptions.
- Choose a format that is easy to read.
- Be consistent in using the format.

Don't

- Include on the résumé the date the résumé was written.
- Include a physical description of yourself (e.g., height, weight, age).
- Include race or religion.
- Mention your health status.
- Include salary information (unless specifically requested; then include it in the cover letter).
- Use abbreviations or acronyms that may not be understood.

or special achievements. Courses that you took when completing the dental assistant program may also be listed (e.g., dental science, dental laboratory procedures, clinical practice, dental radiography, and dental practice management).

Work Experience

A chronological résumé begins with your most recent job or experience and includes the dates of employment, the name and address of the employer, the position held, and a brief description of the job. Summer and part-time jobs may be lumped in a single category; however, if work experiences have been limited, you may want to list them separately. Box 18-8 presents the advantages and disadvantages of a chronological résumé. If using a functional résumé, you will list your skills first and then your work experience. Box 18-9 lists the advantages and disadvantages of the functional résumé.

In some cases, if your work experience is more recent than your education, the work experience should be listed before your education. At this point in your career, work experience is of greater value to a prospective employer than education.

BOX 18-8

Advantages and Disadvantages of a Chronological Résumé

Advantages

- Highlights titles and company/dental practice names, which is advantageous when the names or titles are relevant or impressive
- Highlights consistent progress from one position to another
- Highlights the length of time with each organization

Disadvantages

- Readily shows gaps in the work history
- Shows frequent job changes
- Does not show the most impressive or relevant work experience first if it is not the most recent

BOX 18-9

Advantages and Disadvantages of a Functional Résumé

Advantages

- Highlights your strengths, such as key skills, capabilities, and community service
- If you are looking for a career in a field that you do not have specific qualifications in, highlights some transferable and marketable skills that you do have.
- When you have had extensive experience in a variety of areas, expresses this experience with terms such as *exceptional customer service, highly responsible and ethical,* and *adaptable to new technology—proficient in Microsoft Office.*

Disadvantages

- Not effective for inexperienced persons
- Does not indicate chronology of job history

Optional Areas

Affiliations and Activities

If you have participated in school or community activities or received awards or honors, this information would be valuable to the prospective employer, and it should be included. Activities and hobbies are optional, but they can indicate that you are a well-rounded individual and that you get along well with others.

Volunteer or community work is helpful to mention because it indicates areas in which the practice may be promoted. In addition, include the types of people with whom you have worked (e.g., children, older adults, those with special needs).

References

Generally references are provided upon request and not before the personal interview. Be prepared to supply the names, addresses, and telephone numbers of at least two people who are willing to verify your abilities and skills, and you will also want to include one character reference. If your work experience has been limited, list instructors or clinical supervisors who can evaluate your abilities. Always obtain the individual's permission to use his or her name as a reference, and be sure that person is willing to give you a good recommendation.

Remember, do not give information on the résumé that might be detrimental to you. Details can be given when you are interviewed. At the interview, be prepared to discuss your weaknesses honestly, confidently, and in a way that puts your present self in the best light.

Figures 18-5, *B,* 18-6, *B,* and 18-7, *B,* show the ways in which résumés were designed to accompany each of the letters in Figures 18-5, *A,* 18-6, *A,* and 18-7, *A,* respectively.

COMPLETING THE JOB APPLICATION FORM

The type of job for which you are applying determines the detail and complexity of the application form. The job application form is a series of questions designed to request comprehensive data about you and your past education, work, and professional experience. It often may require you to complete a narrative statement about yourself and to give the reasons you are seeking a particular job. You may have had the opportunity to complete the application form before arriving for the interview, or you may be asked to complete the form when you arrive. Figure 18-8 presents an example of an application used for a private practice.

Regardless of the job for which you are applying, you must keep several things in mind when completing the application form:

- If possible, try to obtain two forms, one to use as a working copy and the other to submit to the employer.
- Before entering data on the application form, read through the application very thoroughly, and avoid asking unnecessary questions. The application form is often used as the first employment test: it tests your ability to follow directions.
- The directions may indicate that the form can be keyed on a computer or handwritten. If you are required to complete the form in your own handwriting, this may be another test of neatness, and it also gives the employer a sample of how well or poorly you write.
- Answer all of the questions. If the question does not relate to you, write "N/A" (not applicable), or draw a line through the question. The employer then realizes you have read the question and have not overlooked it.
- Be truthful when answering interview questions. Dates, names, and places must be accurate. Make a list of your former addresses, schools, family names, and references to take along when going for the interview. It is better to have the information available, even if it is not needed. Be sure that no discrepancies exist between your reported date of birth and your age. If you are residing at a temporary address, be sure to give a permanent address. Be particularly careful with your spelling. A small pocket dictionary or a smartphone is a great item to take along for a handy reference.

PRACTICE NOTE

Be truthful when answering interview questions.

PREPARING FOR AN INTERVIEW

The day that you receive a response from a prospective employer, you will be elated to know that someone is interested in your qualifications after reviewing your résumé and now wishes to meet you in person. This elation is immediately followed by a feeling of fear of the unknown. You may or may not know anything about this prospective position, but one thing is certain: you do know yourself. The following steps can be used to prepare for an interview. At a later time, you should go through each of these steps and apply them to your situation:

1. *Learn about the dental practice or clinic.* After you have identified the dental practice or clinic to which you are interested in applying, spend time learning more about the office or clinic, its mission, and its vision. Find out about its reputation and how it treats its employees. This can be done in several ways:
   a. Ask friends, relatives, and acquaintances what they know about this office or clinic.
   b. Check the office or clinic website, if one is available. For example, dental schools have a website from which you could learn about staffing and the various types of jobs and clinics at the institution.
   c. Search dental society websites to identify professional memberships.
   d. If you are a student, consult with local professional contacts or dental faculty.
   e. Search the state Board of Dentistry website to identify any possible disciplinary action against the practice.
2. *What do I wear?* Wear something that looks businesslike. You may have a new outfit that you would like to wear but cannot decide if it is appropriate. If you question whether an outfit is right, do not wear it. Your hair should be worn up and off of the shoulders, with natural-looking makeup and minimal jewelry. Avoid a fragrance that is too heavy. Your well-groomed and polished image shows that you value and respect your patients and the practice. You may even want to look at photos or video footage of yourself to see what the prospective employer will view with an objective eye. Do you look the part of a confident and up-to-date health professional? It is prudent to follow the old adage, "First appearances are lasting ones." You may know all the answers and have a lot of skill, but you must win the approval of the dentist before you will ever have an opportunity to display those skills.
3. *What do I take with me?* The day that you receive the call for the interview, write down the time, place, and name of the interviewer. Prepare the materials to take with you to the interview. These should include a ballpoint pen, a pencil, an eraser, a small spiral notebook, a pocket dictionary, and a copy of your college transcripts and your résumé. In the notebook, list many of your outstanding characteristics that

you may wish to bring to the attention of the dentist, a list of questions that you hope to cover during the interview, and the names, addresses, and telephone numbers or e-mail addresses of your references.

PRACTICE NOTE

You may know all the answers and have a lot of skill, but you must win the approval of the dentist before you will ever have an opportunity to display those skills.

Depending on the type of job for which you are applying, you may want to take a portfolio, which is a compilation of samples of your work. If you are applying for an administrative assistant position, your portfolio may include the following:

- Letters that you have written, which show your writing style
- Spreadsheets that you have prepared
- Reports, including graphics
- PowerPoint slides

Preparing a portfolio and presenting it during the job interview allows you to show what you can do rather than merely talk about it.

The Personal Interview

Plan to arrive a few minutes early at the office. Your first contact may be with the office manager. The office manager plays an important role in the office; therefore, it is important to be friendly and courteous to this person. You may want to introduce yourself by saying, "Good morning, I am Jennifer Ellis, and I have a 10:30 appointment for an interview with Dr. Lake." The office manager will acknowledge you and may ask you to complete an application form similar to that shown in Figure 18-9. After the form is completed, the office manager may review your résumé and application and then escort you to meet the interviewer. If you are not introduced, take the time to introduce yourself by saying, "Good morning, Dr. Lake, I am Jennifer Ellis." At this point, the interviewer will ask you to be seated, and the interview will begin. Look directly at the interviewer, and respond to the questions clearly and distinctly; do not be evasive. An evasive answer leaves doubt in the interviewer's mind.

In general, the applicant should be responsive and answer in complete sentences. Box 18-10 presents helpful hints regarding things to avoid during an interview. Box 18-11 provides a series of commonly asked interview questions.

There are times when the staff might take the candidate to lunch to provide for a more relaxed atmosphere and to offer an opportunity to discuss topics that might not be able to be discussed during a formal interview. Exposed tattoos, facial and oral jewelry, signs of smoking, and social graces are all being examined during this interviewing process.

After the series of questions, salary and job responsibilities are generally discussed. If the salary that the dentist offers you is lower than you are willing to accept, you may reply that you had hoped to start at a higher salary but that you are willing to

BOX 18-10

Missteps to Avoid During a Job Interview

- Being too aggressive
- Talking about salary and hours immediately
- Chewing gum
- Lacking enthusiasm
- Lacking a neat appearance
- Using little or no eye contact
- Appearing preoccupied
- Using poor grammar
- Being vague
- Wearing too much makeup
- Lacking curiosity

BOX 18-11

Commonly Asked Interview Questions

Initial Questions

- How did you learn about this position?
- What do you know about our practice?
- Why are you interested in this practice?
- Tell me about yourself.
- Why do you think you are qualified for this position?
- Describe your most significant accomplishment.
- What is your definition of "being on time"?
- What qualities are important to you in your work environment?
- If you make a decision and it is questioned, how do you react?

Interest in the Job

- Are you currently employed? If so, does your current employer know you are seeking a new position?
- What would your current employer say makes you most valuable to him or her?
- Why do you want to change jobs?
- What do you consider the ideal job for you?
- What are your long- and short-range goals?

Education

- What formal education have you had?
- Why did you choose to study dental assisting?
- What was your academic average when you were in school?
- What do you consider your greatest strength? Your greatest weakness?

Experience

- Have you ever been fired or asked to resign from a position?
- Which duties performed in the past have you liked the best? The least? Why?
- Why should I hire you?
- What salary do you expect?

Future on the Job

- What would you like to know about this practice?
- Describe how you would demonstrate compassion in this practice.
- How would you want to integrate into this practice?

EMPLOYMENT APPLICATION

All information listed on this application will be considered and handled as personal and confidential. Please write or print legibly.

AN EQUAL OPPORTUNITY EMPLOYER

This employer provides equal opportunity to all persons without regard to handicap, race, color, religion, sex, age, or national origin.

Name:			Date of Application:
Address:	City:	State:	Zip:
Home Phone:	Cell Phone:	Social Security Number:	

GENERAL INFORMATION

Position applied for: ______________________________

Available to work: ☐ Full-Time ☐ Part-Time ☐ Temporary

Date available to start work: ______________

Are you over 18 yrs. of age? ☐ Yes ☐ No   Will transportation be a problem for you? ☐ Yes ☐ No

If you are not a U.S. Citizen, do you have the right to work in the United States? ☐ Yes ☐ No

Have you ever been convicted of a felony? ☐ Yes ☐ No

(A conviction is not an automatic bar to employment. Each case will be considered on its own merits.)

Does the sight of blood bother you? ☐ Yes ☐ No

EDUCATION

	Name and address of School	Major/Degree(s)	No. of Years Completed	Did you Graduate?
High School				
Community College				
4 Year Institution				
Vocational				
Other (specify)				

Describe Specialized Training, Apprenticeship, Skills, Seminars, Courses, Extra-Curricular Activities

SKILLS

Task	Circle One		Task	Circle One	
Keyboarding WPM ______	Yes	No	Pour Models	Yes	No
Bookkeeping	Yes	No	Cavitron	Yes	No
Computer Operations	Yes	No	Cast Onlays	Yes	No
Handling Group Insurance	Yes	No	Plaque Control Instruction	Yes	No
Expose, Process, and Mount X-rays	Yes	No	Oral Evacuator	Yes	No
Panoramic X-Rays	Yes	No	Knowledge of Dental Instruments	Yes	No
Have you used insurance software?	Yes	No	Knowledge of Dental Terms	Yes	No
Other: (Describe if yes)					

EMPLOYMENT RECORD

Beginning with your current employer, please list your work experience over the past ten years. You may include pertinent volunteer activities.

Name of Employer		Start Date	End Date
Address	Phone	Start Salary	End Salary
Job Title	Supervisor	Phone	
Duties			
Reason for Leaving			

Name of Employer		Start Date	End Date
Address	Phone	Start Salary	End Salary
Job Title	Supervisor	Phone	
Duties			
Reason for Leaving			

Name of Employer		Start Date	End Date
Address	Phone	Start Salary	End Salary
Job Title	Supervisor	Phone	
Duties			
Reason for Leaving			

FIGURE 18-9 A sample application for employment.

REFERENCES

Please provide the name, address, and phone number of at least two non employer/relatives as references.

NAME	ADDRESS	PHONE

EMERGENCY CONTACT

Name	Relationship	
Address	Phone	Alt. Phone

DUTY PERFORMANCE

Are you able to perform the essential duties of the position for which you are applying, either with or without reasonable accommodations? ☐ Yes ☐ No

If yes, please indicate what type(s) of reasonable accommodations are needed:

In the course of making an employment decision, this employer makes it a practice to verify with previous employers information such as dates of employment, description of job duties, attendance records, reason for leaving, etc. If there are any employers you want us to contact, please indicate their names below and reasons why:

____

____

____

____

I understand that if I am employed and any statement herein is not true, I may be released immediately, I will be paid only through the day of release and this employer may cancel any rights to accrued benefits.

Date Signature

FIGURE 18-9, cont'd

accept an opportunity to demonstrate your ability and value to the practice. This situation may arise with any one of the dental healthcare providers, be it the administrative or clinical assistant or the dental hygienist. This undoubtedly will result in further discussion, whereupon you should be prepared to give firm answers on what you will accept. In addition, you should inquire as to what benefits may offset the lower salary.

There will come a time in the interview—usually toward the end—when the employer or office manager gives you the opportunity to ask questions. However, not everyone takes this opportunity, and candidates may freeze or be caught off guard when this occurs. Sometimes the candidate feels that he or she has all of the information needed to determine whether the job is for them. It is also possible that, by this time, the candidate may feel that she or he does not want to be viewed as being annoying by asking too many questions. Alternatively, some candidates realize by the end of the interview that they are not interested in the job and therefore do not need to ask any more questions. If you are not interested in the job, it is perfectly acceptable not to ask any final questions. However, if you are interested in the job and do not have any final questions, the interviewer may think you are not interested in the position. Therefore, it is wise to have a series of prepared questions to ask during the final part of the interview. Box 18-12 includes a list of questions that a person might pose during an interview. Be cautious to not be redundant if a topic has already been discussed during the interview, and do not make salary and benefits the primary question.

After an interview that included many of the questions in Boxes 18-11 and 18-12, a prospective applicant for a position as an administrative assistant, Jennifer Ellis, was offered an acceptable salary, although it was lower than her initial request. She replied, "I feel I have the skills you need, and it is going to save you a great deal of time in not having to teach me about all the technical skills. I would be willing to start at the lower salary for a minimal amount of time if you will explain to me what the total salary scale is and how I will be evaluated for salary raises. I would like the opportunity to advance by merit or production, since I am certain you will be pleased with my ability and production in your office." The employer explained the numerous benefits and outlined the salary system to Jennifer. Remember, as discussed previously, salary is not the primary aspect of the job, but you must be able to earn enough to adequately support yourself in a comfortable lifestyle. In

BOX 18-12

Questions for a Potential Employee to Ask and Not to Ask During an Interview

Questions to Ask During an Interview

- How would you describe the practice culture and leadership philosophy?
- What specific qualities and skills are you looking for in the job candidate?
- What would you say are the three most important skills needed to excel in this position?
- What does a typical day or week look like for the person in this position? Is there travel, flextime, and so on?
- How much time is allotted for each patient, for a new patient, for a child, for obtaining radiographs, and for charting?
- Who is in charge of recall?
- Who is in charge of scheduling recall patients?
- What type of laboratory duties are required of the assistant?
- How can I best contribute to the office?
- What is your ideal communication style with your staff? Do you meet regularly with your team or work primarily through other means?
- Do you have satellite offices? Will I be expected to work at all of the sites?
- Do you have any concerns about me or about my qualifications that may prevent you from selecting me for the job?
- What is the next step? When do you think you will be making a decision?

Questions Not to Ask During an Interview

- Never ask for information you could have easily found with a quick Google search.
- Never ask if you can change the job details, the schedule, or the salary.
- Never ask many questions about the interviewer's background.
- Never ask about things such as pay, time off, benefits. (Wait until later in the process to inquire about these things.)
- Never ask about gossip you have heard.
- Never ask if the office monitors e-mail or Internet usage.

addition, the benefits offered with a job often outweigh the basic salary, so do not overlook this aspect.

A similar response could occur with a clinical assistant or a dental hygienist. When these candidates possess a license to practice in the state, it is obvious that they have had training in an accredited program and thus have achieved all of the basic skills, so it is necessary for the clinical assistant or hygienist to point out the skills that go beyond the scope of their license. For example, in the case of the dental hygienist, a candidate may explain that he or she has additional skills in computer software, the use of an intraoral camera, the use of digital radiography, the placement of antimicrobial agents (e.g., Arestin), or the administration of local anesthesia.

Likewise, the clinical assistant could enumerate additional skills in expanded functions, the use of computer software, insurance management, and any additional experience in digital radiography. In all of these situations, the candidate who is bilingual brings an additional skill to the practice. For the dentist, all of these additional skills in any of these candidates will be time savers and thus increase the productivity of the practice.

Other Formats for Interviewing

Some dentists like to have team interviews during which several members of the staff who will work with the applicant participate in the interview. Generally a team interview in a private practice setting involves three or four people. Although this type of interview may sound intimidating, it may not be. Pay attention to the individuals' names as they are introduced so that later you can refer to them by name. Listen carefully, answer questions succinctly, and give your attention to the individual who asked the question. Make eye contact with all participants if the question or statement is meant for the group. As mentioned previously, several members of the staff may take you to lunch, and this can become a form of a team interview.

Working Interview

Often a dentist uses the working interview format to assess an administrative, clinical assistant, or hygiene applicant. The dentist will invite you for a day of work at the office, for which some form of compensation is prearranged. This would serve as an opportunity to observe the office activity and give you a sense of how well the office is organized.

Virtual Interview

Virtual interviews are not common in small dental practices, but some situations may warrant them. For example, if you are applying for a job in Torrance, California, and you live in Biltmore, New Jersey, it might be feasible to conduct a virtual interview. In other words, rather than having you fly to California for the interview, the dental clinic would make arrangements for you to go to a facility that has a teleconferencing center. This allows the interviewer from California to see you and for you to see him or her. It is possible to accomplish a similar type of interview, if necessary, by using a web camera system or even video conferencing via your computer. This concept enables you to send pictures and sound files that say more than a résumé or telephone conversation. Two companies that provide such a format are www.livehire.com and www.hirevue.com. Virtual interviews enable the prospective employer and employee to interact and to have an opportunity to visually meet each other.

If you are going to participate in a virtual interview, careful planning must be done in advance. Be certain that the setting is clear of clutter and that it is a quiet professional setting that will not be interrupted by external noises.

Many of us get a little nervous when we know we are going to be videotaped or observed on camera, but a virtual interview is a two-way system that allows you to communicate with the other person as if you were in the same room. You still greet the interviewer warmly and with a smile, just as you would in person. Sit in the chair provided, and avoid nervous habits. Try to forget that the camera is present, and concentrate on the interviewer and the questions. Avoid wearing black, gray, white, or distracting patterns because they do not come across well on camera. Also, avoid wearing jewelry that is distracting or that makes noise on camera.

Concluding the Interview

An interview is not a lengthy process, and it is often terminated with a tour of the office. Do not be overly flattering to the staff, but thank them for their time before you leave. You may not receive a job offer during the interview because the dentist may have other applicants to interview. However, you may inquire as to when the dentist anticipates arriving at a decision. Remember, do not be discouraged if you do not get the job. Each interview is a learning experience, regardless of whether it produces a job offer, and it should not be treated as a disappointment.

Following Up After the Interview

A good follow-up letter (Figure 18-10) should be written 1 or 2 days after the interview. This is an indication to the interviewer that you are interested in the position, and it may make you a priority applicant. The follow-up letter does not have to be long. It simply restates your interest in the job and mentions some of the facts that interested you about the position.

Another type of follow-up may be necessary if you have not had a reply from the prospective employer. If the job is still available and you are interested, it is permissible to call the interviewer a day or two after the interview. A telephone call lets the interviewer know of your continued interest; however, too many telephone calls can be annoying.

If you decide later that you are not interested in the position, you should send a letter explaining your decision. This is a thoughtful thing to do, and a time may come when you find yourself in a position to go back to this employer.

Regular Self-Evaluation on the Job

Regular self-evaluation is necessary to retain your position in the dental office. People often carefully evaluate themselves before they are hired, but they may become careless after working in the office for a time.

Do not become negligent about evaluating yourself. As a clinical or administrative assistant, you are constantly in the public eye, and you must maintain a good image in your employer's office. In addition, after you have obtained the

Jennifer M. Ellis
JE
1913 Hall Road
East Grand Rapids, MI 49506

Home: 616.111.2817
Work: 616.111.2345
FAX: 616.121.2468
E-mail: jme@juad.org

November 7, 20—

Joseph W. Lake, DDS
611 Main Street SE
Grand Rapids, MI 49502

Dear Dr. Lake:

Thank you for the interview you gave me yesterday. It was a privilege to see such a well-organized dental team. I was especially impressed with your facility and the infection control program you have implemented in the office.

Because of my education, I am confident that I can become an efficient dental assistant and an asset to your dental practice. After you have had a chance to review my application, you will see that I have had considerable work experience. The references I provided you yesterday will validate my reliability and quality of work.

I am available to begin work immediately. You may contact me any day of the week by calling 616.111.2817 after 3:00 p.m.

Sincerely,

Jennifer M. Ellis, RDA

Enclosure

FIGURE 18-10 A sample follow-up letter.

position, you must maintain your skills and acquire new ones as changes occur in dentistry through the expanded use of auxiliary staff. You should promptly join your professional organizations, which offer information about educational activities in relevant techniques.

HINTS FOR SUCCESS AS PART OF THE DENTAL TEAM

When you begin your new job on the dental health team, you should gear yourself for success. The following sections can help make this experience more pleasant and result in personal success. These suggestions are summarized in Box 18-13.

Learn the Names of Staff Members

Learning and remembering the names of your immediate associates should not be difficult. If the staff is large, learning the names of those not in your immediate department may be more difficult. It is wise to learn the names as quickly as possible. It may even be wise to maintain a list of names and the position of each employee until you are able to remember them.

Listen Attentively

You will be eager to learn as much as possible about your new position as quickly as possible. Listen carefully to directions, and avoid talking persistently. If you relax and listen well, often the questions you are eager to ask will be answered. If not, do not hesitate to ask for the clarification of a procedure.

Establish Meaningful Social Friendships

Most employers do not object if employees develop personal friendships with other employees. However, many traps can develop during your first days on a new job. One of these is developing a close relationship with one or two people too quickly, which can cost you friendships with others at a later time. Office cliques frequently create rivalry. Although you must have a friendly attitude toward other employees in the office, you need not think that you must participate in all of the social activities or interests the others have. However, you should avoid a superior attitude that could be interpreted as snobbish. You do not need to become friends with your coworkers, but you do need to get along with them during the workday.

BOX 18-13

Hints for Success in a New Job

- Learn the names of staff members.
- Listen attentively.
- Establish meaningful social friendships.
- Use a notebook and calendar to record important activities and procedures.
- Use judgment when working overtime and taking breaks.
- Do not flaunt your education and abilities.
- Seek honest evaluations.
- Maintain office policies.
- Observe office hours.
- Be yourself.

Use a Notebook and Calendar to Record Important Activities and Procedures

When you begin your new job, many unfamiliar rules and regulations as well as other information will be given to you. To avoid misunderstandings or neglecting important information, develop the "notebook habit," and write down or record each bit of information. It is surprising how many successful people use this system.

Observe Office Hours

In most cases, the office hours have been determined before your arrival. The efficiency of an office depends on your being prompt at all times; your tardiness delays the work processes for which you are responsible. You should ensure your means of transportation at all times. It is your responsibility to anticipate inclement weather and to compensate for any potential delay. It is better to be 20 minutes early for work than 2 minutes late. The dentist will not be interested in your excuses.

PRACTICE NOTE
It is better to be 20 minutes early for work than 2 minutes late.

Use Judgment When Working Overtime and Taking Breaks

Employees sometimes try to impress their employers by working extra hours or skipping lunch hours or breaks. However, you should avoid continual overtime and loss of lunch hours because this may cause friction with other employees. Your actions may be misinterpreted, and other employees may make life miserable for you. This does not mean that you cannot use your discretion on days when legitimate emergencies arise and your presence is necessary to maintain office efficiency.

Do Not Flaunt Your Education and Abilities

Nothing is more irritating than a new employee who constantly informs other employees of his or her exceptional abilities. It is better to prove your abilities through your work than to tell everyone about your great potential. Your coworkers may have had many years of experience, and you might learn something from them if you give them a chance to help you.

Seek Honest Performance Evaluations

Most employees want to learn about their performance. Before accepting a new job, you should ask how and when your performance will be evaluated. As time passes, periodic reviews of your performance should be obtained from the employer. You should have an opportunity to discuss the performance evaluation; have a conversation about the ways in which you are performing satisfactorily as well as the areas that need improvement. Figure 18-11 is an example of a performance evaluation form. Such forms are reviewed periodically with you to evaluate your day-to-day performance. It is wise to use this evaluation form first as a self-evaluation, before your employer completes it.

Maintain Office Policies

Most offices have established policies for grooming, uniform styles, lunch hours, use of social media, and other situations. You should carefully review the office policy and adhere to it. In addition, you should take home any other handbooks that the office uses for its employees and read them carefully so that you will be well informed. If you do not understand a policy, ask for clarification to avoid making an embarrassing mistake.

Be Yourself

As you make your first impression in the office, it is wise to be yourself. Remember, you may admire the characteristics of another person, but you cannot be that person. If you attempt to be someone else, you only destroy yourself and all of the finer parts of your character. Be yourself, and you will be a happier person.

Performance Evaluation Form

Employee Name ______________________

Job Title ______________________

Supervisor ______________________

EVALUATION

4 Excellent performance that demonstrates consistent and important contributions that meet and frequently surpass expectations of the position.

3 Performs with a very acceptable degree of skill that demonstrates the expectations of the position.

2 Performance has not met satisfactory level. Makes mistakes but usually corrects errors after further instruction. Improved performance is needed to achieve defined expectations of this position.

1 Performance indicates deficiencies that seriously interfere with attainment of the defined expectations of the position.

	Evaluation			
Attendance				
Adheres to scheduled work hours.	4	3	2	1
Uses leave appropriately.	4	3	2	1
Adjusts work schedule to office needs.	4	3	2	1
Job Knowledge				
Uses required job skills.	4	3	2	1
Updates skills periodically.	4	3	2	1
Demonstrates knowledge of procedures needed to perform the job.	4	3	2	1
Organizational Skills				
Prioritizes tasks.	4	3	2	1
Plans steps in advance to accomplish tasks.	4	3	2	1
Meets deadlines.	4	3	2	1
Work Quality				
Performs work accurately.	4	3	2	1
Demonstrates thoroughness and attention to detail.	4	3	2	1
Demonstrates neatness.	4	3	2	1
Human Relations/Communications				
Demonstrates a sense of humor.	4	3	2	1
Demonstrates good listening skills.	4	3	2	1
Maintains eye contact when speaking to another person.	4	3	2	1
Displays good manners and professional etiquette.	4	3	2	1
Conveys ideas effectively.	4	3	2	1
Responds to ideas conveyed by others.	4	3	2	1
Demonstrates sensitivity to diverse staff and patients.	4	3	2	1
Problem Solving Skills				
Remains calm in stressful situations.	4	3	2	1
Demonstrates ability to identify the problem.	4	3	2	1
Demonstrates ability to select the best solution.	4	3	2	1
Takes action to prevent future problems.	4	3	2	1
Does not require supervision to accomplish routine tasks.	4	3	2	1
Follows through on chosen solution.	4	3	2	1
Gives constructive criticism in a positive manner.	4	3	2	1
Responds to supervision in a positive manner.	4	3	2	1
Cooperation				
Respects responsibilities of others.	4	3	2	1
Provides assistance and guidance to others.	4	3	2	1
Accepts guidance from supervisor/employer.	4	3	2	1
Works as a team member.	4	3	2	1
Initiative				
Seeks work that needs to be done.	4	3	2	1
Seeks new methods and ideas to improve work.	4	3	2	1
Exhibits self-motivation to achieve team goals.	4	3	2	1
Integrity				
Respects other people and their property.	4	3	2	1
Maintains confidentiality.	4	3	2	1
Can be trusted with money that belongs to the office.	4	3	2	1
Refrains from gossip.	4	3	2	1
Is truthful regardless of potential consequences.	4	3	2	1

Supervisor/Employer Comments ______________________

Employee Comments ______________________

Employee's Signature ______________________ **Date** ____________

Supervisor/Employer Signature ______________________ **Date** ____________

FIGURE 18-11 Performance appraisal form.

ASKING FOR A RAISE

Pay increments should be discussed before you begin work, and you may find that raises are given after 6 or 12 months of successful employment. To avoid any misunderstanding, determine how and when these raises can be obtained before accepting the job. Few dentists would consider performing extensive treatment on patients before informing them of the anticipated fees. Similarly, you should not be working unless you are aware of your potential salary and anticipated promotions. It is wise to obtain written verification of employment conditions and responsibilities as well as a salary scale before beginning work. This can be accomplished in an office procedures manual (see Chapter 2). However, if pay increments have not been discussed and you have completed a year of employment, you might wonder when and how the subject can be raised.

Before approaching the dentist about a raise, you should do a self-evaluation to determine that you are justified in making such a request. The questions listed in Box 18-14 may be considered during such an evaluation. A salary conference should be a two-way discussion that allows you to identify your assets for the job and to explain your performance success. It also allows the employer to relate the performance to a monetary amount that will reward your performance and inspire increased productivity.

If you have given serious thought to the factors mentioned previously and you believe that you deserve a raise, how do you approach the dentist? Select an opportunity when the work schedule allows enough time for a discussion of the subject. Do not wait until the end of the day, when the dentist is tired and ready to leave the office. It also is not wise to start the day by asking for a raise, especially if the schedule is rather heavy.

Let the dentist know why you believe you deserve a raise. If he or she asks why you should have one, be prepared to answer; for example, cite the rising cost of living, transportation costs, insurance, increased office production because of your efforts, or simply compensation for good performance.

Very often employees do not assert themselves enough to make the dentist aware that a raise should be given. If you become passive and content with a salary, naturally you will continue to be paid at this rate; however, if your professional skills are an asset and, as a result of these skills, the dentist can perform his or her job with greater efficiency, then you should be given a raise.

If you are unsuccessful at getting a raise, express your appreciation for the dentist's understanding and consideration, and consider your alternatives. Of course, if you receive a raise, be sure to thank the responsible person.

Salary matters should be treated confidentially and not discussed with other members of the team. Salary problems destroy positive attitudes and productivity and should be resolved as quickly as possible.

BOX 18-14

Questions to Consider Before Asking for a Raise

1. Have I performed my duties well enough to deserve a raise?
2. Have I improved or advanced my skills since beginning the job?
3. Have I been cooperative with other members of the dental team?
4. Have I continued to maintain good patient management skills?
5. Can I verify that my attendance and punctuality have been above average?
6. Have I continually maintained professional ethics, safe practice, and quality standards?
7. Can I verify that the practice's productivity has increased because of my performance?
8. Do economic factors in the practice and the economy warrant a raise?

JOB TERMINATION

Terminating a job can be an obstacle for some individuals, especially when the job change is from one private practice to another in the same general locale. When you change jobs, make sure the change is to your advantage. Circumstances over which you have no control may be the reason for a change in jobs. However, an assistant who frequently changes jobs with inadequate notification or reason soon gains a poor professional reputation. Whatever the reason for terminating the job, do it ethically, and remember the following courtesies:

- Give the reason for leaving the job.
- Give sufficient notice of at least 2 weeks if your job requires an extensive training period for a new assistant.
- Write a letter of resignation as a follow-up to your verbal resignation.
- Do not discuss the termination of your job with other members of the team until you are ready to inform the dentist that you will be leaving. The grapevine is a poor method of informing the employer.
- If you terminate a job in which serious conflicts exist, it is best to leave these conflicts where they originated and not carry the feelings to another job. When beginning a new position, you should not make negative comments about a former employer. This is simply good ethics.

ATTITUDES FOR CONTINUED SUCCESS

A highly qualified and educated administrative or clinical assistant or dental hygienist is the key to production, patient management, organization, accuracy, safe operation, and protection from potential litigation. The right individual can significantly reduce stress placed on the dental team. As you grow past your entry-level position on the job, you will discover that your future success depends more and more on your attitude and your human relations skills. Completing a course in dental practice management is only the beginning.

PRACTICE NOTE

A highly qualified and educated dental healthcare provider is the key to production, patient management, organization, accuracy, safe operation, and protection from potential litigation.

Your willingness to be a team player and to cooperate with patients and staff members, as well as your good communication skills, will be assets to the dental practice. Your initiative, self-motivation, creativity, and enthusiasm indicate an eagerness to accept leadership and challenges in the office. Your desire to learn, your curiosity, and your flexibility will enable you to attain new skills and advance your career.

Continue to market your skills, maintain an interest in new technologies, and accept changes, no matter where you are on your career path. Good luck!

LEARNING ACTIVITIES

1. Write a philosophy in which you describe who you are, where you are going, and what you hope to accomplish. This philosophy should include your goals for life, your basic values, and your strengths and weaknesses.
2. List six areas of potential employment, and explain briefly the benefits of each.
3. Choose one of the advertisements in Figure 18-2 or 18-3. Respond to the advertisement by writing a letter of application for the position. In addition, prepare a résumé to accompany the letter. Make a copy of the letter and the résumé for your personal files. Pretend that you have been interviewed for the position, and write an appropriate follow-up letter.
4. List five assets that you have to offer and that you think would attract the favorable attention of a future employer.
5. Give five ways that an application form may attract unfavorable attention from the interviewer.
6. List 10 questions that you might be asked during an interview that pertain to your personal skills and needs.

Please refer to the student workbook for additional learning activities.

BIBLIOGRAPHY

Dental Assisting National Board: 2012 salary survey. <http://www.danb.org/The-Dental-Community/Dental-Assistants/Salary-and-Benefits.aspx/>, 2012 (Accessed 25.07.14.)

Hartley M: Income power of hygienists and dental assistants in 100 U.S. cities. <http://www.dentistryiq.com/articles/2014/03/>.

Hartley M, Cheesman V, De Shazer L, et al: Dental hygienists? Salaries keep the bills paid. <http://www.dentaleconomics.com/articles/print/volume-89/issue-11/features/>.

Henry K: A look at the latest dental assistant salary figures. <http://www dentistryiq.com/articles/2012/05/>.

U.S. Department of Labor, Bureau of Labor Statistics: Occupational outlook handbook. U.S. Bureau of Labor and Statistics, Washington, DC, 2014.

RECOMMENDED WEBSITES

American Dental Association (www.ada.org)
American Dental Hygienist's Association website (www.adha.org)
American Dental Assistant's Association (www.dental assistant.org)
Dental Assistant National Board (www.danb.org)

APPENDIX **A**

Composition Basics

GRAMMAR

Subject and Verb Agreement

1. When the subject consists of two singular nouns or pronouns connected by *or, either ... or, neither ... nor,* or *not only ... but also,* a singular verb is required.
   Sophia or *Rex has* the letter.
   Either *Ruth* or *Marnie plans* to attend.
   Not only a *book* but also *paper is* needed.
2. When the subject consists of two plural nouns or pronouns connected by *or, either ... or, neither ... nor,* or *not only ... but also,* a plural verb is required.
   Neither the *secretaries* nor the *typists have* access to that information.
3. When the subject is made up of both singular and plural nouns or pronouns connected by *or, either ... or, neither ... nor,* or *not only ... but also,* the verb agrees with the last noun or pronoun mentioned before the verb.
   Either *Ms. Rodriquez* or the *assistants have* access to that information.
   Neither the *men* nor *Jo is* working.
4. Disregard intervening phrases and clauses when establishing agreement between subject and verb.
   One of the men *wants* to go to the convention.
5. The words *each, every, either, neither, one,* and *another* are singular. When they are used as subjects or as adjectives modifying subjects, a singular verb is required.
   Each person *is* deserving of the award.
   Neither boy *rides* the bicycle well.
6. The following pronouns are always singular and require a singular verb: *anybody, everybody, nobody, somebody, anyone, everyone, nothing, something, anything, everything, no one,* and *someone.*
   Everyone plans to attend the meeting.
   Anyone is welcome at the concert.
7. *Both, few, many, others,* and *several* are always plural. When these five words are used as subjects or adjectives modifying subjects, a plural verb is required.
   Several members *were* asked to make presentations.
   Both women *are* going to apply.
8. *All, none, any, some, more,* and *most* may be singular or plural, depending on the noun to which they refer.
   Some of the *supplies are* missing.
   Some of that *paper is* needed.
9. A collective noun is a word that is singular in form but that represents a group of people or things. Some examples of collective nouns are *committee, company, department, public, class,* and *board.* The following rules determine the form of the verb to be used with a collective noun:
   - When the members of a group are thought of as one unit, the verb should be singular.
     The *committee has voted* unanimously to begin the study.
   - When members of the group are thought of as separate units, the verb should be plural.
     The *staff are* not in agreement regarding the decision that should be made.
10. The term *the number* has a singular meaning and requires a singular verb; the term *a number* has a plural meaning and requires a plural verb.
    The number of requests *is* surprising.
    A number of people *are* planning to attend.

PRONOUNS

1. A pronoun agrees with its antecedent (the word for which the pronoun stands) in number, gender, and person.
   Richard wants to know if *his* book is at your house.
2. A plural pronoun is used when the antecedent consists of two nouns joined by *and.*
   Mary and *Felipe* are bringing *their* stereo.
3. A singular pronoun is used when the antecedent consists of two singular nouns joined by *or* or *nor.* A plural pronoun is used when the antecedent consists of two plural nouns joined by *or* or *nor.*
   Neither *Eunice* nor *Johanna* wants to do *her* part.
   Either the *men* or the *women* will do *their* share.
4. Do not confuse certain possessive pronouns and contractions that sound alike.
   its (possessive) *it's* ("it is")
   their (possessive) *they're* ("they are")

theirs (possessive) *there's* ("there is")
your (possessive) *you're* ("you are")
whose (possessive) *who's* ("who is")

As a test for the use of a possessive pronoun or a contraction, try to substitute *it is, they are, it has, there has, there is,* or *you are*. Use the corresponding possessive form if the substitution does not make sense.

Your wording is correct.
You're wording that sentence incorrectly.
Whose book is it?
Who's the owner of this typewriter?

5. Use *who* and *that* when referring to people.
   He is the boy *who* does well in keyboarding.
   She is the type of person *that* we like to employ.
6. Use *which* and *that* when referring to places, objects, and animals.
   The *card that* I sent you was mailed last week.
   The *fox, which* is very sly, caught the skunk.

PLURALS

For most English words, the plural versions are formed by merely adding an *-s* or *-es*. However, for words with Greek or Latin origins, the plural may be designated by changing the ending.

-ae, as in *fasciae* (singular form: *fascia*)
-ia, as in *crania* (singular form: *cranium*)
-i, as in *glomeruli* (singular form: *glomerulus*; when the singular form ends in *-us*, the plural form is made by adding *-i* and dropping the *-us*)
-ata, as in *adenomata* (singular form: *adenoma*)

SPELLING

The aforementioned rules for pronunciation and for the formation of plurals are essential for spelling, but it is important that you consult a dental or medical dictionary if you are not sure. Phonetic spelling has no place in medicine or dentistry because a misspelled word may give the wrong meaning to a diagnosis. Furthermore, some terms are pronounced alike but spelled differently; for example, the *ileum* is a part of the intestinal tract, but the *ilium* is a pelvic bone.

BIBLIOGRAPHY

Fulton-Calkins PJ, Rankin DS, Shumack KA: The administrative professional, ed 14, Mason, OH, 2011, Thomson South-Western.

Straus J, Kaufman L, Stern T: The book of grammar and punctuation, ed 10, San Francisco, 2014, Josey-Bass.

APPENDIX **B**

Numbers

1. Spell out numbers 1 through 10; use figures for numbers greater than 10.
   We ordered *ten* coats and *four* dresses.
   About *60* letters were keyed.
2. If there are numbers greater than and less than 10 in a piece of correspondence, be consistent; either spell out all numbers or place all numbers in figures. If most of the numbers are less than 10, spell them out. If most are more than 10, express them all in figures.
   Please order *12* memo pads, *2* reams of paper, and *11* boxes of envelopes.
3. Numbers in the millions or greater may be expressed in the following manner to aid comprehension:
   3 billion (rather than *3,000,000,000*)
4. Always spell out a number that begins a sentence.
   Five hundred books were ordered.
5. If the numbers are large, rearrange the wording of the sentence so that the number is not the first word of the sentence.
   We had a good year in *1976.*
   Not: Nineteen hundred and seventy-six was a good year.
6. Spell out indefinite numbers and amounts.
   There were a *few* hundred voters.
7. Spell out all ordinals (e.g., *first, second, third*) that can be expressed in words.
   The store's *twenty-fifth* anniversary was held this week.
8. When adjacent numbers are written in words or in figures, use a comma to separate them.
   On Car *33, 450* cartons are being shipped.
9. House or building numbers are written in figures. However, when the number *one* appears by itself, it is spelled out. Numbers one through ten in street names are spelled out; numbers greater than ten are written in figures. When figures are used for both the house number and the street name, use a hyphen that is preceded and followed by a space.
   101 Building
   2301 Fifth Avenue
   One Main Place
   122-33rd Street
10. Ages are usually spelled out except when the age is stated exactly in years, months, and days. When ages are presented in tabular form, they are written in figures.
    She is *18 years* old.
    He is *2 years, 10 months, and 18 days* old.
    Jones, Edward 19
    King, Ruth 21
11. Use figures to express dates that are written in normal month-day-year order. Do not use *th, nd,* or *rd* after the date.
    May 8, 1987
    Not: May 8th, 1987
12. Fractions should be spelled out unless they are part of mixed numbers. Use a hyphen to separate the numerator and denominator of fractions that are written in words when the fraction is used as an adjective.
    three-fourths inch
    $5\frac{1}{2}$
13. In legal documents, numbers may be written in both words and figures.
    One hundred thirty-four and 30/100 dollars ($134.30)
14. Amounts of money are usually expressed in figures. Indefinite amounts of money are written in words.
    $100
    $3.27
    several hundred dollars
15. Express percentages in figures.
    10%
16. To form the plural of figures, add *s*.
    Technological advances will increase during the *1980s*.
17. When giving times of day, use figures with *A.M.* and *P.M.*; spell out numbers with the word *o'clock*. In formal usage, all times are spelled out.
    9 A.M.
    10 P.M.
    eight o'clock in the evening

BIBLIOGRAPHY

Fulton-Calkins PJ, Rankin DS, Shumack KA: The administrative professional, ed 14, Mason, OH, 2011, Thomson South-Western.

APPENDIX C

Prefixes and Suffixes

PREFIXES

Prefixes, which are the most frequently used elements in the formation of medical and dental words, are one or more syllables placed before words or roots to show various kinds of relationships. They are never used independently, but, when they are added before verbs, adjectives, or nouns, they modify the meaning. Most prefixes are a part of words in ordinary speech and do not refer specifically to medical-dental or scientific terminology, but many do occur frequently in medical terminology. Studying them is an important step in learning medical terms and building a medical-dental vocabulary.

Prefix	Translation	Examples
a- (an- before a vowel)	Without, lack of	Apathy (lack of feeling), anemia (lack of blood)
ab-	Away from	Abductor (leading away from), aboral (away from the mouth)
ad-	To, toward, near to	Adductor (leading toward), adhesion (sticking to)
ambi-	Both	Ambidextrous (ability to use both hands equally), ambilaterally (both sides)
amphi-	About, on both sides, both	Amphibious (living on both land and water)
ampho-	Both	Amphogenic (producing offspring of both sexes)
ana-	Up, back, again, excessive according to	Anatomy (a cutting up)
ante-	Before, forward	Antecubital (before the elbow), anteflexion (forward bending)
anti-	Against, opposed to, reversed	Antisepsis (against infection)
apo-	From, away from	Aponeurosis (away from the tendon), apochromatic (abnormal color)
arthro-	Joint	Arthroscope (an instrument used to see a joint)
bi-	Twice, double	Bilateral (two sides), bifurcation (two branches)
cata-	Down, according to, complete	Catabolism (breaking down), catalepsy (complete seizure)
circum-	Around, about	Circumference (surrounding), circumscribe (to draw around)
com-	With, together	Commissure (sending or coming together)
con-	With, together	Conductor (leading together), concentric (having a common center)
contra-	Against, opposite	Contraception (prevention of conception), contraindicated (not indicated)
de-	Away from	Dehydrate (remove water from), decompensation (failure of compensation)
dent-, odont-	Tooth or teeth	Odontoma (tumor composed of tooth structure)
di-	Twice, double	Diplopia (double vision), dichromatic (two colors)
dia-	Through, apart, across, completely	Diaphragm (wall across), diapedesis (ooze through), diagnosis (complete knowledge)
dis-	Reversal, apart from, separation	Disinfection (apart from infection), dissect (cut apart)
dys-	Bad, difficult, disordered	Dyspepsia (bad digestion), dyspnea (difficult breathing)
e-, ex-	Out, away from	Enucleate (remove from), exostosis (outgrowth of bone)
ec-	Out from	Ectopic (out of place), eccentric (away from center)
ecto-	On the outside, situated on	Ectoderm (outer skin), ectoretina (outer layer of retina)
em-, en-	In	Empyema (pus in), encephalon (in the head)
endo-	Within	Endodontic (within the tooth)
epi-	Upon, on	Epidural (upon the dura), epidermis (on the skin)
exo-	Outside, on the outer side or outer layer	Exogenous (produced outside)
extra-	Outside	Extracellular (outside of the cell)
gingiv-	Pertaining to the gums	Gingivitis (inflammation of the gums)

Continued

Prefix	Translation	Examples
glyc-	Sugar	Glycolysis (sugar dissolving)
hemi-	Half	Hemiplegia (partial paralysis), hemianesthesia (loss of feeling on one side of the body)
hyper-	Over, above, excessive	Hyperemia (excessive blood), hypertrophy (overgrowth), hyperplasia (excessive formation)
hypo-	Under, below, deficient	Hypotension (low blood pressure)
im-, in-	In, into	Immersion (act of dipping in), injection (act of forcing liquid into)
im-, in-	Not	Immature (not mature), involuntary (not voluntary), inability (not able)
infra-	Below	Infraorbital (below the eye), infraclavicular (below the clavicle or collarbone)
inter-	Between	Intercostal (between the ribs), intervene (come between)
intra-	Within	Intracerebral (within the cerebrum), intraocular (within the eyes)
intro-	Into, within	Introversion (turning inward), introduce (lead into)
lingu-	Pertaining to the tongue	Lingual surface (the surface closest to the tongue)
muc-	Mucous	Mucositis (inflammation of the mucous membrane)
meta-	Beyond, after, change	Metamorphosis (change of form), metastasis (beyond the original position)
neo-	New	Neoplasm (new growth)
opistho-	Behind, backward	Opisthotic (behind the ears), opisthognathous (behind the jaws)
para-	Beside, by side	Paraplegia (paralysis of both sides), paracentesis (puncture along the side of)
per-	Through, excessive	Permeate (pass through), perforate (bore through)
peri-	Around	Periosteum (around the bone), periatrial (around the atrium)
perio-	Supporting structures of the teeth	Periodontal (supporting structures of the teeth)
post-	After, behind	Postoperative (after operation), postocular (behind the eye)
pre-	Before, in front of	Premolar (in front of the molars), preoral (in front of the mouth)
py-	Pus	Pyogenic (pus-producing)
pro-	Before, in front of	Prognosis (foreknowledge), prophase (appear before)
re-	Back, again, contrary	Reflex (bend back), revert (turn again to)
retro-	Backward, located behind	Retrograde (going backward), retrolingual (behind the tongue)
semi-	Half	Semicartilaginous (half-cartilage), semiconscious (half-conscious)
sial-	Saliva	Sialorrhea (excessive flow of saliva)
sub-	Under	Subcutaneous (under the skin), subungual (under the nail)
super-	Above, upper, excessive	Supercilia (upper brows), supernumerary (excessive number)
supra-	Above, upon, on	Suprarenal (above the kidney), suprascapular (on the upper part of the scapula)
sym-, syn-	Together, with	Symphysis (growing together), synapsis (joining together)
trans-	Across, through	Transection (cut across), transmit (send beyond)
ultra-	Beyond, in	Ultraviolet (beyond the violet end of the spectrum), ultrasonic (sound waves beyond the upper frequency of what can be heard by the human ear)

From Mosby's dental dictionary, ed 2, St. Louis, 2008, Mosby.

SUFFIXES

Suffixes are one or more syllables or elements added to the root of a word (the part that indicates the essential meaning) to alter the meaning or to indicate the intended part of speech.

To make the word pronounceable, the last letter or letters of the root to which the suffix is attached may be changed. The last vowel may be changed to an *o* or an *o* may be inserted if it is not already present before a suffix that begins with a consonant, such as *-logy* to create *cardiology*. The final vowel in the root may be dropped before a suffix that begins with a vowel, such as *-itis* to create *neuritis*.

Most suffixes are in common use in English, but some are peculiar to medical science. The suffixes most commonly used to indicate disease are *-itis,* meaning "inflammation," *-oma,* meaning "tumor", and *-osis,* meaning "a condition" (usually morbid). The following suffixes occur often in medical-dental terminology, but they are also used in ordinary language:

Suffix	Use	Examples
-ise, -ize, -ate	Add to nouns or adjectives to make verbs expressing to use and to act like, to subject to, to make into	Visualize (to see), hypnotize (to put into a state of hypnosis)
-ist, -or, -er	Add to verbs to make nouns expressing agent or person concerned or instrument	Anesthetist (one who practices the science of anesthesia), donor (giver)
-ent	Add to verbs to make adjectives or nouns of agency	Recipient (one who receives), concurrent (happening at the same time)
-sia, -y	Add to verbs to make nouns expressing action, process, or condition	Therapy (treatment), anesthesia (process or condition of feeling)
-ia, -ity	Add to adjectives or nouns to make nouns expressing quality or condition	Septicemia (blood poisoning), disparity (inequality), acidity (condition of excess acid), neuralgia (pain in nerves)
-ma, -mata, -men, -mina, -ment, -ure	Add to verbs to make nouns expressing result of action or object of action	Trauma (injury), foramina (openings), ligament (tough, fibrous band holding bone or viscera together), fissure (groove)
-ium, -olus, -olum, -culus, -culum, -cule, -cle	Add to nouns to make diminutive nouns	Bacterium, alveolus (air sac), follicle (little bag), cerebellum (little brain), molecule (little mass), ossicle (little bone)
-ible, -ile	Add to verbs to make adjectives expressing ability or capacity	Contractile (able to contract), edible (capable of being eaten), flexible (capable of being bent)
-al, -c, -ious, -tic	Add to nouns to make adjectives expressing relationship, concern, or pertaining	Neural (referring to nerve), neoplastic (referring to neoplasm), cardiac (referring to heart), delirious (suffering from delirium)
-id	Add to verbs or nouns to make adjectives expressing state or condition	Flaccid (state of being weak or lax), fluid (state of being fluid or liquid)
-tic	Add to verbs to make adjectives showing relationships	Caustic (referring to burn), acoustic (referring to sound or hearing)
-oid, -form	Add to nouns to make adjectives expressing resemblance	Polypoid (resembling a polyp), plexiform (resembling a plexus), fusiform (resembling a fusion), epidermoid (resembling the epidermis)
-ous	Add to nouns to make adjectives expressing material	Ferrous (composed of iron), serous (composed of serum), mucinous (composed of mucin)

The following verbs or combining forms of verbs are derived from either Greek or Latin. They may be attached to other roots to form words, or suffixes and prefixes may be added to them to form words. In the following examples, the part or root of the word to which the verb is attached is underlined; the meaning, if it is not clear, is given in parentheses.

Root	Translation	Examples
-algia-	Pain	Cardialgia (heart), gastralgia (stomach), neuralgia (nerve)
-audi-, -audio-	Hear, hearing	Audiometer (measure), audiophone (voice instrument for deaf individuals)
-bio-	Live	Biology (study of living), biogenesis (origin)
-cau-, -caus-	Burn	Caustic (suffix added to make an adjective), cauterization, causalgia (burning pain), electrocautery
-centesis-	Puncture, perforate	Thoracentesis (chest), pneumocentesis (lung), arthrocentesis (joint), enterocentesis (intestine)
-clas-, -claz-	Smash, break	Osteoclasis (bone), odontoclasis (tooth)
-duct-	Lead	Ductal (suffix added to make an adjective), oviduct (egg, uterine tube, or fallopian tube), periductal (around)
-dynia-	Pain	Mastodynia (breast), esophagodynia (esophagus)
-ecta-, -ectas-	Dilate	Venectasia (vein), cardiectasis (heart), ectatic (suffix added to make an adjective)
-ectomy	Excision	Gingivectomy (gingiva)
-edem-	Swell	Myoedema (muscle), lymphedema (lymph) (*-a* is a suffix added to make a noun)
-emia	Blood	Hyperemia (more than the normal amount)
-esthes-	Feel	Esthesia (suffix added to make a noun), anesthesia (*an-* is a prefix)
-flex-, -flec-	Bend	Flexion (suffix added to make a noun), flexor (suffix added), anteflect (forward)
-fiss-	Split	Fissure, fission (suffixes added to make nouns)
-flu-, -flux-	Flow	Fluctuate, fluxion, affluent (abundant flowing)

Continued

Root	Translation	Examples
-geno-, -genesis-	Produce, origin	Genotype, homogenesis (same origin), pathogenesis (disease), heterogenesis (alteration of generation)
-ia, -iasis	Condition	Odontalgia (tooth pain)
-iatro-, -iatr-	Treat, cure	Geriatrics (old age), pediatrics (children)
-itis	Inflammation	Periodontitis (periodontium)
-kine-,-kino-,-kineto-,-kinesio-	Move	Kinetogenic (producing movement), kinetic (suffix added to make an adjective), kinesiology (study)
-liga-	Bind	Ligament (suffix added to make a noun) ligate, ligature
-logy-	Study	Parasitology (parasites), bacteriology (bacteria), histology (tissues)
-lysis-	Breaking up, dissolving	Hemolysis (blood), glycolysis (sugar), autolysis (self-destruction of cells)
-morph-, -morpho-	Form	Morphology, amorphous (not definite form), pleomorphic (more, occurring in various forms), polymorphic (many)
-olfact-	Smell	Olfactophobia (fear), olfactory (suffix added to make an adjective)
-oma	Tumor	Odontoma (composed of tooth structures)
-op-, -opto-	See	Amblyopia (dull, dimness of vision), presbyopia (old, impairment of vision in old age), optic myopia (*myo-* means "to wink or to half-close the eyes")
-osis	Condition, disease	Periodontosis (periodontium)
-palpit-	Flutter	Palpitation (Irregular, trembling)
-pep-	Digest	Dyspepsia (bad, difficult), peptic (suffix added to make an adjective)
-phag-, -phago-	Eat	Phagocytosis (eating of cells), phagomania (madness, mad craving for food or to eat), dysphagia (difficulty eating or swallowing)
-phan-	Appear, visible	Phanerosis (act of becoming visible), phantasia, phantasy
-pexy-	Fix	Mastopexy (breast), nephrosplenopexy (kidney and spleen)
-phas-	Speak, utter	Aphasia (unable to speak), dysphasia (difficulty speaking)
-phobia-	Fear	Hydrophobia (water), claustrophobia (fear of close places)
-phil-	Like, love	Hemophilia (blood, a hereditary disease characterized by the delayed clotting of blood), acidophilia (acid stain, liking or staining with acid stains), philanthropy (love of humankind)
-phrax-, -phrag-	Fence off, wall off	Diaphragm (across, partition separating thorax from abdomen), phragmoplast (formed)
-plast-	Form, grow	Neoplasm (new growth), rhinoplasty (operation for formation of nose), otoplasty (ear)
-plegia-	Paralyze	Paraplegia (lower limbs), ophthalmoplegia (eye), hemiplegia (partial paralysis)
-pne-, -pneo-	Breathe	Dyspnea (difficult breathing), apnea (lack of breathing), hyperpnea (excessive breathing)
-poie-	Make	Hematopoiesis (blood), erythropoiesis (red blood cells), leukopoiesis (white blood cells)
-rrhagia-	Burst forth, pour	Menorrhagia (abnormal bleeding during menstruation), hemorrhage (blood)
-rrhaphy-	Suture	Herniorrhaphy (hernia), hepatorrhaphy (liver), nephrorrhaphy (kidney)
-rrhea-	Flow, discharge	Leukorrhea (white discharge from vagina), rhinorrhea (nasal discharge)
-rrhexis-	Rupture	Enterorrhexis (intestines), metrorrhexis (uterus)
-schiz-	Split, divide	Schizophrenia (mind, split personality), schizonychia (nails), schizotrichia (hair)
-scope-	Examine	Microscope, cardioscope, endoscope (*endo-* means "within"; an instrument for examining the interior of a hollow internal organ)
-stasis-	Stop, stand still	Hematostasis (pertaining to stagnation of blood), epistasis (checking or stopping of any discharge)
-stazien-	Drop	Epistaxis (nosebleed)
-stomia	Mouth	Xerostomia (dry mouth)
-teg-, -tect-	Cover	Tegmen, tectum (rooflike structure), integument (skin covering)
-therap-	Treat, cure	Therapy, neurotherapy (nerves), chemotherapy (chemicals), physiotherapy
-tomy-	Cut, incise	Phlebotomy (vein), arthrotomy (joint), appendectomy (*-ectomy* means "to cut out"; excision of appendix)
-topo-	Place	Topography, toponarcosis (numbing of a part or localized anesthesia)
-tropho-	Nourish	Hypertrophy (enlargement or overnourishment), atrophy (undernourishment), dystrophy (difficult or bad)

From Mosby's dental dictionary, ed 2, St. Louis, 2008, Mosby.

The following roots and combining forms are derived from Greek or Latin adjectives. Adjectives appear most often in compound words, and they are joined to either nouns or verbs. Suffixes may be added to make them into nouns. In the following examples, the part or root of the word that the adjective modifies is underlined, and the meaning is given in parentheses if it is not clear.

Root	Translation	Examples
-auto-	Self	Autoinfection, autolysis, autopathy (disease), autopsy (view, postmortem examination)
-brachy-	Short	Brachycephalia (head), brachydactylia (fingers), brachychelia (lip), brachygnathous (jaw)
-brady-	Slow	Bradypnea (breath), bradypragia (action), bradyuria (urine), bradypepsia (digestion)
-brevis-	Short	Brevity, breviflexor (short flexor muscle)
-cavus-	Hollow	Cavity, cavernous, vena cava (vein)
-coel-	Hollow	Coelarium (lining membrane of body cavity), coelom (body cavity of embryo)
-cryo-	Cold	Cryotherapy, cryotolerant, cryometer
-crypto-	Hidden, concealed	Cryptorchid (testis), cryptogenic (origin obscure or doubtful), cryptophthalmos (eye)
-dextro-	Right	Ambidextrous (using both hands with equal ease), dextrophobia (fear of objects on the right side), dextrocardia (heart)
-dys-	Difficult, bad, disordered, painful	Dysarthria (speech), dyshidrosis (sweat), dyskinesia (motion), dystocia (birth), dysphasia (speech), dyspepsia (digestion)
-eu-	Well, good	Euphoria (well-being), euphagia, eupnea (breath), euthyroid (normal thyroid), eutocia (normal birth)
-eury-	Broad, wide	Eurycephalic (head), euryopia (vision), eurysomatic (body; squat, thick-set body)
-glyco-	Sugar, sweet	Glycohemia (sugar in blood), glycopenia (deficiency of sugar, low blood sugar level)
-gravid-	Heavy	Gravida (pregnant woman), gravidism (pregnancy)
-haplo-	Single, simple	Haploid (having a single set of chromosomes), haplodermatitis (simple inflammation of skin), haplopathy (simple uncomplicated disease)
-hetero-	Other, different	Heterogeneous (kind; dissimilar elements), heteroinoculation, heterology (abnormality of structure), heterointoxication
-homo-	Same	Homogeneous (same kind of quality throughout), homozygous (possessing an identical pair of genes), homologous (corresponding in structure)
-hydro-	Wet, water	Hydronephrosis (kidney; collection of urine in kidney and pelvis), hydrophobia (fear of water)
-iso-	Equal	Isocellular (similar cells), isodontic (all teeth alike), isocytosis (equality of size of cells), isochromatic (having same color throughout)
-latus-	Broad	Latitude, latissimus dorsi (muscle adducting humerus)
-leio-	Smooth	Leiomyosarcoma (smooth muscle, fleshy malignant tumor), leiomyofibroma (tumor of muscle and fiber elements), leiomyoma (tumor of unstriped muscle)
-lepto-	Slender	Leptosomatic (body), leptodactylous (fingers)
-levo-	Left	Levocardia (heart), levorotation (turning to the left)
-longus-	Long	Adductor longus (muscle of the thigh), longitude
-macro-	Large, abnormal size	Macrocephalic (head), macrochiria (hands), macromastia (breast), macronychia (nails)
-magna-	Large, great	Magnitude, adductor magnus (thigh muscle)
-malaco-	Soft	Malacia (softening), osteomalacia (bones)
-mal-	Bad	Malady, malaise, malignant, malformation
-medius-	Middle, median, medium	Gluteus medius (femur muscle)
-mega-	Great	Megacolon (large colon), megacephaly (head)
-megalo-	Huge	Megalomania (delusion of grandeur), hepatomegaly (enlarged liver), splenomegaly (enlarged spleen)
-meso-	Middle, mid	Mesocarpal (wrist), mesoderm (skin), mesothelium (a lining membrane of body cavities)
-micro-	Small	Microglossia (tongue), microblepharia (eyelids), microorganism, microphonia (voice)
-minimus-	Smallest	Gluteus minimus (smallest muscle of the hip), adductor minimus (muscle of the thigh)
-mio-	Less	Mioplasmia (plasma; abnormal decrease in plasma in blood), miopragia (perform; decreased activity)
-mono-	One, single, limited to one part	Monochromatic (color), monobrachia (arm)
-multi-	Many, much	Multipara (bear; woman who has borne more than one child), multilobar (numerous lobes), multicentric (many centers)
-necro-	Dead	Necrosed, necrosis, necropsy (postmortem examination), necrophobia (fear of death)
-neo-	New	Neoformation, neomorphism (form), neonatal (first 4 weeks of life), neopathy (disease)
-oligo-	Few, scanty, little	Oligophrenia (mind), oligopnea (breath), oliguria (urine), oligodipsia (thirst)
-ortho-	Straight, normal, correct	Orthodont (teeth, normal), orthogenesis (progressive evolution in a given direction), orthograde (walk, carrying body upright), orthopnea (breath; unable to breathe unless in an upright position)

Continued

Root	Translation	Examples
-oxy-	Sharp, quick	Oxyesthesia (feel), oxyopia (vision), oxyosmia (smell)
-pachy-	Thick	Pachyderm (skin), pachysulemia (blood), pachypleuritis (inflammation of pleura), pachycholia (bile), pachyotia (ears)
-paleo-	Old	Paleogenetic (origin in the past), paleopathology (study of diseases in mummies)
-platy-	Flat	Platybasia (skull base), platycoria (pupil), platycrania (skull)
-pleo-	More	Pleomorphism (forms), pleochromocytoma (tumor composed of different-colored cells)
-poikilo-	Varied	Poikiloderma (skin mottling), poikilothermal (heat, variable body temperature)
-poly-	Many, much	Polyhedral (many bases or faces), polymastia (more than two breasts), polymelia (supernumerary limbs), polymyalgia (pain in many muscles)
-pronus-	Face down	Prone, pronation
-pseudo-	False, spurious	Pseudostratified (layered), pseudocirrhosis (apparent cirrhosis of the liver), pseudohypertrophy
-sclero-	Hard	Sclerosis (hardening), arteriosclerosis (artery), scleronychia (nails), sclerodermatitis (skin)
-scolio-	Twisted, crooked	Scoliodontic (teeth), scoliosis, scoliokyphosis (curvature of the spine)
-sinistro-	Left	Sinistrocardia, sinistromanual (left-handed), sinistraural (hearing better with the left ear)
-supinus-	Face up	Supine, supination, supinator longus (muscle in the arm)
-steno-	Narrow	Stenosis, stenostomia (mouth), mitral stenosis (mitral valve in the heart)
-stereo-	Solid, three dimensions	Stereoscope, stereometer
-tachy-	Fast, swift	Tachycardia (heart), tachyphrasia (speech)
-tele-	End, far away	Telepathy, telecardiogram
-telo-	Complete	Telophase
-thermo-	Heat, warm	Thermal, thermometer, thermobiosis (ability to live in high temperature)
-trachy-	Rough	Trachyphonia (voice), trachychromatic (deeply staining)
-xero-	Dry	Xerophagia (eating of dry foods), xerostomia (mouth), xeroderma (skin)

From Mosby's dental dictionary, ed 2, St. Louis, 2008, Mosby.

PRONUNCIATION OF MEDICAL-DENTAL TERMS

Medical terms are hard to pronounce, especially if you have read them but have never heard them spoken. The following are some helpful shortcuts.

ch is sometimes pronounced like *k*. Examples: *chromatin, chronic*.

ps is pronounced like *s*. Examples: *psychiatry, psychology*.

pn is pronounced with only the *n* sound. Example: *pneumonia*.

c and *g* are given the soft sound of *s* and *j*, respectively, before *e, i,* and *y* in words of both Greek and Latin origin. Examples: *cycle, cytoplasm, giant, generic*.

c and *g* have a harsh sound before other letters. Examples: *gastric, gonad, cast, cardiac*.

ae and *oe* are pronounced *ee*. Examples: *coelom, fasciae*.

e and *es*, when forming the final letter or letters of a word, are often pronounced as separate syllables. Examples: *rete (reetee), nares (nayreez)*.

i at the end of a word (to form a plural) is pronounced *eye*. Examples: *alveoli, glomeruli, fasciculi*.

APPENDIX D

Abbreviations

A ampule
@ at
aa of each (F., ana)
a.c. before meals (L., *ante cibum*)
ad Latin preposition, -to, up to
a.d. alternating days (L., *alternis diebus*)
ad lib at pleasure, as needed or desired (L., *ad libitum*)
adm admission
Ag silver (L., *argentum*)
alt. dieb. every other day (L., *alternis diebus*)
alt. hor. every other hour (L., *alternis horis*)
alt. noct. every other night (L., *alternis noctibus*)
a, am, ag amalgam
AM, a.m., A.M. before noon (L., *ante meridiem*)
amp ampule
amt amount
anat anatomy, anatomical
anes anesthesia
ant anterior
AP anteroposterior
appl applicable, application, appliance
approx approximate
aq water (L., *aqua*)
av average
bact bacterium, bacteria
BF bone fragment
bib drink (L., *bibe*)
b.i.d. twice a day (L., *bis in die*)
biol biological, biology
BP blood pressure
BS blood sugar
BW bite-wing radiograph
Bx biopsy
C centigrade; one hundred (L., *centum*)
c̄ with (L., *cum*)
CA cardiac arrest, chronological age
Ca calcium, carcinoma
cal calorie
caps capsules
cav cavity
CBC complete blood count
CC chief complaint
cc cubic centimeter
CDA Certified Dental Assistant
cent centigrade
CHD childhood disease
CHF congestive heart failure
chr chronic
cm centimeter
c.m. tomorrow morning (L., *cras mane*)
CO_2 carbon dioxide
comp compound
conc concentrated
cond condition
CP centric position
cpd compound
Cu copper (L., *cuprum*)
cu cubic
cur curettage
CV cardiovascular
CVA cerebrovascular accident
Cx convex
CY calendar year
d dose (L., *dosis*)
D, dist distal
dbl double
dc direct current
DDS Doctor of Dental Surgery/Science
deg degree
dev develop, development
Dg diagnosis
diag diagnosis
dil dilute (L., *dilue*)
DO disto-occlusal
dis disease
disp dispensary
dist distal
DMF decayed, missing, and filled (teeth)
DOA dead on arrival
DOB date of birth
doz dozen
Dr. doctor
d.t.d. give of such a dose (L., *datur talis dosis*)
dwt pennyweight

Dx diagnosis
EAC external auditory canal
ed effective dose
EDDA Expanded Duties Dental Assistant (auxiliary)
EENT ears, eyes, nose, and throat
EFDA expanded (extended) function dental assistant (auxiliary)
e.g. for example (L., *exempli gratia*)
EKG elektrokardiogram (German)
emerg emergency
EMT emergency medical treatment
ENT ears, nose, and throat
epith epithelial
equiv equivalent
esp especially
est estimate, estimation
et and, (Latin conjunction)
et al. and others (L., *et alia*)
etc. and so on, and so forth, and others (L., *et cetera*)
eval evaluate, evaluation
ext extract, external
F Fahrenheit
F female
F field (of vision)
F formula
FB foreign body
FBS fasting blood sugar
FD fatal dose
ff following
FH family history
fl fluid
FLD full lower denture
fld field
fl. dr. fluid dram
fl. oz. fluid ounce
FMX full mouth x-ray examination
frac fracture
frag fragment
freq frequent, frequency
ft foot
ft let it be made (L., *fiat/fiant*)
FUD full upper denture
func function
Fx fracture
g gram
gal gallon
ging gingiva, gingivectomy
glob globulin
gm gram
GP general practitioner
gr grain
gt drop (L., *gutta*)
gtt drops (L., *guttae*)
H, h, hr hour (L., *hora*)
H_2O water
Hb, hgb hemoglobin
Hdpc handpiece
h.d. at hour of lying down at bedtime (L., *hora decubitus*)
hosp hospital
hr hour
h.s. hour of sleep (L., *hora somni*)
ht. height
Hx history
I&D incision and drainage
IA incurred accidentally
ibid. in the same place (L., *ibidem*)
id the same (L., *idem*)
i.e. that is (L., *id est*)
IH infectious hepatitis
IM intramuscular
imp impression
in inch
inc incisal, incisive, incise
in d. daily (L., *in dies*)
inf infected, inferior, infusion
inj injection, injury
inop inoperable, inoperative
int internal
IQ intelligence quotient
i.q. the same as (L., *idem quod*)
IS interspace
IV intravenous
kg, kgm kilogram
kilo kilogram
kV kilovolt
L Latin
L, l liter
lab laboratory
lac laceration
LASER (laser) light amplification by stimulated emission of radiation
lat lateral
lb pound (L., *libra*)
lig ligament
ling lingual
liq liquid, liquor
LN lymph node
lt left
m murmur
m meter
m. dict. as directed (L., *modo dictu*)
m male
m, mes mesial
ma milliampere
mand mandibular
MASER (maser) microwave amplification by stimulated emission of radiation
max maximum, maxillary
MDR minimum daily requirement
med medical, medicine
mg, mgm milligram
micro microscopic

min minute, minimum
ML midline
ml milliliter
MM mucous membrane
mm millimeter
MO mesio-occlusal
MOD mesio-occluso-distal
mo month
MS multiple sclerosis
msec millisecond
N_2O nitrous oxide
narc narcotic, narcotism
neg negative
non. rep. do not repeat
norm normal
NPC no previous complaint
NPH no previous history
n.p.o. nothing by mouth (L., *nil per os*)
NR normal record
n.r. not to be repeated (L., *non repetatur*)
N/S normal saline
O oxygen
O_2 oxygen gas
obl oblique
occ occlusal
ODC oral disease control
o.d. every day (L., *omni die*)
o.d. right eye
OH oral hygiene
o.h. every hour (L., *omni hora*)
o.m. every morning (L., *omni mane*)
o.n. every night (L., *omni nocte*)
op operation
OPC outpatient clinic
OPD outpatient department
opp opposite, opposed
OR operating room
org organism, organic
oz ounce
P pulse
P after (L., *post*)
p- para-
PA posteroanterior
Pan panoral x-ray examination
PATH pituitary adrenotropic hormone
path pathology
p.c. after meal (L., *post cibum*)
PCN penicillin
PDR *Physicians' Desk Reference*
perf perforating
PLD partial lower denture
P.M. PM, p.m. after noon (L., *post meridiem*)
PM after death (L., *post mortem*)
PO postoperative
p.o. by mouth (L., *per os*)
POH personal oral hygiene
pos positive
postop postoperative
prep preparation, prepare (for surgery)
p.r.n. as required, as the occasion arises (L., *pro re nata*)
prog prognosis
pt patient
PUD partial upper denture
Px prophylaxis
q every (L., *quaque*)
q.d. every day (L., *quaque die*)
q.h. every hour (L., *quaque hora*)
q.2h every two hours. (L., *quaque secunda hora*)
q.i.d. four times a day (L., *quater in die*)
q.l. as much as pleased (L., *quantum libet*)
q.n. every night (L., *quaque nocte*)
q.p. at will (L., *quantum placeat*)
q.4.h. every 4 hours (L., *quaque quarta hora*)
qt quart
q.v. as much as liked (L., *quantum vis*)
r roentgen
R respiration
RX take (thou) a recipe
rad radiograph
RC retruded contact position
RC root canal
RDA Registered Dental Assistant
RDH Registered Dental Hygienist
reg regular
rem roentgen equivalent man
req requires, required, requisition
rep roentgen equivalent physical
resp respiration
Rh Rh factor in blood (L., *Rhesus*)
RHD rheumatic heart disease
RN Registered Nurse
rt right
Rx treatment (L., *recipe*)
s without (L., *sine*)
SBE subacute bacterial endocarditis
SD sterile dressing
sec second, secondary
Sig. write on label
sol solution
spec specimen
ss one half signs and symptoms (L., *semis*)
stat immediately (L., *statim*)
std standard
stim stimulator, stimulate
strep *Streptococcus* organisms
sup superior
surg surgeon, surgery
Sx symptom
sym symmetric
symp symptom
sys system
T temperature

tab tablet
TB, TBC tuberculosis
tbsp tablespoon
temp temperature
t.i.d. three times a day (L., *ter in die*)
tinc tincture
TLC tender loving care
TM temporomandibular
TMJ temporomandibular joint
TPR temperature, pulse, respiration
tsp teaspoon
U, u unit
ung ointment (L., *unguentum*)
unk unknown
USP *United States Pharmacopeia*
ut. dict. As directed
V, v volt
VD venereal disease
vert vertebra, vertical
visc viscous
VIT vitamin
viz that is, namely (L., *videlicet*)
VO verbal order
vol volume
vs versus
WF white female
wh white
WM white male
w-n well-nourished
wnd wound
wt weight
x times, 4x, four times; x4, times four yard
xt extract, extracted
xyl, xylo Xylocaine
yd yard
YOB year of birth
yr year

SYMBOLS

& and
* birth
† death
↓ decrease
° Degree
= equal
′feet, minutes
♀ Female
> greater than or indicating an increase
" inches, seconds
↑ increase
< less than or indicating a decrease
♂ male
− minus, negative
number, pound
i, ii, iii one, two, or three (as in number of grams)
ʒiss one and one-half drams
℥T one ounce
℥ss one-half ounce
/ per
% percent
+ plus, positive

Modified from Zwemer TJ: Boucher's clinical dental terminology, ed 4, St Louis, 1993, Mosby.

APPENDIX **E**

Dental Terminology

abrasion Mechanical wearing away of teeth by abnormal stressors. This could result from abnormal toothbrushing habits or other abnormal stresses on the teeth.

accessional Permanent teeth that do not replace deciduous teeth but rather become an accession (addition) to the deciduous teeth, the succedaneous teeth, or both types.

accessory root canals Extra openings into the pulp; usually located on the sides of the roots or in the bifurcations.

acquired Pertaining to something obtained by oneself; not inherited.

ala Latin word for "wing." Referring to the sides of the nostrils of the nose; plural *alae*.

alignment Arrangement of teeth in a row.

allergenic Being hypersensitive to something.

allergic reaction Body's reaction to an allergen; an example of such a reaction is hives.

alveolar bone Bone that forms the sockets for the teeth.

alveolar crest Highest part of the alveolar bone closest to the cervical line of the tooth.

alveolar eminences Bulges on the facial surface of the alveolar bone that outline the position of the roots.

alveolar mucosa Mucosa between the mucobuccal fold and the gingiva.

alveolar process Part of the bone in the maxillae and the mandible that forms the sockets for the teeth.

alveolus (alveoli) Cavity or socket in the alveolar process in which the root of the tooth is held.

anatomic crown The part of the tooth that is covered by enamel.

angle of the mandible Point at the lower border of the body of the mandible where it turns up onto the ramus.

Angle's classification System of dental classification based primarily on the relationship of the permanent first molars to each other and, to a lesser degree, on the relationship of the permanent canines to each other.

ankyloglossia See *tongue-tie*.

ankylosis Fusion of the cementum of a tooth with the alveolar bone.

anodontia The absence of teeth in the jaw.

anomaly Any noticeable difference or deviation from that which is ordinary or normal.

anterior Situated in front of; a term commonly used to denote the incisor and canine teeth or the area toward the front of the mouth.

anterior pillar Fold of tissue that extends down in front of the tonsil.

antihistamine Drug that controls the body's histamine reaction, which causes the congestion of tissues.

apex (apices) End point or furthest tip, as of the tooth root.

apical foramen Aperture or opening at or near the apex of a tooth root through which the blood and nerve supply of the pulp enters the tooth.

arch, dental See *dental arch*.

atrophic Pertaining to the wasting away of a tissue, organ, or part from disease, defective nutrition, or lack of use.

atrophy Wasting away of a tissue, organ, or part from disease, defective nutrition, or lack of use.

attached gingiva Tightly adherent gingiva that extends from the free gingiva to the alveolar mucosa.

attrition Process of normal wear on the crown.

autonomic nervous system The part of the nervous system of the body that is not willfully controlled. It controls the functions of the glands and of the smooth and cardiac muscle.

bicuspid See *premolars*.

bifurcation Division into two parts or branches, as any two roots of a tooth.

body of the mandible Horizontal portion of the mandible, excluding the alveolar process.

bone Hard connective tissue that forms the framework of the body. The hardness is attributable to the hydroxyapatite crystal.

bruxism Abnormal grinding of the teeth.

bucca Latin word for "cheek."

buccal Pertaining to the cheek; toward the cheek or next to the cheek. Also called *facial*.

buccal development groove Groove that separates the buccal cusps on a buccal surface.

buccal glands Small minor salivary glands in the cheek.

buccinator Muscle of facial expression that extends from the back buccal portion of the maxilla and mandible and the pterygomandibular raphe forward in the cheek to the corner of the mouth.

calcification Process whereby organic tissue becomes hardened by a deposit of calcium salts within its substance. The term, in a liberal sense, connotes the deposition of any mineral salts that contribute to the hardening and maturation of hard tissue.

canal Long tubular opening through a bone.

canines Third teeth from the midline, at the corner of the mouth; used for grasping; also called *cuspids*.

capsule Fibrous band of tissue surrounding a joint.

cell Basic functioning component of the body; capable of reproducing itself in most instances. Tissues are made up of groups of cells.

cementoenamel junction (CEJ) Junction of the enamel of the crown and the cementum of the root. This junction forms the cervical line around the tooth.

cementoma Cementum tumor at the root tip that destroys the surrounding bone.

cementum Layer of bonelike tissue covering the root of the tooth.

central developmental groove Developmental groove that crosses the occlusal surface of a tooth from the mesial to the distal side; divides the tooth into buccal and lingual parts.

centric occlusion (central occlusion) Relationship of the occlusal surfaces of one arch to those of the other when the jaws are closed and the teeth are in maximum intercuspation.

centric relation Arch-to-arch relationship of the maxilla to the mandible when the condyles are in their most upward position, the mandible is in its most posterior position, and the jaw is most braced by its musculature.

cervical Portion of a tooth near the junction of the crown and root; pertaining to the neck region (e.g., the nerves of the neck).

cervical line Line formed by the junction of the enamel and the cementum on a tooth.

cervical third Portion of the crown or root of a tooth at or near the cervical line.

cervicoenamel ridge Prominent ridge of enamel immediately near the cervical line on the crown of a tooth.

cervix Constricted structure; the narrow region at the junction of the crown and root of the tooth.

circumvallate papillae Large V-shaped row of papillae lying on the posterior dorsum of the tongue; also called *vallate papillae*.

class I occlusal relationship Normal relationship between maxillary and mandibular molars.

class II occlusal relationship Relationship in which a mandibular molar is posterior to its normal position.

class III occlusal relationship Relationship in which a mandibular molar is anterior to its normal position.

cleft lip Gap in the upper lip that occurs during development.

cleft palate Lack of joining together of the hard or soft palates.

clinical crown Part of the tooth protruding from the gingiva.

clinical root Part of the tooth embedded in the gingiva and socket.

concavity Depression in a surface.

congenital Occurring at or before birth; may or may not be hereditary.

contact area Area of contact of one tooth with another in the same arch.

contact point Specific point at which a tooth from one arch occludes with another tooth from the opposing arch.

cross-bite Condition in which the cusps of a tooth in one arch exceed the cusps of a tooth in the opposing arch, buccally or lingually.

cross-section Cutting through a tooth perpendicular to the long axis.

crown Part of the tooth that is covered with enamel.

cusp Major pointed or rounded eminence on or near the occlusal surface of a tooth.

cusp of Carabelli Fifth lobe of a maxillary first molar.

cyst Sac of fluid lined by epithelium that may grow to varying sizes.

cytoplasm Fluid substance of cells.

débrided To have accomplished the removal (débridement) of nerve tissue and other debris from the pulp cavity to leave a surgically cleaned area.

deciduous That which will be shed; specifically, the first dentition of humans or animals.

deglutition The action of swallowing.

dental arch All teeth in either the maxillary or mandibular jaw that form an arch.

DCHP dental health care personnel

dentin (formerly *dentine*) Calcified tissue that forms the inside body of a tooth, underlying the cementum and enamel and surrounding the pulpal tissue.

dentinal tubule Space in the dentin occupied by the ontoblastic process.

dentinocemental junction Location in the root where the dentin joins the cementum.

dentinoenamel junction Line marking the junction of the dentin and the enamel.

dentinogenesis imperfecta Hereditary imperfect dentin formation.

dentition General character and arrangement of the teeth, taken as a whole, as in carnivorous, herbivorous, and omnivorous dentitions. *Primary dentition* refers to the deciduous teeth, and *secondary dentition* refers to the permanent teeth. *Mixed dentition* refers to a combination of permanent and deciduous teeth in the same dentition.

depression Lowering of the mandible or opening of the mouth.

developmental depression Noticeable concavity on the formed crown or root of a tooth; occurs at the junction of two lobes (e.g., on the mesial surface of the maxillary first premolars) or at the furcation of the roots.

developmental grooves Fine depressed lines in the enamel of a tooth that mark the union of the lobes of the crown.

diastema Any spacing between the teeth in the same arch.

distal Distant; farthest from the median line of the face or from the origin of a structure.
distal proximal surface Proximal surface on the posterior side of a tooth.
distal third Viewed from the facial or lingual surface, the third of the surface farthest from the midline.
distobuccal developmental groove Developmental groove that extends on the buccal surface of a lower first or third molar between the distobuccal and distal cusps.
distoclusion See *class II occlusal relationship.*
dorsum of the tongue Top surface of the tongue.
edema Swelling of tissue.
edge, incisal See *incisal edge.*
embrasure Open space between the proximal surfaces of two teeth where they diverge buccally, labially, or lingually and occlusally from the contact area.
enamel Hard calcified tissue that covers the dentin of the crown portion of a tooth.
enamel dysplasia Abnormalities of enamel growth.
enamel hypocalcification Enamel that is not as dense as regular enamel.
enamel hypoplasia Enamel that is thin or pitted.
endocrine Gland or type of secretion that is carried away from the producing cells by the blood vessels. The secretion is used in other parts of the body to control certain functions; these secretions have no duct system.
enzyme Agent capable of producing chemical changes in processes such as the digestion of food.
epiglottis Cartilage that helps to cover the laryngeal opening.
epinephrine Substance produced by the body or synthetically produced that causes many reactions; in dentistry, it is used to constrict blood flow in tissues.
epithelial Pertaining to the epithelium.
epithelial attachment Substance produced by the reduced enamel epithelium that helps to secure the attachment epithelium at the base of the gingival sulcus to the tooth.
epithelium Layer or layers of cells that cover the surface of the body or that line the tubes or cavities inside the body; one of the four basic tissues.
equilibrium Sense of balance.
eruption Movement of the tooth as it emerges through surrounding tissue so that the clinical crown gradually appears longer.
eruptive stage Period of eruption from the completion of crown formation until the teeth come into occlusion.
exfoliation Shedding or loss of a primary tooth.
facial Term used to designate the outer surfaces of the teeth collectively (i.e., buccal or labial).
facial surface See *facial.*
facial third From a proximal view, the third of the surface closest to the facial side.
fauces Space between the left and right palatine tonsils.
FDI system The Fédération Dentaire Internationale (International Dental Federation) system for tooth identification.
filiform papillae Small pointed projections that heavily cover most of the dorsum of the anterior two thirds of the tongue.
fissure Deep cleft; developmental line fault usually found in the occlusal or buccal surface of a tooth, commonly the result of imperfect fusion of the enamel of the adjoining dental lobes.
flange Projecting edge; the edge of the denture.
fluorosis Discolored enamel resulting from excessive fluoride intake during crown development.
foliate papillae Poorly developed papillae that appear as small vertical folds in the posterior part of the sides of the tongue.
foramen Short circular opening through a bone.
fossa Round, wide, relatively shallow depression in the surface of a tooth as commonly seen in the lingual surfaces of the maxillary incisors or between the cusps of molars. This can also be a shallow depression in bone.
free gingiva Gingiva that forms the gingival sulcus.
frenulum Little frenum or fold of tissue.
frontal sinus Air sinus in the frontal bone above the eye that opens into the hiatus semilunaris in the middle meatus.
fungiform papillae Small circular papillae scattered throughout the anterior two thirds of the dorsum of the tongue.
fusion Two teeth that fuse at their dentin while developing.
gingiva Part of the gum tissue that immediately surrounds the teeth and the alveolar bone.
gingival crest Most occlusal or incisal extent of the gingiva.
gingival crevice Subgingival space that under normal conditions lies between the gingival crest and the epithelial attachment.
gingival papillae Portion of the gingiva found between the teeth in the interproximal spaces gingival to the contact area; also called *interdental papillae.*
gingival sulcus Space between the free gingiva and the tooth surface.
gingivitis Inflammation involving the gingival tissues only.
hematoma Escape of blood from an injured blood vessel into the tissue spaces.
hemoglobin Component of red blood cells that carries oxygen.
hereditary Inherited through the genes of the parents or grandparents.
immunity The body's resistance to certain organisms or diseases.
impacted Teeth that are not completely erupted and that are fully or partly covered by bone or soft tissue.
incisal edge Edge formed at the labioincisal line angle of an anterior tooth after an incisal ridge has worn down.
incisal ridge Rounded ridge form of the incisal portion of an anterior tooth.
incisal third From a proximal, lingual, or labial view of an anterior tooth, the third of the surface closest to the incisal edge.
incisive papilla Small, rounded, oblong mound of tissue directly behind or lingual to the maxillary central incisors and lying over the incisive foramen.
incisors The four center teeth in either arch. These are essential for cutting.
inflammatory reaction The body's mechanism to combat harmful organisms by bringing more plasma and blood cells to the injured area.

inherited Passed on from the parents or grandparents.
interdental Located between the teeth.
interdental papilla Projection of the gingiva between the teeth.
interproximal Between the proximal surfaces of adjoining teeth in the same arch.
interproximal space Triangular space between adjoining teeth. The proximal surfaces of the teeth form the sides of the triangle; the alveolar bone, the base, and the contact area of the teeth form the apex.
ISO International Standards Organization System Tooth numbering system based on the FDI system.
labia Latin word for "lips"; singular, *labium*.
labial Of or pertaining to the lips; toward the lips.
labial frenum Fold of tissue that attaches the lip to the labial mucosa at the midline of the lips.
larynx Voice box; the trachea begins just below it.
lingual Pertaining to or affecting the tongue; next to or toward the tongue.
lingual frenum Fold of tissue that attaches the undersurface of the tongue to the floor of the mouth.
lingual glands Minor salivary glands of the tongue.
lingual groove Developmental groove on the lingual side of the tooth.
lingual surface See *lingual.*
lingual third From a proximal view, the third of the surface closest to the lingual side.
macrodontia Condition in which the teeth are too large for the jaw.
malocclusion Abnormal occlusion of the teeth.
mamelon One of the three rounded protuberances of the incisal surface of a newly erupted incisor tooth.
mandible Lower jaw.
mandibular Pertaining to the lower jaw.
mandibular arch First pharyngeal arch that forms the area of the mandible and the maxilla; the lower dental arch.
mandibular condyle Rounded top of the mandible that articulates with the mandibular fossa.
mandibular foramen Opening on the medial surface of the ramus of the mandible for the entrance of nerves and blood vessels to the lower teeth.
mandibular process Portion of the mandibular pharyngeal arch that forms the mandible.
mandibular tori Bony growths on the lingual cortical plate of bone opposite the mandibular canines.
marginal ridge Ridge or elevation of enamel forming the margin of the surface of a tooth, specifically at the mesial and distal margins of the occlusal surfaces of the premolars and molars and at the mesial and distal margins of the lingual surfaces of the incisors and canines.
mastication Act of chewing or grinding.
maxilla Paired main bone of the upper jaw.
maxillary Pertaining to the upper arch.
maxillary arch Upper dental arch.
maxillary sinus Largest of the paired paranasal sinuses, located in the maxilla.
maxillary tuberosity Bulging posterior surface of the maxilla behind the third molar region.
median line Vertical (central) line that divides the body into right and left; the median line of the face.
mesial Toward or situated in the middle (e.g., toward the midline of the dental arch).
mesial drift Phenomenon of the permanent molars continuing to move mesially after eruption.
mesial third From a facial or a lingual view, the third of the surface closest to the midline.
microdontia Condition in which the teeth are too small for the jaw.
mixed dentition State of having the primary and permanent teeth in the dental arches at the same time.
molars Large posterior teeth used for grinding.
mucosa Moist epithelial lining of the oral cavity and the respiratory and digestive systems.
mucous Pertaining to mucus, the thick viscous secretion of a gland.
mulberry molars Molars with multiple cusps that are caused by congenital syphilis.
multiple root Root with more than one branch.
muscle One of the four basic tissues. Muscle has the property of contraction or shortening of the fibers, which accomplishes work. The three types of muscle are skeletal, cardiac, and smooth muscle.
nasal septum Wall between the left and right sides of the nasal cavity, which is made up of the ethmoid and vomer bones.
nervous tissue One of the four basic tissues. Groups of cells (neurons) carry messages to and from the brain and perform many other tasks.
neuron Nerve cell.
nonsuccedaneous Permanent teeth that do not succeed or replace deciduous teeth.
occluding Contacting opposing teeth.
occlusal Articulating or biting surface.
occlusal plane Side view of the occlusal surfaces.
occlusal relationship Way in which the maxillary and mandibular teeth touch each other.
occlusal third From a proximal, lingual, or buccal view of a posterior tooth, the third of the surface closest to the occlusal surface.
occlusal trauma Injury brought about by one tooth prematurely hitting another during closure of the jaws.
occlusion Relationship of the mandibular and maxillary teeth when closed or during excursive movements of the mandible, when the teeth of the mandibular arch come in to contact with the teeth of the maxillary arch in any functional relationship.
odontoma Tumor made up of enamel, dentin, cementum, and pulp.
opaque Not easily able to transmit light.
open bite Space left between the teeth when the jaws close.
open contact Space between adjacent teeth in the same arch; an interproximal opening instead of a contact area where the teeth touch.

overbite Relationship of the teeth in which the incisal ridges of the maxillary anterior teeth extend below the incisal ridges of the mandibular anterior teeth when the teeth are in a centric occlusal relationship.

overhanging restoration Excess of filling material extending past the confines of the tooth preparation; an overextension of filling material.

overjet Relationship of the teeth in which the incisal ridges or buccal cusp ridges of the maxillary teeth extend facially to the incisal ridges or buccal cusp ridges of the mandibular teeth when the teeth are in a centric occlusal relationship.

palatal Pertaining to the palate or roof of the mouth.

Palmer notation system System of coding teeth that involves the use of brackets, numbers, and letters.

papillary gingiva Gingiva that forms the interdental papillae.

paramolar Small supernumerary tooth located buccally or lingually to a molar.

parasympathetic nervous system Part of the autonomic (automatic) nervous system that originates from some of the cranial nerves and some of the sacral nerves. It controls a number of functions, including stimulation of the salivary glands.

parathyroid gland Small gland embedded in the thyroid gland that helps to control calcium metabolism in the body.

passive eruption Condition in which the tooth does not move but the gingival attachment moves farther apically.

peg-shaped lateral Poorly formed maxillary lateral incisor with a cone-shaped crown.

periapical Around the tip of the root of a tooth.

periodontal Surrounding a tooth.

periodontium Supporting tissues surrounding the teeth.

periosteum Fibrous and cellular layer that covers bones and contains cells that become osteoblasts.

periphery Circumferential boundary; outer border.

pharynx Throat area, from the nasal cavity to the larynx.

philtrum Small depression at the midline of the upper lip.

pillars Folds of tissue appearing in front of and behind the palatine tonsils.

pit Small pointed depression in the dental enamel, usually at the junction of two or more developmental grooves; a small hole anywhere on the crown.

posterior Situated toward the back (e.g., premolars, molars).

posterior pillars Folds of tissue behind the tonsil that contain the palatopharyngeus muscle.

posterior teeth Teeth of either jaw located to the rear of the incisors and canines.

pre-eruptive stage Period when the crown of the tooth is developing.

premature contact area Area in which an upper and a lower tooth touch and hit each other before the rest of the teeth occlude.

premaxilla Bony area of the upper jaw that includes the alveolar ridge for the incisors and the area immediately behind it.

premolars Permanent teeth that replace the primary molars.

primary dentin Dentin formed from the beginning of calcification until tooth eruption.

primary dentition First set of teeth; also called *baby teeth, milk teeth,* and *deciduous teeth.*

primary palate The early developing part of the hard palate that originates from the medial nasal process and forms a V-shaped wedge of tissue that runs from the incisive foramen forward and laterally between the lateral incisors and canines of the maxilla.

primary teeth See *deciduous.*

prosthetic appliance Any constructed appliance that replaces a missing part.

protrusion Condition of being thrust forward (e.g., protrusion of the anterior teeth, which refers to the teeth being too far labial); the forward movement of the mandible.

proximal Nearest, next, immediately adjacent to; distal or mesial.

proximal contact area Proximal area of a tooth that touches an adjacent tooth on the mesial or distal side.

pulp canal Canal in the root of a tooth that leads from the apex to the pulp chamber; contains dental pulp tissue under normal conditions.

pulp cavity Entire cavity within the tooth, including the pulp canal and pulp chamber.

pulp chamber Cavity or chamber in the center of the crown of a tooth that normally contains the major portion of the dental pulp. The pulp canals lead into the pulp chambers.

pulp, dental Highly vascular and innervated connective tissue contained within the pulp cavity of the tooth. It is composed of arteries, veins, nerves, connective tissues and cells, lymph tissue, and odontoblasts.

pulp horn (horn of pulp) Extension of pulp tissue into a thin point of the pulp chamber in the tooth crown.

pulp stones Small, dentinlike calcifications in the pulp.

quadrants One fourth of the dentition. The four quadrants are the right, left, maxillary, and mandibular quadrants.

ramus of the mandible Vertical portion of the mandible.

recession Migration of the gingival crest in an apical direction, away from the crown of the tooth.

referred pain Pain that seems to originate in one area but that actually originates in another.

reparative dentin Localized formation of dentin in response to local trauma, such as occlusal trauma or caries.

resorption Physiological removal of tissues or body products (e.g., roots of deciduous teeth) or of some alveolar process after the loss of the permanent teeth.

retromolar pad Pad of tissue behind the mandibular third molars.

retromolar triangle Triangular area of bone just behind the mandibular third molars.

retrusion Act or process of retraction or moving back, as when the mandible is placed in a posterior relationship to the maxilla.

ridge Long and narrow elevation or crest, such as on the surface of a tooth or bone.

root Portion of a tooth that is embedded in the alveolar process and covered with cementum.

root canal See *pulp canal.*

root planing Process of smoothing the cementum of the root of a tooth.

rugae Small ridges of tissue extending laterally across the anterior of the hard palate.
sebaceous glands Small, oil-producing glands that are usually connected to and lubricate the hairs.
secondary dentin Dentin formed throughout the pulp chamber and pulp canal from the time of eruption.
secondary dentition Permanent dentition.
single root Root with one main branch.
slough Loss of dead cells from the surface of tissue; pronounced *sluff.*
soft tissue Noncalcified tissue, such as nerves, arteries, veins, and connective tissue.
spasm Constant contraction of a muscle.
submucosa Supporting layer of loose connective tissue under a mucous membrane.
succedaneous Permanent teeth that succeed, or take the place of, deciduous teeth after the latter have been shed (i.e., the incisors, canines, and premolars).
sulcus Long V-shaped depression or valley in the surface of a tooth between the ridges and the cusps. A sulcus has a developmental groove at the apex of the "V" shape. The term *sulcus* also refers to the trough around the teeth that is formed by the gingiva.
supplemental groove Shallow linear groove in the enamel of a tooth. It differs from a developmental groove in that it does not mark the junction of the lobes; it is a secondary and smaller groove.
supplemental tooth Supernumerary tooth that resembles a regular tooth.
supraeruption Eruption of a tooth beyond the occlusal plane.
taste buds Small structures in the vallate, fungiform, and foliate papillae that detect taste.
temporomandibular ligament Thickened part of the temporomandibular joint capsule on the lateral side.
tongue-tie, tongue-tied Condition in which the lingual frenum is short and attached to the tip of the tongue, which makes normal speech difficult; also called *ankyloglossia.*
tonsillar pillars Vertical folds of tissue that lie in front of and behind the palatine tonsils in the lateral throat wall.
tooth germ Soft tissue that develops into a tooth.
tooth migration Movement of the tooth through the bone and gum tissue.
torus palatinus Large bony growth in the hard palate.
transverse ridge Ridge formed by the union of two triangular ridges that traverses the surface of a posterior tooth from the buccal side to the lingual side.
trauma Wound; bodily injury or damage.
trifurcation Division of three tooth roots at their point of junction with the root trunk.
Universal Numbering System, Universal Code System of coding teeth using the numbers 1 through 32 for the permanent teeth and the letters A through T for the deciduous teeth.
uvula Small hanging fold of tissue at the back of the soft palate.
vallate papillae See *circumvallate papillae.*
vascular Relating to blood supply.
vasoconstrictor Substance that constricts blood vessels.
vermilion zone Red part of the lip where the lip mucosa meets the skin.
vestibule Space between the lips or cheeks and the teeth.

From Brand RW, Isselhard DE: Anatomy of orofacial structures, ed 7, St. Louis, 2003, Mosby.

Index

Page numbers followed by "f" indicate figures, "t" indicate tables, and "b" indicate boxes.

D

Q

R

U

V

W

Y

Z